Electrocardiography of the dog and cat

DIAGNOSIS OF ARRHYTHMIAS

2nd edition

Electrocardiography of the dog and cat

DIAGNOSIS OF ARRHYTHMIAS

2nd edition

Roberto Santilli
N. Sydney Moïse
Romain Pariaut
Manuela Perego

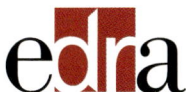

Senior Editor: Alessandra Muntignani

Project Manager: Mercedes González Fernández de Castro

Design and layout: Grupo Asís Biomedia, S.L.

Cover artwork: Federica Farè, Veronica Santilli, and Roberto Santilli

Paper, Print and Binding Manager: Michele Ribatti

© 2018 Edra S.p.A.* – All rights reserved

ISBN: 978-88-214-4784-6

eISBN: 978-88-214-4785-3

No part of this publication may be reproduced, stored in a retrieval system, or transmitted, in any form or by any means, electronic, mechanical, photocopying, recording, or otherwise, without prior written permission from the publisher.

Knowledge and best practice in this field are constantly changing: as new research and experience broaden our knowledge, changes in practice, treatment, and drug therapy may become necessary or appropriate. Readers are advised to check the most current information provided (i) or procedures featured or (ii) by the manufacturer of each product to be administered, to verify the recommended dose or formula, the method and duration of administration, and contraindications. It is the responsibility of the practitioners, relying on their own experience and knowledge of the patient, to make diagnoses, to determine dosages and the best treatment for each individual patient, and to take all appropriate safety precautions. To the fullest extent of the law, neither the Publisher nor the Editors assume any liability for any injury and/or damage to persons, animals or property arising out of or related to any use of the material contained in this book.

Edra S.p.A.
Via G. Spadolini 7, 20141 Milano
Tel. 02 881841
www.edizioniedra.it

Printed in Italy by "Printer Trento" S.r.l. - Trento (Italy), May 2018

(*) Edra S.p.A. is part of LSWR GROUP

The authors

Roberto A. Santilli, Dr. Med. Vet., PhD, DECVIM-CA (Cardiology)

Roberto Santilli graduated from the College of Veterinary Medicine of the University of Milan in 1990. He became a diplomate of the European College of Veterinary Internal Medicine-Companion Animals (Specialty of Cardiology) in 1999. Between 2004 and 2006, he completed a Master in Electrophysiology and Electrical Stimulation at the University of Medicine of Insubria. He then obtained a PhD at the University of Turin, College of Veterinary Internal Medicine in 2010. Roberto Santilli is the head of the cardiology departments of the Clinica Veterinaria Malpensa in Samarate, Varese (Italy) and of the Ospedale Veterinario I Portoni Rossi, Bologna (Italy). Since 2014, he has been an Adjunct Professor of Cardiology at the Cornell University College of Veterinary Medicine, where he is actively involved in the development of a cardiac electrophysiologic laboratory. His main research activities include the diagnosis and treatment of arrhythmias in dogs and cats.

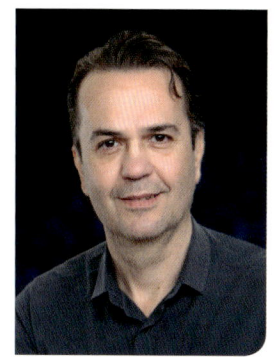

N. Sydney Moïse DVM, MS, DACVIM (Cardiology and Internal Medicine)

Sydney Moïse graduated from the College of Veterinary Medicine, Texas A&M University (DVM) and Cornell University (MS). She became a diplomate of the American College of Internal Medicine in 1982 and the subspecialty of Cardiology in 1986. She established the Cardiology Service at Cornell University and is currently Professor in the Department of Clinical Sciences. She has been involved in the clinical practice of cardiology, teaching and research. Her research has primarily focused on arrhythmias and their underlying mechanisms. For six years she served as Editor-in-Chief for the Journal of Veterinary Cardiology. Throughout her career she has been involved in international veterinary medicine with regards to teaching and collaboration. For her work she has been awarded the American Veterinary Medical Association Research Award (American Kennel Club) and the British Veterinary Medical Association Bourgelat Award.

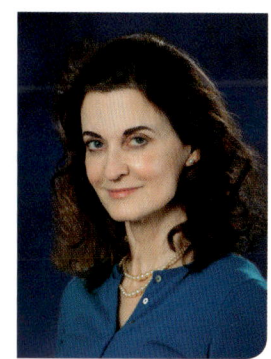

Romain Pariaut Dr. Vre., DACVIM (Cardiology), DECVIM-CA (Cardiology)

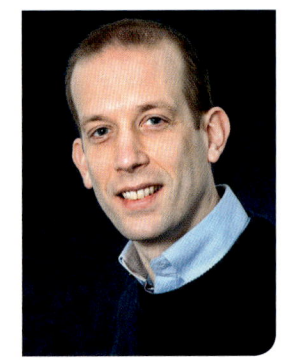

Romain Pariaut graduated from the School of Veterinary Medicine of Lyon, France, in 1999. He became a diplomate of the American College of Internal Medicine (Cardiology Subspecialty) in 2005, and a diplomate of the European College of Internal Medicine-Companion Animals (Specialty of Cardiology) in 2006. Between 2007 and 2015, he was a faculty member in the School of Veterinary medicine at Louisiana State University. He then joined Cornell University as an Associate Professor in the Department of Clinical Sciences and is actively involved in the development of a cardiac electrophysiology laboratory. Since 2007, Romain Pariaut has been an Associate Editor for the Journal of Veterinary Cardiology.

Manuela Perego, Dr. Med. Vet.

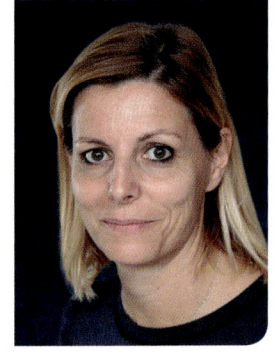

Manuela Perego graduated from the College of Veterinary Medicine of the University of Milan in 2003. She completed a residency program of the European College of Veterinary Internal Medicine-Companion Animals (Specialty of Cardiology) between 2010 and 2013 under the supervision of Dr. Roberto Santilli. She currently works in the Cardiology Departments of the Clinica Veterinaria Malpensa in Samarate, Varese (Italy) and the Ospedale Veterinario I Portoni Rossi, Bologna (Italy). Her main research activities include the diagnosis and treatment of arrhythmias in dogs and cats.

Preface

"It is the theory which decides what we can observe."
Albert Einstein

The main objective of this book is to give both clinical and theoretical information to interpret simple and complex electrocardiograms in dogs and cats. Detailed description of normal rhythm variations and arrhythmias is provided to meet the readers' needs whether they are just beginners or experts. Consequently, veterinary students and busy general practitioners will find the information sought to categorize electrocardiograms, while cardiology residents and specialists will discover additional depths for understanding the complexities of the electrophysiology behind the electrocardiogram. For all, the goal of this book is to increase knowledge to meet the challenge of electrocardiographic interpretation. We have made the deliberate choice to use the same terminology and electrocardiographic planes used for the analysis of the human electrocardiogram. We have done so because the main source of information concerning the clinically applicable electrophysiologic studies of arrhythmias is from those performed in people.

In recent years, research to understand the electrophysiological mechanisms behind cardiac arrhythmias in veterinary patients has increased. Although these studies remain limited, the advancements are real and give us a better understanding of the clinical arrhythmias we commonly and uncommonly diagnose. Such information improves not only our ability to make an accurate diagnosis, but to deliver better treatment.

The first three chapters of this book include a detailed description of the anatomy and electrophysiology of the conduction system, the theory behind the formation of the electrocardiographic waveforms, and the recording techniques available to the clinician. The following chapters first focus on the characteristics of normal rhythm in dogs and cats, the impact of cardiac chamber enlargement on electrocardiogram, and then detail the portfolio of atrial and ventricular arrhythmias described in veterinary medicine. Specifically, chapters 7 to 10 are dedicated to ectopies and tachyarrhythmias. Chapters 11 and 12 describe bradyarrhythmias and conduction abnormalities. Chapter 13 is an overview of the effects of systemic diseases and drugs on the electrocardiogram. Finally, chapter 14 describes the electrocardiogram in the presence of an artificial pacemaker, and the signs of device malfunction. We have included at the end this book a series of electrocardiograms that readers can use to test their knowledge.

Initially published in Italian, this publication is now accessible to the English-speaking readership in an expanded and updated version. This project was possible by the addition of two co-authors. Notably this work stems from a common passion for the fascinating complexity of arrhythmias and it is the product of friendship, collaboration and mutual academic respect.

We hope that the readers will find it helpful in their daily clinical activities, and rather than feeling overwhelmed by the intricacies of electrocardiography, will develop their interest in deciphering the tracings they record.

Finally, we would like to thank all the individuals who have directly or indirectly contributed to this book: architect Federica Farè who designed several new figures; architect Federica Farè and Veronica Santilli for the ideation and realisation of the cover; Dr. Lucia Ramera and Dr. Maria Mateos Panero who prepared the material needed to proceed with the first translation from Italian to English; Dr. Gianmario Spadacini and Dr. Paolo Moretti from the Instituto Clinico Humanitas Mater Domini Castellanza (Varese) for their guidance and leadership in the field of clinical cardiac electrophysiology; Dr. Alberto Perini for his expertise in anesthesiology and his assistance during electrophysiologic studies and pacemaker implantation procedures; Dr. Silvia Scarso and the Anesthesia Section of Cornell University for consulting on the effects of sedatives and anesthetics on the cardiac rhythm; our colleagues of the Veterinary Clinic Malpensa for their help in the management of our canine and feline patients with arrhythmias; Shari Hemsley for extensive Holter analysis at Cornell University; the cardiology residents at Cornell University; the many veterinarians who continue to refer us cases and help us expand our database of electrocardiograms and Holters by using the cardiology services of the Veterinary Clinic Malpensa and Cornell University; finally, Edra Publishing House for technical support, and Dr Carlo Scotti for believing in this work and supporting its development.

Roberto A. Santilli, N. Sydney Moïse, Romain Pariaut, Manuela Perego

Table of contents

Chapter 1
ANATOMY AND PHYSIOLOGY OF THE CONDUCTION SYSTEM ... 1

Anatomy of the conduction system ... 1
Anatomical substrates for arrhythmias ... 8
The action potential ... 9
Correlation between the phases of the action potential and electrocardiographic waves ... 12
Electrical properties of the myocardium and their relationship with the action potential ... 13
Spontaneous automaticity of pacemaker cells ... 14
Atrioventricular conduction ... 16
Propagation of the cardiac electrical impulse ... 17
Cardiac nervous control ... 18
Other factors that influence cardiac activity ... 19

Chapter 2
PRINCIPLES OF ELECTROCARDIOGRAPHY ... 21

Historical notes ... 21
The surface electrocardiogram ... 21

Chapter 3
FORMATION AND INTERPRETATION OF THE ELECTROCARDIOGRAPHIC WAVES ... 35

The electrocardiograph ... 35
Recording and calibration of the electrocardiographic tracing ... 35
Formation of the electrocardiographic waves ... 39
Electrocardiographic analysis ... 47
Tools for interpreting the electrocardiogram ... 62
Electrocardiography during the first weeks of life ... 63
Artifacts ... 64

Chapter 4
NORMAL SINUS RHYTHMS ... 71

Sinus rate ... 71
Sinus rhythm ... 72
Sinus arrhythmia ... 72
Sinus rhythms with other arrhythmias ... 81

Chapter 5
CHAMBER ENLARGEMENT ... 83

Atrial enlargement ... 83
Ventricular enlargement ... 86

Chapter 6
BACKGROUND TO THE DIAGNOSIS OF ARRHYTHMIAS ... 93

Mechanisms of arrhythmias ... 93
Abnormalities of impulse formation: automaticity and triggered activity ... 94
Abnormalities of impulse conduction ... 97
Classification of arrhythmias ... 102
Hemodynamic consequences of arrhythmias ... 105
Arrhythmia-related clinical signs ... 119
Diagnosis of arrhythmias ... 119

Chapter 7
SUPRAVENTRICULAR BEATS AND RHYTHMS ... 131

Ectopic atrial beats and rhythms ... 131
Junctional ectopic beats and rhythms ... 135
Patterns of ectopic supraventricular beats ... 139
Relationship between atrial and ventricular activation ... 140
Atrial parasystole ... 141
Atrial dissociation ... 142

Chapter 8
SUPRAVENTRICULAR TACHYCARDIAS — 145

- Sinus tachycardia — 145
- Atrioventricular nodal reciprocating tachycardia — 146
- Focal junctional tachycardia and non-paroxysmal junctional tachycardia — 149
- Atrioventricular tachycardias mediated by accessory pathways — 151
- Focal atrial tachycardia — 163
- Multifocal atrial tachycardia — 166
- Macro-reentrant atrial tachycardia (atrial flutter) — 166
- Atrial fibrillation — 174
- Differential diagnosis of narrow QRS complex tachycardias in the dog — 181

Chapter 9
VENTRICULAR ECTOPIC BEATS AND RHYTHMS — 189

- Ventricular ectopic beats — 189
- Ventricular parasystole — 200

Chapter 10
VENTRICULAR ARRHYTHMIAS — 203

- Defining tachycardia — 203
- Describing tachycardia — 204
- Monomorphic ventricular tachycardias — 206
- Polymorphic ventricular tachycardia — 216
- Bidirectional ventricular tachycardia — 220
- Ventricular fibrillation — 220
- Ventricular tachycardia without structural cardiac disease — 222
- Ventricular tachycardia during familial dilated cardiomyopathy — 226
- Ventricular tachycardias during arrhythmogenic cardiomyopathy — 227
- Ventricular tachycardias during myocarditis — 228
- Ventricular tachycardia during ischemic cardiomyopathy — 230
- Ventricular tachycardia during ventricular hypertrophy — 230
- Ventricular tachycardia during congestive heart failure — 231
- Ventricular tachycardias during systemic diseases — 231
- Differential diagnosis of wide QRS complex tachycardia — 231
- Determining the danger of ventricular tachycardias — 234

Chapter 11
BRADYARRHYTHMIAS — 239

- Sinus bradycardia — 239
- Sinus arrest — 245
- Sinus standstill — 246
- Sinus node dysfunction or sick sinus syndrome — 247
- Atrial standstill or atrioventricular muscular dystrophy — 252
- Sino-ventricular rhythm — 253
- Asystole or ventricular arrest — 254
- Pulseless electrical activity or electromechanical dissociation — 256

CHAPTER 12
CONDUCTION DISORDERS 259

Disorders of atrial conduction 259
Inter-atrial conduction block 262
Atrioventricular blocks.. 262
Intraventricular conduction disorders
or bundle branch blocks.. 272
Aberrant conduction 286
Linking or sustained aberrant conduction 288
Gap phenomenon and supernormal conduction 289

CHAPTER 13
ELECTROCARDIOGRAPHIC CHANGES SECONDARY TO SYSTEMIC DISORDERS AND DRUGS 293

Hypoxia 293
Electrolytic disorders 293
Pericardial diseases 297
Abdominal diseases 297
Chronic respiratory diseases.. 298
Endocrine diseases 299
Intracranial diseases 300
Hyperthermia and hypothermia.. 301
Electrocution 301
Autoimmune diseases 301
Drugs.. 302

CHAPTER 14
ELECTROCARDIOGRAPHY AND PACING 313

Basic components of the pacemaker............................... 313
Pacing modes... 314
Pacemaker malfunction 318

GUIDED INTERPRETATION OF ELECTROCARDIOGRAPHIC TRACINGS 325

ALPHABETICAL INDEX 341

CHAPTER 1

Anatomy and physiology of the conduction system

Under normal conditions, the electrical impulse generated by the pacemaker cells of the sinus node propagates to the atria, atrioventricular node and ventricles along bundles of specialized cardiomyocytes and triggers muscle contraction, a mechanism known as electro-mechanical coupling.

Anatomy of the conduction system

The cardiac conduction system is not directly visible on gross examination of the heart. In order to identify its various components, it is necessary to combine detailed histological studies and molecular techniques that can reveal the differences between myocytes responsible for the initiation and propagation of electrical impulses and myocytes involved in force generation. The cardiac conduction system consists of two types of tissues with different anatomical and electrophysiological characteristics: the nodal tissue and the conduction tissue. The nodal tissue contains cells that can spontaneously depolarize (*spontaneous automaticity*) and act as pacemakers. The conduction tissue is made of cells organized in bundles and usually separated from the working myocardium by a sheath of connective tissue. These cells are responsible for the rapid propagation of electrical impulses to the rest of the atrial and ventricular myocardium. The conduction system can be divided into three major components:
- the sinus node (or sino-atrial node),
- the atrioventricular junction, which includes the atrioventricular node, and
- the intraventricular conduction system.

Electrical impulses originate in the sinus node. They propagate through the atrial myocardium, the inter-atrial bundles (inferior fascicle and Bachmann's bundle), and possibly internodal tracts (anterior, middle and posterior tracts). The existence of internodal tracts remains controversial. There are likely several reasons behind this controversy: interspecies variations regarding the organization of the conduction system, difficulties in clearly identifying the path of thin bundles in serial histological sections of atrial tissue, and the lack of consistency in the terminology used to describe the various components of the conduction system. Internodal tracts between the sinus node and the atrioventricular conduction axis have been described in detail in the dog by a single investigator (DK Racker, et al.). Although other experts refute the existence of these tracts, they do agree that preferential pathways, defined by myofiber orientation, ridges, valve annuli and venous ostia, exist between the sinus node and the atrioventricular junction in all mammals commonly studied. As they approach the atrioventricular junction, impulses sequentially reach the atrionodal bundles (superior, medial and lateral bundles), the proximal atrioventricular bundle (or *inferior nodal extension*) and the compact atrioventricular node. The latter is located on the floor of the right atrium at the level of the atrioventricular fibrous skeleton. The compact atrioventricular node is in continuity with the distal atrioventricular bundle. The penetrating portion of the distal atrioventricular bundle, or *His bundle*, crosses the right fibrous trigone at the inferior part of the membranous septum, and connects the specialized conduction system of the atrioventricular junction with the specialized ventricular conduction system. Once it reaches the ventricles, the distal atrioventricular bundle divides into left and right branches.

The left branch further subdivides into an antero-superior fascicle and a postero-inferior fascicle, which lead electrical impulses from the interventricular septum to the cardiac apex. The Purkinje network finally connects the bundle branches to the working myocardium, enabling rapid and coordinated activation of the entire ventricular mass (Fig. 1.1). All cardiomyocytes are connected by gap junctions. Gap junctions are one component of the intercalated disc and are responsible for electrical coupling of myocytes; in other words, they allow cell-to-cell propagation of electrical impulses. The number of gap junctions is small within the nodes, which are regions of slow impulse velocity. These gap junctions are formed by the assembly of connexin 40 and 45 molecules. Conversely, in the specialized bundles of the conduction system, in which impulse propagation is rapid, there is a large number of gap junctions made of connexin 43.

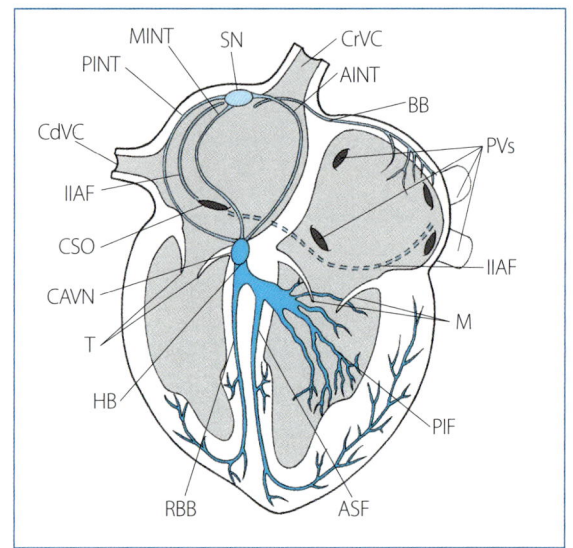

Figure 1.1. The specialized cardiac conduction system in the dog. *CrVC*: cranial vena cava; *CdVC*: caudal vena cava; *PVs*: pulmonary veins; *CSO*: coronary sinus ostium; *SN*: sinus node; *PINT*: posterior internodal tract; *MINT*: medial internodal tract; *AINT*: anterior internodal tract; *IIAF*: inferior inter-atrial fascicle; *BB*: Bachmann's bundle; *CAVN*: compact atrioventricular node; *HB*: His bundle; *RBB*: right bundle branch; *PIF*: postero-inferior fascicle; *ASF*: antero-superior fascicle; *T*: tricuspid leaflets; *M*: mitral leaflets.

Sinus node

The *sinus node* (or *sino-atrial node*) is a complex structure. Fortunately in recent years the canine sinus node has been studied, providing a more accurate appreciation of its structure and function. The sinus node is located below the epicardial surface at the junction of the cranial vena cava and the right atrium. This positioning is near the upper portion of the sulcus terminalis/crista terminalis. The sulcus terminalis is the name given to the epicardial landmark that corresponds to the endocardial landmark of the crista terminalis. These two landmarks (epicardial view versus endocardial view), which extend between the cavae (intercaval strip), represent the junction of the embryonic sinus venosus and the pectinate muscles of the right auricle. This line of demarcation, which is composed of fibrous tissue, is important in the function of the sinus node. Parallel to the sulcus terminalis/crista terminalis is the sinus node artery. This artery has two branches which surround the central sinus node. Each of these anatomical structures serves to insulate the sinus node from the atrium (Fig. 1.2).

Although the sinus node is represented in books as a well-defined nodule, it should only be seen as a schematic representation of a very complex structure (Fig. 1.2). Recent studies in dogs and humans reveal that the sinus node should really be thought of as a *sinus node complex* composed of the compact sinus node, exit pathways, and transitional cells. The compact sinus node is defined anatomically and functionally today with the aid of immunofluorescence staining for specific connexins. As explained above, specific areas of the heart have different concentrations of different types of connexins. The atrial myocardial cells have connexin 43; however, this connexin is absent in the sinus node. Therefore, staining for this protein aids in the proper identification of the sinus node. In addition to the central or compact sinus node there is a transitional region which has a mixture of cell types and varying densities of fibrous tissue and myocardial cells. In mid-size dogs, the length of the compact sinus node ranges between 15 and 20 mm, its width is between 5 and 7 mm and it is approximately 200-µm thick. A layer of atrial myocardium separates the sinus node from the endocardium. In cats, the sinus node is approximately 7-mm long, 2-mm wide and it is approximately 300- to 500-µm

Anatomy of the conduction system

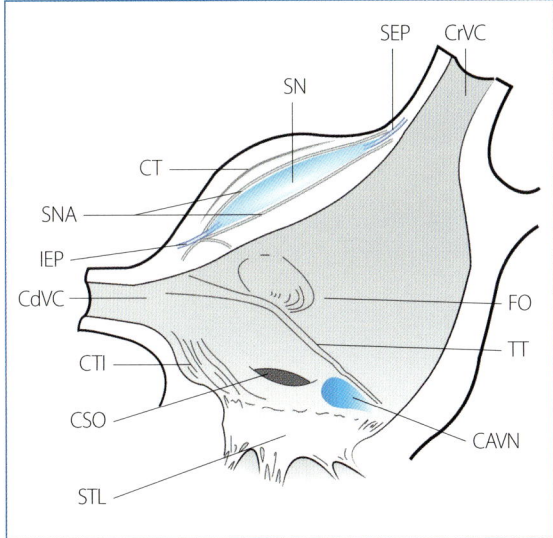

Figure 1.2. Anatomical section of the right atrial cavity and the entrance of the venae cavae after removal of part of the right atrial free wall and the right appendage to show sinus node complex anatomy. *CrVC*: cranial vena cava; *SEP*: superior exit pathway; *SN*: sinus node; *CT*: crista terminalis; *SNA*: sinus node arteries; *IEP*: inferior exit pathway; *CdVC*: caudal vena cava; *CTI*: cavotricuspid isthmus; *CSO*: coronary sinus ostium; *STL*: septal tricuspid leaflet; *CAVN*: compact atrioventricular node; *TT*: tendon of Todaro; *FO*: fossa ovalis.

The sinus node is formed by a large amount of connective tissue, and two types of specialized atrial myocytes: the P (pacemaker or "typical" nodal) cells and the T (or transitional) cells.

The *P cells* are at the center of the sinus node (compact sinus node) and account for approximately 45 % to 50 % of the cell population of the sinus node. P cells are small and sometimes called "empty cells" because they contain fewer myofilaments, mitochondria and sarcoplasmic reticulum than working atrial myocytes. Moreover, they are connected by a low number of gap junctions. At least three morphologies of P cells have been described: the first type is made of ovoid cells containing scattered myofibrils; the second type (or *spindle* cell) is characterized by an elongated shape with numerous myofibrils; finally, the third type (spider-shaped cell) consists of cells with a central body from which three or more extensions branch out.

T cells are organized at the periphery of the P cells and form a transition zone between the compact sinus node and the working atrial myocardium. T cells have an intermediate morphology between P cells and regular atrial myocytes. All degrees of intermediate morphology can be found, with some cells having almost all the characteristics of the P cells and others resembling working atrial myocytes.

There are interspecies variations regarding the vascularization of the sinus node. Two-thirds of the blood supply is provided by the sinus node artery, which is a terminal branch of the right coronary artery in 90 % of dogs, although it is a branch of the left coronary artery in 10 % of dogs. The remaining one-third is provided by collateral vessels. Venous drainage of the sinus node depends on small veins, called Thebesian veins, which, after traveling through endocardium, open into the right atrium.

Sinus node automaticity is modulated by autonomic tone, and at rest vagal tone predominates. Vagal innervation is provided by discrete vagal efferents and a local (or intrinsic) network of autonomic nerves concentrated in several epicardial fat pads. Sympathetic innervation to the sinus node travels via the left and right subclavian loops, which project from the stellate ganglia. The sinus node mainly receives input from right sympathetic fibers.

thick. Importantly, the entire sinus node complex including the sino-atrial exit pathways encompasses a much larger region. In the dog the sinus node complex can extend from the cranial vena cava to near the coronary sinus. It is this large size that permits the wandering pacemaker. It should be emphasized however that a wandering pacemaker is a reflection of atrial depolarization. The excitation of the atrium is dependent on which exit pathway is used for a given sinus impulse. Studies in the dog reveal that there are at least two such pathways with one located near the cranial vena cava (superior) and the other more inferior and lower on the atrial floor (inferior). The autonomic nervous system largely determines which pathway is used by electrical impulses to exit the sinus node. They exit from the superior exit pathway with high sympathetic tone and from the inferior exit pathway with high parasympathetic tone. It is also important to note that portions of the atria can be depolarized before the sinus node complex itself has completely depolarized.

Internodal tracts

As previously stated, the existence of anatomically distinct bundles of specialized myocytes between the sinus and atrioventricular nodes remains controversial, although detailed histopathologic studies of the atrioventricular conduction axis (DK Racker) have provided convincing evidence that they are present at least in the dog. In other species, preferential conduction pathways between the sinus and atrioventricular nodes have been recognized but do not appear to be clearly separated from the adjacent myocardium.

Based on Racker's description of the intra-atrial conduction system in dogs, there are three internodal tracts (Fig. 1.3):
- an anterior internodal tract,
- a middle internodal tract, and
- a posterior internodal tract.

The *anterior internodal tract* arises from the anterior aspect of the sinus node, runs along the anterior margin of the cranial vena cava, crosses Bachmann's bundle and then continues along the anterior part of the atrial septum. Finally, it joins the superior atrionodal bundle.

The *middle internodal tract* originates from the sinus node, runs parallel to the posterior internodal tract, anteriorly contours the region of the *fossa ovalis* and continues in the medial atrionodal bundle.

The *posterior internodal tract* originates from the sinus node, runs along the crista terminalis and travels along the posterior part of the inter-atrial septum, to reach the coronary sinus ostium. Finally, it continues in the lateral atrionodal bundle.

Inter-atrial bundles

In dogs, inter-atrial conduction occurs along two preferential pathways formed by Bachmann's bundle and the inferior inter-atrial fascicle. *Bachmann's bundle* extends from the region of the sinus node on the right to the left auricle and forms a discrete subepicardial bundle of myocytes where it straddles the inter-atrial groove (Figs. 1.1 and 1.3). The myocytes that form Bachmann's bundle have some of the characteristics of Purkinje fibers: they conduct impulses at a higher velocity than working atrial myocytes, and they are more resistant to hyperkalemia.

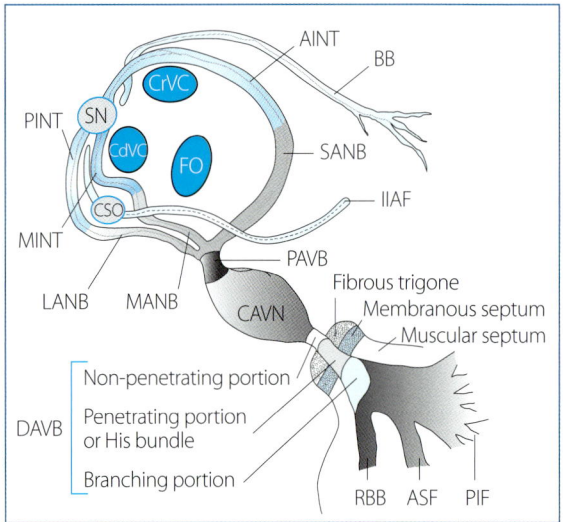

Figure 1.3. Detailed anatomy of the atrial, junctional and ventricular conduction system in the dog. See text for explanation. *SN*: sinus node; *CdVC*: caudal vena cava; *CrVC*: cranial vena cava; *CSO*: coronary sinus ostium; *FO*: fossa ovalis; *BB*: Bachmann's bundle; *IIAF*: inferior inter-atrial fascicle; *AINT*: anterior internodal tract; *MINT*: middle internodal tract; *PINT*: posterior internodal tract; *LANB*: lateral atrionodal bundle; *MANB*: medial atrionodal bundle; *SANB*: superior atrionodal bundle; *PAVB*: proximal atrioventricular bundle; *CAVN*: compact atrioventricular node; *DAVB*: distal atrioventricular bundle; *RBB*: right bundle branch; *ASF*: antero-superior fascicle; *PIF*: postero-inferior fascicle.

The *inferior inter-atrial fascicle* connects the right and left atrium along the path of the coronary sinus. The distal portion of the inferior fascicle terminates in the left atrial myocardium, at the level of the *ligament of Marshall* (Figs. 1.1 and 1.3). The ligament of Marshall is the remnant of the left cranial vena cava, and extends between the upper and lower left pulmonary veins.

The epicardial portion of the coronary sinus represents another inter-atrial connection between the lower right and left atrium.

Atrioventricular junction

The *atrioventricular junction* (or *atrioventricular conduction axis*) includes: 1) preferential pathways (*nodal approaches*) along the right atrial wall and inter-atrial septum, and possibly discrete atrionodal bundles in dogs; 2) a proximal atrioventricular bundle (or *inferior nodal extension*); 3) the compact atrioventricular node; and 4) the non-penetrating and penetrating portions of the distal atrioventricular bundle. The membranous interventricular septum represents the distal boundary of the atrioventricular junction.

Atrionodal bundles and proximal atrioventricular bundle (inferior nodal extension)

Controversies remain about the exact nature of these pathways, and whether discrete tracts (*atrionodal and proximal atrioventricular bundles*) of specialized cells proximal to the compact atrioventricular node exist. DK Racker's detailed studies of the conduction system in the canine heart support the existence of several atrionodal bundles (superior, medial and lateral) that converge into a proximal atrioventricular bundle, whereas other investigators refute the existence of specialized myocytes insulated from surrounding tissue leading to the compact atrioventricular node. Instead, their results are consistent with functional pathways formed by transitional cells (T cells) and delineated by vein ostia, intra-atrial ridges and the tricuspid valve annulus.

According to DK Racker's observations these atrionodal bundles (also called *nodal approaches*) represent the distal continuation of the internodal tracts, and constitute, together with the proximal atrioventricular bundle, the atrionodal region (AN) of the atrioventricular node (Fig. 1.3). Three atrionodal bundles have been described and classified as:
- the superior atrionodal bundle,
- the medial atrionodal bundle, and
- the lateral atrionodal bundle.

The *superior atrionodal bundle* is the distal continuation of the anterior internodal tract. It runs in the supero-anterior portion of the medial wall of the right atrium, close to the interventricular septal ridge.

The *medial atrionodal bundle* is the distal continuation of the medial internodal tract. It runs along the supero-medial portion of the coronary sinus ostium, under the epicardial layer of the right atrial medial wall, at the opposite site of the medial portion of the tendon of Todaro.

The *lateral atrionodal bundle* is the distal continuation of the posterior internodal tract. It runs along the infero-lateral portion of the coronary sinus ostium, under the epicardial layer of the infero-posterior portion of the right atrial medial wall.

The three atrionodal bundles converge to form the proximal atrioventricular bundle (or *inferior nodal extension*) which is in continuity with the compact node (Fig. 1.3).

Atrioventricular node

The *atrioventricular node* consists of a proximal portion formed by the atrionodal bundle and the proximal atrioventricular bundle, a central portion also called the *compact node*, located to the right of the fibrous trigone (or central fibrous body), and a distal portion corresponding to the non-penetrating portion of the distal atrioventricular bundle.

In dogs, the compact atrioventricular node has an elongated shape with its concave surface facing the central fibrous body and the mitral annulus. On average it is 2- to 4- mm long, with a width of 2 mm and a thickness of 0.5 to 1 mm. It is located on the floor of the right atrium approximately 1 mm below the epicardium in the triangle of Koch. The triangle of Koch is bordered by the coronary sinus ostium and its sides are delineated by the tendon of Todaro (an extension of the Eustachian valve) and the attachment of the septal leaflet of the tricuspid valve; its apex corresponds to the penetrating portion of the distal atrioventricular bundle (*bundle of His*) (Fig. 1.4).

Based on the electrophysiological characteristics of the cells, the atrioventricular node can be divided into three regions: atrionodal (AN), nodal (N) and nodo-Hisian (NH).

The *AN region* results from the convergence of the atrionodal bundles and the proximal atrioventricular bundle. This region is composed of large cells with a similar morphology to that of Purkinje cells, separated by transitional cells that have an elongated shape. These transitional cells are mixed with P cells, adipocytes, atrial myocytes, collagen and nerve fibers.

The *N region* is composed of transitional cells closely connected with each other without interposition of connective tissue. For this reason, this region is also called compact node.

The *NH region* is characterized by P cells and transitional cells connected with the Purkinje cells originating at the atrioventricular distal bundle.

Because of the very different cell populations within the AN, N and NH regions, the atrioventricular node is a site of anisotropic conduction (see p. 99).

In dogs, although the majority of the myofibers direct the electrical impulse along the proximal atrioventricular bundle, preferential pathways also exist in the anterior atrial septum. The presence of these normal pathways represents the anatomical substrate for a property of the atrioventricular node called longitudinal dissociation (Fig. 1.13).

In dogs, the atrioventricular node receives two arterial branches from the circumflex left coronary artery and from the terminal branches of the septal artery. The latter also supplies the His bundle and the proximal part of the bundle branches. Venous drainage occurs via the Thebesian system, which opens into the right atrial chamber through the Thebesian's ostium, although a small portion of blood also flows into the coronary sinus distal to its opening into the right atrium.

The atrioventricular node is densely innervated by vagal and adrenergic fibers. The atrioventricular node is predominantly influenced by the left vagal and sympathetic nerves.

Distal atrioventricular bundle

This bundle is the distal prolongation of the compact node and is the only connection between the atrial and ventricular conduction systems. Atria and ventricles are indeed electrically insulated along the entire circumference of the atrioventricular junction and semilunar rings by the fibrous skeleton. The central portion of this structure, known as the *central fibrous body*, corresponds to a triangle of fibrous tissue situated between the mitral, tricuspid and aortic valve rings. The *central fibrous body* is crossed posteriorly by the penetrating portion of the distal atrioventricular bundle, also known as the *bundle of His*.

The distal atrioventricular bundle can be divided into three segments (Fig. 1.3):
- a non-penetrating portion,
- a penetrating portion or *bundle of His*, and
- a branching portion.

The *penetrating portion* of the distal atrioventricular bundle, or *bundle of His*, is the continuation of the non-penetrating bundle, and is believed to start at the point where the cells of the specialized conduction system lose their reticulated distribution to form parallel fascicles, and ends at the point of its first branch, after crossing the right fibrous trigone at the level of the non-coronary aortic cusp. In medium-sized dogs, the His bundle is approximately 5- to 10- mm long.

The *branching segment* of the distal atrioventricular bundle starts where the postero-inferior fascicle of the left bundle branch branches off the main bundle, and ends at the emergence of the right bundle branch and the left antero-superior fascicle. Its proximal end, which is a direct continuation of the penetrating portion, is located on the posterior side of the non-coronary aortic cusp, while its distal end is located at the junction between the non-coronary and the right coronary cusps of the aortic valve when examined from the left ventricle. The branching segment of the distal atrioventricular bundle

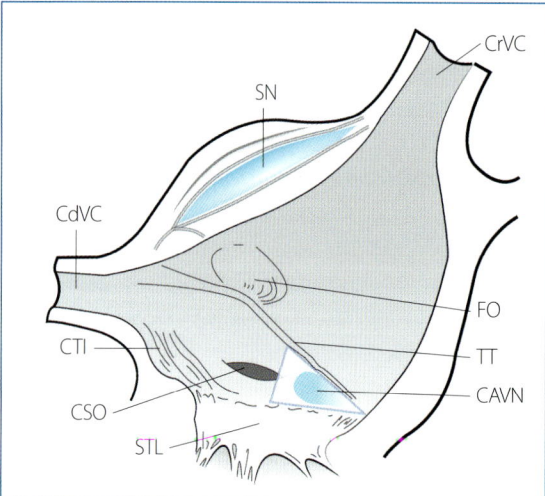

Figure 1.4. Anatomical landmarks of the junctional area and Koch's triangle. The sides of the triangle, which delimit the location of the atrioventricular node, are formed by the tendon of Todaro and the septal leaflet of the tricuspid valve. The apex of the triangle is formed by the membranous portion of the interventricular septum at the point where the penetrating portion of the distal atrioventricular bundle, or His bundle, enters the atrioventricular junction. The base of the triangle is represented by the coronary sinus ostium. *CrVC*: cranial vena cava; *SN*: sinus node; *CdVC*: caudal vena cava; *CTI*: cavotricuspid isthmus; *CSO*: coronary sinus ostium; *STL*: septal tricuspid leaflet; *CAVN*: compact atrioventricular node; *TT*: tendon of Todaro; *FO*: fossa ovalis.

is located below the insertion of the septal leaflet of the tricuspid valve when viewed from the right ventricle.

The His bundle is perfused by a small artery arising from the right coronary artery, or less frequently by the circumflex artery, which is a branch of the left coronary artery. The innervation of the His bundle is similar to that of the atrioventricular node.

Intraventricular conduction system

In dogs, the intraventricular conduction system is trifascicular in nature. The right bundle branch is an extension of the His bundle. The left bundle branch has two divisions that fan out from the branching segment of the distal atrioventricular bundle, separately or as a common trunk (Fig. 1.5).

Right bundle branch

The *right bundle branch* is in direct continuation with the His bundle. It forms a cord-like bundle that travels subendocardially down the interventricular septum to the anterior papillary muscle. A fibrous sheath insulates it from the surrounding myocardium. It then divides into several intra-cavitary false tendons (anterior, medial, posterior) that terminate in the right ventricular free wall where they ramify into a subendocardial Purkinje network. Electrical activation of the interventricular septum is not initiated by the right bundle branch (Fig. 1.5). The length of the right bundle branch in medium-size dogs is 35 to 40 mm.

Left bundle branch

The *left bundle branch* fans out of the branching portion of the distal atrioventricular bundle, and then, immediately below the aortic leaflets, forms a postero-inferior fascicle and an antero-superior fascicle, which then travel towards the base of the postero-medial and antero-lateral papillary muscles, respectively. In dogs, the initial truncular portion of the left bundle branch is short (6-8 mm in medium-size dogs) and wide (approximately 5 mm), and its path is subendocardial. It continues to widen until it divides into the two fascicles. Unlike the right bundle branch that has a cord-like aspect, the truncular portion of the left bundle branch is flat and ribbon-shaped.

The number of fascicles that emerge from the common trunk, and their divisions and paths are highly

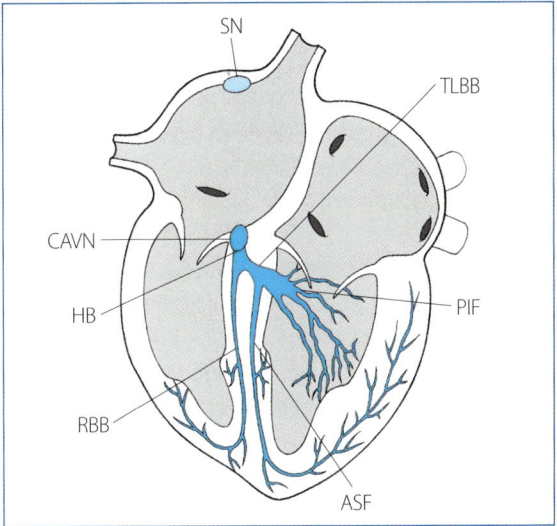

Figure 1.5. Anatomy of the atrioventricular and intraventricular conduction system. *SN*: sinus node; *CAVN*: compact portion of the atrioventricular node; *HB*: His bundle; *RBB*: right bundle branch; *TLBB*: truncular portion of the left bundle branch; *PIF*: postero-inferior fascicle; *ASF*: antero-superior fascicle.

variable. In the human heart, a discrete third branch, positioned between the two other fascicles and called the septal fascicle is commonly present. Nevertheless, for the purpose of electrocardiographic interpretation, two main fascicles are described, one in an antero-superior position and the other in a postero-inferior position (Fig. 1.5).

The *antero-superior fascicle* appears as a direct continuation of the trunk of the left bundle branch and is oriented supero-inferiorly and postero-anteriorly. In dogs, the antero-superior fascicle is thin and measures 3.5 to 4 cm in medium-size animals.

The *postero-inferior fascicle* emerges almost perpendicularly from the truncular portion of the left bundle. In dogs, the postero-inferior fascicle is thick and measures approximately 3.5 cm in medium-size animals.

Purkinje network

The *Purkinje fibers* connect the terminal portion of the conduction system to the endocardial surface of the ventricles. The myocytes that form the Purkinje fibers are connected by a high number of intercalated discs, which facilitate rapid propagation of electrical impulses (approximately 2 m/s).

On the left side, the Purkinje fibers form a subendocardial network that is denser around the papillary muscles and less developed at the base of the ventricles. Some fibers travel directly inside the cavity of the ventricles, and are called "false tendons". The Purkinje network of the anterior wall of the left ventricle depends on the antero-superior division of the left bundle branch, while the network of the posterior wall is associated with the postero-inferior division. It is more difficult to identify the origin of the septal and apical left Purkinje network, although, in most cases, the interventricular septum and the apical region are activated by fibers in continuity with the postero-inferior division. The distribution of the Purkinje network in the right ventricular wall and on the right surface of the interventricular septum is connected to the major ramifications of the right bundle branch. The concentration of Purkinje fibers is greater in the antero-apical region of the right ventricular wall and in the apical third of the interventricular septum. Purkinje fibers are mostly absent in the ventricular outflow region.

Anatomical substrates for arrhythmias

Several cardiac anatomical structures are involved in the genesis of arrhythmias. The main anatomical substrates that have been identified in dogs are shown in Table 1.1.

Atrial tachycardias originate from foci distributed within the atria, particularly in the region of the crista terminalis, the coronary sinus ostium and the ostia of the pulmonary veins, which have been recognized as a trigger for atrial fibrillation.

Atrial myocardial fiber stretch, fibrosis and electrical remodeling secondary to atrial dilation can promote atrial tachycardia, atrial flutter and atrial fibrillation. Atrioventricular muscular dystrophy or atrial standstill is another rhythm disturbance linked to severe atrial fibrosis.

The *cavotricuspid isthmus* is a small region of the right atrium that forms the slow conduction area of an atrial flutter circuit. Specifically, it is at the level of the posterior right atrium and delimited by the ostium of the caudal vena cava, the Eustachian ridge and the annulus of the tricuspid valve. The complete circuit of atrial flutter is a ring of myocardium that includes the septal and posterior walls of the right atrium, joined dorsally by the roof of the right atrium. The wavefront of depolarization can travel in a counterclockwise direction, resulting in an arrhythmia called typical flutter, or it can rotate clockwise, resulting in a reverse typical flutter.

Occasionally, the electrical insulation of the fibrous skeleton between the atrium and ventricle is interrupted by an accessory atrioventricular pathway. This muscular bundle is also known as a bypass tract because it allows electrical impulses to bypass the atrioventricular node, and travel from atrium to ventricle, or retrogradely from ventricle to atrium. Accessory pathways are responsible for the occurrence of atrioventricular reciprocating tachycardia.

Various forms of ventricular tachycardia circuits are associated with the presence of myocardial fibrosis secondary to cardiomyopathies, including dilated cardiomyopathy, hypertrophic cardiomyopathy and arrhythmogenic right ventricular cardiomyopathy (Fig. 1.6).

TABLE 1.1. Anatomical structures involved in the genesis of rhythm disturbances in the dog.

Anatomical structure	Rhythm disturbance
Atrial myocardium Crista terminalis Coronary sinus Pulmonary veins Caval veins Ligament or vein of Marshall	Focal atrial tachycardia
Atrial remodeling	Focal atrial tachycardia Atrial fibrillation Atrial flutter
Cavotricuspid isthmus	Typical and reverse typical atrial flutter
Accessory pathway (Kent fibers)	Atrioventricular tachycardia
Myocardial fibrosis in structural heart disease	Focal atrial tachycardia Atrial fibrillation Ventricular tachycardia Ventricular fibrillation Atypical atrial flutter
Fibrous and/or fatty myocardial replacement	Atrial standstill Ventricular tachycardia

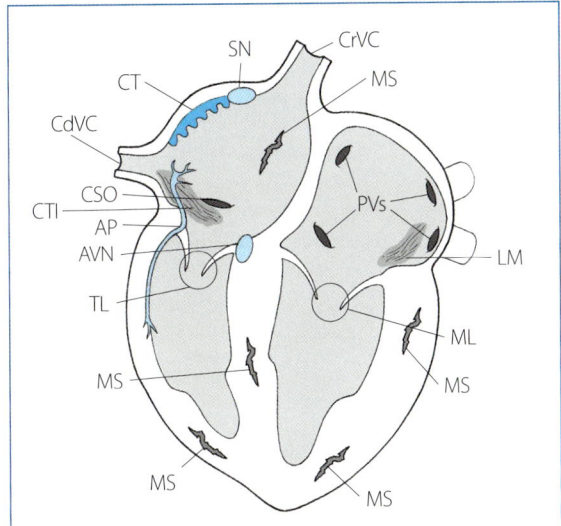

Figure 1.6. Anatomy of the principal sites involved in the genesis of cardiac arrhythmias. *SN*: sinus node; *CT*: crista terminalis; *CrVC*: cranial vena cava; *CdVC*: caudal vena cava; *PVs*: pulmonary veins; *CTI*: cavotricuspid isthmus; *CSO*: coronary sinus ostium; *AVN*: atrioventricular node; *LM*: ligament of Marshall; *TL*: tricuspid leaflets; *ML*: mitral leaflets; *AP*: accessory pathway; *MS*: myocardial scars.

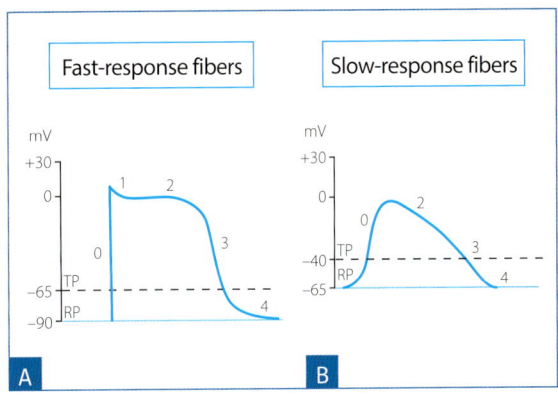

Figure 1.7. Changes in the transmembrane potential value of the fast-response fibers (A) and the slow-response fibers (B). Note how the fast-response fibers show lower values of the resting transmembrane potential (RP) and the threshold potential (TP), a steeper phase 0 of the action potential and a larger amplitude compared to the action potential characteristics of the slow-response fibers. Phase 1 is absent in the slow-response fibers.

The action potential

Resting membrane potential

All cell membranes are polarized. The *resting membrane potential* of cardiomyocytes corresponds to a difference in electrical charge between the intracellular and extracellular space in the absence of an electrical impulse. At rest, the cell membrane is impermeable to Na^+ and partially permeable to K^+ and Cl^- ions. The Na^+ concentration is lower in the intracellular space in part because of the continuous activity of the Na^+/K^+ pump, which hydrolyses ATP to pump Na^+ out of the cell and move K^+ into the cell. Potassium concentration therefore remains higher in the intracellular space. Chloride concentration is higher in the extracellular compartment, which promotes the passive diffusion of Cl^- into the cell. As a result of the increased permeability to K^+, the *resting transmembrane potential* of most cardiomyocytes (working myocardium and Purkinje cells) varies between −80 mV and −90 mV, which approaches the Nernst potential for K^+. A true resting potential does not exist in the P (pacemaker) cells of the sinus node and the atrioventricular node, as these cells continuously depolarize between two action potentials. The lowest transmembrane potential varies from −50 mV to −70 mV in the P cells because of a different expression of ion channels on their surface compared with that of other myocytes (Fig. 1.7).

Any stimulus, whether it is from a P cell or an external electrical impulse that is able to alter the transmembrane potential to a critical value, called the *threshold potential*, can trigger an action potential in the neighboring cells. The threshold potential of the nodal cells is −40 mV, while it is −65 mV to −70 mV in the Purkinje cells and working myocardium.

Phases of the action potential

There are two types of action potentials: "fast response" and "slow response" (Fig. 1.7). The fast response action potential is found in atrial and ventricular working cardiomyocytes and in the cells of the atrioventricular conduction axis, with the exception of the compact node. The slow response action potential is characteristic of the P cells of the sinus node and the compact node (Figs. 1.7 and 1.8).

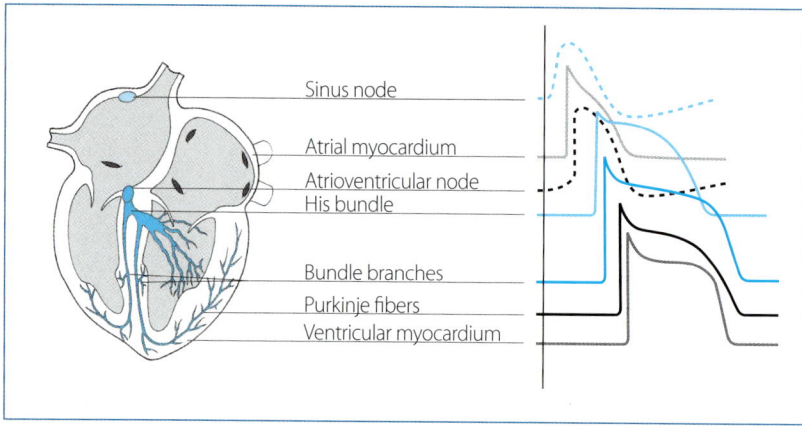

Figure 1.8. Morphology of the action potential in different regions of the conduction tissue, the atrial and ventricular working myocardium. Note the absence of phase 1, the reduction in the slope and amplitude of phase 0, the shorter action potential duration, and spontaneous phase 4 depolarization in the pacemaker cells of the sinus node and the atrioventricular node, compared to the working atrial and ventricular myocardium.

Phases of the fast response action potential

The *action potential* is divided into five phases:

Phase 0 or rapid depolarization. Because the cell membrane is polarized at rest, the first phase of the action potential is depolarization (a change from more negative to less negative and even positive values). It starts with a rapid rise of the transmembrane potential (rate of depolarization of 100-200 V/s in the atrial and ventricular myocytes, and 500-1000 V/s in the fibers of the His-Purkinje system) to a peak voltage of approximately +30 mV that corresponds to a Na$^+$ (I_{Na}) current caused by the rapid influx of Na$^+$ through voltage-gated Na$^+$ channels (Na$_v$1.5) and the simultaneous decreased permeability of the membrane to K$^+$. The structure of the Na$^+$ channels includes two "gates", described by Hodgkin and Huxley; one called the *m or activation gate*, and the other called the *h or inactivation gate*. During the resting phase between two action potentials (phase 4, also called diastolic interval), the flux of Na$^+$ across the membrane is blocked because *m* gates are closed. The voltage-dependent gating of the Na$^+$ channels means that the *m* gates quickly open when the threshold potential of −65 mV is reached, allowing the rapid influx of Na$^+$ into the cell driven by the concentration gradient. The transmembrane voltage rapidly reaches a value between 0 mV and +40 mV. The transition from a negative transmembrane voltage to a positive one is called the *overshoot phase*. At this point the flux of Na$^+$ ions stops as a result of the closure of the *h* gates, which reflects the time-dependent gating property of the channel. The *h* gates remain closed until the transmembrane potential returns to resting values, preventing any further exchange of Na$^+$ across the membrane until the end of the action potential.

Phase 1 or early repolarization phase. This phase is a brief period of repolarization associated with a potassium current (transient outward current or I_{to}) corresponding to an efflux of K$^+$. The transmembrane potential returns to approximately 0 mV at the end of phase 1. The transient outward current is stronger in the epicardium than the endocardium. When phase 1 is amplified the action potential duration is prolonged, and it is shortened if phase 1 is attenuated. Indeed, the transmembrane voltage at the end of phase 1 determines the magnitude of the Ca^{2+} current during the subsequent phase of the action potential (phase 2). A calcium-activated chloride current also contributes to phase 1. Of special note in the dog is the ion channel I_{to}. I_{to} can be prominent in the epicardium of the dog and is responsible for the J wave that is seen in the terminal portion of the downstroke of the R wave particularly in leads II, III and aVF. The expression of this particular ion channel is not fully mature in the dog until approximately 4 to 5 months of age. Consequently, J waves are most commonly seen in mature dogs. Moreover, this particular deflection varies in breeds. In human beings this may be an indication of an ominous electrophysiologic situation or induced by hypothermia, and although such situations can exaggerate the J wave in the dog, it is a normal finding (Figs. 1.9 and 1.10).

Phase 2 or plateau. This phase is characterized by an influx of Ca^{2+} through voltage-gated L (*long-lasting*)-type Ca^{2+} channels. L-type Ca^{2+} channels open when the transmembrane potential is approximately −10 mV. The depolarizing current I_{Ca-L} secondary to the influx of Ca^{2+} is rapidly balanced by the contribution of two outward currents (a larger current I_{Ks} and a smaller current I_{Kr}). The small influx of Ca^{2+} during the plateau phase triggers the release into the cytoplasm of large amounts of Ca^{2+} stored in the sarcoplasmic reticulum, which subsequently triggers myocardial contraction, a phenomenon known as excitation-contraction coupling. During the final phase of the plateau, the transmembrane potential value decreases gradually in response to a reduction in the conductance for Ca^{2+}, and a simultaneous increase in the conductance for K^+, thus initiating phase 3 of the action potential, or repolarization.

Phase 3 or final repolarization. This phase results from at least three K^+ currents (I_{Ks}, I_{Kr}, I_{K1}) associated with an efflux of K^+. I_{Kr} is the major contributor of phase 3, which ultimately brings the transmembrane potential back to resting values. I_{Kur} is a potassium current only measured in the atrial myocytes which contributes to repolarization and is responsible for the shorter action potential duration in the atrial myocytes than in the ventricular myocytes.

Phase 4 or resting phase. During this phase, the membrane potential is back to resting values. The intracellular concentration of ions is restored by ionic pumps (Na^+/K^+-ATPase, Ca^{2+}-ATPase) and the Na^+/Ca^{2+} exchanger. In the atrial, His-Purkinje and ventricular cells, the value of the resting membrane potential is mainly determined by the high conductance for K^+ ions through I_{K1} channels.

Phases of the slow response action potential

The slow response action potential is a characteristic of not only myocytes in the sinus and atrioventricular nodes but also many other regions of the heart. These myocytes have in common the expression of the transcriptional inhibitor Tbx3. There are several major differences between the slow response and the fast response action potential:

- The membrane potential is less negative during phase 4 of the action potential because of the absence of the potassium channel $K_{ir}2$ that is associated with the I_{K1} current and is responsible for maintaining the resting membrane potential at –90 mV.
- A stable resting membrane potential does not exist during phase 4, as slow depolarization starts immediately after the end of the preceding action potential (*diastolic depolarization*). Two mechanisms are responsible for the spontaneous depolarization that characterizes the slow response action potential: the "membrane or voltage clock" and the "calcium clock". The "voltage clock" corresponds to the progressive reduction in repolarizing currents via the closure of potassium channels at the end of an action potential and several depolarizing currents: I_f current from the activation of HCN channels leading to an influx of Na^+; and $I_{Ca,T}$ and $I_{Ca,L}$ currents from the activation of calcium channels leading to an influx of Ca^{2+}. The "calcium clock" is initiated by the spontaneous release of Ca^{2+} from the sarcoplasmic reticulum through the ryanodine receptor which triggers an influx of Na^+ and an efflux of Ca^{2+} in a 3:1 ratio (3 Na^+ for 1 Ca^{2+}) through the transmembrane Na^+/Ca^{2+} exchanger. The "calcium clock" mainly contributes to the final portion of phase 4.
- Phase 0 is dependent on a calcium current ($I_{Ca,L}$), and due to the absence of voltage-gated Na^+ channels ($Na_v1.5$) the upstroke of phase 4 is not as steep as it is in regular myocytes. The threshold potential of phase 0 is –40 mV and its slow upstroke results in a low conduction velocity.
- There is no phase 1.

Finally, pathologic states, especially ischemia, can lead any cardiomyocyte to develop the characteristics of slow response cells and depolarize spontaneously (*abnormal enhanced automaticity*).

The pacemaker current If is a major contributor of spontaneous automaticity in the sinus node and the atrioventricular junction. It also appears to participate in the diastolic depolarization of Purkinje cells, although this complex process likely involves other factors, including intracellular Ca^{2+} cycling and a K^+ current called I_{Kdd}. It is possible, however, that I_{Kdd} and I_f represent the same current.

Transmural dispersion of action potential

Epicardial myocytes exhibit an action potential with a prominent phase 1 and a doming shape. Myocytes in the mid-myocardium, referred to as M cells, have a prominent and clearly visible phase 1 and a longer action potential compared to the myocytes of the epicardium and the endocardium. Finally, endocardial myocytes have an action potential with a small phase 1 and a duration intermediate between epicardial and mid-myocardial cells.

These differences in duration and morphology of the action potentials reflect different expressions of I_{to} and I_{Ks} potassium channels: I_{to} channels are present in large numbers in epicardial myocytes, to a lesser extent in the M cells and are almost absent in the endocardial myocytes. The reduced number of I_{Ks} channels in M cells explains their prolonged phase 2.

The differences in amplitude and duration of the action potentials generate a transmural electrical gradient during repolarization of the heart. The resulting electrical heterogeneity between layers of myocardium can serve as the substrate for arrhythmias, via a mechanism called reentry (see p. 99).

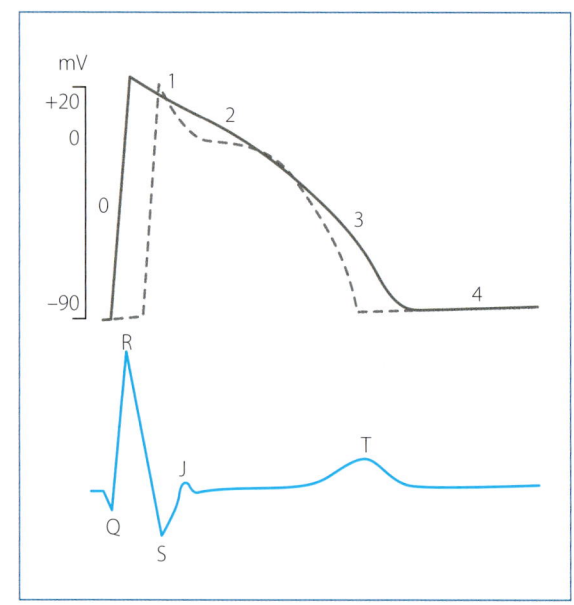

Figure 1.9. Correlation between the phases of the transmembrane action potential and electrocardiographic waves. The solid line represents an action potential in the subendocardial cells, while the dotted line corresponds to an action potential recorded from the subepicardial cells.

Correlation between the phases of the action potential and electrocardiographic waves

The QRS complex of the surface electrocardiogram represents the manifestation on the body surface of the algebraic sum of two action potentials with different morphology, one deriving from the activation of the subendocardial myocytes and one resulting from the activation of subepicardial myocytes. The action potential of the subendocardial cells starts and ends earlier than the action potential of the subepicardial cells since depolarization follows an endocardium to epicardium direction, while repolarization progresses from the epicardium to the endocardium. The correlation between the monophasic action potential and electrocardiographic waves is as follows (Fig. 1.9):
- Phase 0 - beginning of the QRS complex;
- Phase 1 - J point;
- Phase 2 - S-T segment;
- Phase 3 - T wave;
- Phase 4 - electrical diastole.

On the electrocardiogram, the duration of the action potential of ventricular epicardial cells is approximately from the onset of the QRS complex to the peak of the T wave and for the mid-myocardial cells, it is from the onset of the QRS complex to the end of the T wave. The transmural dispersion of repolarization can be approximated by the interval from the peak to the end of the T wave. As described previously, the heterogeneity of repolarization within the ventricles can become the substrate for arrhythmias. The risk of arrhythmias is maximum during a brief portion of ventricular repolarization, called the *vulnerable period*, which corresponds to the peak of the T wave in lead II of the surface electrocardiogram in dogs. A stimulus of adequate intensity delivered during the vulnerable period can trigger ventricular fibrillation. There is also a vulnerable period for the atria which corresponds to the descending branch of the R wave or the S wave.

Electrical properties of the myocardium and their relationship with the action potential

Several properties characterize the myocardium: excitability, automaticity, refractoriness and conduction velocity.

Excitability is the ability of a cell to generate an action potential as a result of a stimulus equal to or above the membrane threshold potential. Excitability depends on the availability of Na^+ channels to open in response to a stimulus.

Automaticity is the ability of a cell to spontaneously generate an action potential. Automaticity is a characteristic of the sinus node (the *leading pacemaker*) and subsidiary pacemakers, including various areas in the atria, the ostia of pulmonary veins, the coronary sinus, atrioventricular valves, portions of the atrioventricular conduction axis and the His-Purkinje system. These subsidiary pacemakers are usually latent because they are inhibited by the faster rate of the sinus node (*overdrive suppression*). Working atrial and ventricular myocytes do not have the property of automaticity, and only generate an action potential if triggered by an adequate stimulus.

Refractoriness or refractory period is a period of time when myocytes are non-excitable, and it extends from phase 0 to the end of phase 3 of the action potential. The refractory period is due to the inactivation of the Na^+ channels soon after the onset of the action potential (Fig. 1.10). The total refractory period can be divided into effective and relative refractory periods:

- The *effective refractory period* is defined as the period beginning with phase 0 of the action potential and ending during the repolarization phase (approximately halfway during phase 3), when an appropriate electrical stimulus cannot evoke another action potential. Indeed, when the membrane is depolarized to a value of −50 mV or less, all Na^+ channels are inactivated, and therefore an action potential cannot be initiated. Electrocardiographically the effective refractory period of the ventricles begins with the QRS complex and ends at the beginning of the T wave.
- The *relative refractory period* is the time between the end of the effective refractory period and the end of the action potential. It, therefore, extends from the mid-portion to the last portion of phase 3. This period corresponds to the progressive re-activation of the Na^+ channels that occurs when the membrane potential returns below −50 mV. Na^+ channels have fully recovered when the membrane potential reaches −90 mV. During the relative refractory period, myocytes can respond to very intense stimuli that initiate action potentials with a decreased upstroke velocity (phase 0) due to the low number of Na^+ channels available. As a result, impulse conduction is slower within the myocardium. On the electrocardiogram, the relative refractory period of the ventricles corresponds to the initial portion of the T wave.

The *phase of supernormal excitability* is a short period after the relative refractory period when a sub-threshold stimulus can elicit an action potential. The action potential generated is not "better" than normal, but instead unexpected, because the same stimulus would fail to initiate an action potential if delivered just before or just after the supernormal phase. The phase of supernormal excitability corresponds to the period when the membrane potential is close to the membrane threshold potential, as it returns to diastolic values.

The sum of the effective refractory period and the relative refractory period represents the *total refractory period*. The difference in refractory period between cardiac cells within the conduction system and the different layers of the myocardium limits the risk of retrograde conduction.

Changes of the cardiac cycle length (heart rate) alter the duration of the action potential, and therefore the refractory period: an increase of the cycle length (slower heart rate) results in an increase of the action potential duration; conversely, a shortening of the cycle length (faster heart rate) is associated with a decrease of the action potential duration. The potassium currents responsible for this mechanism are I_{KS} and I_{to}.

Conduction is the property of cells to propagate an impulse from one cell to another. The conduction characteristics vary between fast response fibers and slow response fibers. In the fast response fibers, conduction velocity is proportional to the intensity of the Na^+ current during phase 0 of the action potential (slope of phase 0) and the maximum diastolic potential value (or resting

Chapter 1. Anatomy and physiology of the conduction system

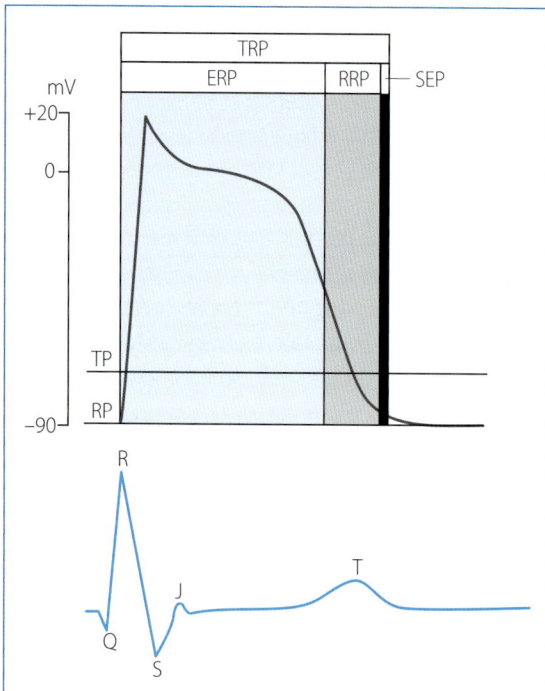

Figure 1.10. Ventricular action potential, refractory periods and relationship with the surface electrocardiogram. *ERP*: effective refractory period; *RRP*: relative refractory period; *SEP*: supernormal excitability period; *TP*: threshold potential; *RP*: resting potential; *TRP*: total refractory period.

potential). The slope of phase 0 corresponds to the rate of change of the membrane voltage over time (dVm/dt). An increase in the slope of phase 0 causes an increase in conduction velocity along the cell. The value of the resting membrane potential determines the number of Na⁺ channels available at the onset of phase 0 (100 % for a resting membrane potential of –90 mV, 50 % for a resting membrane potential of –75 mV and 0 % for a resting membrane potential of –40 mV). A more negative resting potential results in a larger amplitude phase 0 and higher conduction velocity along the myofiber. In addition to the slope and amplitude of phase 0 of the action potential, other factors that contribute to conduction velocity include the diameter of the cells, the number of intercalated discs between cells, and the type of connexin that forms the gap junctions. Conduction velocity of the fast fibers varies from 0.8 to 1 m/s for the atrial and ventricular myocytes, and reaches 1 to 5 m/s in specialized conduction tissue.

Conduction in the nodal tissue (slow-response action potential) is much slower, between 0.05 and 0.1 m/s. It results from the slow depolarization phase associated with an influx of calcium, the large amount of connective tissue with nodal tissue, the small diameter of the intranodal myocytes, the low number of intercalated discs between cells and the composition of the gap junctions (mostly connexin 45).

Spontaneous automaticity of pacemaker cells

Pacemaker cells present in the sinus node, AN and NH regions of the atrioventricular node, the bundle of His and the Purkinje fibers have the ability to spontaneously depolarize and generate a regenerative action potential in the absence of an external stimulus. The membrane potential progressively changes to less negative values during phase 4 until it reaches the threshold potential for the initiation of an action potential.

The rate of spontaneous depolarization is modulated by three main factors: the slope of phase 4 depolarization, the threshold potential and the membrane potential at the initiation of phase 4 (Fig. 1.11A):

- An increase in the slope of phase 4 allows the membrane potential to reach the threshold potential sooner, which leads to an increase in the discharge rate of the pacemaker (increased heart rate); conversely, a decrease in the slope of phase 4 prolongs the time needed to reach threshold, causing a reduction in the discharge rate of the pacemaker (Fig. 1.11B).
- A shift of the threshold potential towards less negative values delays the onset of phase 0 of the action potential, causing a reduction in the pacemaker discharge rate, while a shift of the threshold potential towards more negative values results in an earlier onset of phase 0, causing an increase in the rate of the pacemaker (Fig. 1.11C).
- A less negative membrane potential at the initiation of phase 4 makes it easier to reach the threshold value, and results in an increase of the discharge rate of the pacemaker. Alternatively, if the membrane potential

is more negative at the beginning of phase 4 (hyperpolarized), the discharge rate of the pacemaker decreases (Fig. 1.11D).

Under normal conditions, the rate of discharge of the sinus P cells is higher than the intrinsic rate of the P cells in other parts of the heart (i.e. atrioventricular node, bundle of His and Purkinje network). In dogs, the rate of spontaneous depolarization of the P cells is 70 to 160 bpm in the sinus node, 40 to 60 bpm in the AN and NH regions of the atrioventricular node, and 15 to 40 bpm in the Purkinje fibers (Fig. 1.12).

The P cells with the higher discharge rate at a given moment govern the cardiac rhythm, and become the *dominant pacemaker*. During physiological conditions, the dominant pacemaker is the sinus node. The mechanism by which the spontaneous automaticity of other P cells with a slower firing rate is depressed by those that have a higher discharge rate is called *overdrive suppression*. This suppression of automaticity seems to be dependent on the increased activity of the ATPase Na^+/K^+ pump, which removes an excess of positively charged Na^+ ions from the intracellular space, and as a result hyperpolarizes the cell membrane. This hyperpolarization prolongs the time needed for the cell membrane potential to reach threshold, limiting the competition between the dominant and the slower subsidiary pacemaker sites. Recovery from overdrive suppression is delayed, as the increased activity of the ATPase Na^+/K^+ pump continues for some time after cessation of the dominant pacemaker.

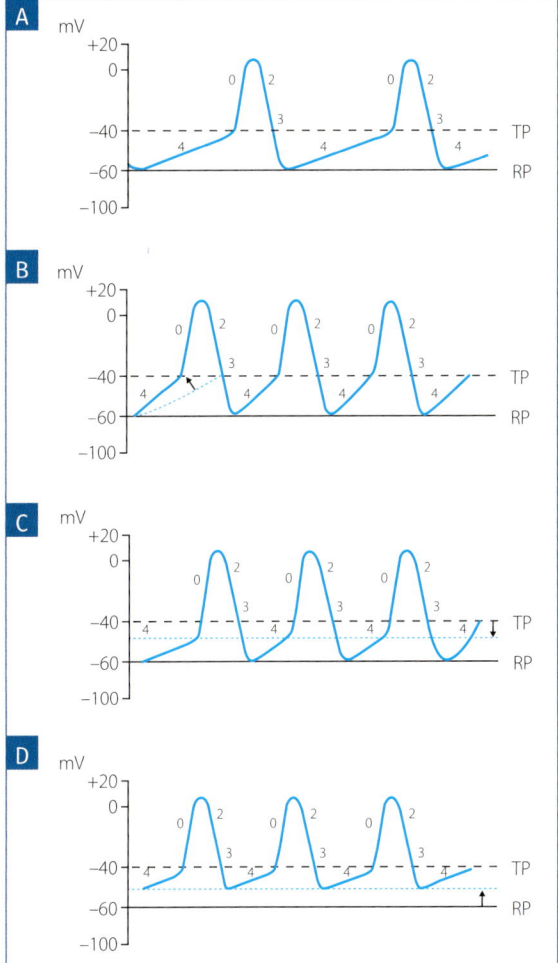

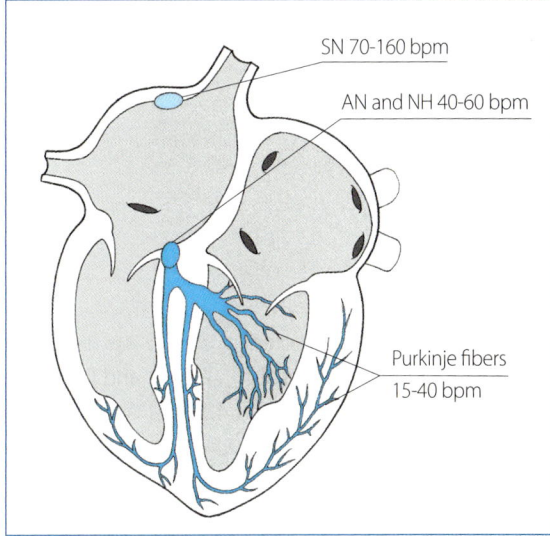

Figure 1.11. Mechanisms involved in the control of the firing rate of the pacemaker cells of the sinus node. A) Normal firing rate of the sinus node. B) An increase in the slope of phase 4. C) A lower (more negative value) threshold potential. D) A less negative membrane voltage at the onset of phase 4 depolarization. The increase of the depolarization rate of the pacemaker cells is usually caused by a combination of these three mechanisms.
TP: threshold potential; *RP*: resting potential.

Figure 1.12. Normal values of the depolarization rate of pacemaker cells in different regions of the conduction system in dogs. *SN*: sinus node; *AN*: atrionodal region; *NH*: nodal-His region.

Atrioventricular conduction

Conduction along the atrioventricular node can occur in either an anterograde (*atrioventricular conduction*) direction or a retrograde (*ventriculo-atrial conduction*) direction. Impulse propagation through the atrioventricular conduction axis usually takes approximately 110 ms: the impulse travels through the atrionodal segment (AN) during the first 30 ms, then through the compact node for approximately 60 ms, and finally through the nodo-hissian (NH) segment for the last 20 ms. Although it is generally accepted that maximum reduction in the velocity of impulse propagation occurs in the region of the compact node, a few studies localize this effect to the proximal atrioventricular bundle (*inferior nodal extension*).

Conduction through the atrioventricular node involves, both in humans and dogs, a fast pathway and a slow pathway (*longitudinal dissociation*). The slow pathway starts in the postero-inferior region of the right atrium by the ostium of the coronary sinus. It is bordered by the tendon of Todaro and the insertion of the tricuspid valve as it extends along the proximal atrionodal bundle (also referred to as the inferior nodal extension) towards the compact node (Fig. 1.13). The fast pathway starts in the antero-superior right atrial region and travels anteriorly down the inter-atrial septum towards the compact node (Fig. 1.13).

The atrioventricular junction is one of the structures of the conduction system in which *decremental conduction occurs*. The others described in the dog are the postero-septal atrioventricular accessory pathways responsible for permanent junctional reciprocating tachycardia and the sinus node from the leading pacemaker site to its terminal parts. Decremental conduction corresponds to a progressive delay of impulse propagation across the atrioventricular junction with increasing heart rate. As the rate increases, myocytes have only time to recover partially from the previous action potential before they are depolarized again, which affects the slope of the subsequent action potential and the propagation of electrical impulses. The cumulative effect of repetitive depolarizations can lead to complete block of the electrical impulse in the atrioventricular junction. The property of decremental conduction gives the atrioventricular node the

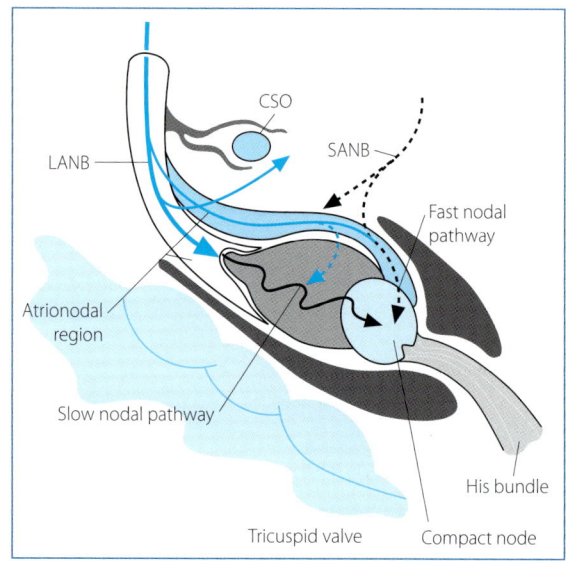

Figure 1.13. Anatomy of the junctional region according to the theory of longitudinal dissociation. The picture shows the location of the slow nodal pathway which, starting from the lateral atrionodal bundle crosses longitudinally the proximal atrioventricular bundle and the compact portion of the atrioventricular node, following the typical slow conduction pathway. The fast nodal pathway proceeds along the inter-atrial septum from the antero-superior region of the right atrium to enter and cross through the distal portion of the compact node in a transverse direction. The direction of the impulse as it crosses the compact node through the fast pathway avoids the slowing of conduction. *SANB*: superior atrionodal bundle; *LANB*: lateral atrionodal bundle; *CSO*: coronary sinus ostium.

important role of a "filter" during rapid supraventricular arrhythmias, by reducing the number of supraventricular impulses that can activate the ventricles (*ventricular response*).

Although impulse propagation within the atrioventricular node is not directly detectable on the surface electrocardiogram, it can affect a subsequent impulse by delaying atrioventricular conduction. Concealed *conduction* is a term used to describe the characteristics of the surface electrocardiogram that reveal an alteration of the properties of the atrioventricular node by a previous event that was hidden to the observer. A detailed examination of the electrocardiogram can reveal the presence of concealed atrioventricular conduction by identifying an apparently unexplained prolongation of the PQ interval, due to the fact that the node is in a state of partial refractoriness. Anterograde atrioventricular conduction can be influenced by concealed conduction following an atrial ectopy, during atrial tachycardia, atrial flutter and atrial fibrillation. Concealead conduction in the atrioventricular node can also result from retrograde (ventriculo-atrial) conduction of a ventricular ectopic beat.

Ventriculo-atrial conduction typically occurs along the normal nodal conduction tissue (*concentric ventriculo-atrial conduction*), but occasionally through atrioventricular accessory pathways (*eccentric ventriculo-atrial conduction*).

Concentric ventriculo-atrial conduction corresponds to the passage of electrical impulses in a retrograde direction, i.e. from the ventricles to the atria, along the atrioventricular conduction axis. In this case, atrial depolarization starts at the level of the inter-atrial septum, proximal to the anterior junctional region, and then propagates simultaneously to the two atrial chambers (Fig. 1.14A). Concentric ventriculo-atrial conduction occurs with ventricular ectopic beats, ventricular tachycardia, ventricular escape rhythm, junctional rhythms and tachycardia, common nodal atrioventricular reciprocating tachycardia or in animals with cardiac pacemakers.

Eccentric ventriculo-atrial conduction is defined as the passage of impulses from the ventricles to the atria through a pathway other than the atrioventricular node, usually an atrioventricular accessory pathway. In this type of conduction, the atria are activated sequentially, starting from a point more or less distant from the atrioventricular node, which corresponds to the atrial insertion of the accessory pathway. This type of conduction is present during orthodromic atrioventricular reciprocating tachycardia and during ventricular rhythms with retrograde conduction through the accessory pathway (Fig. 1.14B).

Propagation of the cardiac electrical impulse

Electrical impulses generated by the P cells of the sinus node propagate through the atrial myocardium and preferential pathways to depolarize the entire atrial mass, with a velocity within the sinus node of approximately 0.05 m/s and in the atrial myocardium of approximately 0.8 to 1 m/s. The wavefront proceeds from the sinus node to the atrioventricular node. Within the node, normal slowing of conduction occurs, which allows mechanical atrioventricular synchrony.

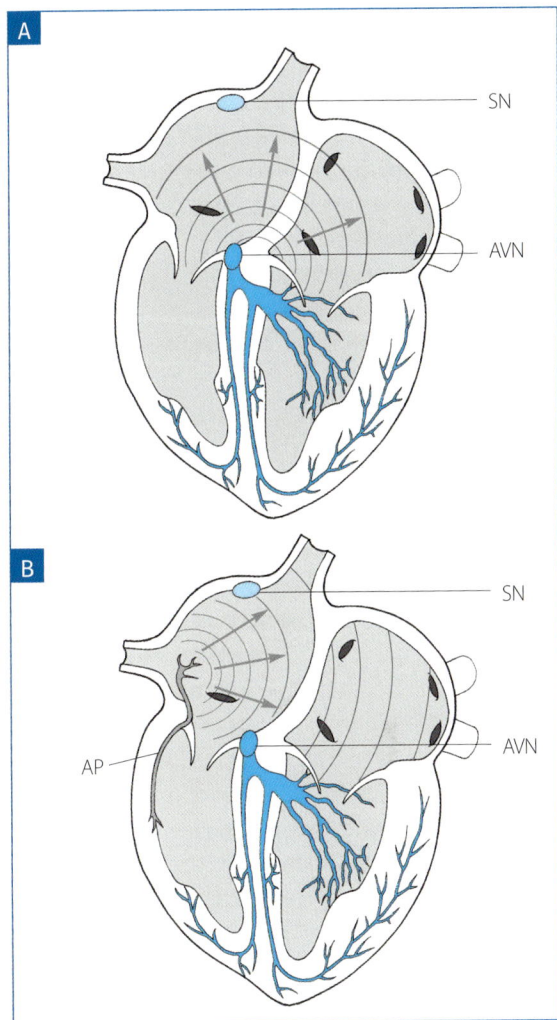

Figure 1.14. Direction of the wavefront in the frontal plane during concentric ventriculo-atrial conduction (A) and eccentric ventriculo-atrial conduction (B). Note that during concentric ventriculo-atrial conduction, the simultaneous activation of the two atria from the atrioventricular node occurs in an inferior-to-superior direction. In the case of retrograde eccentric ventriculo-atrial conduction, characteristic of the orthodromic atrioventricular reciprocating tachycardia associated with an accessory pathway, the wave-front coming from the ventricle activates the atria sequentially, starting from a point more or less distant from the atrioventricular node depending on the site of the atrial insertion of the atrioventricular accessory pathway. *SN*: sinus node; *AVN*: atrioventricular node; *AP*: accessory pathway.

In this area, impulse velocity is approximately 0.01 to 0.1 m/s. At the level of the His bundle, velocity gradually increases from 0.05 m/s to 5 m/s in the Purkinje fibers, and then decreases again at the junction between the Purkinje network and the working ventricular myocardium (0.8-1 m/s) (Fig. 1.15). Ventricular depolarization starts along the interventricular septum with a left-to-right, inferior-to-superior and posterior-to-anterior direction. The right ventricular myocardium is activated from left-to-right, posterior-to-anterior and inferior-to-superior direction; the left ventricle is activated in a right-to-left, anterior-to-posterior and superior-to-inferior direction (see p. 43). Full activation of the Purkinje network takes about 15 to 23 ms and is followed by the activation time of the ventricular myocardial mass lasting another 25 to 27 ms.

Cardiac nervous control

The effects of the autonomic nervous system on the heart are more pronounced on the automaticity of the sinus node and the velocity of impulse propagation in the atrioventricular conduction axis. In the resting dog, the effect of the vagal tone on the sinus node is dominant. As a result, during periods of inactivity, heart rate is lower, sinus arrhythmia is evident, and the site of origin of the dominant nodal pacemaker or the exit pathway of the impulse leaving the sinus node varies over time (*wandering pacemaker*) (see p. 78). The vagal tone is responsible for the beat-to-beat control of the sinus node. Cholinergic fiber ends are rich in cholinesterase which can metabolize acetylcholine at a fast rate (50 - 100 ms).

Vagal stimulation causes a decrease in heart rate and a reduction in conduction velocity through the atrioventricular node. The primary effects of the activation of muscarinic receptors include an increase in K+ conductance, a decrease of calcium current (I_{CaL}) and a shift of the I_f channel activation potential towards more negative values. The increase in the conductance for K+ occurs through the opening of acetylcholine-gated channels, resulting in an efflux of K+ (I_{KAch} current) which hyperpolarizes the membrane potential of P cells to approximately −90 mV and makes it more difficult for the membrane potential to reach threshold. The decrease in I_{CaL} current

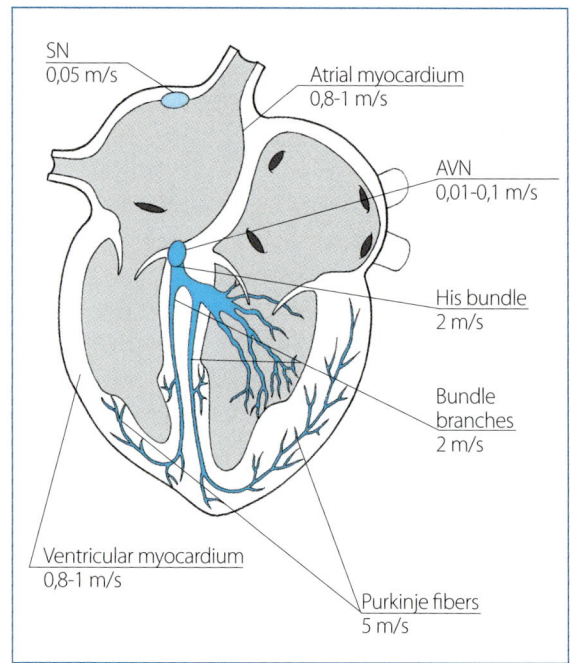

Figure 1.15. Electrical impulse conduction velocity along the different regions of the specialized conduction system. *SN*: sinus node; *AVN*: atrioventricular node.

and the shift of the activation potential of the channels responsible for the I_f current lead to a reduction of the sinus discharge rate and the electrical impulse propagation velocity, because the I_{CaL} current is also responsible for the onset of the action potential in P cells. The working atrial myocytes are sensitive to the effect of vagal tone, which causes a shortening of their action potential duration through an activation of the I_{KAch}.

Sympathetic stimulation is mediated by the release of norepinephrine and epinephrine. It activates the cardiac β_1 and β_2 receptors, which results in an increase in sinus discharge rate associated with an increase of the conduction velocity through the atrioventricular node, and the atrial and the ventricular myocardium. Sympathetic stimulation increases Ca^{2+} currents via phosphorylation of calcium channels, which increases the rate of phase 4 depolarization. In the working myocytes, the increase in Ca^{2+} influx is counter-balanced by an increase in K+ currents, which leads to a shortening of the action potential duration at increased heart rate.

Other factors that influence cardiac activity

An increase in body temperature influences the activity of spontaneous diastolic depolarization of the sinus node, increasing the slope of phase 4 of the action potential, and consequently the heart rate. Usually, a 1°C rise in temperature is accompanied by an increase in heart rate of approximately 10 bpm. Cooling of body tissues causes the opposite effect, and in extreme cases it can result in cardiac arrest.

Electrolytic disorders, particularly those involving Ca^{2+} and K^+ ions, can induce important effects on cardiac function. Hypercalcemia shortens the duration of the action potential and accelerates the phase of repolarization, while hypocalcemia prolongs the duration of the action potential. The presence of a normal concentration of Ca^{2+} is also essential to maintain adequate myocardial contraction. Hyperkalemia increases the value of the resting potential, and slows conduction velocity and the velocity of voltage increase during phase 0 of the action potential. As a result, the atrial cells can reach a state of constant depolarization and lose their excitability. Under these conditions the sinus impulse reaches the atrioventricular node directly through preferential pathways (*sinoventricular conduction*), which are less affected by high potassium concentration (see p. 293). Hypokalemia is responsible for more negative resting potential values, making the myocytes less excitable. It also leads to a prolongation of action potential duration associated with a reduction in I_{Kr} and I_{K1}.

Suggested readings

1. Alanis J, Benitez D. Two preferential conducting pathways within the bundle of His of the dog heart. *Jpn J Physiol* 1975; 25:371-385.
2. Anderson RH, Ho SY, Becker AE. Anatomy of the human atrioventricular junction revisited. *Anat Rec* 2000; 260:81-91.
3. Anderson RH, Yanni J, Boyett MR. The anatomy of the cardiac conduction system. *Clin Anat* 2009; 22:99-113.
4. Boineau JP, Schuessler RB, Mooney, et al. Multicentric origin of the atrial depolarization wave: the pacemaker complex. Relation to dynamics of atrial conduction, P-wave changes and heart rate control. *Circulation* 1978; 58:1036-1048.
5. Boyden PA, Robinson RB. Cardiac Purkinje fibers and arrhythmias; The GK Moe Award Lecture 2015. *Heart Rhythm* 2016; 13:1172-1181.
6. Boyett MR. "And the beat goes on". The cardiac conduction system: the wiring system of the heart. *Exp Physiol* 2009; 94:1035-1049.
7. Dobrzynski H, Anderson RH, Atkinson A, et al. Structure, function and clinical relevance of the cardiac conduction system, including the atrioventricular ring and outflow tract tissues. *Pharmacol Ther* 2013; 139:260-288.
8. Elizari MV, Acunzo RS, Ferreiro M. Hemiblocks revisited. *Circulation* 2007; 115:1154-1163.
9. Fedorov CC, Schuessler RB, Hemphill M, et al. Structural and functional evidence for discrete exit pathways that connect the canine sinoatrial node and atria. *Circ Res* 2009; 104:915-923.
10. Fedorov VV, Chang R, Glukhov AV, et al. Complex interactions between the sinoatrial node and atrium during reentrant arrhythmias in the canine heart. *Circulation* 2010; 24; 122:782-789.
11. Geis WP, Kaye MP, Randall WC. Major autonomic pathways to the atria and S-A and A-V nodes of the canine heart. *Am J Physiol* 1973; 224:202-208.
12. Hara T. Morphological and histochemical studies on the cardiac conduction system of the dog. *Arch Histol Jpn* 1967; 28:227-246.
13. Hayashi S. Electron microscopy of the heart conduction system of the dog. *Arch Histol Jpn* 1971; 33:67-86.
14. Hocini M, Loh P, Ho SY, et al. Anisotropic conduction in the triangle of Koch of mammalian hearts: electrophysiologic and anatomic correlations. *J Am Coll Cardiol* 1998; 1:629-636.
15. Hoffman BF. Atrioventricular conduction in mammalian hearts. *Ann N Y Acad Sci* 1965; 127:105-112.
16. Hogan PM, Davis LD. Evidence for specialized fibers in the canine right atrium. *Circ Res* 1968; 23:387-396.
17. Isaacson R, Boucek RJ. The atrioventricular conduction tissue of the dog. Histochemical properties; influence of electric shock. *Am Heart J* 1968; 75:206-214.
18. James TN. Anatomy of A-V node of the dog. *Anat Rec* 1964; 148:15-27.
19. James TN, Sherf L, Fine G, et al. Comparative ultrastructure of the sinus node in man and dog. *Circulation* 1966; 34:139-163.
20. Lavee J, Smolinsky A, David I, et al. Functional anatomy of the right bundle of His ramifications in the canine heart. *Isr J Med Sci* 1982; 18:1060-1064.
21. McKibben JS, Getty R. A comparative morphologic study of the cardiac innervation in domestic animals. II. The feline. *Am J Anat* 1968; 122:545-553.
22. Meijler FL, Janse MJ. Morphology and electrophysiology of the mammalian atrioventricular node. *Physiol Rev* 1988; 68:608-647.

23. Opthof T, Jonge B, Jongsma HJ, et al. Functional morphology of the mammalian sinuatrial node. *Eur Heart J* 1987; 8:1249-1259.
24. Qayyum MA. Anatomy and histology of the specialized tissues of the heart of the domestic cat. *Acta Anat* 1972; 82:352-367.
25. Racker DK. Atrioventricular node and input pathways: a correlated gross anatomical and histological study of the canine atrioventricular junctional region. *Anat Rec* 1989; 224:336-354.
26. Racker DK. The AV junction region of the heart: a comprehensive study correlating gross anatomy and direct three-dimensional analysis. Part I. Architecture and topography. *Anat Rec* 1999; 256:49-63.
27. Racker DK, Kadish AH. Proximal atrioventricular bundle, atrioventricular node, and distal atrioventricular bundle are distinct anatomic structures with unique histological characteristics and innervation. *Circulation* 2000; 101:1049-1059.
28. Racker DK. The AV junction region of the heart: a comprehensive study correlating gross anatomy and direct three-dimensional analysis. Part II. Morphology and cytoarchitecture. *Am J Physiol Heart Circ Physiol* 2004; 286:H1853-H1871.
29. Rudling EH, Schlamowitz S, Pipper CB, et al. The prevalence of the electrocardiographic J wave in the Petit Basset Griffon Vendéen compared to 10 different dog breeds. *J Vet Cardiol* 2016; 18:26-33.
30. Sakamoto S, Nitta T, Ishii Y, et al. Inter-atrial electrical connections: the precise location and preferential conduction. *J Cardiovasc Electrophysiol* 2005; 16:1077-1086.
31. Scherlag BJ, Yeh BK, Robinson MJ. Inferior inter-atrial pathway in the dog. *Circ Res* 1972; 31:18-35.
32. Sicouri S, Fish J, Antzelevitch C. Distribution of M cells in the canine ventricle. *J Cardiovasc Electrophysiol* 1994; 5:824-837.
33. Shen MJ, Zipes DP. Role of the autonomic nervous system in modulating cardiac arrhythmias. *Circ Res* 2014; 114:1004-1021.
34. Temple IP, Inada S, Dobrzynski H, et al. Connexins and the atrioventricular node. *Heart Rhythm* 2013; 10:297-304.
35. Truex RC, Smythe MQ. Comparative morphology of the cardiac conduction tissue in animals. *Ann N Y Acad Sci* 1965; 127:19-33.
36. Tse WW. Evidence of presence of automatic fibers in the canine atrioventricular node. *Am J Physiol* 1973; 225:716-723.
37. Wagner ML, Lazzara R, Weiss RM, et al. Specialized conducting fibers in the inter-atrial band. *Circ Res* 1966; 8:502-518.
38. Woods WT, Urthaler F, James TN. Spontaneous action potentials of cells in the canine sinus node. *Circ Res* 1976; 39:76-82.

CHAPTER 2

Principles of electrocardiography

The electrocardiogram records the variations of electric potentials in an electrical field generated by the heart during the different phases of the cardiac cycle. These changes can be detected by a device called an *electrocardiograph* using electrodes attached to the surface of the body. To produce an electrocardiogram an electrical circuit must be established between the heart muscle and the electrocardiograph. This electrical circuit is created by interposing clips (or adhesive patches) and cables between the animal and the machine. The placement of the electrodes at specific points on the body surface has been standardized to display various lead systems.

Historical notes

In 1856, Rudolph von Koelliker and Heinrich Muller determined that cardiac contractions were initiated by electric currents. In their experiment they demonstrated that a twitch of the ventricle occurred just before systole and another one soon after. These twitches were subsequently identified to correspond to the QRS and T waves of the electrocardiogram. In 1872, Gabriel Lippmann developed the *capillary electrometer*, which could detect changes in electrical potentials in the heart muscle from the body surface. The term *electrocardiogram* was later invented to describe the graphical representation of the cardiac electrical activity recorded by Augustus D. Waller in 1887 using the capillary electrometer. On Waller's electrocardiogram, the changes in electrical potential appeared as two deflections for each heart beat. A detailed analysis of the cardiac electrical activity was done in 1902 by Willem Einthoven using a *string galvanometer*.

Einthoven developed a triaxial bipolar lead system that displayed an electrocardiographic recording consisting of five successive waves that he named P, Q, R, S and T (later on he identified the U wave). The first clinical use of this lead system was reported by Thomas Lewis in 1913. The system was improved in 1931 by Franck N. Wilson, who developed the unipolar leads by combining a so-called exploring electrode and an indifferent, or reference electrode. Although Waller and Einthoven conducted their first experiments in dogs, the first clinical study in veterinary medicine was finally carried out by Norr in 1922.

The surface electrocardiogram

In order to understand the formation of the electrocardiographic waves, it is not only necessary to understand the phases of the cardiac action potential (see p. 9), but also the equivalent dipole theory, the concept of cardiac vectors and the lead systems.

The equivalent dipole theory and cardiac vectors

The equivalent dipole theory states that the heart can be approximated to a dipole (it is "equivalent" to a dipole when studied from a distance, at the surface of the body), and the force it generates has a direction and a magnitude that can be represented by a vector. The electrocardiogram records this vector from the body surface as it changes in direction and magnitude. The magnitude of the vector depends on the position of the recording electrodes relative to its direction, as well as the distance of the electrode from the dipole. Specifically, the magnitude is proportional to the angle of intersection between the direction of the vector and the axis of the bipolar or unipolar leads, and inversely proportional to the cube of the distance between the dipole and the recording electrode.

A dipole is defined as a pair of electrical charges of equal magnitude and opposite polarity that are separated by a very small distance. If a dipole is placed in a conducting medium, such as water, it generates an electrical field that propagates and is distributed symmetrically in the medium. The electrical potential generated by the dipole can therefore be measured with a galvanometer, which consists of two exploring electrodes positioned on each side of the medium that contains the dipole. The electrical potential measured by the galvanometer depends on the intensity of the electrical force generated by the dipole, the distance of the electrodes to the dipole and by the position of the exploring electrode relative to the orientation of the dipole.

The variations of electrical charges during depolarization and repolarization in the myocardial cells and muscle bundles act as dipoles that create an electric field in the body of the animal, which serves as the conducting medium. The electrical forces generated by the heart constantly change in magnitude and direction, and can be represented by consecutive vectors. Electrodes placed on the surface of the body can record these changes (Fig. 2.1).

When the myocardium is at rest (i.e. it is polarized), the intracellular compartment is negatively charged compared to the extracellular compartment (Fig. 2.1A). At the time of depolarization, the outside surface of the cell membrane becomes negative compared to the inside (Fig. 2.1B). In working myocytes, depolarization does not take place spontaneously but, once induced, it propagates across the cell membrane and then spreads from cell to cell. Depolarization spreads to adjacent cells as a result of the interaction between an area of depolarized membrane and an area of polarized membrane, which act respectively as a cathode and an anode, and create an electric field sufficient to propagate the depolarization to the neighboring cell. At the end of depolarization, the outer surface of the cell membrane is negative compared to the intracellular space (Fig. 2.1C). This is followed by repolarization, which restores the transmembrane potential to baseline value, i.e. the inside of the cell is negative relative to the outside (Fig. 2.1D).

By convention, the electrical activation within the myocardium is represented by arrows that have a magnitude and a direction. Each arrow represents a *vector of electrical activation*. By convention, the arrowhead of the vector points towards the positive pole, and the length of the arrow is proportional to the magnitude of the vector, which is directly proportional to the excitable myocardial mass available and opposing forces.

If two or more vectors of activation occur simultaneously, the resulting vector (*summation vector*) is represented by the sum of the individual vectors. Depending on their direction, they can be added or subtracted according to the parallelogram law of vector addition (Fig. 2.2).

The magnitude of the vector detected on the body surface depends on the angle of intersection between the recording site (exploring electrode) and the direction of the vector. Figure 2.3 shows the variations of the

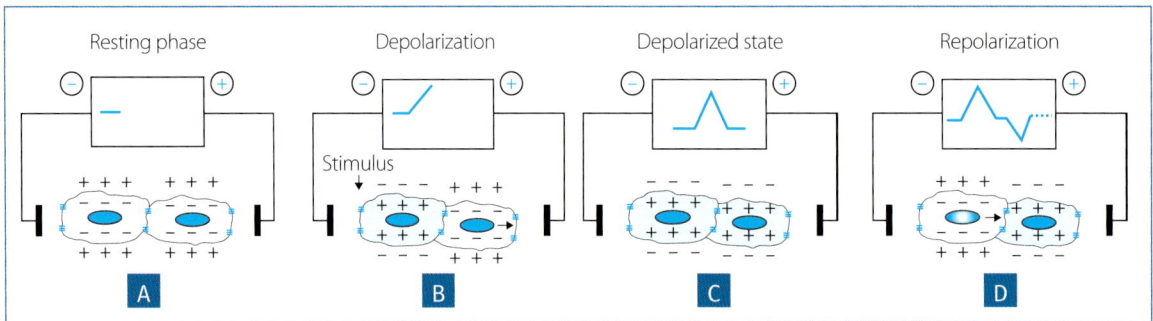

Figure 2.1. Electric potential difference recorded with a galvanometer at the two ends of the dipole formed by a strip of myocardial tissue. See text for further details.

magnitude of the cardiac vector in relation to the position of the recording electrode. Only the electrodes placed on a line parallel to the direction of the vector are able to record the maximum amplitude of the electric front (A and E). The positive exploring electrode (E) sees the front of cardiac activation approaching and, consequently, generates a wave with positive polarity. Contrariwise, the negative exploring electrode (A) sees the front of cardiac activation moving away, resulting in the formation of a wave which has the same amplitude but opposite polarity as the wave recorded from point E. In contrast, recording electrodes placed on a line perpendicular to the direction of the vector record the smallest wave amplitude (C and G). The observation points B, D, F and H display waves with an intermediate amplitude according to the angle between the exploring electrode and the vector, and with variable polarity depending on the direction of the vector relative to the position of the electrode.

The magnitude of the cardiac vectors, measured on the body surface, also depends on the interaction of the electric forces with thoracic structures. The heart can be seen as being surrounded by concentric spheres consisting from the inside towards the outside of the lungs, thoracic muscles, fat and skin. Each sphere can vary in diameter and conductivity. The electrical forces are gradually attenuated as they propagate through these layers. Due to its structure, the body does not act as a homogeneous conducting medium, and therefore the electrical potentials that are measured in volts (V) on the surface of the heart, are only measured in millivolts (mV) on the surface of the body.

For the above reasons, the true magnitude of a vector of activation can only be obtained by placing an exploring electrode in direct contact with the cardiac surface. The magnitude recorded at the surface of the body is an approximation of the actual voltage generated by the heart.

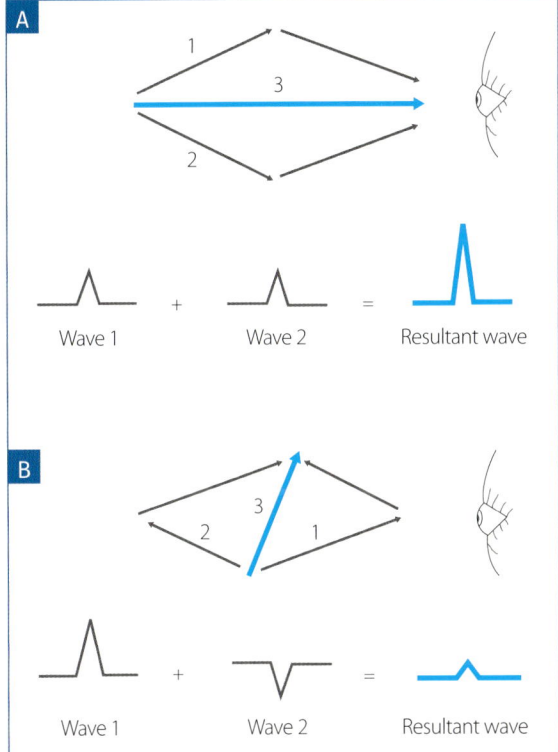

Figure 2.2. Summation (A) and subtraction (B) of the vectors according to the parallelogram rule. A) The magnitude, direction, and polarity of vector 3 is the result of the summation of two simultaneous vectors of activation (1 and 2) that have the same direction. B) The magnitude, direction, and polarity of vector 3 is the result of the subtraction of two simultaneous vectors of activation (1 and 2) that have opposite directions.

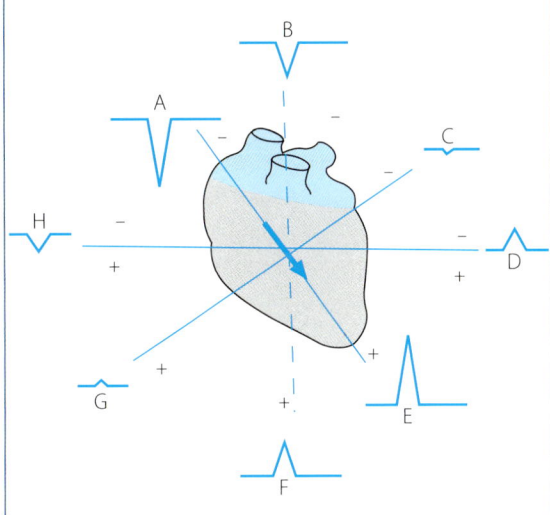

Figure 2.3. Magnitude of a vector of activation when recorded from different observation points. See text for details.

Volume and linear conductor theory

In accordance with the equivalent dipole theory, the precise position of the exploring electrode is crucial to record the cardiac electrical activity on the surface of the thorax. This is because the thorax behaves as a *volume conductor*; therefore, the voltage of the deflections will differ according to the position of the exploring electrode on the thoracic surface. On the other hand, a limb behaves as a *linear conductor*, comparable to an electric cable and, therefore, the voltage does not vary from the base to the extremity of the limb. Practically, this means that the exploring electrodes of the precordial leads must be positioned precisely on the chest wall, whereas the limb lead electrodes can be placed at any point along the limbs, without the risk of altering the characteristics of the recorded waves.

Lead systems

By applying several exploring electrodes on the body surface at a fixed distance from the heart, it is possible to record the magnitude and direction of the cardiac vectors. In reality, the electrocardiogram detects the variations of the electric potential over time between a point on the body surface and an indifferent (or reference) electrode, or between pairs of recording electrodes. The lines joining pairs of electrodes on which the cardiac vector are called *leads* (Fig. 2.4). The leads are called *unipolar* if the potential difference is recorded between an electrode on the body surface (exploring electrode) and an indifferent (or reference) electrode; the leads are called *bipolar* if the potential difference is recorded between two recording electrodes. Unipolar leads, therefore, detect variations of electrical potential at a specific point on the body surface, while bipolar leads record the differences of electrical potential between two points on the body surface.

The voltage change recorded by the leads is displayed graphically as a wave of variable amplitude, polarity and duration. A recording from a lead parallel to the direction of the main vector of cardiac activation produces a wave with maximum amplitude, whereas the wave is very small or absent if the lead is oriented perpendicular to the vector of activation (Fig. 2.3). By convention, a depolarizing vector pointing towards the positive electrode of the lead is represented by a positive wave, and a vector directed towards the negative electrode is represented

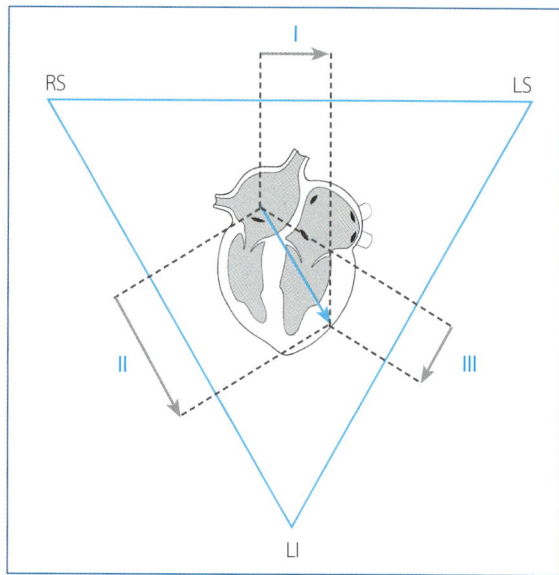

Figure 2.4. Projection of the cardiac vector on the axes formed by the bipolar limb leads. The magnitude of the vector recorded from different leads depends on the angle between the cardiac vector of activation and the lead. The vector with the largest magnitude is recorded in the lead that is oriented almost parallel to it (lead II). *RS*: right superior limb; *LS*: left superior limb; *LI*: left inferior limb; I: Lead I; II: Lead II; III: Lead III.

by a negative wave. The duration of the wave depends on the cardiac activation time and the mass of excitable myocardium.

The electrocardiogram can be studied from three different anatomical planes (Fig. 2.5):
- the *frontal plane* (X-axis of the Cartesian system),
- the *sagittal plane* (Y-axis of the Cartesian system), and
- the *horizontal or transverse plane* (Z-axis of the Cartesian system).

Each of these planes divides the body in two halves: the *frontal plane* divides the body in an anterior half and a posterior half; the *sagittal plane* divides the body in a right half and a left half; the *horizontal plane* divides the body in a superior half and an inferior half. Although dogs and cats are quadrupeds, the authors of this book prefer to consider these anatomical planes as if the animals were standing on their hind limbs and adopt the terminology used by human cardiologists (Fig. 2.5). If the veterinary nomenclature is used instead, the frontal plane divides the body in a cranial half and a caudal half; the sagittal plane is divided in a right half and a left half; the horizontal or transverse plane divides the body in a ventral and dorsal half.

These planes serve as the basis for three main lead systems (Fig. 2.6):
- Bailey's hexaxial system, which records the electrical activity in the frontal plane;
- the precordial or chest lead system, which records the electrical activity in the horizontal plane;
- the bipolar orthogonal system, which records the electrical activity in all three planes.

Bailey's hexaxial system

Bailey's hexaxial system records the heart's electrical activity in the frontal plane through the use of the three bipolar leads, known as *standard, classical* or *differential leads* (I, II and III), and three *augmented unipolar limb leads* also known as *peripheral unipolar leads* (aVR, aVL, aVF).

The first lead system used in clinical practice was developed by Einthoven in 1902. This system involved the use of three bipolar leads positioned on the limbs of the patient so as to form an equilateral triangle, at the center of which the cardiac dipole was located (*Einthoven triangle*) (Fig. 2.4).

Even if the Einthoven triangle is considered equilateral, in reality the placement of the exploring electrodes on the limbs does not allow the three sides of the triangle to be of equal length. However this small variation is not important, since the distance between the small cardiac dipole and the recording electrodes at the surface of the body can be considered to be infinite.

Under normal conditions, the wavefront of cardiac depolarization assumes a right-to-left and superior-to-inferior direction. For this reason, the positive electrodes are positioned on the left and lower (inferior) part of the

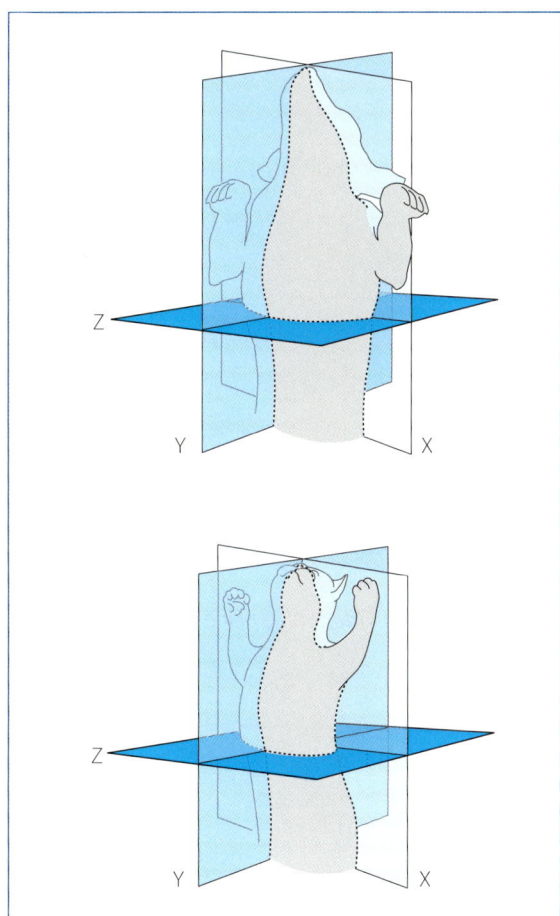

Figure 2.5. Division of the body by the three anatomical planes. X: frontal plane; Y: sagittal plane; Z: horizontal or transverse plane.

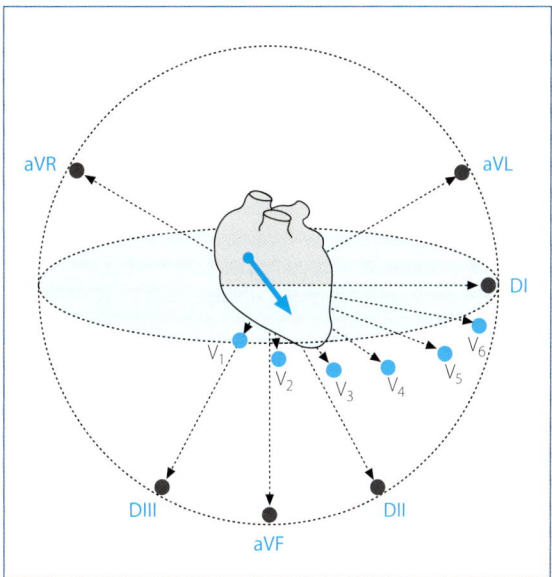

Figure 2.6. Position of the exploring electrodes of the bipolar and unipolar limb leads in the frontal plane (leads I, II, III, aVR, aVL, aVF) and of the precordial leads (leads $V_1, V_2, V_3, V_4, V_5, V_6$) in the horizontal (or transverse) plane.

body to record a positive wave when the cardiac vectors of activation are approaching.

The three leads of the Einthoven system were called *lead I* (I), *lead II* (II) and *lead III* (III) (Table 2.1).

Lead I records the differences in potential between the positive electrode on the left superior limb and the negative electrode on the right superior limb. Since vectors typically propagate from right-to-left and superior-to-inferior during cardiac depolarization, and therefore towards the positive electrode, lead I records an electrocardiographic wave with positive polarity.

Lead II records the potential difference between the positive electrode on the left inferior limb and the negative electrode on the right superior limb. In this lead, a wave with a positive deflection is also recorded, given the direction of the cardiac vector that is left-to-right and superior-to-inferior. Since this lead is mostly parallel to the direction of the main cardiac vector of activation, it displays the wave with the largest amplitude of all three leads.

Lead III records the potential difference between the positive electrode on the inferior left limb and the negative electrode on the superior left limb. Since the heart's normal vector of activation is right-to-left and superior-to-inferior, the waveform recorded in this derivation has a positive polarity (Fig. 2.7).

TABLE 2.1. Electrocardiographic lead systems for the detection of vectors of cardiac activation in the different anatomical planes.

Bipolar limb leads, standard or differential leads	C_5: fifth right intercostal space at the level of the costochondral junction.
I: left superior limb (+) - right superior limb (−).	C_6: third right intercostal space at the level of the costochondral junction.
II: left inferior limb (+) - right superior limb (−).	M_1: third left intercostal space at the widest point of the chest.
III: left inferior limb (+) - left superior limb (−).	M_2: sixth left intercostal space at the level of the widest point of the chest.
Unipolar augmented limb leads or peripheral leads	M_3: just to the left of the xiphoid process of the sternum.
aVR: right superior limb (+) - indifferent reference electrode (−) consisting of left superior and left inferior limbs.	M_4: just to the right of the xiphoid process of the sternum.
aVL: left superior limb (+) - indifferent reference electrode (−) consisting of right superior and left inferior limbs.	M_5: seventh right intercostal space at the widest point of the chest.
aVF: left inferior limb (+) - indifferent reference electrode (−) consisting of left superior and right superior limbs.	M_6: third right intercostal space at the widest point of the chest.
Unipolar precordial leads or chest leads	**Modified Wilson precordial system**
Modified Lannek precordial lead system (Detweiler and Patterson)	V_1: first (Santilli, et al.) or fifth (Kraus, et al.) right intercostal space at the level of the sternochondral junction respectively.
CV_5RL (rV_2): fifth right intercostal space at the level of the sternochondral junction.	V_2: sixth left intercostal space at the level of the sternochondral junction.
CV_6LL (V_2): sixth left intercostal space level of the sternochondral junction.	V_3: sixth left intercostal space and equidistant from V_2 and V_4.
CV_6LU (V_4): sixth left intercostal space at the level of the costochondral junction.	V_4: sixth left intercostal space at the costochondral junction.
V_{10}: dorsal to the spinous process of the seventh thoracic vertebra, along a vertical line that joins V_4.	V_5: sixth left intercostal space above V_4, keeping the same distance between V_5 and V_4 as between V_4 and V_3.
Precordial Takahashi lead system	V_6: sixth left intercostal space above V_5 keeping the same distance between V_6 and V_5 as between V_5 and V_4.
C_1: cranial to the first left rib at the level of the costochondral junction.	**Modified bipolar orthogonal lead system**
C_2: second left intercostal space at the level of the costochondral junction.	X: positive electrode at the fifth left intercostal space, negative electrode at the fifth right intercostal space; both electrodes at the level of the cardiac base.
C_3: fifth left intercostal space at the level of the costochondral junction.	Y: positive electrode at the level of the xiphoid process of the sternum, negative electrode at the manubrium.
C_4: seventh right intercostal space at the level of the costochondral junction.	Z: positive electrode at the seventh thoracic vertebra, negative electrode at a point on the sternum just opposite to the positive electrode.

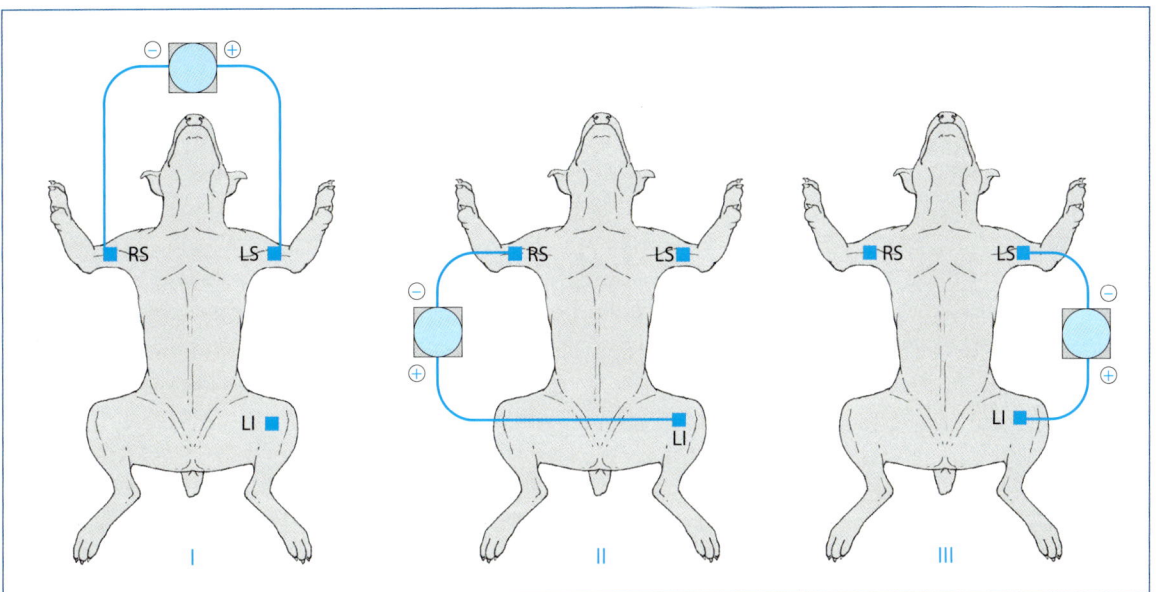

Figure 2.7. Detection of the differences in electrical potential between the electrodes of the bipolar limb leads. I: lead I; II: lead II; III: lead III; *RS*: right superior limb; *LS*: left superior limb; *LI*: left inferior limb.

The three standard leads of the bipolar or Einthoven's triaxial system represent the three sides of the triangle, and can display the cardiac vector and its temporal variations as seen from three different angles. Leads II and III form an angle of +60 ° and +120 ° with lead I, respectively. Lead I is by convention considered to be the horizontal line that splits the frontal plane into two semicircles. The lower half is numbered clockwise with positive degrees from 0 ° to +180 °, and the upper half counterclockwise from 0 ° to –180 ° (Fig. 2.8).

In order to increase the number of viewpoints to study the cardiac vector accurately in the frontal plane, three

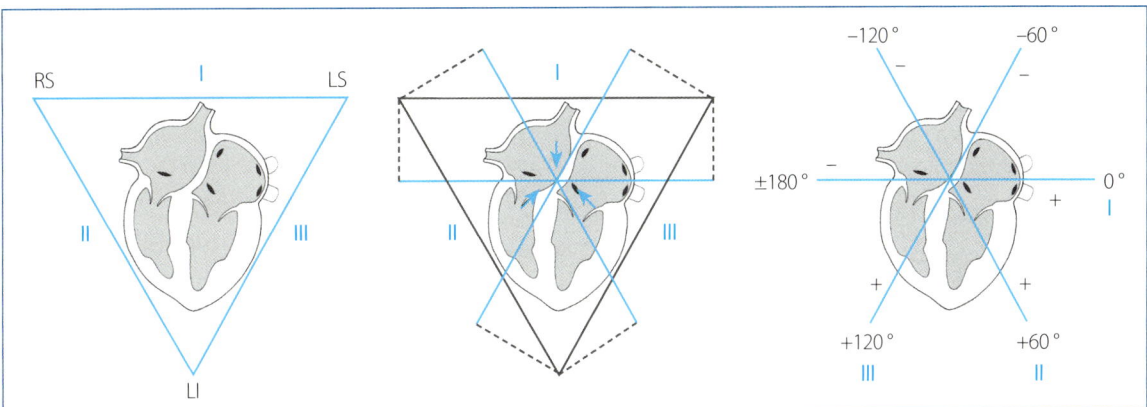

Figure 2.8. Triaxial system of bipolar limb leads. Starting from Einthoven's triangle, the bipolar limb leads are projected to intersect the center of the triangle and make the triaxial system. Lead I is by convention considered to be the line that divides the frontal plane in a lower (inferior) semicircular half numbered clockwise from 0 ° to +180 ° and in a upper (superior) semicircular half numbered counterclockwise from 0 ° to –180 °. Lead II forms an angle of + 60 ° with lead I. Lead III forms an angle of +120 ° with lead I. *RS*: right superior limb; *LS*: left superior limb; *LI*: left inferior limb; I: lead I; II: lead II; III: lead III.

unipolar leads were added to the three leads of Einthoven's triaxial system to form Bailey's hexaxial system. These leads bisect the angles defined by the bipolar leads (R –150 °, L –30 ° and F +90 °). Leads R, L and F therefore point towards the apices of Einthoven's equilateral triangle (Fig. 2.9).

The letters "R", "L" and "F" describing the three unipolar leads mean *right arm*, *left arm* and *left foot*, respectively, which correspond to the placement of the exploring positive electrode on the superior right limb, on the superior left limb and on the inferior left limb. Although defined as unipolar, leads R, L and F measure the difference in electrical potential between the exploring electrode of the considered limb and a *reference electrode*. The reference electrode does not record a change in electrical potential during the cardiac cycle; it can be made by connecting leads R, L and F together to form the *indifferent electrode* or *Wilson's central terminal*, which is connected to the negative port of the galvanometer. Any lead that uses the indifferent electrode as the negative one and the exploring electrode as the positive one is described by the letter "V" for voltage (VR, VL, VF for the limbs leads, V_1 to V_6 for precordial leads).

Recordings of the electrical activity from the three unipolar limb leads are obtained as indicated below in Table 2.1.

The *VR lead* records potential differences between the right superior limb (exploring positive electrode) and the reference electrode. Lead VR makes an angle of –150 ° with lead I (Fig. 2.9). Given the direction of the normal cardiac activation from right-to-left and superior-to-inferior, the resulting cardiac vector propagates away from the exploring electrode, producing a large negative wave.

The *VL lead* records potential differences between the left superior limb (exploring positive electrode) and the reference electrode. Lead VL makes an angle of –30 ° with lead I (Fig. 2.9). Given the direction of the normal cardiac activation from right-to-left and superior-to-inferior, the resulting cardiac vector propagates away from the exploring electrode, resulting in a diphasic or negative wave. Although this lead records the cardiac vector moving away, the waveform is typically less negative than that recorded from lead VR.

The *VF lead* records potential differences between the left inferior limb (exploring positive electrode) and the reference electrode. Lead VF makes an angle of +90 ° with lead I and bisects lead II and III (Fig. 2.9). Given the direction of the normal cardiac activation from right-to-left and superior-to-inferior, the wave is positive when recorded from VF.

The original Wilson's central terminal was later on modified to increase the voltage of the signals recorded from the unipolar limb leads. It consisted in excluding one exploring electrode from Wilson's central terminal (Fig. 2.10), which allowed the voltage to be amplified by 50 %. This is the reason why unipolar limb leads are called *augmented* and the prefix "a" is added to the abbreviation that identifies them (aVR, aVL, aVF).

Bailey's hexaxial system is the combination on the frontal plane of the triaxial system of bipolar limbs leads and the triaxial system of unipolar limb leads (Fig. 2.11). The axis of each lead is identified by successive increments of 30 °, from 0 ° to +180 ° and from 0 ° to –180 °.

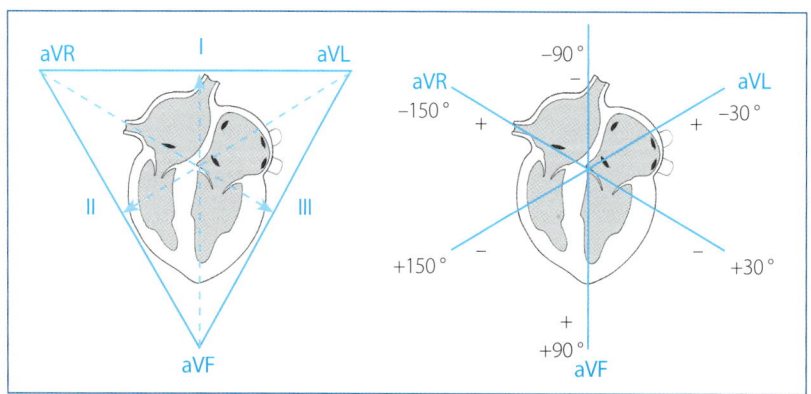

Figure 2.9. Triaxial lead system of unipolar limb leads. The unipolar limb leads represent the apices of the equilateral triangle of Einthoven, and bisect the angles formed by the bipolar limb leads (I, II, III).

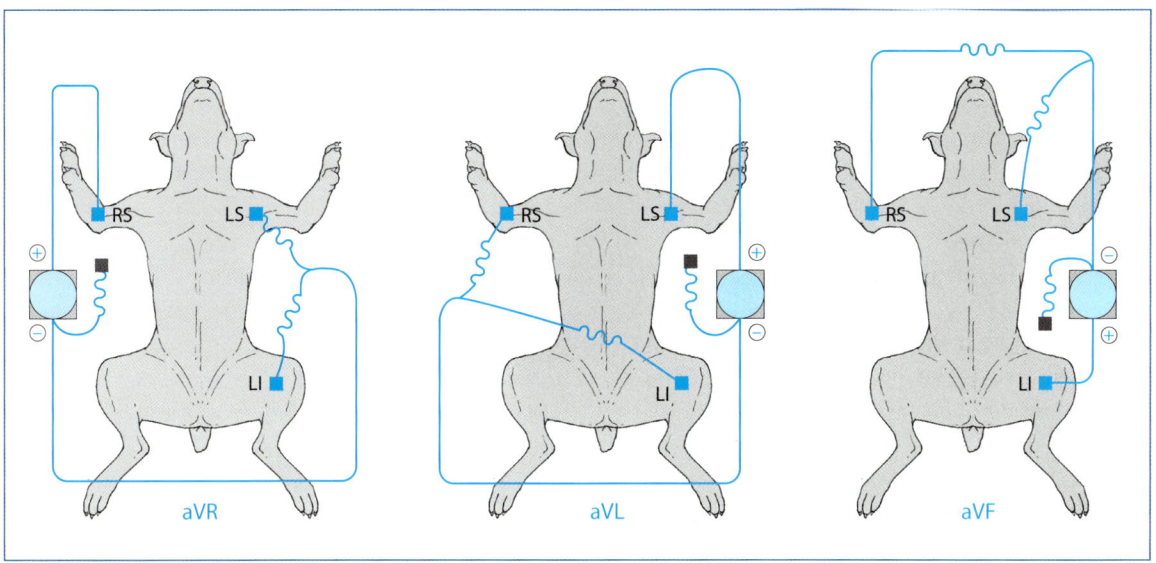

Figure 2.10. Circuitry used to record the unipolar limb leads (aVR, aVL, aVF). The three leads VR, VL and VF are joined and connected to the negative terminal of the galvanometer to form the indifferent electrode or Wilson's central terminal. To obtain augmented unipolar limb leads, the limb which is connected to the positive exploring electrode is disconnected from Wilson's central terminal. *RS*: right superior limb; *LS*: left superior limb; *LI*: left inferior limb.

The positive exploring electrode of each lead is identified with a "+" sign, and the negative or indifferent electrode is marked with a "−" sign. Leads I, II, aVF and III positive exploring electrodes point towards the lower (inferior) half of the body, with an axis of 0 °, +60 °, +90 ° and +120 °, respectively. Conversely, aVL and aVR positive exploring electrodes point towards the upper (superior) half of the body, with an axis of −30 ° and −150 °, respectively. Bailey's hexaxial system can be used for the calculation of the mean electrical axis of the P wave, QRS complex and T wave in the frontal plane.

Lead orientation in the frontal plane relative to the orientation of the vectors of electrical activation explains the morphology of the recorded wave in each electrocardiographic lead. In particular, leads II, aVF and III examine cardiac activation wavefronts from an inferior position, while aVL and I record electrical activation from a left lateral position. aVR displays electrocardiographic waves with a very different morphology from all other leads of the Bailey system, since it records cardiac electrical activation from a right superior position (Fig. 2.11).

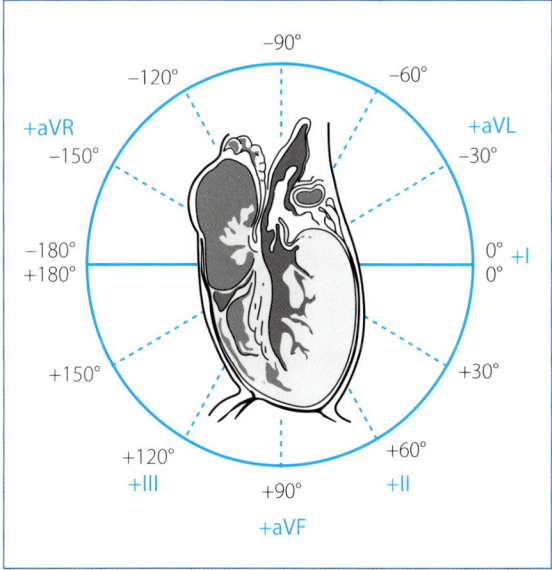

Figure 2.11. Bailey's hexaxial lead system representing the combination of the triaxial bipolar and unipolar limb lead systems in the frontal plane. The axis of each lead is identified by successive increments of 30 ° from 0 ° to +180 ° (I: 0 °; II: +60 °; aVF: +90 °; III: +120 °) and from 0 ° to −180 ° (aVR: −150 °; aVL: −30 °).

Precordial or chest lead system

The *precordial (or chest)* leads are recorded by placing the exploring positive electrode at pre-defined positions on the surface of the chest. The precordial lead system only uses unipolar leads. The indifferent electrode is the same that is used to obtain the unipolar limb leads in the hexaxial system. The chest leads record changes of electrical potential in the transverse (or horizontal) plane (Fig. 2.6). These leads are identified by the letter "V" followed by a number that corresponds to the position of the exploring positive electrode on the chest (V_1 to V_6). On occasion, the letter "V" is preceded by the letter "r" to indicate that the exploring electrode is placed on the right hemithorax (for example rV_2).

The unipolar precordial leads detect changes in cardiac electrical potential according to the solid angle theory; this theory describes the existence of an imaginary structure of conical shape interposed between the exploring positive electrode and the heart. In this system the electrode is the apex of the cone, while the base is constituted by the epicardial surface explored. For this reason, the chest leads are similar to leads placed directly on the epicardium since they analyze the variations of potential confined to a narrow region of the myocardium.

Precordial leads can be helpful to confirm a diagnosis of cardiac chamber enlargement or intraventricular conduction abnormalities, and to detect P waves, if they are difficult to identify in the frontal plane. Due to the position of atrial chambers with respect to the horizontal plane, in the dog and the cat, the precordial leads are not useful to determine the direction of the atrial cardiac vector and predict the site of origin of an atrial depolarization.

In veterinary medicine, and particularly in dogs, variations in chest conformation and the variable relationship between the heart and surrounding structures make it difficult to have a single chest lead system that can be used in all animals in a repeatable way.

The precordial (chest) lead systems used in veterinary medicine (Table 2.1) are:
- Lannek's lead system, later modified by Detweiler and Patterson,
- Takahashi's lead system, and
- Wilson's lead system, later modified by Kraus, et al.

Modified Lannek's precordial lead system

The first chest lead system in dogs was developed by Lannek in 1949 and was based on three unipolar precordial leads called CR_{6L}, CR_{6U} and CR_5, recorded with the animal in right lateral recumbency.

The exploring electrode for lead CR_{6L} was placed at the sixth left intercostal space, at the level of the sternochondral junction.

The exploring electrode for lead CR_{6U} was placed at the sixth left intercostal space, at the level of the costochondral junction.

The exploring electrode for lead CR_5 was placed at the fifth right intercostal space, at the level of the sternochondral junction.

In 1965, Detweiler and Patterson modified Lannek's precordial system (Fig. 2.12). This modified system uses four exploring electrodes placed at different points of the chest and identified by the following letters and numbers: "C" (*chest*), "V" (*voltage*), 5 or 6 (*intercostal space*), "R" (*right*) or "L" (*left*), "L" (*lower*) or "U" (*upper*).

The exploring electrode for lead CV_5RL, also called rV_2, is positioned at the fifth right intercostal space at the level of the sternochondral junction.

The exploring electrode for lead CV_6LL, also called V_2, is positioned at the sixth left intercostal space at the level of the sternochondral junction.

The exploring electrode for lead CV_6LU, also called V_4, is positioned at the level of the sixth left intercostal space at the level of the costochondral junction.

The exploring electrode for lead V_{10} is positioned dorsally on the spinous process of the seventh thoracic vertebra, along a vertical line that joins V_4.

Takahashi's precordial lead system

A more complex lead system was developed in 1964 by Takahashi on the basis of experimental studies conducted in dogs. This system is based on twelve precordial leads, six of which are placed on the left hemithorax and six on the right hemithorax (Fig. 2.13).

The exploring electrodes C_1, C_2 and C_3 are placed on the left hemithorax at the costochondral junction. C_1 is positioned cranial to the first rib, C_2 in the second intercostal space and C_3 in the fifth intercostal space.

The exploring electrodes C_4, C_5 and C_6 are placed on the right hemithorax, at the level of the costochondral

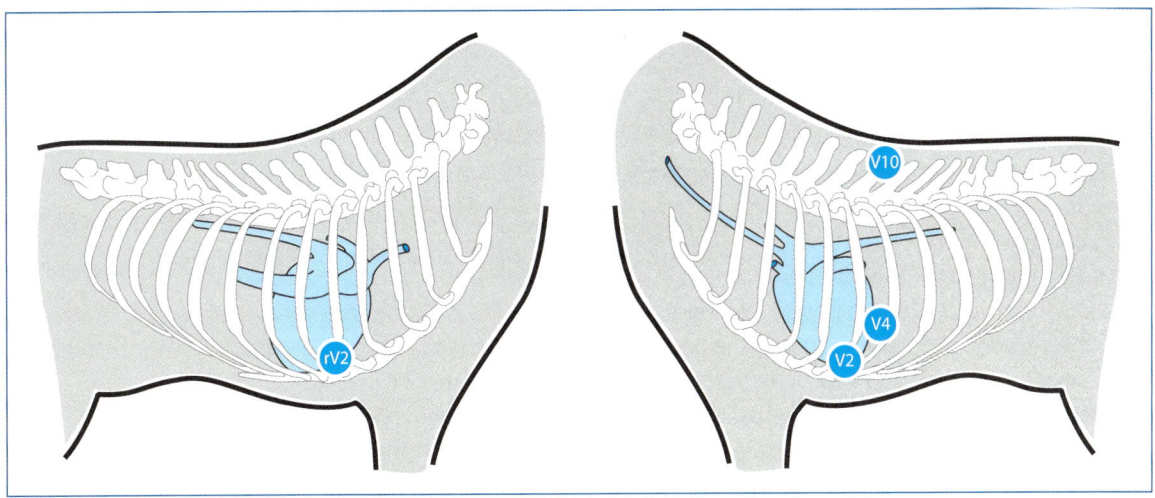

Figure 2.12. Exploring electrodes positioned according to the modified Lannek precordial lead system (Detweiler and Patterson, 1965).

junction. C_4 is positioned in the seventh intercostal space, C_5 in the fifth and C_6 in third intercostal space.

The exploring electrodes M_1 and M_2 are placed on the left hemithorax where the thorax is widest. M_1 is positioned at the third intercostal space and M_2 at the sixth intercostal space.

The exploring electrode M_3 is placed immediately to the left of the xiphoid process of the sternum.

The exploring electrode M_4 is placed immediately to the right of the xiphoid process of the sternum.

The exploring electrodes M_5 and M_6 are placed on the right hemithorax where the thorax is widest. M_5 is positioned at the seventh intercostal space, and M_6 at the third intercostal space.

In 1966, the Japanese Association of Animal Electrocardiography added two new precordial leads to the system developed by Takahashi: a positive (electrode A) and a negative (electrode B) electrode positioned at the costochondral junction of the sixth left rib, and on the scapula of the right shoulder, respectively.

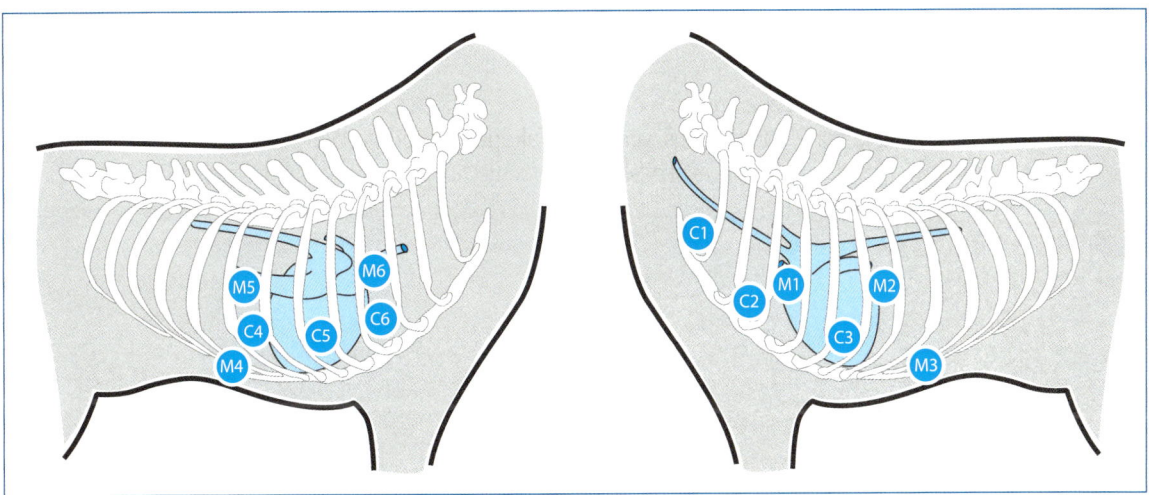

Figure 2.13. Exploring electrodes positioned according to Takahashi's precordial lead system (1964).

Modified Wilson's chest lead system

In 2002 Kraus, et al., adapted Wilson's precordial lead system, which was developed in 1931 and is in use in human cardiology (Fig. 2.14).

Despite the limitations related to the differences between humans and dogs in chest conformation and the relationship of the heart with surrounding tissues, this system is the most commonly used in veterinary medicine.

It is based on six unipolar exploring electrodes (V_1 to V_6) that are positioned on the left and right hemithorax.

The exploring electrode of lead V_1 is placed on the right hemithorax, in the fifth intercostal space at the level of the sternochondral junction. A more cranial placement of lead V_1 in the first right intercostal space at the level of costocondral junction has been proposed by Santilli to obtain a more reliable recording of right ventricular activation in all canine thoracic morphotypes.

The exploring electrode of lead V_2 is placed on the left hemithorax, in the sixth intercostal space at the level of the sternochondral junction.

The exploring electrode of lead V_3 is placed on the left hemithorax, in the sixth intercostal space and midway between V_2 and V_4.

The exploring electrode of lead V_4 is placed on the left hemithorax, in the sixth intercostal space at the level of the costochondral junction.

The exploring electrode of lead V_5 is placed on the left hemithorax, in the sixth intercostal space dorsally to V_4. The distance between V_5 and V_4 is the same as the distance between V_4 and V_3.

The exploring electrode of lead V_6 is placed on the left hemithorax, in the sixth intercostal space dorsally to V_5. The distance between V_6 and V_5 is the same as the distance between V_5 and V_4, or V_4 and V_3.

All twelve-lead electrocardiograms displayed in this book were recorded using the hexaxial limb lead system and the modified Wilson's precordial lead system.

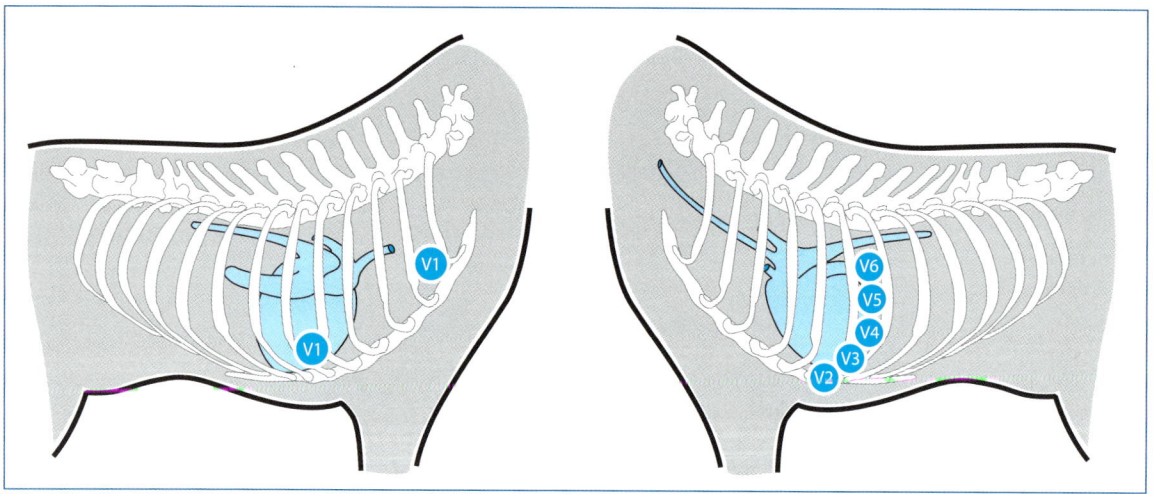

Figure 2.14. Exploring electrodes positioned according to Wilson's precordial lead system (1931) modified for dogs by Santilli, et al. (2017) (V_1 at the first right intercostal space) and Kraus, et al. (2002) (V_1 at the fifth right intercostal space).

Orthogonal bipolar lead system

The orthogonal bipolar lead system was designed to simultaneously record the vector of cardiac activation from three perpendicular planes: the frontal (X), sagittal (Y) and horizontal (Z) planes (Fig. 2.5). The X lead of the orthogonal system records a projection of the cardiac vector in the frontal plane and from right to left; it is similar to lead I. The Y lead records a projection of the cardiac vector in the sagittal plane in a superior to inferior direction; it is comparable to lead aVF. The Z lead records a projection of the cardiac vector in the horizontal plane in an anterior to posterior direction; it is similar to V_{10}.

Various orthogonal lead systems have been described by McFee and Parungao, Schmidt, as well as Frank and Simonson. The position of the electrodes on the body surface is different in each system. In veterinary medicine, the most commonly used orthogonal bipolar lead system is based on the placement of the electrodes at the following locations:

The X lead is obtained by positioning the positive electrode at the level of the fifth left intercostal space and the negative electrode at the level of the fifth right intercostal space, roughly at the level of the heart base.

The Y lead is obtained by positioning the positive electrode at the level of the xiphoid process of the sternum and a negative electrode on the manubrium.

The Z lead is obtained by positioning the positive electrode at the level of the seventh thoracic vertebra and the negative electrode at a point on the sternum opposite to the positive electrode.

The bipolar orthogonal lead systems are used in clinical practice for the study of cardiac vectors in the three anatomical planes (a technique called vectorcardiography) and for recording high-definition electrocardiograms to study late potentials. They are also used when placing electrodes for 24-hour Holter recordings.

Suggested readings

1. Abildskov JA, Wilkinson RS. The relation of precordial and orthogonal leads. *Circulation* 1963; 27:58-63.
2. Bayer AK. Determination of the electrical heart axis in animals. *Zentralbl Veterinarmed B* 1980; 27:534-543.
3. Bojrab MJ, Breazile JE, Morrison RD. Vectorcardiography in normal dogs using the Frank lead system. *Am J Vet Res* 1971; 32:925-934.
4. Breathnach CS, Westphal W. Early detectors of the heart's electrical activity. *Pacing Clin Electrophysiol* 2006; 29:422-424.
5. Burger HC, Van Milaan. Heart vector and leads. *Br Heart J* 1946; 8:157-161.
6. Coleman MG, Robson MC. Evaluation of six-lead electrocardiograms obtained from dogs in a sitting position or sternal recumbency. *Am J Vet Res* 2005; 66:233-237.
7. Detweiler DK. The dog electrocardiogram: a critical review. In: Macfarlane PW, Veitch Lawrie TD, eds. *Comprehensive Electrocardiology. Theory and Practice in Health and Disease*. New York, NY: Pergamon Press. 1993; 1267-1329.
8. Dubin S, Beard R, Staib J, et al. Variation of canine and feline frontal-plane QRS axes with lead choice and augmentation ratio. *Am J Vet Res* 1977; 38:1957-1962.
9. Eckenfels A. On the variability of the direction of the cardiac vector and of the T-, Q- and S-waves in the normal ECG of the conscious beagle dog. *Arzneimittelforschung/Drug Res* 1980; 30:1626-1630.
10. Frank E. The image surface of a homogeneous torso. *Am Heart J* 1954; 47:757-768.
11. Gompf RE, Tilley LP. Comparison of lateral and sternal recumbent positions for electrocardiography of the cat. *Am J Vet Res* 1979; 40:1483-1486.
12. Horan LG. Manifest orientation: the theoretical link between the anatomy of the heart and the clinical electrocardiogram. *J Am Coll Cardiol* 1987; 9:1049-1056.
13. Hurst JW. Naming of the waves in the ECG, with a brief account of their genesis. *Circulation* 1998; 98:1937-1942.
14. Kar AK, Roy D, Sinha PK. Electricity and the heart. *J Assoc Physicians India* 2005; 53:1055-1059.
15. Katzeff IE, Gathiram P, Edwards H, et al. Dynamic electrocardiography V. The "imaginary cardiac vector" hypothesis: experimental evaluation. *Med Hypotheses* 1981; 7:863-884.
16. Kraus MS, Moïse NS, Rishniw M, et al. Morphology of ventricular arrhythmias in the Boxer as measured by 12-lead electrocardiography with pace-mapping comparison. *J Vet Intern Med* 2002; 16:153-158.
17. Lannek N. Clinical and Experimental Study on the Electrocardiogram in Dogs (Thesis). Stockholm: Royal Veterinary College. 1949, Dissertation.
18. McFee R, Purangao A. An orthogonal lead system for clinical electrocardiography. *Am Heart J* 1961; 62:93-100.
19. Moss AJ. The electrocardiogram: from Einthoven to molecular genetics. *Ann Noninvasive Electrocardiol* 2001; 6:181-182.
20. Norr J. Uber Hertzstromkurvenaufnahmen an Haustieren. Zur Einfuhrung der Elektrokardiographie in die Veterinärmedizin. *Arch Wiss Prakt Tierhdikd* 1922; 48:85.
21. Pipberger HV, Goldman MJ, Littman D, et al. Correlations of the orthogonal electrocardiogram and vectorcardiogram with constitutional variables in 518 normal men. *Circulation* 1967; 35:536-551.
22. Porteiro Vázquez DM, Perego M, Lombardo S, Santilli RA. Analysis of precordial lead system in dogs with different thoracic conformations. *J Vet Intern Med* 2017; 31:208.
23. Rosenbaum SH, Fleisher LA. Was Einthoven a 21st century visionary? *J Clin Anesth* 1992; 4:263-264.
24. Silverman ME, Grove D, Upshaw CB Jr. Why does the heart beat? The discovery of the electrical system of the heart. *Circulation* 2006; 113:2775-1781.
25. Smith CR, Hamlin RL, Crocker HD. Comparative electrocardiography. *Ann NY Acad Sci* 1957; 65:155-169.
26. Spach MS, Kootsey JM, Sloan JD. Active modulation of electrical coupling between cardiac cells of the dog. A mechanism for transient and steady state variations in conduction velocity. *Circ Res* 1982; 51:347-362.
27. Takahashi M. Experimental studies on the electrocardiogram of the dog. *Jpn J Vet Sci* 1964; 24:191-210.
28. Waller AD. A demonstration on man of electromotive changes accompanying the heart's beat. *J Physiol Lond* 1887; 8:229.
29. Wilson FN, Johnston FD, Macleod AG, et al. Electrocardiograms that represent the potential variations of a single electrode. *Am Heart J* 1934; 9:477.
30. Wilson FN, Johnston FD, Rosenbaum FF, et al. On Einthoven's triangle, the theory of unipolar electrocardiographic leads and the interpretation of the precordial electrocardiogram. *Am Heart J* 1946; 32:279.

Suggested links

Electrical system of the heart video
https://www.khanacademy.org/science/health-and-medicine/circulatory-system/heart-depolarization/v/electrical-system-of-the-heart

Formation and interpretation of the electrocardiographic waves

Since the introduction of the galvanometer by W. Einthoven, the electrocardiogram has become a diagnostic procedure that is widely used in human cardiology to identify rhythm abnormalities, intraventricular conduction disturbances and signs of myocardial ischemia.

In veterinary medicine, the electrocardiogram is an essential diagnostic tool in the evaluation of animals with cardiovascular disorders, when combined with other clinical findings obtained through the history, physical examination, chest radiographs, laboratory tests and echocardiography.

The main indications for an electrocardiogram in animals include the analysis of the heart rhythm with syncope (*transient loss of consciousness*), intermittent weakness (*transient loss of posture*), structural cardiac diseases, irregular heart beats on auscultation and an inherited predisposition to rhythm abnormalities. The electrocardiogram may also have some value as a pre-anesthetic test, in the presence of electrolyte, acid-base or hormonal disorders, and systemic conditions, including shock, pancreatitis, hyperthyroidism, cranial trauma and neoplasia. Despite its clinical utility, the electrocardiogram has several limitations including a lack of sensitivity for the identification of chamber enlargement, wall hypertrophy and, because of the short duration of the recording, for the detection of intermittent (paroxysmal) arrhythmias.

The electrocardiograph

The electrocardiograph is a galvanometer, which is able to record electrical events generated rhythmically by the cardiac dipole from several electrodes attached to the surface of the body. The differences in electrical potential measured between the electrodes are then converted into electrocardiographic waves and displayed on calibrated paper.

Depending on the modality of acquisition and signal processing, electrocardiographs are classified as analog or digital. *Analog electrocardiographs* acquire the signal, which is then printed as electrocardiographic waves on calibrated paper. *Digital electrocardiographs* allow for post-processing of the signal after the recording has been obtained and stored in the hard drive of the device or a computer. Digital electrocardiographs have some advantages over their analog counterparts, including the ability to record 12 leads simultaneously, to measure electrocardiographic waves manually or automatically using varying degrees of signal amplification, to reduce the non-respiratory beat-to-beat variability normally present during cardiac electrical activity, to export the recording to other computers, which facilitates data sharing, and finally to store recordings in the long-term, without the risk of seeing the tracings printed on thermal activated paper fading over time (the lifespan of these tracings is usually limited to 3 to 5 years).

Recording and calibration of the electrocardiographic tracing

The electrocardiogram should be performed with the animal placed in right lateral recumbency with the head and neck lying on the table's surface and aligned with the thoracic and lumbar spine. The forelimbs must be maintained parallel, slightly separated and perpendicular to the spine, so that the shoulder joints overlap (Fig. 3.1).

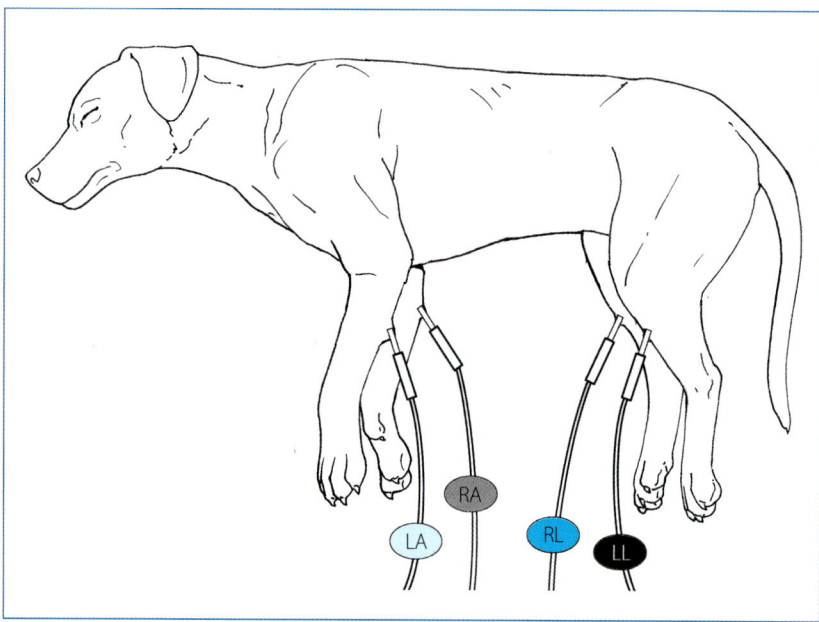

Figure 3.1. Correct positioning of the patient to record an electrocardiogram. The animal should be gently restrained in right lateral recumbency, with the head and the neck resting on the surface of the table and aligned with the thoracic and lumbar spine. The anterior limbs must be positioned parallel to each other, slightly separated and perpendicular to the spine. The electrodes of the bipolar and unipolar limb leads must be applied according to the standardized color coding (American system): left thoracic limb (LA) black electrode, right thoracic limb (RA) white electrode, the left pelvic limb (LL) red electrode and right pelvic limb (RL) green electrode.

All the reference values for electrocardiographic measurements in the dog and the cat have been obtained with the animals gently restrained in this position. One should, therefore, be careful when using these reference values on electrocardiographic recordings obtained with animals placed in other positions, including left lateral recumbency, sternal, sitting and standing positions. Indeed, changes in body position can alter the direction of the cardiac vectors with respect to the exploring electrodes, which results in variations of the morphology and polarity of the electrocardiographic waves in the frontal plane. With respect to these guidelines of positioning it should also be understood that when the major goal of the electrocardiographic recording is to assess rhythm in a distressed animal, the electrocardiogram can be recorded with the body in any position to obtain the basic information regarding rhythm.

To connect the electrocardiograph to the animal's body surface, connectors called electrodes are used. The most common electrodes used in veterinary medicine are alligator clips and adhesive patches (Fig. 3.2). Alligator clips are easy to use because they can be secured directly to the skin without removing hair. Clipping is however required before placing adhesive patches, which are used for long-term electrocardiographic monitoring (Intensive Care Unit telemetry, Holter recording). In order to ascertain good contact between the electrodes and the skin, conducting gel or alcohol must be applied.

The electrodes of the bipolar and unipolar limb lead systems are identified with a standard code of colors.

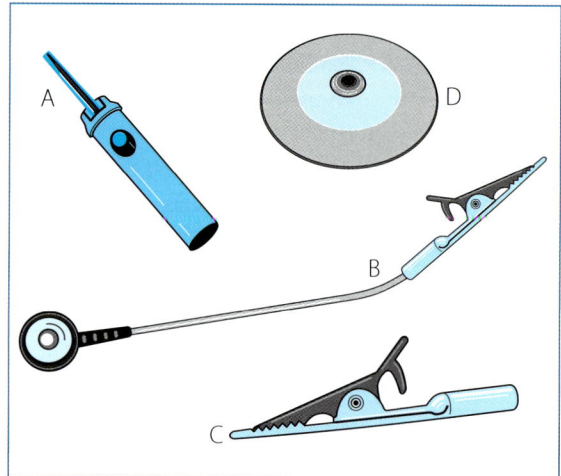

Figure 3.2. Electrode connectors. The electrode that is most widely used in veterinary medicine is the alligator clip (A, B, C), which is directly connected to the animal's skin. Adhesive patches (D) are used for longer term electrocardiographic monitoring (Intensive Care Unit, 24-hour Holter or external event recorder).

In most countries, the yellow electrode is connected to the left thoracic limb (LA), the red electrode to the right thoracic limb (RA), the green electrode to the left pelvic limb (LL) and the black electrode to the right pelvic limb (RL). In the United States of America, a different color coding is used: the black electrode is connected to the left thoracic limb (LA), the white electrode to the right thoracic limb (RA), the red electrode to the left pelvic limb (LL) and the green electrode to the right pelvic limb (RL) (Fig. 3.1). Considering that the animal's limbs behave as linear conductors, the amplitude of the electrocardiographic waves remains constant along their entire length. The level at which electrodes are attached on the limbs does not, therefore, affect the recording. However, in order to limit artifacts caused by respiratory movements, it is preferable to attach the forelimb electrodes away from the chest, halfway between the carpus and the olecranon.

In dogs, the electrodes of the precordial leads are placed on the chest surface. Several lead systems have been developed in dogs (see p. 26). The correct positioning of the electrodes on the chest wall is extremely important as the chest behaves as a volume conductor, which means that the value of the electrical potentials and the resulting electrocardiographic waves are different at every point.

Following placement of the electrodes, the next step is to select the recording parameters, including the number of leads to be recorded, the recording speed and amplitude, and finally the filter settings.

Electrocardiographic tracings are recorded on calibrated paper composed of vertical and horizontal lines 1 mm apart (Fig. 3.3). The intersection of these lines form squares that are 1 mm on each side. Every fifth horizontal and vertical line is thicker. These thick lines form squares that are 5 mm on each side.

The amplitude of the electrocardiographic waves is measured on the vertical axis of the calibrated paper, and is expressed in millivolts (mV). The duration of the waves is measured on the horizontal axis, and expressed in milliseconds (ms).

The standard calibration is an amplitude of 10 mm/1 mV, i.e. an electrical signal with an amplitude of 1 mV produces a vertical deflection of 10 mm = 1 cm, and each millimeter on the vertical axis represents 0.1 mV.

Whenever the amplitude of the waves displayed on the recording is too large or too small, the amplitude can be halved or doubled. In the first case, the amplitude is decreased to 5 mm/1 mV (1 mm corresponds to 0.2 mV); in the second case, the amplitude is increased to 20 mm/1 mV (1 mm corresponds to 0.05 mV). Whenever an electrocardiogram is recorded, the tracing displays first a calibration waveform (Fig. 3.4) that confirms the current settings.

An electrocardiogram can be recorded at a speed of 12.5 mm/s to 500 mm/s depending on the capability of the electrocardiograph, although in clinical practice the speed most commonly used is 25 mm/s or 50 mm/s. It should be mentioned that these speeds were developed primarily because electrocardiographs were designed for use in humans and it may actually be important in small animals, especially those with fast heart rates, that the recordings are done at 100 mm/s to improve the accuracy of measurements. The flexibility in recording in clinical practice has now expanded because of the many digital electrocardiographic systems that are available. At a speed of 25 mm/s, 1 mm in the horizontal axis on the calibrated paper represents $1/25^{th}$ of a second, or 40 ms; at a speed of 50 mm/s, 1 mm represents $1/50^{th}$ of a second, or 20 ms.

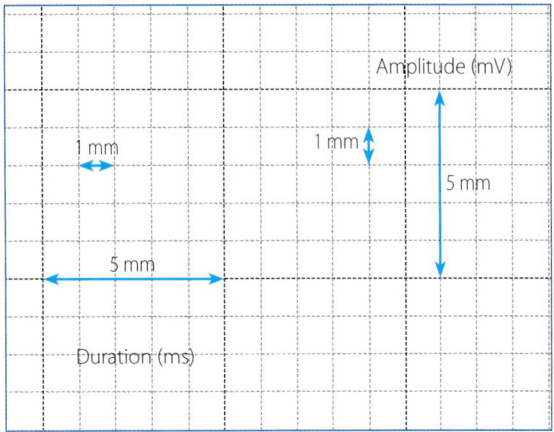

Figure 3.3. Electrocardiographic paper. Vertical and horizontal lines spaced 1 mm apart form a grid. The intersection of these lines forms small squares that have a side-length of 1 mm. Every fifth horizontal or vertical line is thicker, which forms squares that have a side-length of 5 mm. On this graph paper, the amplitude (expressed in mV) of the electrocardiographic waves can be measured on the vertical axis, and the duration of the waves is measured on the horizontal axis (expressed in ms).

The calibration waveform present at the beginning of each recording will have a width of 10 mm if the speed is 50 mm/s and 5 mm if the speed is 25 mm/s (Fig. 3.4).

The last parameter to adjust to obtain a good quality recording is the filter settings in order to minimize artifacts.

Three main types of interference have been recognized: electromyographic interference, breathing-induced fluctuations of the isoelectric line, and electrical interference from the powerline. Electromyographic interference and the oscillations induced by respiratory movements are generated by the animal's skeletal muscles, while the electromagnetic interference from the powerline originates from the power cord that connects the electrocardiograph to the electrical outlet. Many of these interferences can be mitigated with the use of various filters. A filter receives an incoming signal composed of a large number of frequencies, and eliminates a pre-selected range of frequencies from the signal that is transmitted and displayed as the electrocardiogram. Therefore, a filter eliminates signals that have a frequency below or above a pre-determined cut-off value. Filters are classified as *low-pass* (LP) filters, *high-pass* (HP) filters and notch filters. Low-pass filters only eliminate signals with a frequency above their cut-off value (frequencies below the cut-off value are allowed to "pass", i.e. be transmitted and displayed). High-pass filters eliminate signals with frequencies below their cut-off frequency. Finally, *notch* filters eliminate signals within a narrow range of frequencies. In most electrocardiographs, a notch filter is included to eliminate signals with frequencies between 50 and 60 Hz, which correspond to the frequencies of the alternating electric current from the powerline. It should be noted that in the examination of electrocardiographic recordings from animals with pacemakers it may be necessary to adjust filtering in order to see the pacing artifact. Such adjustments may cause the electrocardiographic recording of the waveforms to have additional artifacts, but if it is important to identify the spike from the pacemaker they may be required.

Most analog electrocardiographs activate filters to exclude signals with a frequency below 0.05 Hz and above 100 Hz from the recording. This setting eliminates the most common causes of interference. Digital electrocardiographs however give the option to adjust the low-pass

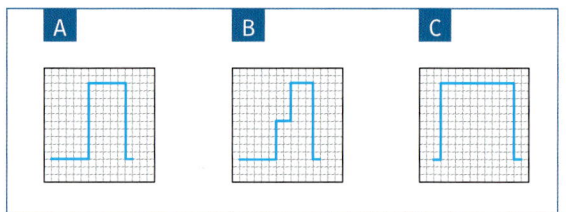

Figure 3.4. Electrocardiogram calibration. At the beginning of each electrocardiographic recording, the electrocardiograph performs automatic calibration by generating a 1 mV electrical signal for 0.2 s that appears as a rectangular waveform. If an amplitude setting of 10 mm/1 mV is selected, the calibration deflection measures 10 mm in height (A). If the amplitude setting is 5 mm/mV, the signal measures 5 mm in height (B). As for speed, a calibration waveform measuring 5 mm on the horizontal axis indicates a paper speed of 25 mm/s (A-B); if the length of the signal is 10 mm, the paper speed is 50 mm/s (C).

and high-pass filters independently. With these systems, the low-pass filter cut-off frequency should be set at 70 Hz for dogs, and 150 Hz for cats. This higher cut-off in cats is necessary because of the higher frequency of the signals that form the QRS complex on the tracing. It should be noted that the use of low-pass filters with cut-off frequencies selected below 150 Hz results in a reduction of the amplitude of the QRS complex and eliminates any indentations caused by low amplitude depolarizations that usually have frequencies above 500 Hz. If the recorded band of frequencies is comprised between 1 and 30 Hz, the electrocardiogram is free of artifacts but the components of the electrocardiogram become distorted, especially when rapid variations in voltage occur (Q wave, R wave), and the amplitude of electrocardiographic waves are underestimated (Fig. 3.5A-B). The effect of the filter setting on the amplitude of the R wave is inversely related to the size of the dog and the duration of the QRS complex.

Ideally, the high-pass filter should be set at 0.05 Hz. Its role is to eliminate oscillations of the isoelectric line due to breathing (Fig. 3.5C-D). If a higher cut-off (0.5 Hz) value is used for this filter, it can alter the morphology of the electrocardiogram at the level of the J point and the ST segment.

An electrocardiogram should be recorded for at least 3 to 5 minutes if the 12 leads are recorded simultaneously. When the leads are recorded in sequence, each one should be recorded for at least 10 seconds.

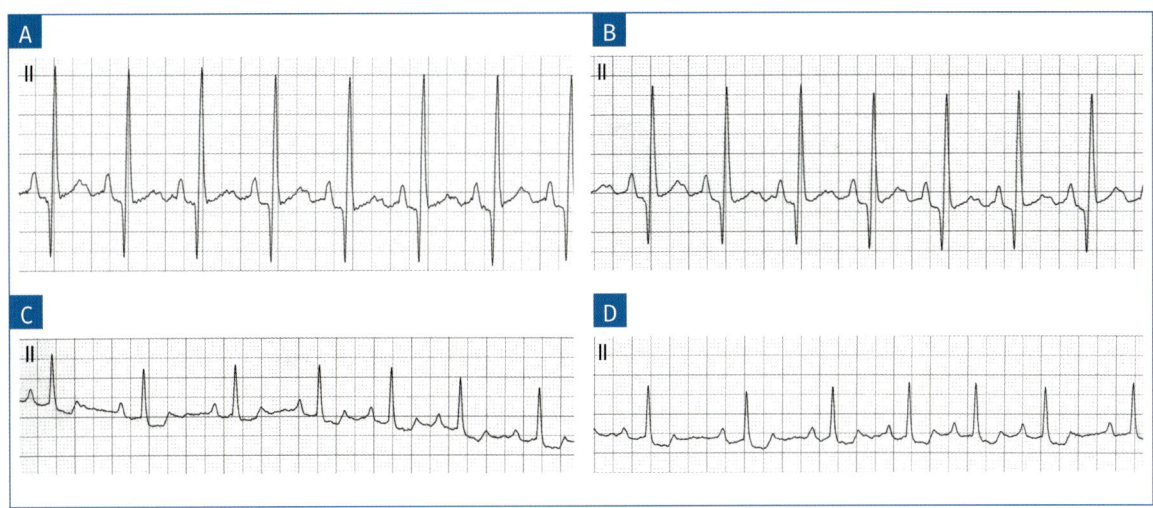

Figure 3.5. Examples of low-pass (A-B) and high-pass (C-D) filter adjustment during the recording of an electrocardiogram for the elimination of the most common artifacts.

A) Dog, Great Dane, male, 8 months. Lead II - speed 50 mm/s - calibration 10 mm/1 mV. Recording made using a low-pass filter with a cut-off frequency of 250 Hz. Note the presence of artifacts due to skeletal muscle tremors that are responsible for irregular oscillations of the baseline with an amplitude ranging from 0.03 to 0.2 mV.

B) Dog, Great Dane, male, 8 months. Lead II - speed 50 mm/s - calibration 10 mm/1 mV. Recording obtained in the same dog as Fig. 3.5A after adjusting the low-pass filters to a cut-off value of 30 Hz. Note the absence of the irregular oscillations that are typical of muscle tremor, and the distortion and decrease in the amplitude of the high frequency signals, where rapid variations of voltage occur (Q and R waves).

C) Dog, mixed breed, female, 13 years. Lead II - speed 50 mm/s - calibration 10 mm/1 mV. Recording made without a high-pass filter. Note the presence of oscillations of the isoelectric line due to respiratory movements.

D) Dog, mixed breed, female, 13 years. Lead II - speed 50 mm/s - calibration 10 mm/1 mV. Recording performed in the same dog as Fig. 3.5C with a high-pass filter adjusted to a cut-off value of 0.05 Hz. This filter eliminates respiratory artifacts, and ensures correct alignment of the P-QRS-T complexes.

In order to store digital electrocardiographic signals, various methods of compressions are applied to the signal. A 5-minute uncompressed 12-lead tracing takes 2 to 3 megabytes of storage space, in addition to the space needed to store patient information. Compression methods mainly affect the high frequency components of the recording. The optimal compression method should not alter the original amplitude of the signal by more than 0.01 mV.

Formation of the electrocardiographic waves

During the depolarization and repolarization phases of the atrial and ventricular working myocardium, the electrocardiograph records changes in electrical potential represented by waveforms of variable amplitude and duration. A *wave* represents an electrical event inside the myocardium, and corresponds to a deflection on the tracing above or below the baseline. A *segment* is a line joining two consecutive electrocardiographic waves. The term *interval* refers to the distance, measured in millimeters, between two consecutive cardiac events. The distance can then be converted to a duration (usually in ms) based on the recording speed selected during the recording. Electrocardiographic waves are identified as the P wave, or atrial depolarization wave; T_a wave or atrial repolarization wave; QRS complex or ventricular depolarization wave; J wave or early repolarization wave; T wave and U wave or ventricular repolarization waves. The segment between the end of the T wave and the beginning of the next P wave is defined as the *TP segment*, and the line forming that segment corresponds to the *baseline* or *isoelectric line*. The *PQ segment* is the section between the end of the P wave and the beginning of the Q wave. The segment between the end of the QRS complex and the onset of the T wave is the *ST segment*; the segment between the end of the T wave and beginning of the U wave is the *TU interval*. It should be noted that the U wave is rarely seen in the dog or cat, although it is important to know of its existence because it does develop when excessive doses of potassium channel blockers are used. The time interval between the beginning of the P wave and the beginning of the QRS complex is defined as the *PQ interval*; the time interval between the start of the Q wave and the end of the T wave is the *QT interval* (Fig. 3.6). Other intervals of time that must be taken into account are the *QTU interval*, which is the interval between the onset of the Q wave and the end of the U wave, the P-P interval, which is the interval of time between two consecutive P waves, and finally the R-R interval, which is the time interval between two consecutive R waves. The P-P and R-R intervals represent the time interval between two atrial depolarizations and two ventricular depolarizations (interval or cycle length), respectively.

A few notations are warranted at this point to decrease confusion regarding the names of the waveforms seen on the electrocardiogram. In fact, reviews have been written concerning terminology. Clinicians most commonly refer to the waveform denoting ventricular depolarization as

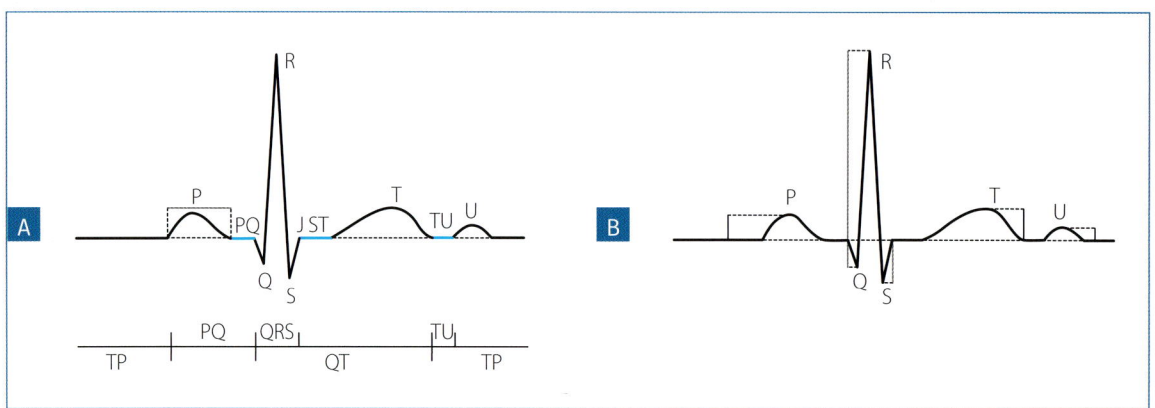

Figure 3.6. Characterization of the electrocardiographic waves, segments and intervals in lead II.
A) The electrocardiographic waves, the various segments and reference marks to measure waveform duration and intervals accurately are represented. The atrial depolarization generates a deflection on the electrocardiogram known as the P wave with a positive polarity in lead II, and the ventricular depolarization produces a complex called QRS. Although infrequently present on the electrocardiogram of normal dogs and cats, the wave of atrial repolarization (T_a) may be seen during the PQ segment, and on occasion extends into or beyond the QRS complex. Ventricular repolarization generates an electrocardiographic wave, called the T wave, which is rarely followed by a concordant deflection (same polarity as the T wave) caused by the repolarization of M (mid-myocardial) cells, known as the U wave. The segment between the end of the T wave and the beginning of the next P wave is called the TP segment, while the line that joins two TP segments is called the isoelectric line or baseline (dotted line). The segment between the end of the P wave and the beginning of the QRS complex is defined as the PQ (PR) segment. The segment between the end of the QRS complex, sometimes identifiable by the presence of a J wave (early repolarization wave), and the onset of the T wave is called the ST segment. The segment between the end of the T wave and the beginning of the rarely seen U wave is defined as the TU interval. The time interval measured from the start of the P wave to the beginning of the QRS complex is called the PQ interval. Depending on the species, lead examined and electrocardiographic diagnosis, the QRS complex may not begin with a Q wave, but an R wave and in this situation it is the PR interval. In clinical discussions PR or PQ interval is commonly used interchangeably, although in a given animal or lead, the specifics of what is beginning the QRS complex may vary. The time interval from the beginning of the QRS complex to the end of the T wave is called the QT interval. The duration of the P wave is measured from the point at which the deflection separates from the isoelectric line to the point where it returns to it. The duration of the QRS complex is measured from the beginning of the Q wave when present to the end of the S wave.
B) Illustration of electrocardiographic wave amplitude measurements. The amplitude is calculated from the isoelectric line to the apex or nadir of the waves. When the heart rate is rapid more accurate measurements can be obtained with faster recording speeds (50 mm/s and up to 100 mm/s with some electrocardiographic systems).

the QRS complex, regardless of whether or not the particular waveform does indeed have each of these components. That is, if in lead II the waveform has only Q and R components it will often still be generically termed the QRS complex. Similarly, if in lead aVR the waveform has only a small R and a deep S, the term QRS complex will be used. Additionally, the term PR interval or PR segment is most commonly used in the literature; however, it is common in the dog when referring to lead II that a small Q wave deflection is seen initially, thus, the term PQ interval. Furthermore, the term QT interval is used to describe the total time of the duration of the ventricular depolarization and repolarization, as reflected on the electrocardiogram; however, not all QRS complexes begin with the Q wave. Nevertheless, the term QT interval is used for this measurement. An understanding of the semantics will, therefore, decrease confusion during discussions of electrocardiography.

The waves can be formed by *positive*, *negative* or *diphasic deflections*. The polarity of the waves is defined as positive if the deflection is above the baseline and negative if it is below. The waves that have both positive and negative components are called *diphasic*; when the summation of the positive and negative components equals zero, the waves are called *isodiphasic*. The electrocardiographic waves are also described as *bifid* or *bimodal* when they include two positive or negative components (i.e. double peaked or notched) (Fig. 3.7).

Atrial depolarization

Under physiological conditions the wavefront of cardiac depolarization originates from the sinus node pacemaker (P) cells and propagates through the preferential inter-atrial, internodal and atrionodal pathways to the atrial working myocardium and the atrioventricular node; it then activates the ventricles in an ordered sequence. The conduction velocity within the sinus node is approximately 0.05 m/s and it is 0.8-1 m/s in the atrial myocardium. From the sinus node, the wavefront of activation can be compared to a wildfire that propagates to the whole atrium in a right-to-left, superior-to-inferior and anterior-to-posterior direction. The atrial activation proceeds parallel to the surface of the atrium, differently from what happens in the ventricular myocardium, where the activation proceeds from

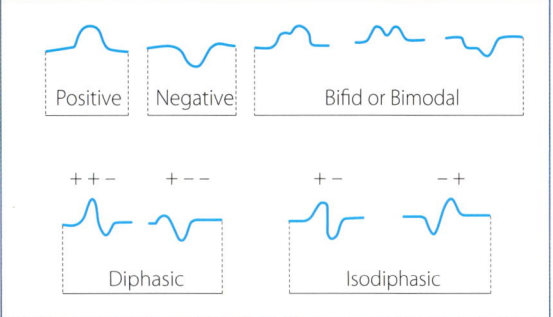

Figure 3.7. Morphology of the electrocardiographic waves. Electrocardiographic waves can be formed by positive, negative or diphasic deflections. The polarity is defined as positive if the deflection extends above the baseline and negative if it extends below the baseline. The waves that have a positive component and a negative component are called diphasic. If the algebraic sum of the positive and negative components of a diphasic wave is equal to zero, it is called isodiphasic. Electrocardiographic waves that have two positive or negative components are called bifid or bimodal.

the endocardium to the epicardium. The position of the heart in the chest, the location of the sinus node and the mode of propagation of the electrical impulses allow atrial depolarization to be described by two major vectors called vector I and vector II. Vector I represents the right atrial depolarization and is directed superior-to-inferior, posterior-to-anterior and slightly to the left. Vector II represents the left atrial activation and assumes an anterior-to-posterior, right-to-left and slightly superior-to-inferior direction.

The sequential activation of the atria starting from the sinus node gives rise to an electrocardiographic deflection called the *P wave or atriogram* (Fig. 3.8). The depolarization of the sinus node pacemaker cells (P cells) does not induce the formation of a visible electrocardiographic deflection and occurs before the onset of the P wave. In dogs, following the formation of the impulse in the sinus node, Bachmann's bundle is activated after approximately 30 ms and after a total of approximately 20 ms the medial terminal sulcus, the right appendage, the lower inter-atrial septum and the lower right atrium are activated. Next, the left atrial working myocardium, initially from the inferior region followed by the left atrial appendage and finally the postero-inferior region is activated. The initial part of the P wave is therefore attributable to the activation of the right atrium, while the final portion of the P wave represents left atrial activation. The mid-portion of the P wave corresponds to the depolarization of both the left and right atria.

The mean vector of atrial activation has a superior-to-inferior, anterior-to-posterior and right-to-left axis, which results in a P wave with positive polarity in the inferior leads (II, III, and aVF), negative polarity in aVR and aVL and finally a positive, diphasic or isodiphasic polarity in lead I. Since the direction of the vector is almost parallel to the direction of lead II and perpendicular to lead I, the P wave is detected with maximum voltage in lead II and a voltage close to 0 in lead I. The vector of atrial depolarization forms a P wave with maximal negativity in aVR (Fig. 3.9).

In the dog, the orientation of the vectors of atrial activation produces a P wave with positive polarity in lead CV_6LU and variable polarity in leads CV_5RL and V_{10} when the lead system of Lannek later modified by Dettweiler and Patterson is used. P waves have variable polarity in lead V_1 and are positive in leads V_2 to V_6 in the lead system established by Wilson and later modified by Kraus, et al.

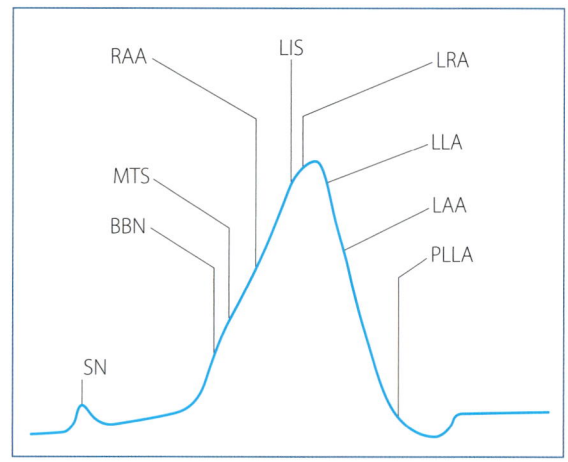

Figure 3.8. Atrial depolarization and P wave formation. The P wave is generated by the sequential activation of the atria starting from the sinus node. The initial portion of the P wave is attributable to the electrical activation of the various parts of the right atrium, and the final portion of the P wave corresponds to the activation of the left atrium. In the central portion of the P wave there is an overlap between left and right atrial activation. *SN*: sinus node; *BBN*: Bachmann's bundle; *MTS*: medial terminal sulcus; *RAA*: right atrial appendage; *LIS*: lower inter-atrial septum; *LRA*: lower right atrium; *LLA*: lower left atrium; *LAA*: left atrial appendage; *PLLA*: posterior lower left atrium (see text for explanations).

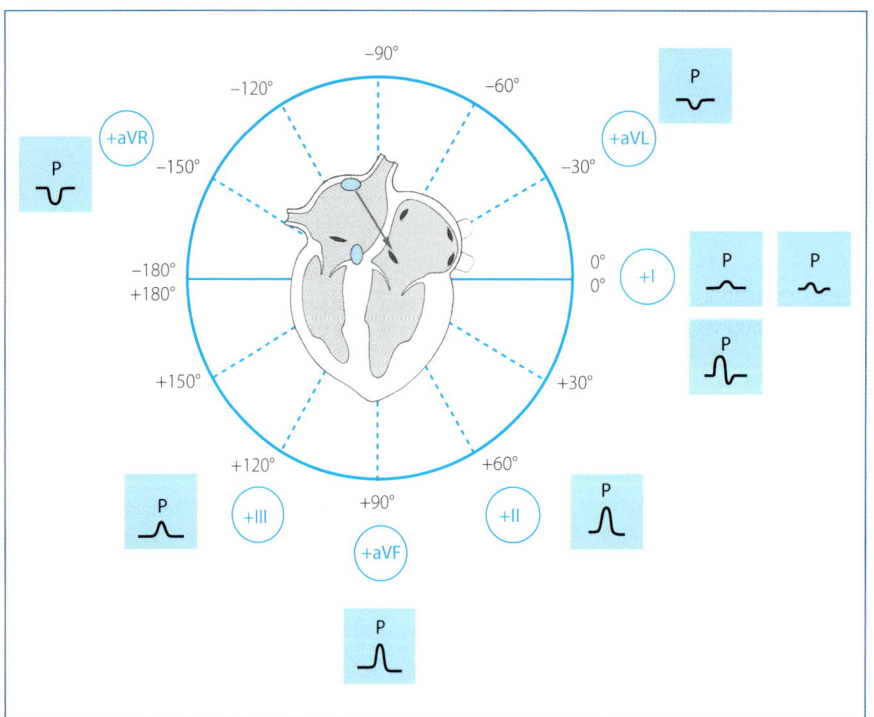

Figure 3.9. Atrial depolarization wavefront and electrocardiographic appearance of the P wave in the six limb leads. The mean vector of atrial activation has a superior-to-inferior, anterior-to-posterior and right-to-left direction. As a result, the P wave appears as a deflection with positive polarity in the inferior leads (II, III, and aVF), with negative polarity in leads aVR and aVL, and positive, diphasic or isodiphasic polarity in lead I. Note how the P wave has the maximum positivity in lead II and the maximum negativity in lead aVR.

Atrial repolarization

Atrial depolarization is followed by atrial repolarization which has a summed vector in the superior-to-inferior, anterior-to-posterior and right-to-left axis. This wave of repolarization travels parallel to the atrial muscle walls. The vector of repolarization is a negative wave approaching the positive pole of lead II, which gives rise to a wave called T_a, with a polarity opposite to that of the P wave. The T_a wave has a smaller amplitude than the P wave but its duration is 2.5 times longer, such that the areas under the curves are approximately equal. Normally, the T_a wave is difficult to recognize because it is a low voltage deflection. Several factors likely play a role in the visualization of the T_a wave. These may include the PQ interval duration, amount of vagal tone and conduction properties of the atrial myocardium (Fig. 3.10A-B). The latter portion of the T_a wave can extend into the QRS complex and under certain situations actually be apparent in the ST segment. (Fig. 3.10B). It is not possible to completely identify the end of T_a in the presence of a QRS complex; data available from dogs have been acquired during atrioventricular block or in experimental conditions.

During second- and third-degree atrioventricular blocks, when not all P waves are followed by a QRS complex, a T_a wave is easier to recognize as a negative polarity deflection in the inferior leads (II, III, and aVF) which begins immediately after the end of the P wave (Fig. 3.10C).

Ventricular depolarization

Depolarization of the ventricle can be thought of in two parts: (1) depolarization through the specialized conduction system (bundle branches and Purkinje system) and (2) depolarization of the working myocardium. The former occurs much more rapidly than the latter. Importantly, the complete electrical depolarization of the heart representing electrical systole occurs before mechanical systole with the generation of myocardial contraction. The initial depolarization through the specialized conduction system, after an impulse emerges from the non-penetrating portion of the distal atrioventricular bundle, accelerates along the bundle of His, and then propagates to the right and left bundle branches and the Purkinje network at a speed of 5 m/sec. Conduction times in this region are shown in Fig. 3.11. This phase of activation

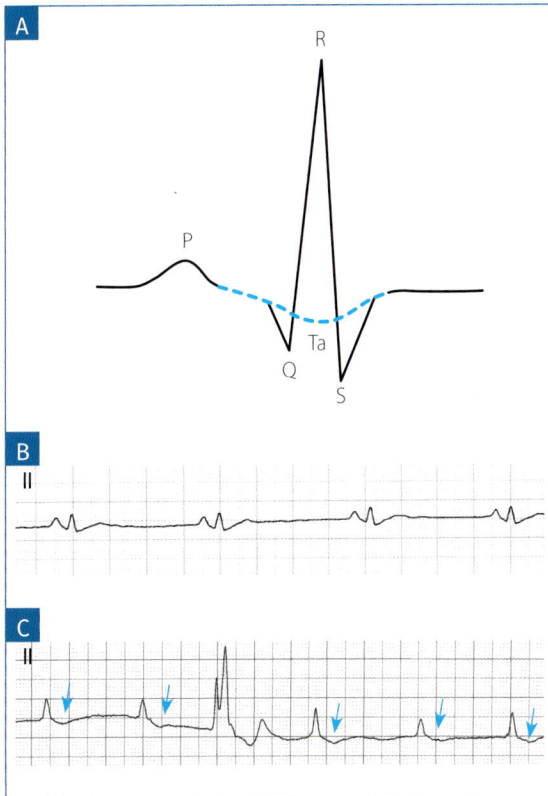

Figure 3.10. Atrial repolarization wave or T_a wave in lead II.
A) The atrial repolarization wave (T_a wave) is shown in blue. T_a has the opposite polarity to that of the P wave and it typically has a very small amplitude, although it is more easily identified in some dog breeds or dogs with atrial enlargement.
B) Dog, Labrador Retriever, male, 12 years. Lead II - speed 50 mm/s - calibration 10 mm/1 mV. Sinus rhythm with T_a that extends from the end of the P wave to 40 ms after the end of the QRS complex.
C) Dog, Rottweiler, female, 5 years. Lead II - speed 50 mm/s - calibration 20 mm/1 mV. Third-degree atrioventricular block with idioventricular rhythm. Note the presence of a deflection with a negative polarity following the P waves and corresponding to the T_a wave (arrows).

of the ventricular conduction tissue corresponds to the electrocardiographic PQ segment. During this period, the depolarization does not involve the working myocardium but exclusively the nodal and intraventricular conduction tissue and, consequently, no deflections are seen on the electrocardiogram; instead it is represented by an isoelectric line that follows the P wave and has a duration of 30-100 ms. The extensive Purkinje system permits the electrical impulse to quickly reach the apical region of the right and left heart. The rapid depolarization in this region permits depolarization of the working myocardium so that the initial contraction of the heart begins in the apex. Such a contraction sequence affords the most efficient ejection of blood from the ventricles. When the depolarization phase of the ventricular working myocardium begins, the isoelectric line is interrupted by the first deflection of the QRS complex. The sequence of myocardial depolarization is described below; however, the entire process is extremely rapid such that from beginning to end it takes 40 to 50 ms in the dog and 25 to 40 ms in the cat.

Ventricular depolarization of the working myocardium starts from the left side of the interventricular septum where the electric impulse propagates with a slower speed of 0.8-1 m/s compared to the speed in the Purkinje fibers. The depolarization of ventricular muscle starts from the postero-inferior and antero-superior divisions of the left bundle branch. The wavefront then activates the right portion of the interventricular septum with a posterior-to-anterior and inferior-to-superior direction, and is followed by depolarization of the ventricular free walls. The apical regions of the ventricles contain a higher concentration of Purkinje fibers compared to the basal regions; therefore, the muscular ventricular apex is activated faster and the direction of the parietal (i.e., wall) depolarization assumes an inferior-to-superior direction, from the apex to the cardiac base. The activation times for the different segments of the ventricular myocardium in dogs are shown in Fig. 3.12.

Ventricular activation can be represented by a sequence of three vectors (Fig. 3.13): the *first vector* (1) represents the activation of the interventricular septum by the divisions of the left bundle branch and predominantly by its posterior portion; at the same time the *second vector* corresponds to right ventricular activation (2); it is followed by the *third vector*, which corresponds to left ventricular activation and can be further subdivided into two vectors (3a and 3b). The first (or septal) vector has a left-to-right, posterior-to-anterior and inferior-or-to-superior direction. The second (or right ventricular depolarization) vector is directed posterior-to-anterior, inferior-to-superior and towards the right. The 3a vector represents the depolarization of the antero-superior

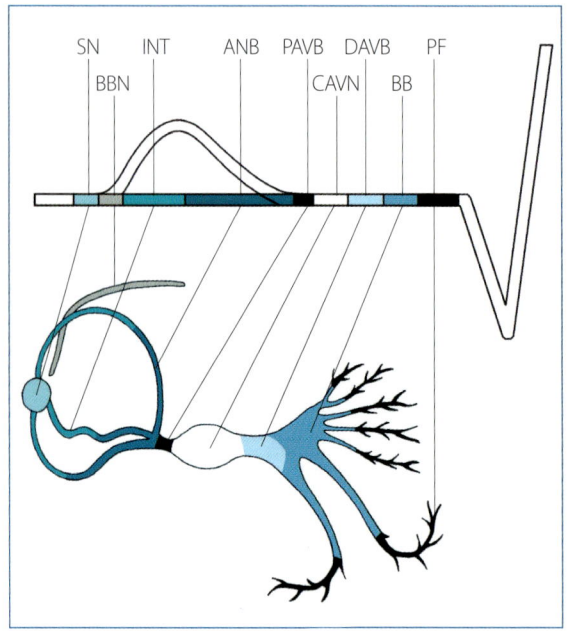

Figure 3.11. Representation of the anatomy of the cardiac conduction system including the atrioventricular and intraventricular activation times with the corresponding electrocardiographic tracing (from Rosenbaum MB, et al., 1976). Depolarization of the sinus node P cells is followed by sequential depolarization of Bachmann's bundle, the internodal tracts, the atrionodal bundles, the atrial myocardium, the proximal atrioventricular bundle, the compact node, the distal atrioventricular bundle, the bundle branches and finally the Purkinje fibers. Depolarization of the atrionodal portion of the atrioventricular conduction axis starts in the middle of the ascending branch of the P wave and is not detectable on the electrocardiogram. The compact node is activated approximately 10 ms after the end of the P wave. The activation of the distal atrioventricular bundle follows after 23 ms, then the bundle branches after 25 ms and finally the Purkinje fibers after 40 ms. This phase of depolarization only involves the specialized conduction tissue and electrocardiographically corresponds to the PQ segment. The isoelectric line of the PQ segment is interrupted by the first deflection of the QRS complex and reflects the depolarization of the ventricular working myocardium. Note that the existence of discrete internodal tracts and atrionodal bundles remains controversial. However, preferential pathways of conduction exist between the sinus node and the atrioventricular junction. *SN*: sinus node; *BBN*: Bachmann's bundle; *INT*: internodal tracts; *ANB*: atrionodal bundles; *PAVB*: proximal atrioventricular bundle; *CAVN*: compact portion of the atrioventricular node; *DAVB*: distal atrioventricular bundle; *BB*: bundle branches; *PF*: Purkinje fibers.

Formation of the electrocardiographic waves | 45

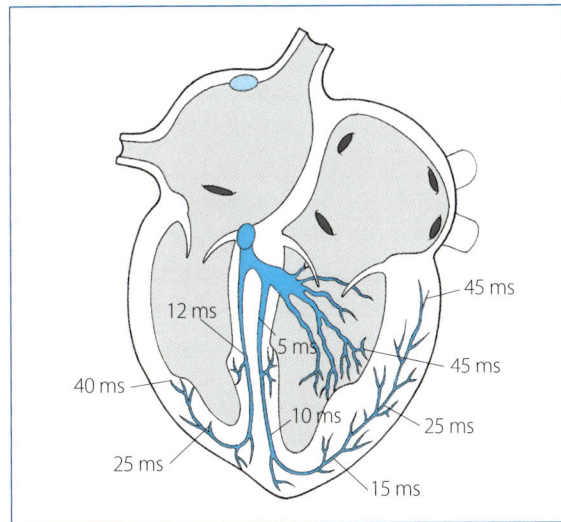

Figure 3.12. Activation times of the left and right ventricular working myocardium (from Rosenbaum MB, et al., 1976).

Understanding the generation of the electrocardiographic waveforms of the ventricles can be confusing when one considers the speed of conduction through the Purkinje system, the rapid depolarization of the ventricular apex, and the electrical and mechanical relationship that results in the apex initiating contraction. The net ventricular vector of depolarization is directed primarily towards lead II in the frontal plane causing a positive complex with a tall R wave in the normal dog and cat. However, this simplistic vision is disturbed when recalling that the Purkinje system does not cause a deflection on the surface electrocardiogram and that the working myocardium of the apex is actually depolarized first to cause the heart to contract from the apex towards the base. Reconciling this conflict may be found in an understanding of the other important component of depolarization. This component concerns myocardial depolarization from endocardium to epicardium. Since the left ventricle has the thicker wall such net vectors are directed primarily towards the positive pole of lead II. Certainly, the compartmentalization of depolarization prevents a complete perspective of this action. Three-dimensional imaging of the process assists in understanding it (see video links).

In the dog, the first vector (interventricular septum) represents electrical forces with an inferior-to-superior and left-to-right orientation in the frontal plane, moving away from the positive poles and approaching the negative poles of leads I, II, III, and aVF. These electrical forces result in the formation of a first negative deflection or Q wave in lead I, and in leads II, III, and aVF in 80 % of dogs. Because this first vector moves toward the positive pole of aVR, it generates an R wave in this lead. Within milliseconds after the onset of interventricular septum depolarization, the electrocardiographic line returns to the level of the isoelectric line. The depolarization of the right and left ventricles then results in electrical forces that are directed toward the positive pole of leads I, II, III, and aVF and therefore an R wave. Commonly in the dog and cat lead II has the largest R wave amplitude. For the same reason the vector of left ventricular depolarization is directed towards the negative pole of aVR and aVL and generates deep S waves in these leads.

Several precordial lead systems for the dog have historically been proposed. That described by Lannek, and later

portion of the left ventricle activated by the antero-superior fascicle, and vector 3*b* corresponds to the depolarization of the infero-posterior portion, the apex and the inflow portion of the left ventricle by the postero-inferior fascicle. The synchronous activation of these portions of the left ventricle can be combined in a single vector that is directed to the left, anterior-to-posterior and superior-to-inferior. The terminal phase of ventricular depolarization is represented by an activation front, called basal, which is directed somewhat perpendicular to the frontal plane and toward the cardiac base. Depending on the position of the heart in the thorax relative to the frontal plane, the electrocardiographic recording of this terminal phase is represented by the S wave of the QRS complex. This deflection in the dog and cat is usually small unless cardiac enlargement or conduction disturbances have caused the S wave to deepen.

The sequence of ventricular depolarization of the various segments produces a succession of negative and positive electrocardiographic waves that follow the PQ segment and that are defined as the *QRS complex* or *ventriculogram*. The first positive deflection is called the R wave and the second positive deflection the R' wave. A negative electrocardiographic wave is defined as Q if it precedes the R wave, and is called S if it follows the R wave.

modified by Dettweiler and Patterson, is characterized by an R wave in lead CV_5RL which corresponds to the septal vector, a Q wave in V_{10} in 100 % of healthy dogs, and Q waves in CV_6LL and CV_6LU in 40 % and 80 % of animals, respectively. The second and third vectors of ventricular activation produce an S wave in CV_5RL and an R wave in leads CV_6LL, CV_6LU and V_{10}. In the system proposed by Wilson, and later modified by Kraus, et al., the first vector appears with an R wave in V_1 and with a Q wave from V_2 to V_6, while the second and third vectors are detected as S waves in V_1 and R waves from V_2 to V_6. The amplitude of the waves in each lead depends of the animal's chest conformation and the position of the heart within the thorax. Clinically, with modern 12-lead electronic digital electrocardiographs, the V_1 to V_6 system is more commonly used today and thus this will be emphasized hereafter.

Ventricular repolarization

Following depolarization, the membrane potential of all cardiomyocytes progressively returns to baseline during the phase of repolarization. Ventricular repolarization begins with phase 1 of the monophasic action potential (J wave) and lasts until the end of phase 3. During phases 1 and 2, the epicardial and endocardial cells have similar membrane potential values, which correspond on the surface electrocardiogram to the isoelectric ST segment. During phase 3, however, the epicardial region repolarizes before the endocardium, which results in a transmural gradient of repolarization from epicardium to endocardium.

Ventricular repolarization lasts two to three times longer than depolarization, because the electrical impulses propagate through the working myocardium

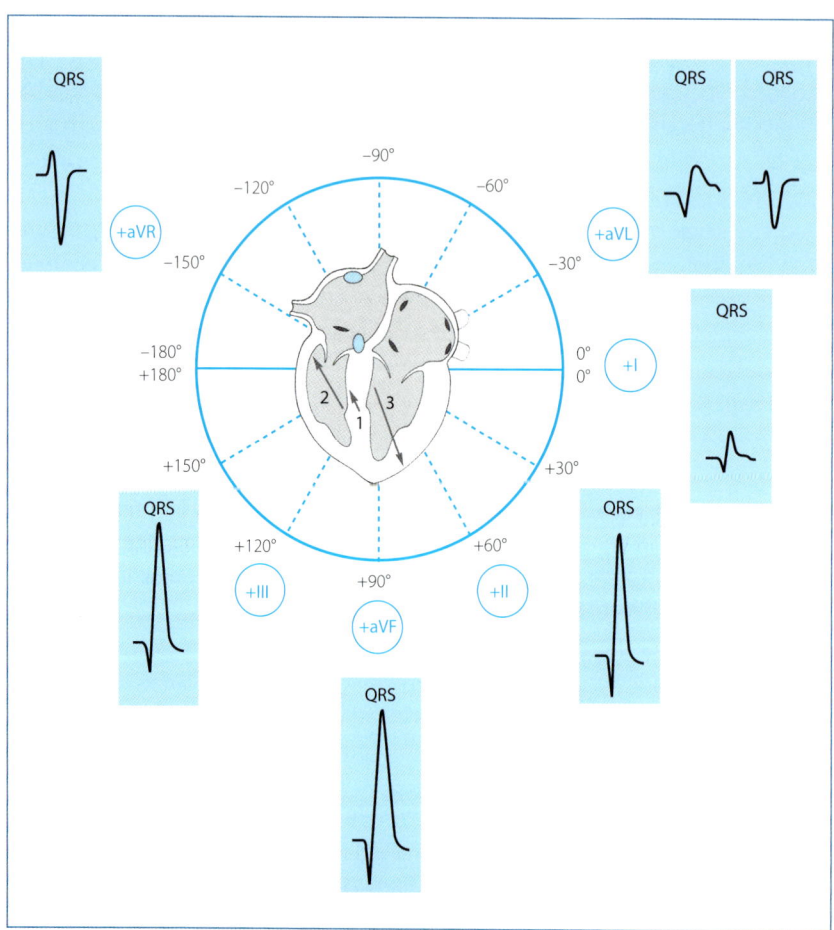

Figure 3.13. Ventricular depolarization wavefront and electrocardiographic appearance of the QRS complex in the six limb leads. Depolarization of the ventricular myocardium can be represented by three vectors: the first (1) vector indicates activation of the interventricular septum, the second (2) activation of the right ventricle and the third (3) activation of the left ventricle. Vector 1 has an inferior-to-superior, posterior-to-anterior and left-to-right direction. Vector 2 is simultaneous to vector 3, and is directed inferior-to-superior, posterior-to-anterior and left-to-right. Vector 3 is the summation of vectors 3*a* and 3*b* that depolarize the antero-superior and postero-inferior portions of the left ventricle, respectively. Vector 3 has a superior-to-inferior, anterior-to-posterior and rigth-to-left direction. This sequence of depolarization generates a sequence of negative and positive waves that end the PQ segment and are defined as the QRS complex or ventriculogram. Typically, the QRS complex displays a maximum positive deflection in the inferior leads (II, III, and aVF) and its maximum negative deflection in lead aVR.

rather than the specialized conduction system. The T wave does, therefore, have a longer duration than the QRS complex, although the areas under the two curves are similar. Repolarization occurs perpendicularly to the ventricular wall from epicardium to endocardium. Ventricular repolarization velocity is slower in the sub-epicardial regions because of their delayed activation, and faster in the sub-endocardial regions. The magnitude of transmural dispersion of repolarization is also due to intrinsic differences in the action potential duration of the endocardial, mid-myocardial (M cells) and epicardial cells. M cells and Purkinje cells have the longest action potential duration while the epicardial cells have the shortest action potential duration. The configuration of the action potential also differs among the layers of the myocardium. For example, phase 1 is more prominent in the epicardial cells due to a high density of transient outward current (I_{to}), particularly in the dog.

Given the characteristics of the repolarization phase and the presence of a transmural gradient of repolarization, the T wave is formed by two asymmetric segments joined by a rounded apex. The ascending portion, which is associated with the sub-epicardial repolarization is not as steep as the descending branch.

In dogs, the T wave can have variable polarity, and is positive, negative or diphasic in the inferior leads (II, III, and aVF). The T wave polarity depends on the direction of the electrical forces, the position of the heart in the chest, the position of the limbs, the heterogeneity of repolarization and differences in action potential duration between the different regions of the ventricular myocardium.

T wave polarity is also variable in all precordial leads except in CV_5RL and V_1 in which it is positive, and in V_{10}, in which it is negative.

Rarely, a prominent electrocardiographic deflection, called the *U wave*, is seen after the T wave in leads CV_5RL, CV_6LL and CV_6LU, V_1, V_2 and V_4. This wave can have variable amplitude, and can appear or disappear in consecutive beats. The genesis of the U wave is still controversial and has been attributed by some authors to the repolarization of the M cells, or of the Purkinje network; others attribute it to the presence of an endocardial to epicardial gradient originating during the isovolumic relaxation phase of the cardiac cycle.

Electrocardiographic analysis

In order to interpret an electrocardiogram correctly, it is important to follow a methodical and systematic approach, which includes determination of the heart rate, rhythm, the amplitude and duration of the various waves, the duration of the PQ and QT intervals, as well as the PQ and ST segments, and finally the mean electrical axis of the P wave and QRS complex in the frontal plane.

Heart rate calculation

The heart rate is usually calculated using lead II and taking into account the recording speed of the electrocardiogram. A separate rate should be calculated for the P waves (atrial rate) and the QRS complexes (ventricular rate or heart rate). These rates are expressed in beats per minute (bpm). The determination of the atrial rate is particularly useful in all types of arrhythmias associated with atrioventricular dissociation, when the number of P waves and QRS complexes differ.

An average heart rate or an instantaneous heart rate can be determined from the electrocardiogram. To obtain the average heart rate, the number of waveforms (P waves or QRS complexes) is counted on a 15-cm portion of the tracing, which corresponds to 3 s if the paper speed is 50 mm/s and 6 s if the paper speed is 25 mm/s. Subsequently, to determine the atrial or ventricular rate per minute, the number of P waves or QRS complexes is multiplied by 20 (3 s × 20 = 60 s or 1 min) if the recording speed is 50 mm/s, and multiplied by 10 (6 s × 10 = 60 s or 1 min) if the recording speed is 25 mm/s (Fig. 3.14). It should be noted that many digital programs, the most common now for purchase, have built-in calipers or rate detectors triggering from the R wave. It is important to realize that many of these give a beat-to-beat rate and this must be taken into consideration with dogs that have a sinus arrhythmia. Furthermore, some systems will mistakenly count T waves if the R wave is small and the T wave is tall. In some situations beats may be missed if the overall complex is small, such as in cats. It is, therefore, important always to verify the rate that the digital readout provides.

The instantaneous heart rate is obtained by dividing the number of milliseconds in one minute (60,000) by the number of milliseconds between two consecutive P waves (P-P interval) or QRS complexes (R-R interval). The interval in millisecond is determined by measuring the distance in millimeters between two consecutive waveforms and multiplying the number by 20 if the recording speed is 50 mm/s, and by 40 if the recording speed is 25 mm/s (Fig. 3.14).

If the atrial and ventricular rhythms are regular, the instantaneous and average heart rates are equal. When the rhythm is irregular, it is recommended that the lowest and fastest instantaneous rates recorded on the electrocardiogram are measured, and that the heart rate is expressed as a range. When several rhythms of different origin are present, and when the relationship between P waves and QRS complexes varies, it is also recommended that the instantaneous rate of the various rhythms is determined rather than the average rate of the electrocardiogram.

Interpretation of the heart rhythm

The normal electrocardiogram of dogs and cats is characterized by the presence of P waves with positive polarity in the inferior leads (II, III, and aVF), negative polarity in aVR and aVL and positive, diphasic or isodiphasic polarity in lead I. Each P wave must be followed by a QRS complex with a normal and usually constant PQ interval. The PQ interval is interrupted by a Q wave in leads I, II, III, and aVF followed by an R wave with maximum amplitude in lead II. In leads aVR and aVL, an S wave is usually present with a maximum amplitude in aVR (Fig. 3.15).

In dogs and cats, the normal cardiac rhythm is called sinus rhythm when the following electrocardiographic characteristics are present: the heart rate determined from lead II is within the reference range for the animal evaluated, P-P and R-R intervals are regular, P waves have a constant morphology, every P wave is followed by a QRS complex and every QRS complex is preceded by a P wave. The relationship between P waves and QRS complexes is proven by measuring PQ intervals, which must remain constant.

The normal cardiac rhythm of the dog can show two variations, which are usually concomitant: respiratory sinus arrhythmia and a wandering pacemaker (see p.72). Respiratory sinus arrhythmia is characterized by the presence of cyclic variations of the R-R intervals in relation to the phases of respiration. It should be emphasized however that respiratory sinus arrhythmia is in fact more complicated than just the mechanics of breathing. Sinus arrhythmias are still present in dogs that are panting and intervals will change if the dog begins to breathe deeply.

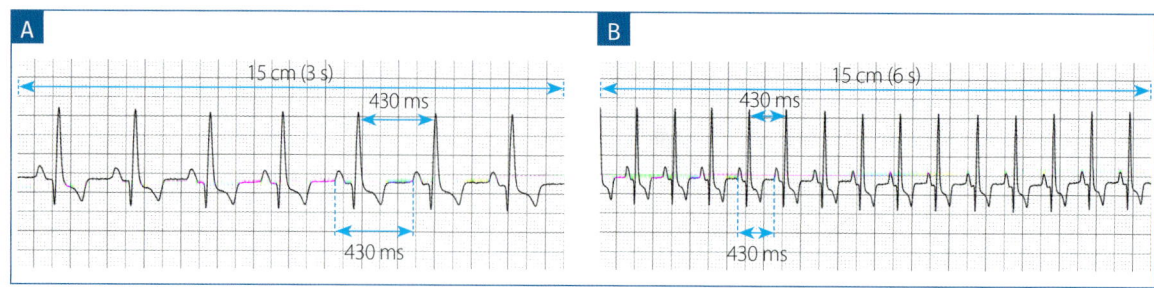

Figure 3.14. Heart rate calculation.
A) Dog, German Shepherd, male, 9 years. Lead II - speed 50 mm/s - calibration 10 mm/1 mV.
The paper speed of the tracing is 50 mm/s, therefore 15 cm correspond to 3 s. To calculate the atrial or ventricular rate per minute, the number of P waves or QRS complexes counted on a 15-cm portion of the tracing must be multiplied by 20. In this example, there are seven P waves and seven QRS complexes visible on a 15-cm segment; therefore, the atrial and ventricular rates are both 140 bpm. Alternatively, the atrial and ventricular rates can be calculated by dividing 60,000 (the number of milliseconds in a minute) by the interval in milliseconds between two P waves or two QRS complexes. In this case: 60,000/430 ms = 139 to 140 bpm. This last method provides an instantaneous heart rate rather than an average heart rate.
B) Dog, German Shepherd, male, 9 years. Lead II - speed 25 mm/s - calibration 10 mm/1 mV.
The paper speed of the tracing is 25 mm/s; therefore, 15 cm correspond to 6 s. To calculate the atrial or ventricular rate per minute, the number of P waves or QRS complexes counted on a 15-cm portion of the tracing must be multiplied by 10. In this example, there are 14 P waves and 14 QRS complexes on a 15-cm segment; therefore, the atrial and ventricular rates are both 140 bpm.

Electrocardiographic analysis | 49

Figure 3.15. Appearance of the P- QRS-T complex in the limb leads and in precordial leads during sinus rhythm.

A) Dog, Dachshund, male, 10 years. Twelve leads (I, II, III, aVR, aVL, aVF, V_1, V_2, V_3, V_4, V_5, V_6) based on Wilson's system modified by Kraus, et al. - speed 50 mm/s - calibration 5 mm/1 mV.

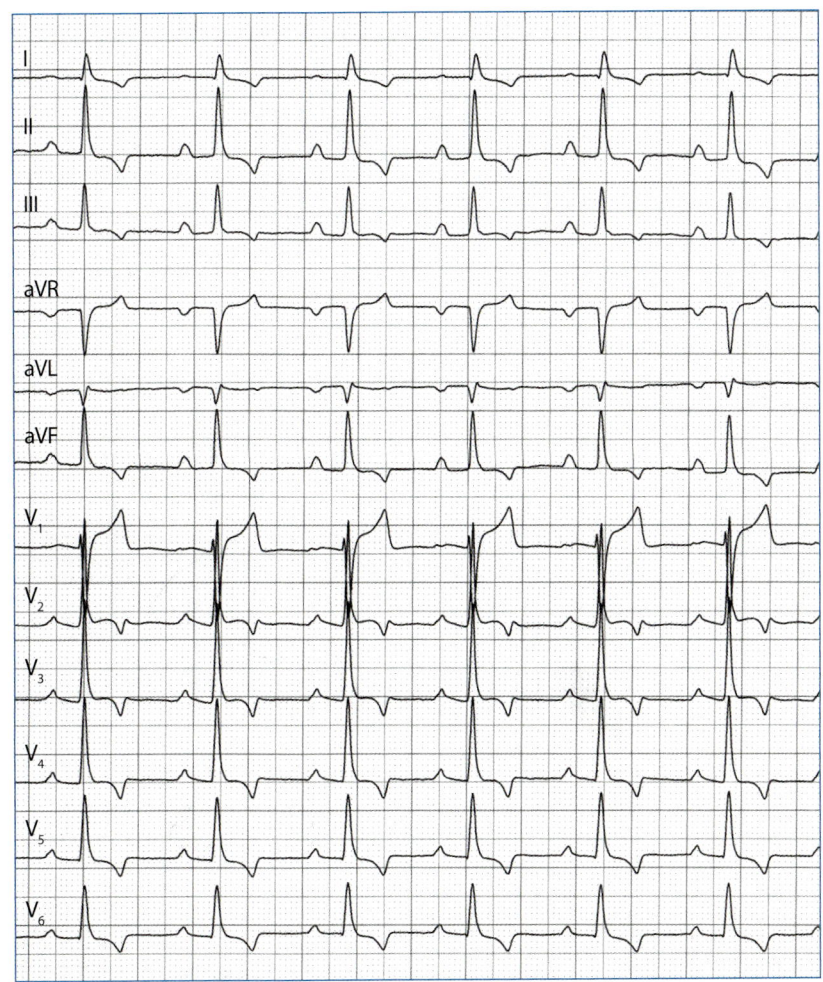

B) Cat, Domestic Shorthair, male, 6 years. Limbs leads (I, II, III, aVR, aVL, aVF) - speed 50 mm/s - calibration 10 mm/1 mV.

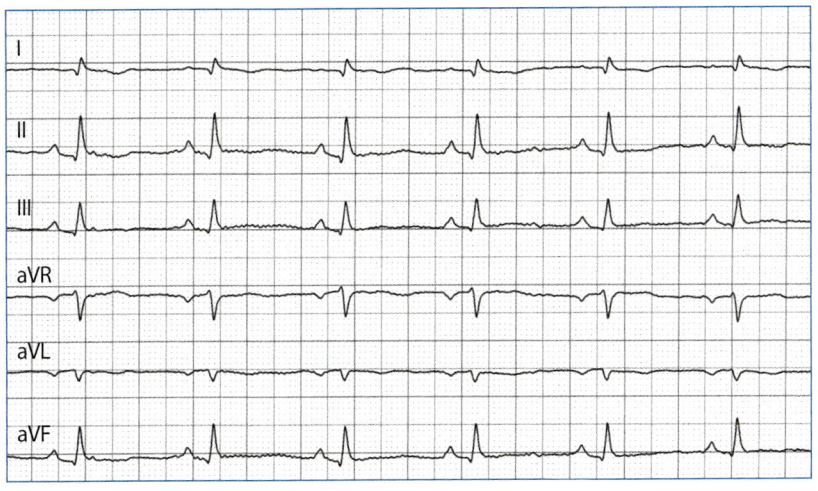

The wandering pacemaker corresponds to variations of the voltage (amplitude) and the polarity of P waves also in relation to respiratory phases. Respiratory sinus arrhythmia has been documented on 24-hour Holter recordings from cats kept in a familiar environment.

Analysis of deflections and measurement of intervals

The duration and amplitude of the electrocardiographic waveforms and the duration of the various intervals should be measured in lead II. In order to determine the duration of the waveforms and intervals in milliseconds, the measurement obtained in millimeters on the horizontal axis of the calibrated paper is multiplied by 20 if the recording speed is 50 mm/s and by 40 if the speed is 25 mm/s. As for the voltage (or amplitude), it is measured from the baseline to the peak (or nadir) of the wave. Whenever a standard calibration of 10 mm/1 mV is used, the voltage (or amplitude) in millivolts is obtained by multiplying the measurement by 0.1. If the calibration is halved (5 mm/1 mV) or doubled (20 mm/1 mV), the amplitude in millivolts is obtained by multiplying the measurement by 0.2 and 0.05, respectively (Fig. 3.16).

The P wave

The *P wave* represents the sequential depolarization of the right atrium and the left atrium and is identified in lead II as a positive deflection during sinus rhythm. It begins where the wave separates from the isoelectric line and ends at the point where the tracing returns back to the isoelectric line. The duration of the P wave is measured from its earliest point of departure from the baseline to its last point of intersection with the isoelectric line. If the older thermal paper analog electrocardiograph is used the thick line should be excluded from the measurement. The amplitude of the P wave is measured from the isoelectric line to its peak (Fig. 3.6). The normal P wave amplitude is less than 0.4 mV in dogs and less than 0.2 mV in cats. The normal P wave duration is less than 40 ms in dogs (less than 50 ms in the giant dog breeds) and less than 35 ms in cats. Usually, the polarity of the P wave should not change in any leads (Table 3.1).

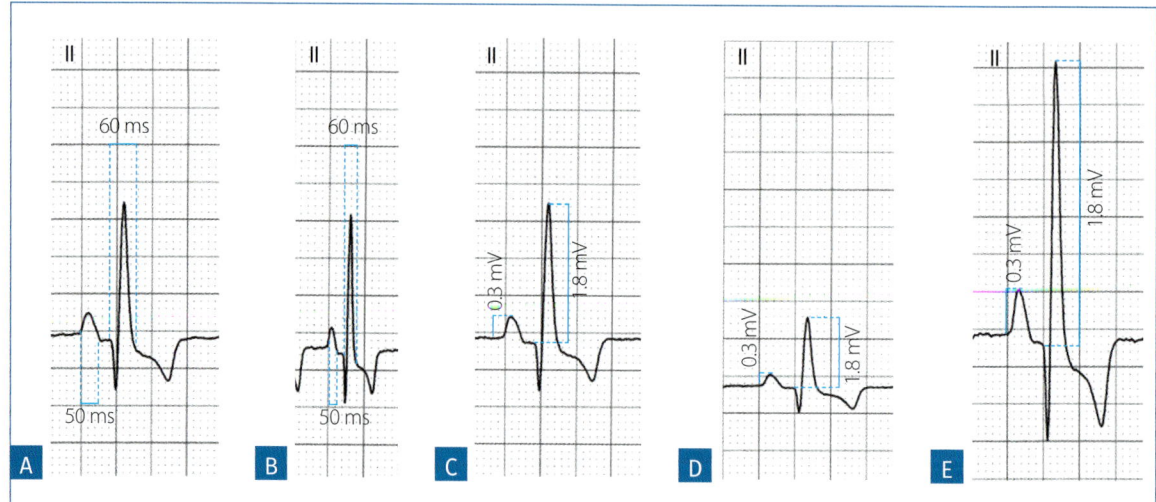

Figure 3.16. Measurement of electrocardiographic waves. The first requisite to measure the duration and amplitude of the electrocardiographic waves and intervals accurately is to know the paper calibration settings. At a speed of 50 mm/s (A) every millimeter on the horizontal axis of the graph paper corresponds to 20 ms, and at a speed of 25 mm/s (B) each corresponds to 40 ms. The duration of the waves and of the intervals is calculated by multiplying the measured number of millimeters on the horizontal axis by 20 (speed at 50 mm/s) or 40 (speed at 25 mm/s) to obtain the value in milliseconds.
With the standard calibration (10 mm/1 mV) (C), every millimeter on the vertical axis of the graph paper corresponds to 0.1 mV; with a 5 mm/1 mV amplitude setting, (D) every millimeter corresponds to 0.2 mV; with a 20 mm/1 mV amplitude setting, (E) each millimeter corresponds to 0.05 mV. The amplitude of the electrocardiographic waves is determined by multiplying the number of millimeters measured on the vertical axis by 0.1, 0.2 or 0.05 depending on the calibration selected to obtain a value in millivolts.

Variations are often observed in healthy dogs, including the wandering pacemaker, bifid P waves, and P waves with an amplitude greater than 0.4 mV in leads II and aVF, particularly in the presence of high sympathetic tone. Consequently, the obvious question is which P wave should be measured? One possible approach is to assess the amplitude and duration of the largest P wave to ensure that it is within the normal limits. The P wave in the cat is much more consistent in size and morphology.

P wave morphology, amplitude and duration may vary with right atrial, left atrial or biatrial enlargement, with inter or intra-atrial conduction delays or blocks, and in the presence of supraventricular ectopic beats or rhythms.

The T_a wave

The T_a wave is the electrocardiographic representation of atrial repolarization; it is a dome-shaped deflection with negative polarity in leads II, III, aVF and positive polarity in leads aVR, aVL, CV_5RL and V_1 during normal sinus rhythm. The T_a wave directly follows the P wave without interposition of an isoelectric line. It is typically hidden within the QRS complex, and in some circumstances can extend after the J point. The amplitude of the T_a wave is calculated from the isoelectric line to its nadir, while its duration is measured from the end of the P wave to the point where the wave's ascending branch intersects the isoelectric line. The mean value of the T_a amplitude in lead II in dogs is 0.09 mV, while its mean duration is 140 ms. The ratio between T_a and P wave amplitude is about 0.35 (range between 0.08 and 0.62); while the ratio between T_a wave duration and P wave duration is about 2.99 (range between 2.18 and 3.8). The P-T_a interval, which is measured from the beginning of the P wave to the end of T_a wave, varies from 149 ms to 227 ms with an average duration of 188 ms (Table 3.1).

The PQ interval and PQ segment

In the medical literature this interval is often called the PR interval. The *PQ interval* represents the time it takes for the electric impulse generated by the sinus node to activate the atrial tissue, travel through the atrioventricular and intraventricular conduction systems, and initiate ventricular depolarization. The depolarization of the atrioventricular node starts approximately in the middle of the ascending branch of the P wave and, consequently, the P wave duration does not affect the duration of the PQ interval. The PQ interval is constituted by the P wave and the isoelectric line that separates the P wave from the QRS complex (*PQ segment*). The PQ interval is measured from the beginning of the P wave to the first deflection of the QRS complex and, since the ventricular depolarization most commonly begins with a Q wave in lead II, this time interval is strictly referred as PQ (Fig. 3.6). Moreover, when this interval is measured in other leads or if the dog or cat does not have a Q wave either because of normal variation due to the position of the heart in the thorax or enlargement or conduction disorders, the term PR interval is used.

The normal PQ interval duration varies from 60 to 130 ms in the dog and from 50 to 90 ms in the cat. It is important to note that the duration of this interval changes with heart rate, increasing with a slower ventricular rate and decreasing with a faster rate. Under physiological conditions, and especially in brachycephalic breeds of dogs, the PQ interval can occasionally be longer than 150 ms (Table 3.1).

In disease states, such as the presence of atrioventricular accessory pathways, electrical stimulation can reach the ventricular myocardium directly, avoiding the normal atrioventricular conduction delay and it is therefore possible to find a PQ interval shorter than 60 ms in dogs and 50 ms in cats. These findings are characteristic of ventricular pre-excitation (see p. 154). Other PQ interval abnormalities include atrioventricular conduction delays, represented by a prolonged PQ interval, and variable PQ interval duration in the presence of ectopic rhythms with atrioventricular dissociation or advanced atrioventricular conduction disturbances.

The *PQ segment*, measured from the end of the P wave to the onset of the QRS complex, is often isoelectric, and therefore lies on the same level as the baseline, which is the line between two consecutive TP segments. A PQ segment deflection below the isoelectric line may reflect the presence of a T_a wave that exists either as a normal variation or because of right atrial enlargement, disturbances of atrial repolarization, atrial infarction or ischemia and pericarditis. In some supraventricular tachycardias that have a negative P wave the PQ segment may actually be elevated due the presence of a positive T_a wave.

TABLE 3.1. Reference range of electrocardiographic measurements in awake dogs and cats. These values apply to animals placed in right lateral recumbency and for measurements made in lead II unless specified otherwise. The table also includes information on normal cardiac rhythms in these species, the mean electrical axis of the P wave, QRS complex and T wave, the most common axis deviations, and ST segment changes.

Electrocardiographic parameter	Dog	Cat
Heart rate	Adult: 60-170 bpm Puppies: 60-220 bpm	140-220 bpm
Normal cardiac rhythms in a clinical setting	Sinus rhythm Respiratory sinus arrhythmia Wandering pacemaker	Sinus rhythm
P wave Amplitude Duration Mean electrical axis in the frontal plane	 <0.4 mV <40 ms (<50 ms in giant breeds) From –18 ° to +90 °	 <0.2 mV <35 ms From 0 ° to + 90 °
T_a wave Amplitude Duration P-T_a interval	 0.06 mV T_a amplitude/P amplitude 0.35 140 ms T_a duration/ P duration 2.99 149 - 227 ms	
PQ interval	60-130 ms	50-90 ms
QRS complex R wave amplitude Duration Mean electrical axis in the frontal plane Right axis deviation Left axial deviation	 >0.5 mV in II, III and aVF <3 mV CV_5RL and V_{10} <5 mV CV_6LL and CV_6LU R/S >0.5 in CV_5RL >0.9 CV_6LL and CV_6LU V_1 <0.5 mV V_2-V_6 >1 mV R / S <1 in V_1 <70 ms From +40 ° to +100 ° From +100 ° to –80 ° clockwise From +40 ° to –60 ° counter-clockwise	 <0.9 mV <40 ms From 0 ° to +160 ° From +160 ° to –0 ° clockwise From 0 ° to –60 ° counter-clockwise
J wave ST segment	0.19 (0.10-0.50) ms in lead II Normal: isoelectric Segment elevation and depression >±0.20 mV in the limb leads >±0.25 mV in the precordial leads	 Normal: isoelectric
QT interval	150-240 ms	160-220 ms
T wave Amplitude Polarity Mean electrical axis in the frontal plane	 <±0.05 to 1 mV in all leads Variable in all leads except CV_5RL, and V_1 (positive) and V_{10} (negative). From –45 ° to –147 °	 From ±0.03 mV Variable
U wave Amplitude Duration Polarity T-U interval	 Absent or <0.05 mV 70-90 ms Concordant with T wave 40 ms	

The QRS complex

The QRS complex is the graphical representation of ventricular depolarization and can be divided into several components, which are named according to their amplitude, position within the ventriculogram and polarity. The onset of the QRS complex coincides with the first electrocardiographic deflection that interrupts the PQ segment. The first positive deflection of the complex is called R wave and a second positive deflection is a R' wave. The negative electrocardiographic waves of the QRS complex are named Q waves if they precede the R wave, and S waves if they follow the R wave. The ventriculogram is named QS if it is made of a single negative wave. The end of the QRS complex can be difficult to identify and, by convention, it corresponds to the point where the last deflection of the ventriculogram intersects the isoelectric line. This point is also called the *J point* or *ST junction* (Fig. 3.6).

The time interval between the beginning of the QRS wave and the beginning of its descending branch is called R-peak time or *intrinsicoid deflection* (Fig. 3.17). In humans this parameter is commonly measured in the precordial leads. This interval corresponds to ventricular depolarization from the endocardium to epicardium. An increase in the duration of the R-peak time may be secondary to an increase of ventricular wall thickness or reflect an intraventricular conduction delay. Additionally, the duration of the intrinsicoid deflection may be of value in the evaluation of concentric versus eccentric hypertrophy of the right versus the left ventricle. The specific lead used for this measurement reflects these abnormalities. Subjectively veterinary clinicians have noted a change in the shape of the QRS complex in cardiomyopathies in both the dog and cat. This parameter might become useful once normal values in dogs and cats are established.

The duration of the QRS complex is calculated from the beginning of the Q wave to the end of the S wave. If the S wave is absent, the measurement is made from the beginning of Q wave to the end of R wave; when the Q wave is absent, the measurement is made from the beginning of the R wave to the end of the S wave; if both the Q and S waves are absent, the measurement is made from the onset to the end of the R wave.

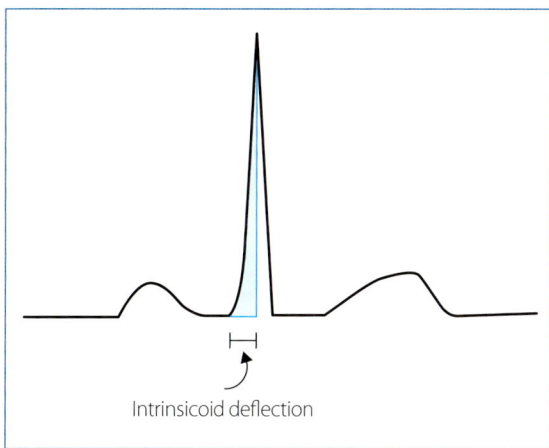

Figure 3.17. R-peak time or intrinsicoid deflection. The intrinsicoid deflection is defined as the slope of the ascending part of the R wave, and its duration is measured as the time interval between the beginning of the QRS wave and the peak or beginning of the descending branch of the R wave.

The amplitude of the components of the QRS complex is measured from the isoelectric line to their peak voltage (positive or negative) (Fig. 3.6).

By convention, the letters (Q, R and S) used to describe the various deflections of the QRS complex should be capitalized (Q, R, S) if their amplitude is greater than 0.5 mV; a lower case letter (q, r, s) is used when their amplitude is less 0.5 mV. The typical morphologies of the QRS complex in the limb leads and precordial lead systems are listed in Table 3.2 (Fig. 3.18).

In dogs, the QRS complex must last less than 70 ms and have an R wave amplitude less than 3 mV in CV_5RL and V_{10}, less than 5 mV in leads CV_6LL and CV_6LU and larger than 0.5 mV in the inferior leads (II, III, and aVF). The ratio between R wave and S wave amplitudes (R/S) must be greater than 0.5 in CV_5RL and greater than 0.9 in CV_6LL and CV_6LU. The R wave should be less than 0.5 mV in lead V_1 and greater than 1 mV in leads V_2, V_3, V_4, V_5 and V_6. The ratio between R wave and S wave amplitude (R/S) in V_1 must be less than 1. In lead I the QRS complex should not show an rs, rS, Rs or RS morphology. In cats, the QRS complex must last less than 40 ms and have an amplitude less than 0.9 mV in lead II (Table 3.1).

TABLE 3.2. Electrocardiographic appearance of the QRS complex in the limb leads and precordial leads in the dog. Reported morphologies are listed in order of frequency.

Lead	QRS complex morphology
I	QR, qR, qRS
II	qR, qRS, Rs, QrS
III	qRs, qR, Rs, rS
aVR	rS, rSr', qRs
aVL	Qr, QR, qRs
aVF	qR, Rs, QrS
CV_5RL or rV_2	RS, Rs
CV_6LL or V_2	Rs, qRs, qR
CV_6LU or V_4	Rs, qRs, qR
V_{10}	Qr, rS, qR, QR
V_1	RS, rS
From V_2 to V_6	qR, qRs, Rs

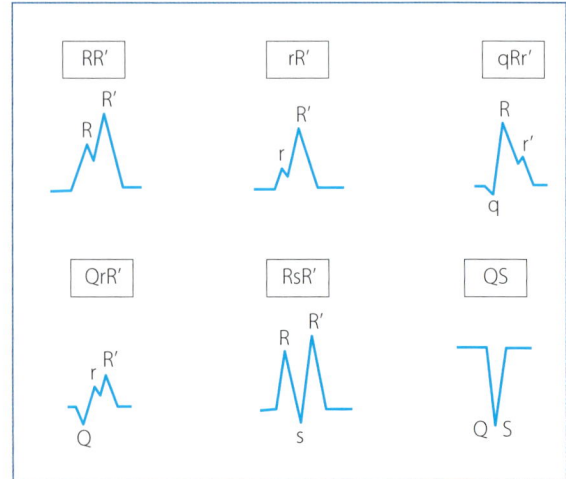

Figure 3.18. Electrocardiographic terminology of the deflections forming the QRS complex. The first positive deflection is called an R wave and any subsequent positive wave is a R' wave. Negative electrocardiographic waves are called Q waves if they precede the R wave, and S waves if they follow the R wave. If there is only one negative wave, the ventriculogram is called QS. Deflections are identified by capital letters (Q, R, S) if they have an amplitude greater than 0.5 mV, and lowercase letters (q, r, s) if they have an amplitude of less than 0.5 mV.

A QR morphology of the QRS complex in lead I can be attributed to a counterclockwise rotation of the vector of ventricular activation. Other deviations of the orientation of the ventricular vector may be present secondary to changes in the animal's position while recording the electrocardiogram (see p. 62). A physiological variant of the morphology of the QRS complex, called "butterfly", is characterized by the presence of a small R wave (qrS and QrS) or by a W shape in which the R wave does not reach the isoelectric line in the inferior leads (II, III, and aVF). Deep Q waves and prominent R waves are usually present in lead I. The R wave can also display a notch on its descending branch at its point of intersection with the isoelectric line. The QRS complex in aVL is usually positive and not altered in the precordial leads. The presence of notches on the descending branch of the R wave, a QRS complex with a Rr' type morphology in leads II, III, aVF, and a Rs or rS type morphology in CV_5RL can be considered normal variants.

The amplitude and the duration of the QRS complex may increase with ventricular enlargement or intraventricular conduction disorders. The amplitude of the QRS complex may decrease in the presence of a pleural effusion, pneumothorax, pericardial effusion or because of the interposition of fat between the heart (dipole) and the surface electrodes (exploring electrodes); this is known as a *damping effect*. The maximum damping effect occurs when this distance is greater than 10 cm and, consequently, the signal attenuation is more visible in the limb lead recordings and less in the precordial leads. The reduction of the voltage of the QRS complex may also be secondary to areas of decreased myocardial tissue that may result, for example, from fibrous tissue which is electrically silent.

The J wave

J waves reflect the early repolarization of the ventricles during phase 1 of the action potential. The exact electrophysiologic mechanism underlying the formation of J waves is not completely understood, although it is generally attributed to a transient repolarization gradient between ventricular endocardium and epicardium, specifically because the transient outward current (I_{to}) is more pronounced in the epicardial myocytes.

J waves are common and considered a normal feature of the dog's QRS complex. One study reported that it is present in more than 90 % of Petit Griffon Vendéen dogs, and in other breeds, it would be identified on at least 40 % of electrocardiographic tracings (Fig. 1.9).

J waves appear as a positive hump on the descending branch of the QRS complex at the R-ST junction (J point). They are usually more pronounced in the inferior leads (II, III and aVF). It is important to note that excessive filtering during recording of the electrocardiogram to remove motion artifacts can also eliminate this small amplitude wave (reported to have a mean amplitude of 0.19 mV with a range of 0.10 to 0.50 mV in veterinary studies). A high-pass filter set a 0.05 Hz and a low-pass filter set at 150 Hz are, therefore, recommended to better detect J waves.

Large amplitude J waves are occasionally seen during hypercalcemia, hypothermia (Osborn wave), and brain injury (see p. 301).

The ST segment

The *ST segment* is included between the end of the QRS complex and the beginning of the T wave (Fig. 3.6). It correlates with phase 2 (or plateau) of the action potential and corresponds to ventricular systole. During this time, the membrane potential of all ventricular myocytes is equal, and therefore no difference in potential is recorded by the surface electrocardiogram, which displays a horizontal segment on the isoelectric line. The point at which the QRS complex ends is identified as the *J point*. It is the intersection of the descending branch of the R wave, or the ascending branch of the S wave when present, and the isoelectric line. In many cases it is difficult to measure the ST segment precisely because the J point and the onset of the T wave cannot be clearly identified.

Deviation of the ST segment describes the displacement of the entire segment above (elevation of the ST segment) or below (depression of the ST segment) the isoelectric line by more than 0.20 mV in the limb leads and more than 0.25 mV in the precordial leads. The degree of ST-segment deviation must be measured at a specific point, which is typically 40 ms after the J point (Table 3.1). It reflects repolarization heterogeneity (heterogeneity of action potential duration and amplitude) within the ventricular myocardium. Deviation of the ST

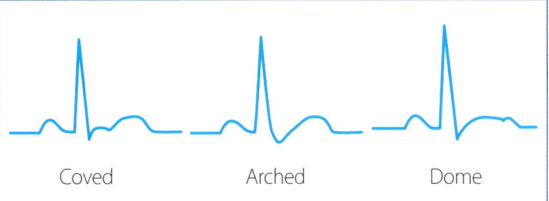

Figure 3.19. ST segment morphology changes commonly found in dogs. A deviation of the ST segment is described as coved when it has a convex shape, arched when it has a lower concavity and dome-shaped when the ST segment and ascending branch of the T wave are fused to form a rounded arc.

segment not only includes obvious elevation and depression, but also a variety of shape alterations described as slurring, coving, arching, and dome-shaped (Fig. 3.19).

In dogs, ST segment or J point deviations are frequently identified, and usually more apparent in leads II, aVF, CV_6LL and CV_6LU. These ST segment alterations are evident in serial tracings, but they can vary or disappear, and have no clinical significance. The degree of ST segment deviation can follow a pattern as it varies over time in relation to changes in R-R intervals, typically during respiratory sinus arrhythmia. In this case, the degree of deviation decreases when the P-QRS-T complex is preceded by a long R-R interval.

Clinically, the most relevant observation in dogs and cats is the presence of ST segment slurring. Slurring of the ST segment is seen with left ventricular enlargement, left bundle branch blocks or tachycardias. This type of appearance is also characteristic of ventricular rhythms. With marked right ventricular enlargement or right bundle branch blocks the ST segment slurs upward towards the T wave. The identification of changes in the ST segment can have very important clinical implications. In the monitoring of the electrocardiogram during anesthetic procedures changes in the ST segment and T wave may indicate critical problems with oxygenation of the myocardium. Therefore, ST segment elevation or depression may be an initial finding or may be recognized as a change that demands immediate assessment to correct the underlying problem (i.e. lack of adequate oxygen flow).

In addition to low oxygen levels, several other conditions can affect the ST segment. A T_a wave (atrial repolarization) that extends beyond the QRS complex can mimic ST segment deviation; a method to distinguish the T_a wave from an ST segment alteration consists in predicting where the T_a wave should end by measuring three times the P wave duration starting from the end of the P wave. An ST segment deviation would extend beyond this point. The presence of a retrograde P' wave during a supraventricular tachycardia can also give the appearance of ST segment deviation.

Limited attention has been given to the study of the ST segment in veterinary medicine because of the low incidence of myocardial infarction and coronary heart disease in domestic species. This contrasts with human cardiology in which the accurate identification of signs of ischemia on the electrocardiogram is critical. Factors that influence the electrocardiographic changes during ischemia include its duration, extent, location and the presence of other conduction abnormalities. Depending on whether the ischemic zone is subendocardial, transmural or subepicardial, ST segment elevation or depression can be observed. In humans, a distinction is made between persistent ST segment elevation in the inferior leads (II, III and aVF) or left precordial leads (V_1-V_6), which indicates myocardial infarction, and transient ST elevation, which is consistent with coronary vasospasm. During the evaluation of the patient with ST segment abnormalities, other conditions that can affect the ST segment must be taken into account, including acute pericarditis, myocarditis, electrical cardioversion (ST segment elevation that resolves within 1 to 2 minutes), hyperkalemia and pulmonary embolism. ST segment depression in inferior leads (II, III and aVF) or left precordial leads (V_1-V_6) can be found in acute coronary syndromes with ischemia and no infarction, reciprocal ST changes (ST segment elevation in some leads and depression in the electrically opposite leads that are distant from the infarct site), intraventricular conduction delays, left ventricular hypertrophy and during digoxin use. The ST segment alteration with digoxin therapy or toxicity ("digitalis effect") is frequently described as a "coving" (or "scooped") depression of the ST segment or dome-shaped ST segment depending on the electrocardiographic lead.

The T wave

The T wave is the electrocardiographic representation of the final phase of ventricular repolarization and follows the ST segment (Fig. 3.6). The amplitude of the T wave is measured from the isoelectric line to the peak of the wave.

The morphology, polarity and amplitude of the T wave should be evaluated. Typically, the T wave has asymmetrical branches, with the ascending branch having a more gradual slope than the descending branch. The T wave can be positive, negative or diphasic and its polarity should not reverse in any leads. The presence of flat T waves is not abnormal, especially if found in leads I, aVR, aVL and V_{10}. The descending branch should not be notched. When the T wave has the same polarity as the predominant direction of the QRS complex, it is described as concordant; if its polarity is opposite to that of the QRS complex, it is called *discordant*. Under normal conditions, in the dog, the T wave amplitude does not exceed 0.05 to 1 mV in all leads, and it should be less than 0.3 mV in cats (Table 3.1).

Alterations of the T wave morphology are usually non-specific and difficult to interpret. One exception is the electrocardiographic changes that occur with hyperkalemia, characterized by T waves with symmetrical branches, usually when potassium concentration is greater than 6 mEq/L. In addition, whenever depolarization is associated with ventricular ectopic beats, bundle branch block or ventricular enlargement, repolarization is also altered, which is reflected by changes in the ST segment and T wave.

The U wave

The U wave can be detected in the inferior leads (II, III, and aVF) as a positive deflection, which is within the TP segment approximately 40 ms after the end of the T wave (Fig. 3.6). It is thought that it corresponds to the repolarization of the M cells, which have longer action potentials than the epicardial and endocardial cells.

It is possible to find U waves in the presence of systemic hypertension, anemia, myocardial ischemia and electrolyte disorders (hypokalemia, hypomagnesemia) and during the administration of drugs that prolong the QT interval.

The QT interval

The QT interval corresponds to the duration of the ventricular monophasic action potential and encompasses the phases of depolarization and repolarization of the ventricular myocardium; for this reason, this interval is also called *electrical systole*. The QT interval is measured from the beginning of the QRS complex to the end of the T wave (Fig. 3.6). The intersection of the descending branch of the T wave and the isoelectric line is often difficult to identify; therefore, the QT interval is best defined if it is evaluated from the 12 leads recorded at a speed of 50 mm/s. In dogs, the end of the T wave is usually more visible in leads aVF, V_1 and V_3. Whenever a U wave is present, it should not be included in the calculation of the QT interval.

The duration of the QT interval varies with heart rate: the slower the heart rate, the longer the QT interval. As a general rule, if the animal is not tachycardic, the QT interval should not be longer than 50 % the duration of the previous R-R interval. Because of changes in the QT interval duration, methods have been developed to determine a *corrected QT* interval (QTc), which is a correction of the QT interval duration based on the previous R-R interval or the average heart rate depending on the formula used. Most of the formulas developed were done so from studies in humans and then applied to dogs. In toxicological research identification of drugs that cause QT prolongation is important because the intake of some drugs is associated with prolonged repolarization, torsade de pointes and sudden death. Because of the necessity to standardize comparisons of the QT interval before and after treatment which may also affect heart rate, various formulas have been used in the studies of dogs and cats. Each of these formulas is flawed because of under- or over-correction: Bazett's formula (QTc = QT/RR$^{1/2}$), Fridericia's formula (QTc = QT/RR$^{1/3}$), Van der Water's formula (QTc = QT − 0.087 [(60/HR) − 1]) and the logarithmic formula (QTc = 600 × log QT/RR log). Extensive research in recent years by Fossa has highlighted the inaccuracy of these formulas.

Publications by Fossa have demonstrated that a more accurate means of assessing the risk of prolonged repolarization, particularly in the dog, is to assess QT/TQ restitution. This assessment gives insight into the ability of the heart to recover from one beat to the next by examining the relationship between the QT interval and the TQ interval. That is, the action potential duration and the diastolic interval, respectively. The restitution on a beat-to-beat basis is measured from the QT interval and the TQ interval as a ratio. Ideally, this relationship is calculated over many beats and may be particularly used in 24-hour Holter monitoring. When the QT/TQ ratio increases, the arrhythmic risk increases. If the QT interval which is reflecting the action potential duration prolongs with tachycardia, the ability of the heart to recover, that is the restitution, decreases. This increases the vulnerability to reentrant arrhythmias. When this parameter is used in the analysis of 24-hour cardiac recordings the number of beats with a QT/TQ greater than one is calculated to give an appreciation of the amount of time whereby restitution may be such to increase the risk of arrhythmias. In the dog sinus arrhythmia is prominent so the QT/TQ is constantly changing. The dog may have a relatively high repolarization reserve. Although the QT interval changes with the previous R-R interval in the dog, the changes are minimal on a beat-to-beat basis.

In dogs, the QT interval should have a duration between 150 and 240 ms. In cats, equations have been developed to predict the QT interval duration as a function of heart rate using the following formula (Ware, et al., 1999):

$$\text{QT interval duration} = 0.41845798 - (0.00181963 \times HR) + (0.00000313 \times HR^2)$$

The QT interval of healthy cats with a heart rate between 160 and 240 bpm has a duration of 160 to 220 ms (Table 3.1).

Through the analysis of QT interval duration in the 12 leads it is also possible to determine the homogeneity of myocardial repolarization in the different segments of the ventricles. *Dispersion of ventricular repolarization* has been noted when neighboring areas are in different states of repolarization and can be estimated by calculating *QT interval dispersion*. It is determined by subtracting the shortest QT interval from the longest QT interval recorded in the 12-lead electrocardiogram. In humans, dispersion of repolarization estimated by QT interval dispersion should be less than 60 ms. Normal values for QT interval dispersion have not been determined in dogs and cats.

Electrical alternans

The presence of beat-to-beat changes in the amplitude of the P wave, the QRS complex, the T wave and the magnitude of the PQ and ST segment deviation should be considered. This phenomenon is known as *electrical alternans*, and can be divided into three categories:
- *repolarization alternans* (ST and T),
- *conduction alternans* (P, PQ and QRS), and
- *alternans due to cardiac movements*.

Only the first two types represent true electrical alternans, while the third is present with pericardial effusion and is an artifact caused by the oscillating movements of the heart within the pericardial sac (see p. 297).

The alternation of repolarization which includes T wave and ST segment alternans is caused by the dispersion of repolarization of the Purkinje fibers and ventricular myocardium. T wave alternans is usually due to sudden changes in heart rate or prolongation of the QT interval. The study of beat-to-beat amplitude and polarity variations of the T wave, whether macroscopic or in the order of microvolts (*micro T wave alternans*), might have some value in predicting the presence of dispersion of repolarization and the risk of the onset of ventricular tachycardias (torsade de pointes). T wave electrical alternans may be secondary to electrolyte disorders (hypocalcemia, hypokalemia, hypomagnesemia), administration of quinidine or amiodarone, hypertrophic cardiomyopathy, congestive heart failure, acute pulmonary thromboembolism and long QT syndrome.

ST segment electrical alternans describes the alternation of different levels of ST segment elevation or depression during myocardial ischemia.

Conduction alternans, also known as depolarization alternans, appears on the electrocardiogram as a beat-to-beat alternation of a depolarization waveform duration or amplitude. It can result from fluctuations of impulse propagation velocity, conduction pathways or tissue excitability. The most frequently recognized form of conduction alternans is QRS complex electrical alternans (beat-to-beat variation of R wave amplitude greater than 0.1 mV in at least one of the 12 leads) during rapid tachycardias, including atrial fibrillation, orthodromic atrioventricular reciprocating tachycardia and focal and macro-reentrant atrial tachycardias. QRS complex electrical alternans is also possible during myocardial ischemia, left ventricular dysfunction and acute pulmonary embolism.

Other factors that may cause R wave amplitude variations include changes in heart volume (Brody effect), the degree of cardiac contractility and changes of the cardiac electrical axis.

Mean electrical axis

The direction and amplitude of the atrial and ventricular depolarization waves continuously change over time and therefore the number of required activation vectors to describe this process is endless. Software developments that permit three-dimensional visualization of the depolarization wave through the Purkinje system and ventricular myocardium is a better way to understand the complete depolarization of the ventricles. Similarly such representation by software models may enable better understanding of atrial depolarization. Historically the variations in time of the activation vector have been represented by a closed line joining the tip of all the vectors that represent the propagation of the electrical impulse and have their origin at the center of the hexaxial reference system. This representation is known as a *vectorcardiogram*. The vectorcardiogram is the vector loop in the two-dimensional frontal plane and indicates the magnitude and the direction of the instantaneous electrical cardiac vector, which is the sum of the dipole vectors located along the instantaneous depolarization wavefront. The largest diameter of the loop corresponds to the *mean electrical axis* on the frontal plane (Fig. 3.20).

The mean electrical axis constitutes, therefore, the overall direction of the excitation wave during the depolarization of the myocardium and is the resultant of the multitude of instantaneous vectors present during the different phases of the cardiac cycle. The orientation of the electrical axis in the frontal plane is defined by the angle of intersection between the mean vector and the horizontal line that corresponds to lead I. On the electrocardiogram a depolarization vector approaching the positive pole of the exploring electrode is represented as a positive waveform (above the baseline), while a vector of depolarization moving away is represented as a negative wave. A waveform is considered positive if the algebraic sum of its components above and below the baseline is positive and, in the same way, it is considered negative if the algebraic sum of the deflections is negative. It is defined as isodiphasic when the algebraic sum of its components is equal to zero.

The mean electrical axis can be calculated in the different anatomical planes (frontal, sagittal and horizontal) for atrial depolarization (P wave), ventricular depolarization (QRS complex) and for ventricular repolarization (T wave). In clinical practice, the electrical axis is determined only in the frontal plane, most frequently for the P wave and QRS complex.

To calculate the mean electrical axis in the frontal plane, Bailey's hexaxial system is used, with the heart placed at its center. Bailey's hexaxial system is the combination of the triaxial bipolar limb lead system and the triaxial unipolar limb lead system. The hexaxial system includes, therefore, all the electrocardiographic limb leads, and each lead divides the circle into a positive half and a negative half. The axes of each lead are identified by successive increments of 30 ° starting from 0 ° up to +180 ° and from 0 ° to –180 °. The six leads are marked with a "+" sign to identify the positive exploring electrode, and with a "–" sign to identify the opposite direction. Leads I, II, III and aVF have their positive electrode in the lower (inferior) hemisphere with positive angles (0 °, +60 °, +90° and +120 °); leads aVL and aVR have their positive exploring electrode in the upper (superior) hemisphere with negative angles (–150 ° and –30 °) (Fig. 3.21).

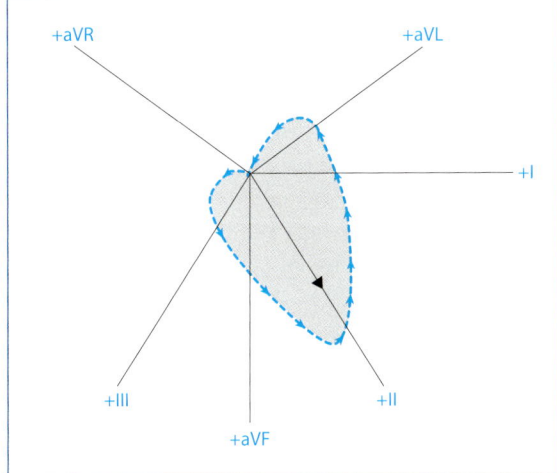

Figure 3.20. Vector loop of ventricular depolarization in the frontal plane. The vector loop is a graphical representation of changes in the intensity and direction of the depolarization vectors. The major vector loop diameter represents the mean electrical axis of the QRS complex in the frontal plane (arrow).

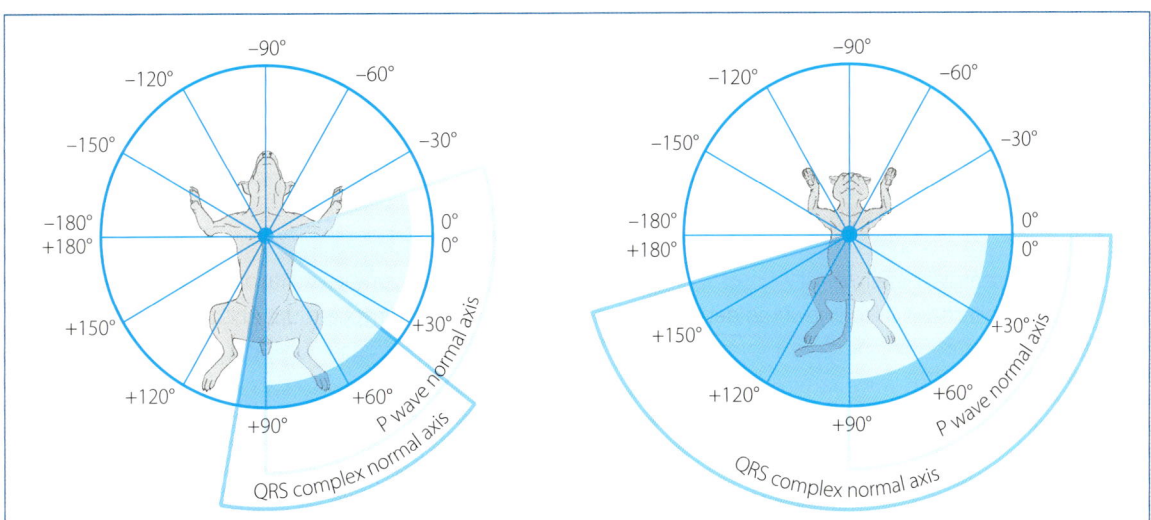

Figure 3.21. Mean cardiac electrical axis of the P wave and the QRS complex in the frontal plane. The normal values for the mean electrical axis of the P wave in the frontal plane vary between –18 ° and +90 ° in the dog and 0 ° and +90 ° in the cat. Normal values for the mean electrical axis of the QRS complex are between +40 ° and +100 ° in the dog and between 0 ° and +160 ° in the cat. A right axis shift corresponds to a clockwise rotation of the electrical axis with values between +100 ° and –80 ° in the dog and between +160 ° and –80 ° in the cat. A left axis shift is a counterclockwise rotation of the electrical axis with values between +40 ° and –60 ° in the dog and 0 ° and –60 ° in the cat.

The heart in dogs and cats is oriented in the frontal plane with the left apical region at the level of the positive pole of lead II, while the free wall of the right ventricle faces the positive pole of leads III or aVR depending on chest conformation. Due to the posterior position of the left ventricle, unlike humans, the positive poles of the lateral leads I and aVL fail to fully explore the free wall of the left ventricle. In the frontal plane, the right atrium and the left atrium are oriented toward the positive pole of aVR and the positive pole of aVL, respectively.

Determination of the mean electric axis of the QRS complex in the frontal plane

The mean electric axis of the QRS complex represents the average direction of the simultaneous depolarization of the right ventricle and the left ventricle. Since the left ventricle is the largest myocardial mass to be depolarized, the mean electrical axis of the QRS complex is oriented toward the positive pole of lead II assuming a right-to-left and the superior-to-inferior direction. It is important to realize that the mean axis is not only related to the mass that is being depolarized but also to the timing of the myocardial depolarization. If there is delay in one part of the heart during depolarization, when this region is depolarized, it will have no opposing vectors. In the absence of opposing vectors to cancel the forces a vector directed towards the delayed region will be appreciated on the electrocardiogram.

There are several ways to calculate the mean electrical axis of the QRS complex in the frontal plane. One method, which provides a rapid determination of the electrical axis, is based on the recognition of the lead of the six-lead system with the highest net positive or negative deflection. To obtain the value of the net deflection, it is necessary to measure the height in millimeters of the positive deflection (R wave) and subtract the negative deflections (Q wave and S wave), also in millimeters. If the number (*net deflection*) is positive, the axis is oriented towards the positive pole of the considered lead; if it is negative, the axis is directed towards the negative pole of the examined lead. With this method, the axis is determined with a precision of ± 30 °, which is usually acceptable in clinical practice (Fig. 3.22A).

A second method consists in evaluating the orientation of the cardiac vector from leads I and aVF. These two orthogonal leads divide the Bailey system into four quadrants: the first quadrant is between 0 ° and +90 °, the second quadrant between +90 ° and +180 °, the third quadrant between +180 ° and –90 °, and the fourth quadrant between –90 ° and 0 °. If the QRS complex has a net positive deflection in lead I, the mean electrical axis is directed towards the left; therefore the axis is included in the first or fourth quadrant; if it is also positive in the aVF lead, the mean electrical axis is within the first quadrant; if it is negative in aVF, the electrical axis is within the fourth quadrant. If the QRS complex is negative in I and aVF, the mean electrical axis is within the third quadrant. Finally if the QRS is negative in lead I and positive in aVF, the electrical axis is within the second quadrant (Fig. 3.22A).

A third method involves the identification of the most isodiphasic lead, which has a net deflection equal or close to zero. The lead perpendicular to the isodiphasic lead represents the orientation of the mean electrical axis. If the QRS complex is mostly positive in this lead, the mean electrical axis is directed towards the positive pole of the lead. Alternatively, if the QRS is negative, the mean electrical axis is directed towards the negative pole. This method also has a precision of ±30 °.

In order to increase the accuracy of the last method, one can closely examine the isodiphasic (or isoelectric) lead, and determine if the summation of the positive and negative components of the waveform is exactly equal to 0, or if it is slightly positive or negative. When the summation of the components of the waveform is exactly zero, it gives a precision of ±15 ° to the determination of the electrical axis. Conversely, if the sum is slightly positive, the "real" axis moves 15 ° towards the positive pole of the isodiphasic lead, while if it is slightly negative, the axis moves 15 ° towards the negative pole of the isodiphasic lead (Fig. 3.22A).

A fourth method, known as the graphic method, consists in measuring the net deflection in leads I and III. After calculating the net deflection in millimeters and reporting it on the axis of the respective leads of the hexaxial system, a line is drawn perpendicular to each lead direction starting from the point determined on the leads. The direction of the mean electrical axis is the line that connects the center of the hexaxial system and the point of intersection of these two perpendicular lines (Fig. 3.22B).

Electrocardiographic analysis

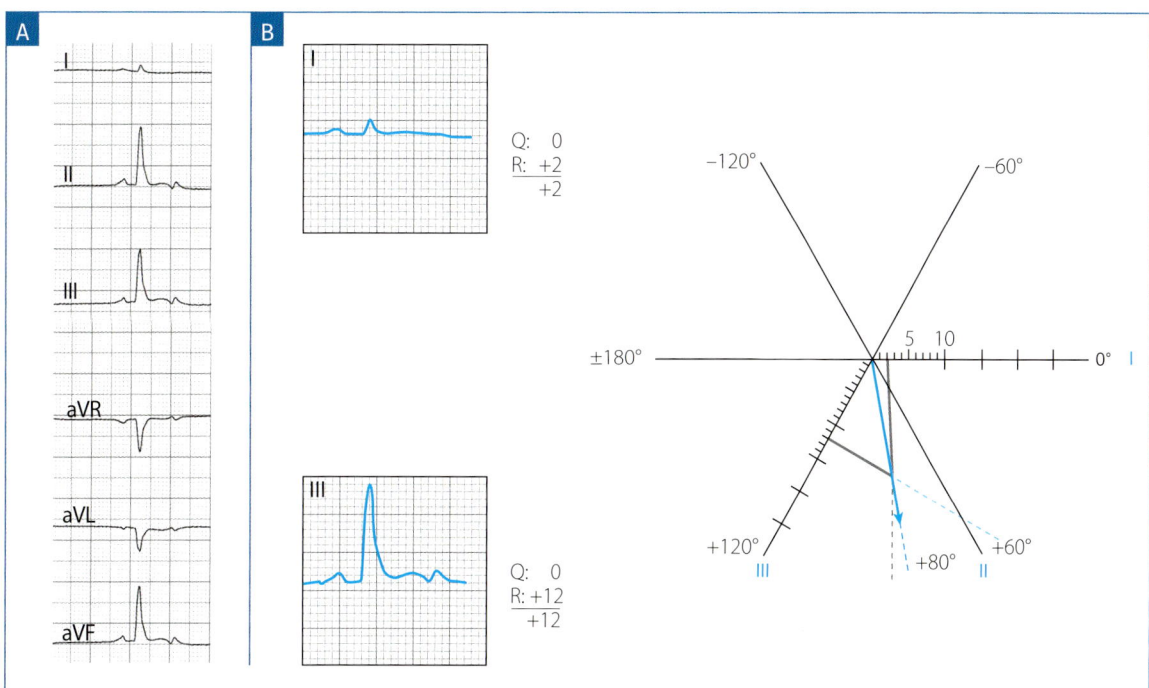

Figure 3.22. There are several methods to determine the mean cardiac electrical axis of the QRS complex in the frontal plane. With the first method, the largest net positive or negative deflection needs to be identified first. Considering tracing A, the lead with the largest net deflection is lead II. Since the QRS complex in lead II has a positive polarity, the mean electrical axis is directed toward the positive pole of this lead, i.e. +60 °. The second method divides the frontal plane into four quadrants: quadrant 1 between 0 and +90 °, quadrant 2 between +90 ° and +180 °, quadrant 3 between +180 ° and −90 ° and quadrant 4 between −90 ° and 0 °. The polarity of the QRS complex is then examined in leads I and aVF. In the example, the QRS complex has a positive polarity in lead I, indicating that the mean electrical axis is within quadrant 1 or 4. The QRS complex also has a positive polarity in the aVF lead, indicating that the mean electrical axis is within quadrant 1. The third method consists in identifying the lead with the most isodiphasic QRS or the most isoelectric QRS. In the example, the most isodiphasic lead is I. This indicates that the mean electrical axis is along the lead perpendicular to lead I, that is aVF. Since the polarity of the QRS complex in the aVF lead is positive, the mean electrical axis points toward the positive pole of this lead, i.e. +90 °. This method provides an estimate which can be improved, by further examining the most isodiphasic QRS and determining whether its net deflection is equal to zero, slightly positive or slightly negative. In the example, the net deflection in lead I is greater than +0.2 mV; therefore, the electric axis is rotated 15 ° towards the positive pole of the isodiphasic lead, which in this example results in an electrical axis close to +75 °. If the net deflection of the isodiphasic lead was negative, the mean electrical axis would have to be rotated 15° toward the negative pole of the isoelectric lead. Finally, the graphical method is shown in panel B. The net deflection of leads I and III is determined first in millimeters. It is then reporting on the hexaxial system on the respective leads. The next step consists in tracing two lines perpendicular to lead I and lead III that originate from the two points previously identified on both leads. The mean electrical axis is the line that joins in the center of the hexaxial system and the point where the two perpendicular lines intersect. In this example, the mean electrical axis is +80 °.

Finally, the most accurate method for measuring the electrical axis of the QRS complex is based on the calculation of the net deflections in leads I and aVF to determine the amplitude of the vector in the two leads and subsequently calculate the mean electrical axis using the following equation:

$$\arctan(I_{amp}, aVF_{amp}) \times 180 / \pi$$

Under normal conditions, since the left ventricle has a myocardial mass about three times larger than that of the right ventricle, the wave of ventricular depolarization assumes a superior-to-inferior, right-to-left and anterior-to-posterior direction, generating prominent R waves in leads I, II, III, and aVF.

The mean electrical axis of the QRS complex in the frontal plane with the animal placed in right lateral recumbency varies, therefore, under physiological conditions from +40 ° to +100 ° in the dog and from ± 0 ° to +160 ° in the cat (Fig. 3.21).

The mean electrical axis of the QRS complex in the frontal plane may be subject to deviations associated with the animal's position during the recording, variations in chest conformation, the presence of intraventricular conduction blocks, and the presence of structural cardiac diseases that induce right ventricular enlargement.

The mean electrical axis in the frontal plane obtained from dogs that are standing varies between +10 ° and +100 °, whereas that of dogs in a sitting position ranges from 0 ° to +71 °. The electrical axis remains within the reference range if the animal is positioned in left lateral or sternal recumbency. Even the position of the thoracic limbs in relation to the trunk can affect the mean axis of the QRS complex in the frontal plane because it changes the position of the exploring electrodes in relation to the cardiac dipole. With the dog in right lateral recumbency, the flexion or misalignment of the forelimbs can induce either clockwise or counterclockwise axis deviation.

In cats, the mean electric axis of the electrocardiogram performed with the animal in sternal recumbency shows no significant differences compared to that recorded with the animal in right lateral recumbency, despite a small reduction in R wave amplitude.

A *right axis deviation* corresponds to a clockwise shift of the mean electric axis in the frontal plane from +100° to −80 ° in the dog and from +160 ° to −80 ° in the cat. A *left axis deviation*, instead, is a counterclockwise shift of the mean electrical axis in the frontal plane from +40 ° to −60 ° in the dog and from 0 ° to −60 ° in the cat.

The right axis deviation occurs with right ventricular enlargement, right bundle branch block and a block of the postero-inferior fascicle. Left axis deviation is associated with antero-superior fascicular block, or right bundle branch block associated with an antero-superior fascicular block.

Similarly, the mean electrical axis in the frontal plane can be calculated for the P wave and for the T wave. The wavefront of the mean atrial depolarization assumes a right-to-left, superior-to-inferior and anterior-to-posterior direction, which usually generates positive P waves in leads II, III, and aVF. The mean electrical axis of the P wave in the frontal plane varies from −18 ° to +90 ° in the dog and from 0 ° to +90 ° in cats (Fig. 3.21). In dogs, the wide range of normal values for the mean electrical axis of the P wave in the frontal plane is due to the presence of sinus node wandering pacemaker and sino-atrioventricular junction wandering pacemaker. The P wave axis is of particular importance for the identification of the site of origin of supraventricular ectopic beats, and if dextrocardia or wrong placement of the electrodes on the limbs is suspected.

In dogs, the electrical axis of the T wave in the frontal plane can range from −45 ° to −147 °. This wide range is attributable to changes in position of the heart in the chest in relation to the exploring electrodes, to the heterogeneity of repolarization and to the differences of action potential duration in different regions of the ventricular myocardium.

Tools for interpreting the electrocardiogram

Different tools can be used to facilitate the evaluation of the electrocardiogram: calipers, an electrocardiographic ruler and a ladder diagram. Nowadays, with most electrocardiographs using electronic recordings and paper recordings being at a minimum, new methods for measuring waveforms and "marching" P waves through the recording or identifying relationships between complexes need to be developed. Until new tools are developed, evaluation of these may actually be quicker and easier with paper recordings.

Calipers are used to measure the intervals and the amplitudes of the electrocardiographic waves in a precise and repeatable way. In order to evaluate the regularity of the P-to-P and R-to-R intervals, the tips of the calipers are adjusted to fit across the first interval to be measured. The tip positioned at the beginning of the next interval to measure is maintained in place, and the calipers are rotated to place the other tip over the next interval. If the tip overlaps with the P or R wave, it indicates that the rhythm is regular (Fig. 3.23). Calipers can also be used to measure and compare the amplitude and duration of the various waveforms.

The *electrocardiographic ruler* is a tool that allows determination of the heart rate, the duration of the electrocardiographic waves and intervals, and the cardiac mean electrical axis in the frontal plane for the P wave and the QRS complex. Most rulers include a standard metric ruler on one side, which allows measurements of the electrocardiographic waves and intervals, and a graduated scale on the opposite side, designed for rapid calculation of the heart rate (Fig. 3.24).

A *ladder diagram* is a useful tool to represent the formation and propagation of electrical impulses along the specialized conduction system. It is made by drawing a vertical line for each P wave and QRS complex. These lines, which must coincide with the onset of the P and QRS complexes are then connected by oblique lines, which represent the electrical conduction through the atrioventricular junction. Typically, the origin of the impulse is represented by a dot. Fig. 3.25 illustrates the propagation of the electrical impulse through the various parts of the heart using a ladder diagram. Fig. 3.26 shows other examples of ladder diagrams.

Electrocardiography during the first weeks of life

In relation to the morphological and functional changes that occur in the cardiovascular system within the first weeks of life, the mean electrical axis of the QRS complex in the frontal plane changes from an inferior-to-superior, posterior-to-anterior and left-to-right direction to superior-to-inferior, anterior-to-posterior and right-to-left. This change of vector orientation is due to the fact that at birth the two ventricles have similar mass. In the first weeks

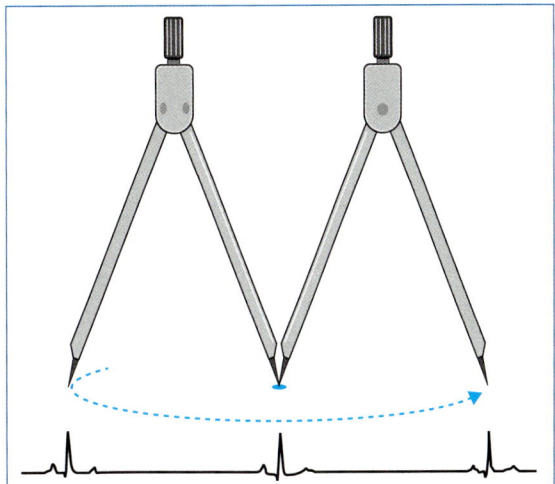

Figure 3.23. Use of calipers to measure the regularity of electrocardiographic intervals. To compare intervals, one of the two tips of the calipers is placed on top of one of the QRS complexes and the other tip is placed above the next one. Then, while holding the second tip of the calipers in place, the calipers are rotated 180 °. If the tip falls on top of the subsequent QRS complex, it indicates that the rhythm is regular.

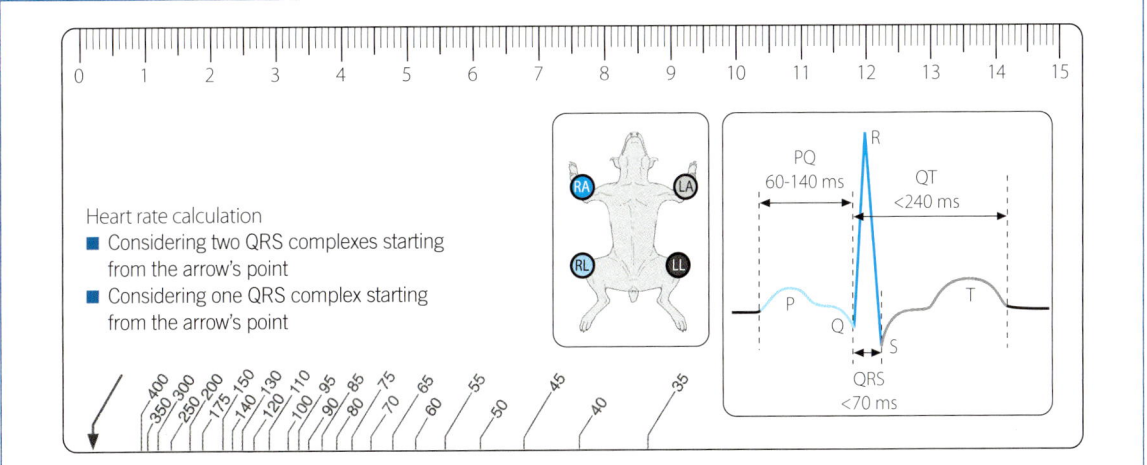

Figure 3.24. Electrocardiographic ruler. This instruments incorporates a ruler, information on correct electrode placement on the limbs, reference values for electrocardiographic wave and interval durations, and a graduated scale for rapid heart rate calculation. In order to determine the heart rate, the arrow on the left of the ruler is aligned to the peak of the QRS complex and the number aligned with the subsequent QRS complex corresponds to the heart rate when the paper speed is 50 mm/s; when the paper speed is 25 mm/s, the heart rate corresponds to the number aligned with the second QRS complex to the right of the arrow, rather than the QRS immediately after the arrow.

of life, after a progressive decrease of the pulmonary resistance, the right ventricle remodels and lose myocardial mass. It changes the ratio of right ventricular mass to left ventricular mass from an initial value of 1:1 to 1:3.

In the first two weeks of life, there is, therefore, an increase in the ratio between the R wave amplitude and the S amplitude (R/S) in the precordial leads. This ratio, with values lower than one at birth, changes progressively to values greater than one before the sixth week of life and, in the following months, increases progressively until it becomes infinite due to the disappearance of the S waves.

Artifacts

The main artifacts that result in alterations of the isoelectric baseline, polarity, morphology and amplitude of the electrocardiographic waves include:
- muscle artifacts,
- breathing artifacts,
- electrical interference from outside sources, and
- errors in electrode placement.

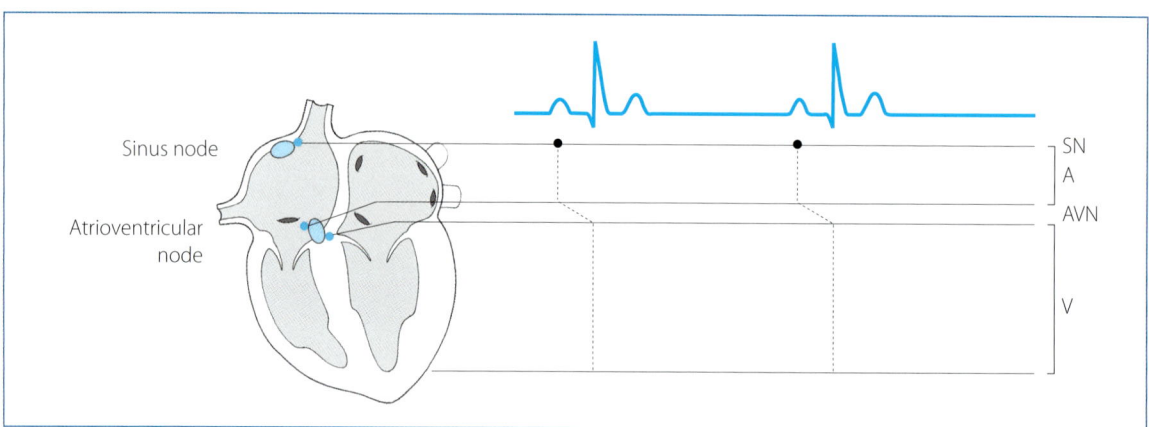

Figure 3.25. Ladder diagram. A ladder diagram with the corresponding segments of the conduction system and the representation of sinus beats. *SN*: sinus node; *A*: atrium; *AVN*: atrioventricular node; *V*: ventricle.

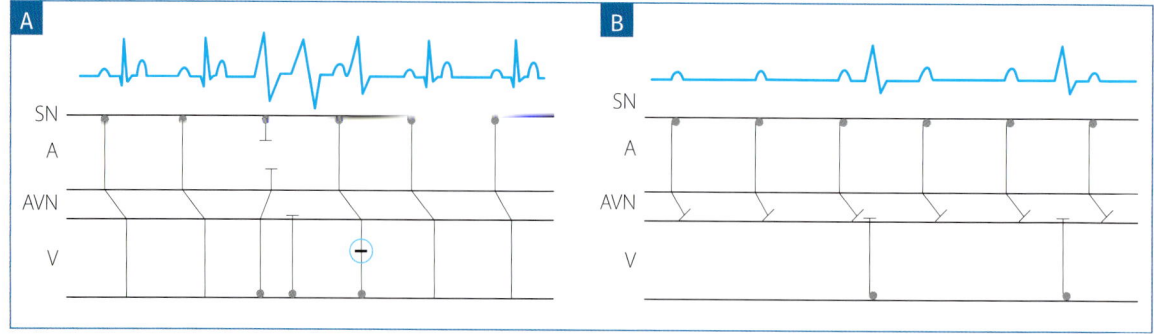

Figure 3.26. Examples of ladder diagrams in the presence of arrhythmias.
A) The first two sinus depolarizations (P waves) travel along the atrioventricular region and are normally conducted to the ventricles. They are followed by three ventricular premature ectopic beats. The first one conducts retrogradely to the atria through the junctional region, and the second is blocked in the atrioventricular node. The next atrial depolarization starting from the sinus node reaches the junctional area and part of the ventricles, where it collides with the wavefront of an ectopic ventricular depolarization (circle). The result is a fusion beat.
B) Third-degree atrioventricular block. P waves blocked within the atrioventricular junction. After the third and the fifth P waves, there is a wide QRS complex originating in the ventricles, which is dissociated from the atrial depolarizations. *SN*: sinus node; *A*: atrium; *AVN*: atrioventricular node; *V*: ventricle.

Muscle artifacts

Skeletal muscle activity can induce artifacts with frequencies ranging from 1 to 35 Hz and amplitudes of 0.03 to 5 mV. They include tremor artifacts and motion artifacts.

Muscle tremors result in irregular artifacts, caused by the rapid stretching of the skin, with a frequency of 15 to 35 Hz and an amplitude of 0.03 to 0.2 mV. These artifacts appear as a fine and irregular oscillation of the isoelectric line that usually intensifies during inspiration and decreases during expiration, or appears and disappears with a periodic pattern (Fig. 3.27A).

Artifacts caused by the movement of somatic muscles with intermediate frequency have a sporadic character, a frequency of about 1 to 15 Hz and an amplitude of 0.1 to 0.5 mV. These artifacts are present in particularly stressed animals and they distort the isoelectric line mimicking the morphology of P waves and are, therefore, frequently misdiagnosed as atrial dissociation (see p. 142) (Fig. 3.27B). This electrocardiographic pattern is called *pseudo-atrial dissociation* and can be caused, in addition to somatic muscle movement, by a loss of contact between the skin and the electrodes or rhythmic movements of the diaphragm. In cats, it has been shown that the diaphragmatic activity induced by stimulation of the phrenic nerve can generate on the surface electrocardiogram waveforms similar to P waves, with positive polarity in the inferior leads. Whenever pseudo-atrial dissociation is due to respiratory artifacts, the rate of the pseudo-P' waves corresponds to the respiratory rate, and disappears during periods of spontaneous apnea.

Motion artifacts from large muscle groups cause deflections of high amplitude (1 to 5 mV) that can mimic "bizarre" QRS complexes. These artifacts can sometimes induce large upward or downward movement of the isoelectric line that extends beyond the borders of the paper recording or computer screen (Fig. 3.27C). Even rhythmic wagging of the tail can result in an artifact that mimics a run of ventricular tachycardia. Rapid and superficial respiratory movements characteristic of panting can cause fluctuations of the isoelectric line with a frequency and amplitude that can be confused with arrhythmias, such as atrial flutter or atrial fibrillation.

Muscle artifacts can be eliminated by activating low-pass filters, by repositioning the electrodes, by avoiding the standing position, by calming the animal and by raising its limbs to minimize tremors. Identification of the lead that is most affected by the artifact can be used to pinpoint the origin of the artifact. If the interference is more evident in leads I and II, the affected limbs are the right thoracic and left pelvic ones. If the artifact mostly affect leads I and III, the electrodes attached to the left thoracic and the left pelvic limbs should be repositioned. If, finally, the artifacts are most visible in leads II and III, the electrode on the left pelvic limb must be repositioned.

Breathing artifacts

Respiratory movements produce low frequency artifacts (less than 0.5 Hz) that appear as rhythmic fluctuations of the isoelectric line. These artifacts can be mitigated by activating the high-pass filter with a cut-off frequency of 0.5 Hz. Digital electrocardiographs have high-pass filters which guarantee the elimination of respiratory artifacts, allowing proper alignment of the P-QRS-T complex sequence with minimum alteration of the ST segment (Fig. 3.28).

Electrical artifacts

Electrical interference originating from the alternating current power source generates regular sinusoidal waves, with a frequency 60 Hz (60-cycles) in the United States of America and 50 Hz in Europe and South Africa, which makes it difficult to evaluate the low-amplitude electrocardiographic waves. These artifacts cause rapid, regular and low voltage undulations of the isoelectric line, and are associated with electromagnetic fields in the room in which the electrocardiogram is recorded (Fig. 3.29). Electromagnetic waves can be transmitted by the operator who is holding the patient and serves as an antenna. These artifacts can also be caused by the cables of the electrocardiograph when there is poor contact between the skin and the electrodes and, finally, they can be associated with excessive alcohol use that causes the formation of an electrical bridge between the limbs or between the limbs and the table.

Electrical interference from the power line can be eliminated by activating a *notch* filter, through appropriate grounding of the electrical system, good electrode-skin contact by the use of a reasonable amount of alcohol or conductive gel, and by wearing latex gloves when holding the animal during the recording.

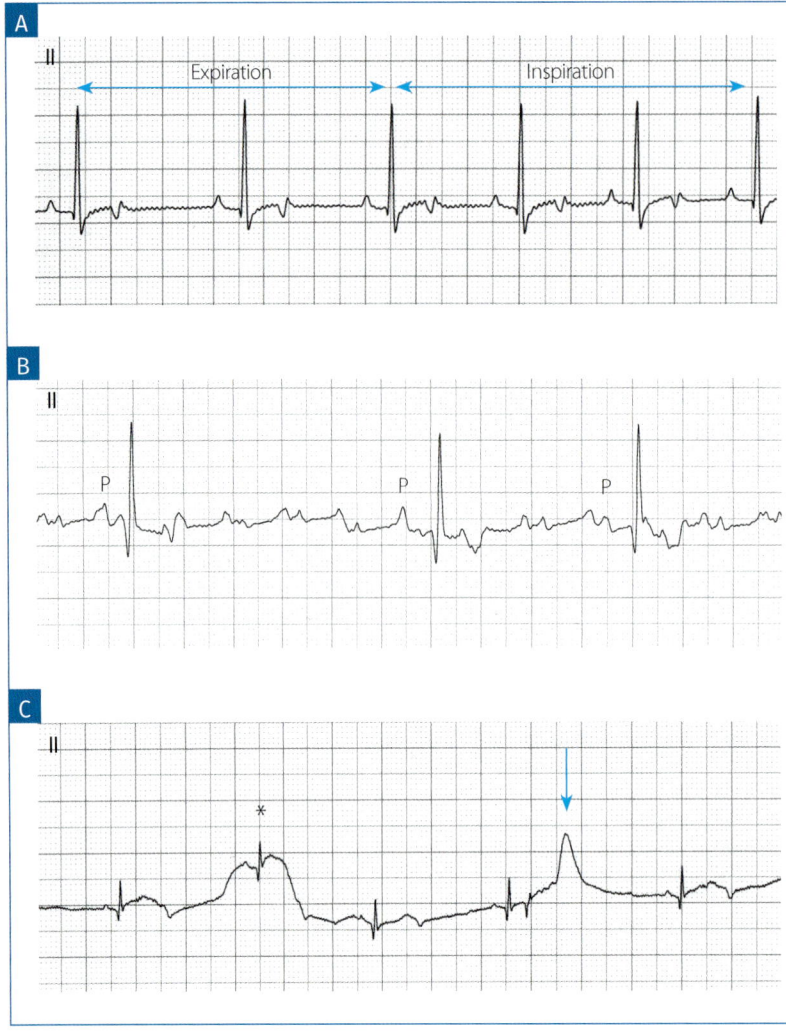

Figure 3.27. Muscle artifacts.
A) Dog, Fox Terrier, female, 9 months. Lead II - speed 50 mm/s - calibration 10 mm/1 mV. Note the fine, irregular fluctuations of the isoelectric line of low amplitude (0.03 to 0.2 mV), which intensify during inspiration and decrease during expiration. They are caused by muscle tremors.

B) Dog, German Bloodhound, male, 8 years. Lead II - speed 50 mm/s - calibration 10 mm/1 mV. Note the artifacts caused by movements of the skeletal muscles. They are intermittent, have intermediate frequency, an amplitude between 0.4 and 0.6 mV, and are intercalated between normal P waves.

C) Dog, mongrel, male, 11 years. Lead II - speed 25 mm/s - calibration 10 mm/1 mV. Note, after the fourth QRS complex, the presence of a high amplitude oscillation (1 mV) of the isoelectric line (arrow) due to movements of a large muscle mass. A similar artifact overlaps with the second QRS complex (1.4 mV) (*).

Errors in electrode placement

Inversion of the limb lead electrodes induces a change in the polarity of the electrocardiographic waves with alterations of the P wave and the QRS complex mean electrical axis. Even the incorrect positioning of the electrodes of the thoracic limbs may cause modifications of the amplitude and duration of the electrocardiographic waves. The position of the precordial electrodes is critical to ensure the reproducibility of the electrocardiographic wave amplitude, while the duration of the waveforms is less influenced by position of the electrodes. The identification of P waves with reversed polarity in leads I and aVL suggests incorrect positioning of the electrodes on the limbs or the presence of dextrocardia (Fig. 3.30). The arrangement of the atrial chambers, and the location of the sinus node in animals with dextrocardia is the mirror of the normal anatomy. As a result, the mean vector of atrial activation assumes a superior-to-inferior, anterior-to-posterior and left-to-right direction. The mean vector of the P waves is +120°, negative P waves are noted in leads aVL and I, and the P waves have the largest positive amplitude in lead III.

Figure 3.28. Respiratory movement artifact (Dog, English Bulldog, female, 3 years. Lead II - speed 25 mm/s - calibration 10 mm/1 mV). Note the slow undulation of the isoelectric line that accompanies the movements of the respiratory muscles. This artifact is usually amplified if the limb electrodes are placed close to the chest wall.

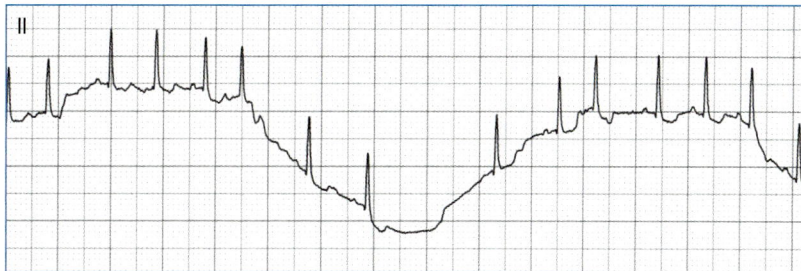

Figure 3.29. Dog, Yorkshire Terrier, male, 15 years (Lead II - speed 50 mm/s - calibration 10 mm/1 mV). Note the alternating current artifact consisting of regular sinusoidal waves with a frequency of 50 Hz. This artifact is characterized by rapid, regular and low voltage deflections.

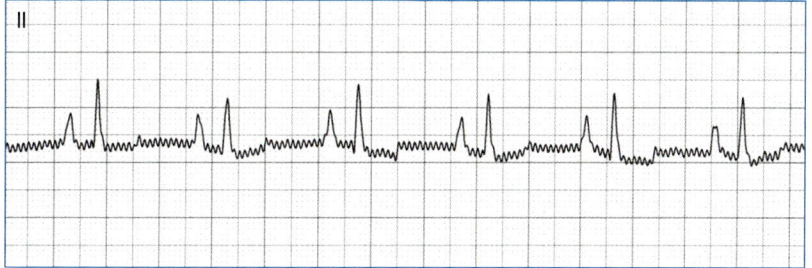

Figure 3.30. Dog, Shih-Tzu, female, 9 years (limb leads - speed 50 mm/s - calibration 10 mm/1 mV). In this example, the P wave and QRS complex polarity are unusual. An error during electrode placement should be suspected first. The presence of an inversion of P wave polarity in leads I and aVL could also be consistent with dextrocardia.

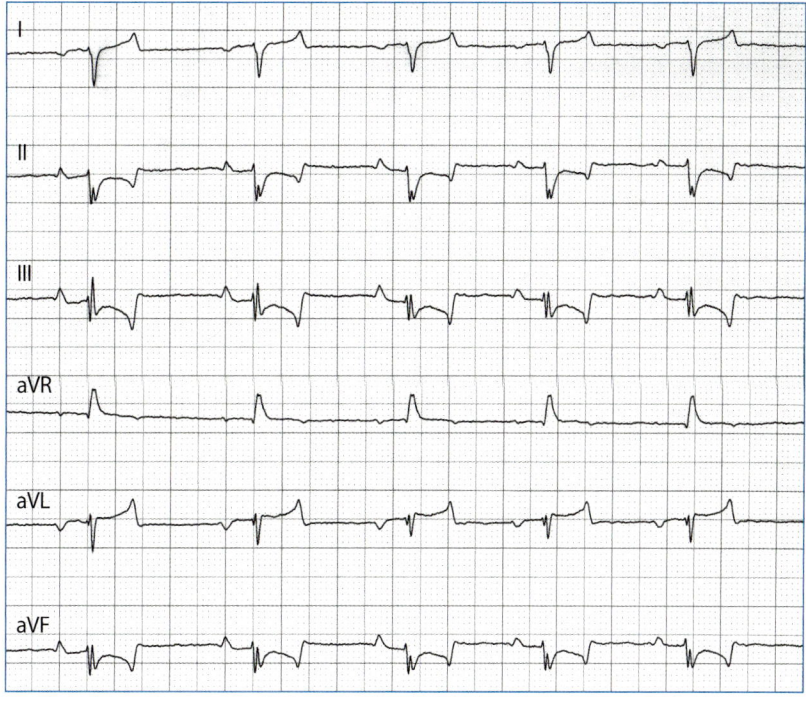

Suggested readings

1. Agudelo CF, Scheer P, Tomenendalova J. How to approach the QT interval in dogs - State of the heart: a review. *Veterinarni Medicina* 2011; 56:14-21.
2. Agudelo CF, Schanilec P. The canine J wave. *Veterinarni Medicina* 2015; 4:208-212.
3. Antzelevitch C, Shimizu W, Yan GX, et al. The M cell: its contribution to the ECG and to normal and abnormal electrical function of the heart. *J Cardiovasc Electrophysiol* 1999; 10:1124–1152.
4. Batey AJ, Doe CPA. A method for QT correction based on beat-to-beat analysis of the QT/RR interval relationship in conscious telemetred Beagle dogs. *J Pharmacol Toxicol Methods* 2002; 48:11-19.
5. Blumenthal SR, Vonderhaar MA, Tilley LP, et al. P-wave duration in a clinically normal hound population. *Lab Anim Sci* 1996; 46:211-214.
6. Burman SO, Panagopoulos P, Kahn S. The electrocardiogram of the normal dog. *J Thorac Cardiovasc Surg* 1966; 51:379-382.
7. Burch GE. History of precordial leads in electrocardiography. *Eur J Cardiol* 1978: 8:207–236.
8. Calvert CA, Coulter DB. Electrocardiographic values for anesthetized cats in lateral and sternal recumbency. *Am J Vet Res* 1981; 8:1453-1455.
9. Cohen I, Giles W, Noble D. Cellular basis for the T wave of the electrocardiogram. *Nature* 1976; 262: 657-661.
10. Coleman MG, Robson MC. Evaluation of six-lead electrocardiograms obtained from dogs in a sitting position or sternal recumbency. *Am J Vet Res* 2005; 66:233-237.
11. Coppola G, Carità P, Corrado E, et al. ST segment elevations: always a marker of acute myocardial infarction? *Indian Heart J* 2013; 65:412-413.
12. Coulter DB, Calvert CA. Orientation and configuration of vectorcadiographic QRS loops from normal cats. *Am J Vet Res* 1981; 42:282-289.
13. Detweiler DK: The dog electrocardiogram: a critical review. In MacFarland PW, Lawrie, TDV, eds: Comprehensive electrocardiography: theory and practice in health and disease, New York, 1998, Pergamon Press.
14. Dubin S, Beard R, Staib J, et al. Variation of canine and feline frontal plane QRS axes with lead choice and augmentation ratio. *Am J Vet Res* 1977; 38:1957-1962.
15. Dvir E, Cilliers PJ, Lobetti RG. Effect of electrocardiographic filters on the R-amplitude of canine electrocardiograms. *Vet Rec* 2002; 150:171-176.
16. Eckenfels A. On the variability of the direction of the cardiac vector and of the T-, Q- and S waves in the normal ECG of the conscious Beagle dog. *Arzneimmittelforschung* 1980; 30:1626-1630.
17. Eckenfels A., Trieb G. The normal electrocardiogram of the conscious Beagle dog. *Toxicol Appl Pharmacol* 1979; 47:567-584.
18. Ferasin L, Ferasin H, Little CJ. Lack of correlation between canine heart rate and body size in veterinary clinical practice. *J Small Anim Pract* 2010; 51:412-418.
19. Fine DM. How to determine and interpret the mean electrical axis. *Vet Med* 2006; 101:28-36.
20. Fossa AA. Assessing QT prolongation in conscious dogs: validation of a beat-to-beat method. *Pharmacol Ther* 2008; 119:133-140.
21. Fossa AA. The impact of varying autonomic states on the dynamic beat-to-beat QT-RR and QT-TQ interval relationships. *Br J Pharmacol* 2008; 154:1508-515.
22. Fossa AA. Assessing QT prolongation in conscious dogs: validation of a beat-to-beat method. *Pharmacol Ther* 2008; 118:231-238.
23. Gitter MJ, Salerno DM, Berry DA, et al. Variability of different methods for measurement of ECG interval temporal variation. *J Electrocardiol* 1989; 22:125-126.
24. Gompf RE, Tilley LP. Comparison of lateral and sternal recumbent positions for electrocardiography of the cat. *Am J Vet Res* 1979; 10:1483-1486.
25. Gönül R, Or ME, Dodurka T. Electrocardiographically determination of cardiac enlargements in dogs. *Turk J Vet Anim Sci* 2002; 26:871-877.
26. Hamlin RL, Smetzer DR, Smith CR. The electrocardiogram, phonocardiogram and derived ventricular activation process of domestic cats. *Am J Vet Res* 1963; 24:792-802.
27. Hamlin RL, Kijtawornrat A, Keene BW. How many cardiac cycles must be measured to permit accurate RR, QT and QTc estimates in conscious dogs? *J Pharm Toxicol Methods* 2004; 50:103-108.
28. Hanås S1, Tidholm A, Egenvall A, et al. Twenty-four hour Holter monitoring of unsedated healthy cats in the home environment. *J Vet Cardiol* 2009; 11:17-22.
29. Hanton G, Rabemampianina Y. The electrocardiogram of the Beagle dog: reference values and effect of sex, genetic strain, body position and heart rate. *Lab Anim* 2006; 40:123-136.
30. Hurst JW. Naming of the waves in the ECG with a brief account of their genesis. *Circulation* 1998: 98:1937-1942.
31. Harvey AM, Faena M, Darke PGG, et al. Effect of body position on feline electrocardiographic recordings. *J Vet Intern Med* 2005; 19:533-536.
32. Hayashi H. The experimental study of normal atrial T wave (T_a) in electrocardiograms. *Jpn Heart J* 1970; 11:91-103.
33. Hezzell MJ, Dennis SG, Humm K, Agee L, Boswood A, et al. Relationships between heart rate and age, body weight and breed in 10,949 dogs. *J Small Anim Pract* 2013; 54:318-324.
34. Hill JD. The electrocardiogram in dogs with standardized body and limb positions. *J Electrocardiol* 1968; 1:175-182.
35. Hill JD. The significance of foreleg positions in the interpretation of electrocardiograms and vectorcardiograms from research animals. *Am Heart J* 1968; 75: 518-527.
36. Hashimoto H, Suzuki K, Miyake S, Nakashima M. Effects of calcium antagonists on the electrical alternans of the ST segment and on associated mechanical alternans during acute coronary occlusion in dogs. *Circulation* 1983; 68:667-672.

37. Kijtawornrat A, Panyasing Y, Del Rio C, Hamlin RL. Assessment of ECG interval and restitution parameters in the canine model of short QT syndrome. *J Pharmacol Toxicol Methods* 2010; 61:231-237.
38. Kligfield P, Gettes LS, Bailey JJ, et al. Recommendations for the standardization and interpretation of the electrocardiogram. Part I: the electrocardiogram and its technology. *Heart Rhythm* 2007; 4:394-412.
39. Mason JW, Hancock WE, Gettes LS. Recommendations for the standardization and interpretation of the electrocardiogram. Part II: electrocardiography diagnostic statement list. *Circulation* 2007; 115:1325-1332.
40. Mirvis DM, Marin-Garcia J. Effects of tachycardia with normal and ectopic ventricular activation on S-T segment potential and patterns in the dog. *J Electrocardiol* 1985; 18:223-232.
41. Moss AJ. The electrocardiogram: from Einthoven to molecular genetics. *Ann Noninvasive Electrocardiol* 2001; 6:181-182.
42. Musselman EE. Digital computer analysis of the QRS complex of the dog, using the McFee axial system. *Am J Vet Res* 1976; 37:417-425.
43. Musselman EE, Church KE. Computer analysis of the non-angular parameters of the QRSA loop and orthogonal lead QRS characteristics in necropsy-verified normal dogs. *J Electrocardiol* 1983; 16:263-268.
44. Oguchi Y, Hamlin RL. Duration of QT interval in clinically normal dogs. *Am J Vet Res* 1993; 54:2145-2149.
45. Oguchi Y, Hamlin RL. Rate of change of QT interval in response to a sudden change in the heart rate in dogs. *Am J Vet Res* 1994; 55:1618-1623.
46. Perego M, Skert S, Santilli RA. Analysis of the atrial repolarization wave in dogs with third-degree atrioventricular block. *Am J Vet Res* 2014; 75:54-58.
47. Pérez-Riera AR, de Abreu LC, Barbosa-Barros R, Nikus KC, Baranchuk A, et al. R-peak time: an electrocardiographic parameter with multiple clinical applications. *Ann Noninvasive Electrocardiol* 2016; 21:10-19.
48. Pollehn T, Brady WJ, Perron AD, et al. The electrocardiographic differential diagnosis of ST segment depression. *Emerg Med J* 2002; 19:129-135.
49. Porteiro Vázquez DM, Perego M, Lombardo S, Santilli RA. Analysis of precordial lead system in dogs with different thoracic conformations. Proceedings 26th ECVIM Congress 2016:1:84.
50. Rishniw M, Porciello F, Erb HN, et al. Effect of body position on the 6-lead ECG of dogs. *J Vet Intern Med* 2002; 16:69-73.
51. Robertson BT, Figg FA, Ewell WM. Normal values for the electrocardiogram in the cat. *Feline Practice* 1976; 7:20-22.
52. Roffi M, Patrono C, Collet JP, et al. 2015 ESC guidelines for the management of acute coronary syndromes in patients presenting without persistent ST-segment elevation. *Eur Heart J* 2016; 37:267-315.
53. Rogers WA, Bishop SP. Electrocardiographic parameters of the normal domestic cat: a comparison of standard limb leads and an orthogonal system. *J Electrocardiol* 1971; 4:315-321.
54. Rosenbaum MB. The hemiblocks: diagnostic criteria and clinical significance. *Am Heart J* 1970; 70:141-146.
55. Rosenbaum MB, Elizari MV, Lazzari JO. *Gli emiblocchi*. Edizioni Piccin Padova (I). 192-134.
56. Rudling EH, Schlamowitz S, Pipper CB, et al. The prevalence of the electrocardiographic J wave in the Petit Basset Griffon Vendéen compared to 10 different dog breeds. *J Vet Cardiol* 2016; 18:26-33.
57. Scher AM. Studies of the electrical activity of the ventricles and the origin of the QRS complex. *Acta Cardiol* 1995; 50:429-465.
58. Schneider HP, Truex RC, Knowles JO. Comparative observations of the hearts of mongrel and Greyhound dogs. *Anat Rec* 1964; 149:173-179.
59. Schober KE, Maerz I, Ludewig E, et al. Diagnostic accuracy of electrocardiography and thoracic radiography in the assessment of left atrial size in cats: comparison with transthoracic 2-dimensional echocardiography. *J Vet Intern Med* 2007; 21:709-718.
60. Schrope DP, Fox PR, Hahn AW, et al. Effects of electrocardiograph frequency filters on P-QRS-T amplitudes of the feline electrocardiogram. *Am J Vet Res* 1995; 56:1534-1540.
61. Spence S, Soper K, Hoe Chao-Min, et al. The heart rate-corrected QT interval of conscious beagle dogs: a formula based on analysis of covariance. *Toxicol Sci* 1998; 45:247-258.
62. Steg PG, James SK, Atar D, et al. ESC guidelines for the management of acute myocardial infarction in patients presenting with ST-segment elevation. *Eur Heart J* 2012; 33:2659-2619.
63. Takahashi M, Nakaya Y, Wada Y, et al. The U wave change during increased blood pressure. *Tokushima J Exp Med* 1985; 32:49-56.
64. Trautvetter E, Detweiler DK, Patterson DF. Evolution of the electrocardiogram in young dogs during the first 12 weeks of life. *J Electrocardiol* 1981; 14:267-274.
65. Van der Linde H, Van de Water A, Loots W, et al. A new method to calculate the beat-to-beat instability of QT duration in drug-induced long QT in anesthetized dogs. *J Pharmacol Toxicol Methods* 2005; 52:168-177.
66. Ware WA, Christensen WF. Duration of the QT interval in healthy cats. *Am J Vet Res* 1999;60:1426-1429.
67. Wilson FN, Johnston FD, Rosenbaum FF, et al. On Einthoven's triangle, the theory of unipolar electrocardiographic leads and the interpretation of the precordial electrocardiogram. *Am Heart J* 1946; 32:279.
68. Wilson FN, Macleod GM, Barker PS, et al. The interpretation of the initial deflections of the ventricular complex of the electrocardiogram. *Am Heart J* 1931; 6:637-664.

Suggested links

https://www.youtube.com/watch?v=EA2DY0tjpFI

CHAPTER 4

Normal sinus rhythms

The sinus node controls the rhythm of the normal heart and contains the cells most resistant to overdrive suppression. The sinus node dominates because in health it is the fastest pacemaker overdrive suppressing subsidiary pacemakers. Importantly, the sinus rhythm can be normal and yet an arrhythmia (e.g. ventricular tachycardia) or conduction disturbance (e.g. third-degree atrioventricular block) can coexist. That is, despite the presence of an arrhythmia the sinus node usually continues to discharge resulting in P waves that may or may not be seen. Visualization of a P wave depends on the actual depolarization of the atria and whether or not the wave is hidden within a ventricular QRS complex. Essentially, regardless of what arrhythmia is diagnosed, the following questions should be posed for every patient: is there an underlying rhythm of sinus origin and what is the rate? This will help to answer the question: what is the *underlying rhythm*?

Autonomic tone has profound influence on sinus rhythm. Consequently, it is important to understand the genesis and modulation of rate and rhythm of the sinus node discharges in response to physiologic and pathologic conditions. In this chapter the normal sinus rate and influences will be addressed along with the characteristics of normal sinus rhythm, sinus arrhythmia and sinus rhythm during arrhythmias.

Sinus rate

The heart rhythms originating from the pacemaker cells of the sinus node are defined as sinus rhythms. Without input from the autonomic nervous system the discharge rate of the sinus node in the dog is approximately 90 to 100 bpm and the interval between successive P waves, the P-P interval, is regular. This is known as the inherent non-modulated heart rate of the sinus node. However, in the dog, the parasympathetic system has a very pronounced effect and normal physiologic responses modulate this inherent regular sinus rhythm. Fundamentally, the heart rate changes to match physiologic demands of activity and rest with the response required and the ability of each individual dog or cat to react. The average daily heart rate declines as a dog matures. Most dogs reach a mature heart rate between 6 and 12 months of age. In humans aging is known to lessen the ability of the sinus node to increase heart rate; however, the effect of aging in the dog is unknown. An adult dog has an average daily heart rate of approximately 80 bpm with a typical range during the 24 hours between 40 and 260 bpm (as determined by 24-hour ambulatory monitoring). Although this range is broad, the majority of dogs in the home environment have a heart rate between 50 and 120 bpm for approximately 85 % of the day. The sinus rate in immature and young dogs may exceed 300 bpm; however, such high rates are usually not sustained for more than a minute.

Until 24-hour electrocardiographic monitoring was performed in cats in the home environment, the true heart rate in the non-hospitalized cat was not known. Cats typically have an average heart rate of approximately 160 bpm with the rate ranging between 120 and 220 bpm over 24 hours.

It is important to appreciate that when evaluating the sinus rate even in a normal dog cardiovascular reflexes must be understood. These reflexes hinge critically on the autonomic nervous system and can have profound effects. Most cardiovascular reflexes result from the interplay of baroreceptors and the balance of the sympathetic and parasympathetic responses to changes in blood pressure. In the most basic terms the baroreceptors respond to a decrease in blood pressure with the enhancement of sympathetic tone and withdrawal of the parasympathetic tone to increase heart rate and initiate vasoconstriction. In contrast, when blood pressure rises, the heart rate falls with decreased sympathetic tone and increased parasympathetic tone. Under certain conditions these responses can result in profound changes in sinus heart rate, which may be detrimental. An example is the vasovagal response, which results in bradycardia and hypotension. Numerous stimuli or circumstances, including, but not limited to, extreme excitement, exercise, coughing, the Valsalva maneuver, micturition, and emotional distress, can evoke a vasovagal response which can result in neurocardiogenic syncope due to severe bradycardia or pauses. One reflex that overlaps vasovagal bradycardia is that known as the Bezold-Jarisch reflex, which follows as a response usually to an extreme tachycardia that stimulates the C fibers in the myocardium resulting in long sinus pauses. Such responses may be confused with sinus node dysfunction. Another cardiovascular reflex that can alter heart rate is the result of increased intracranial pressure, which stimulates the sympathetic tone to increase systemic blood pressure which then stimulates the baroreceptors to increase vagal tone resulting in bradycardia. This reflex has been termed the Cushing response.

When trying to evaluate the sinus rhythm, environmental, situational, and pharmacological factors must be considered. Drugs, physiologic responses (e.g. sleep, excitement), physiologic responses to pathologic conditions (e.g. cardiac tamponade, loss of blood volume) and sinus node disease can result in sinus bradycardia (see p. 239), excessively long sinus pauses (see p. 245), or sinus tachycardia (see p. 145).

Sinus rhythm

The term *sinus rhythm* indicates that the origin of the depolarizing wave is from the cells of the sinus node and that a constant P-P interval exists (<10 % variation). This is the most common rhythm identified in normal cats during an electrocardiographic examination when the heart rate is between 160 and 220 bpm. However, sinus rhythm in dogs is uncommon because parasympathetic tone dominates, even in the hospital environment. In dogs with a normal sinus node, a sinus rhythm is frequently present with heart rates greater than 160 bpm and is often diagnosed as sinus tachycardia. Suspicions of abnormality should be raised if there is no variability in the P-P interval when rates are below 100 bpm in the dog. A constant slower rate may be possible for brief periods of time, but in the normal dog such sequences are broken irregularly because of the influence of the parasympathetic system. It should be noted that sinus rhythm is common in dogs less than 3 months of age.

Waveform characteristics. The sinus rhythm is characterized by the presence of P waves with a superior-to-inferior axis in the frontal plane between $-18°$ and $+90°$ in the dog and between $0°$ and $+90°$ in the cat. The P waves appear positive in leads II, III and aVF; they are positive, biphasic or isodiphasic (positive and negative deflections are equal in amplitude) in lead I, and have maximum negativity in lead aVR (*sinus axis*). In the normal animal each P wave is followed by a QRS complex; however, a sinus rhythm can still be diagnosed even in the presence of an arrhythmia or conduction disturbance characterized by an abnormal QRS complex. That is, a sinus rhythm can exist even if complete heart block is present; a sinus rhythm can exist even with left or right bundle branch block; finally, a sinus rhythm can exist in the presence of ventricular tachycardia. (Boxes 4.1 and 4.2).

Sinus arrhythmia

Respiratory sinus arrhythmia (Box 4.3, Figs. 4.1, 4.2 and 4.3) is characterized by a cyclic variation in heart rate, approximately synchronous with the phases of respiration and with the concomitant fluctuations of vagal tone. Importantly, although the word arrhythmia gives the connotation of an abnormality, it is the normal rhythm in dogs. A sinus arrhythmia in the normal dog most commonly occurs with a heart rate between 60 and 160 bpm. In resting dogs, the sinus discharge rate

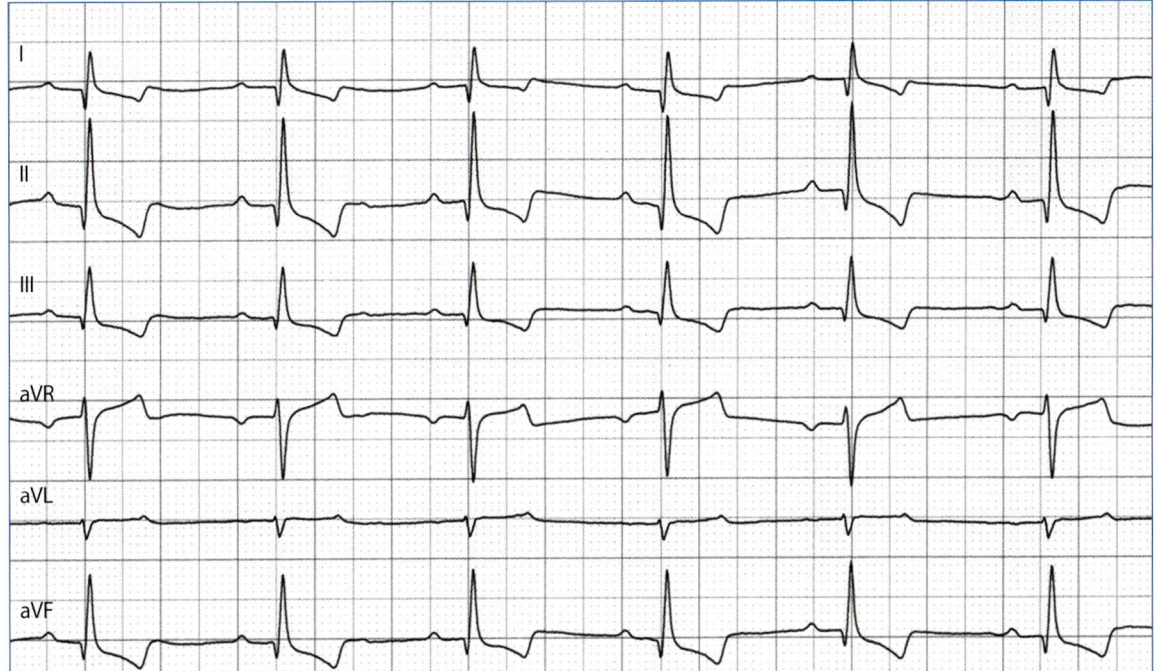

BOX 4.1.
SINUS RHYTHM IN DOGS

HEART RATE: 60-160 bpm. Most dogs have sinus arrhythmia.
R-R INTERVAL: regular.
P WAVE: present, axis in superior-inferior and left direction (between −18° and +90°), positive in leads II, III and aVF, positive, biphasic or isodiphasic in lead I and maximum negativity in lead aVR.

ATRIOVENTRICULAR CONDUCTION: present.
PQ INTERVAL: usually normal (60-130 ms).
QRS COMPLEX: normal (≤70 ms), except in case of pre-existing intraventricular conduction disorders.
VENTRICULO-ATRIAL CONDUCTION: absent.
BLOCKED BEATS: none.

Dog, Cocker Spaniel, female, 3 years.
Six limbs leads (I, II, III, aVR, aVL, aVF) - speed 50 mm/s - calibration 5 mm/1 mV.

Notes: sinus rhythm with a rate of 120 bpm. P waves with sinus axis and regular P-P intervals, normal QRS complexes and PQ intervals are normal.

---

accelerates during inspiration, while it decelerates during expiration. Linking of heart rate and the mechanics of breathing may improve the efficacy of pulmonary gas exchange. At fast heart rates, the typical changing of the R-R intervals with respiratory sinus arrhythmia diminishes until it disappears. The heart rate during the slowing cycle varies considerably from that during the speeding cycle. Moreover, the rate does not change abruptly, there being intermediate P-P intervals. The complex mechanisms responsible for respiratory sinus arrhythmia have been studied extensively in humans and dogs. Respiratory sinus arrhythmia is not only related to cyclic respiratory variations in vagal tone, but also depends on a series of controlling mechanisms which include activation of the cardiovascular centers of the medulla oblongata, the degree of lung inflation, the cardiac acceleration reflex due to right atrial wall distension during inspiration and chemoreceptor and baroreceptor reflexes inducing a rise in blood pressure after a phase of cardiac acceleration. It should be emphasized that although

Chapter 4. Normal sinus rhythms

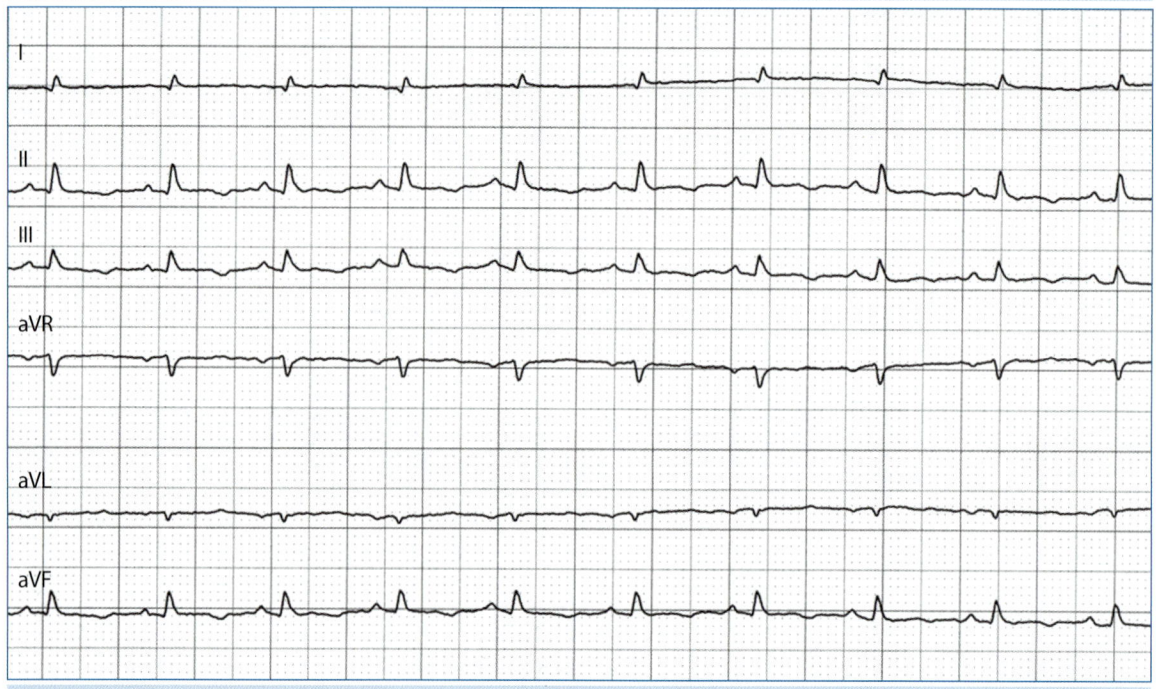

> **BOX 4.2.**
> **SINUS RHYTHM IN CATS**
>
> **HEART RATE:** 160-220 bpm. Slower rates at home.
> **R-R INTERVAL:** regular.
> **P WAVE:** present, sinus axis superior-inferior and left direction (between 0 ° and +90 °), positive in leads II, III and aVF, positive, biphasic or isodiphasic in lead I and maximum negativity in lead aVR.
>
> **ATRIOVENTRICULAR CONDUCTION:** present.
> **PQ INTERVAL:** usually normal (50-90 ms).
> **QRS COMPLEX:** normal (<40 ms), except in case of pre-existing intraventricular conduction disorders.
> **VENTRICULO-ATRIAL CONDUCTION:** absent.
> **BLOCKED BEATS:** none.
>
> Cat, Common European, male, 5 years.
> Six limbs leads (I, II, III, aVR, aVL, aVF) - speed 50 mm/s - calibration 10 mm/1 mV.
>
> Notes: sinus rhythm with a rate of 188 bpm. P waves with sinus axis and regular P-P intervals, normal QRS complexes and PQ intervals are normal.

"clustering features" have been described for respiratory sinus arrhythmia, the precise grouping of the speeding and slowing of the P-P intervals, Holter recordings from normal dogs reveal a variety in the patterns. Such variability is likely due to the multiplicity and complexity of the autonomic input.

Respiratory sinus arrhythmia is strongly dominant in dogs because of the influences of the parasympathetic system, but in cats during electrocardiographic examinations the sympathetic tone is higher and parasympathetic tone is lower causing sinus arrhythmia to be uncommon. Until 24-hour ambulatory electrocardiographic monitoring was performed on cats in their home environment, it was believed that sinus arrhythmia did not exist in the normal cat. However, it is now known that when the feline heart rate falls below 160 bpm, sinus arrhythmia can be identified in the majority of cats in their home environment because of the higher parasympathetic tone in this situation. On occasion a sinus arrhythmia may be identified in very calm, normal cats in a clinical situation.

Sinus arrhythmia

BOX 4.3.
SINUS RESPIRATORY ARRHYTHMIA IN DOGS

HEART RATE: 60-160 bpm. Higher rates usually sinus rhythm.
R-R INTERVAL: variable, increase in rate with inspiration and decrease with expiration. Grouped patterns of beats common.
P WAVE: present, sinus axis except in case of wandering pacemaker which is common with this rhythm.
ATRIOVENTRICULAR CONDUCTION: present.

PQ INTERVAL: normal (60-130 ms) with possible occurrence of first-degree atrioventricular block during heart rate deceleration. Can have second-degree atrioventricular block with underlying rhythm of sinus arrhythmia.
QRS COMPLEX: normal (<70 ms), except in case of pre-existing intraventricular conduction disorders.
VENTRICULO-ATRIAL CONDUCTION: absent.
BLOCKED BEATS: none.

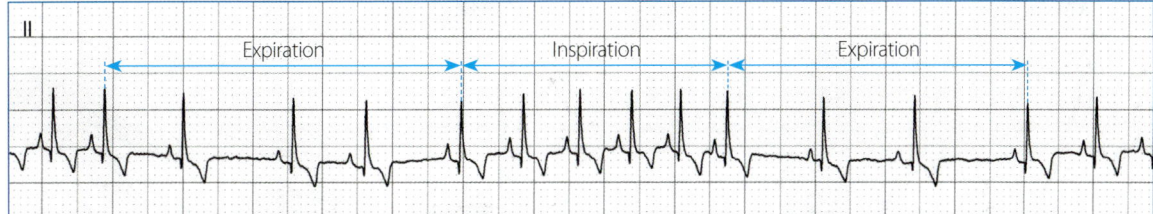

Dog, Pinscher, male, 10 years old.
Lead II - speed 25 mm/s - calibration 5 mm/1 mV.

Notes: respiratory sinus arrhythmia, variable P-P/R-R intervals (heart rate). Note the P waves have a sinus axis and irregular P-P intervals, a gradual acceleration of the sinus rate occurs during inspiration and a sudden deceleration occurs during expiration. The QRS complexes and PQ intervals are normal.

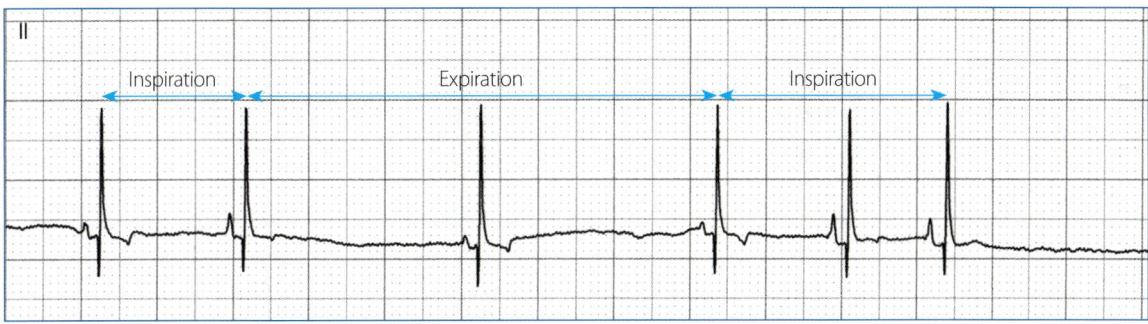

Figure 4.1. Respiratory sinus arrhythmia with sinus node wandering pacemaker (Dog, mongrel, female, 12 years. Lead II - speed 25 mm/s - calibration 10 mm/1 mV).
The dominant rhythm is a respiratory sinus arrhythmia characterized by an increase in heart rate during inspiration and by a decrease during expiration. Note the cyclic variation of the P wave amplitude, the increased voltage during the faster rate (shorter R-R intervals) and the decreased voltage during the slower rate (longer R-R intervals).

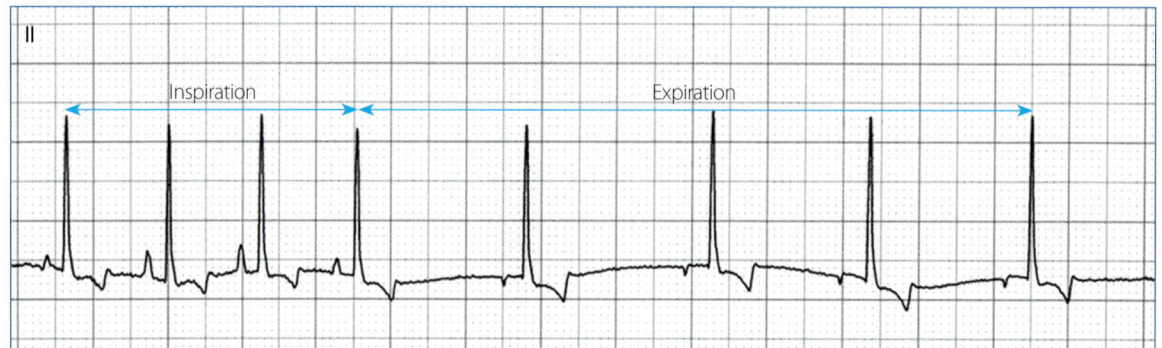

Figure 4.2. Respiratory sinus arrhythmia with a sinus node-atrioventricular junction wandering pacemaker (Dog, Spitz, male, 8 years. Lead II- speed 25 mm/s - calibration 10 mm/1 mV).
The dominant rhythm is a respiratory sinus arrhythmia characterized by an increase of the discharge rate during inspiration (125 bpm) and by a decrease during expiration (60 bpm). Note the cyclic variations of amplitude and polarity of the P wave, which changes from positive to negative when the sinus discharge rate decreases (longer P-P interval). The morphology and polarity of the P wave on the frontal plane in the six-lead system change because the depolarization of the atria is initiating from the sinus node closer to the cranial vena cava during inspiration and lower in the atria during expiration. This results in a different vector of atrial depolarization.

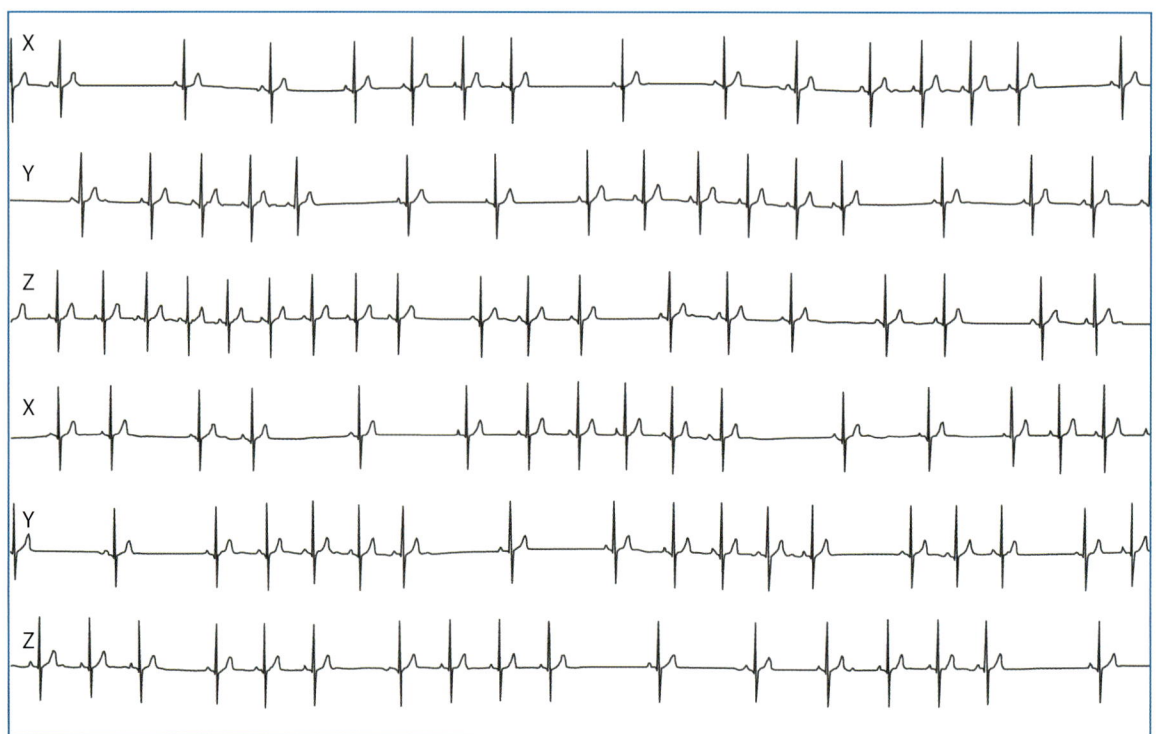

Figure 4.3. Selected continuous segment from a 24-hour ambulatory electrocardiographic recording (Holter recording - Leads X, Y and Z) from a dog. A single lead is represented to demonstrate the variability in the heart rate that can occur spontaneously in a dog. Sinus arrhythmia can be linked to the respiratory rate; however, other autonomic influences that decrease or increase sympathetic and parasympathetic tone can change the heart rate on a beat-to-beat basis.

Non-respiratory sinus arrhythmia (Box 4.4) can be present when the P-P intervals vary but the variation is not linked to breathing or tone of the autonomic nervous system. In humans such variation is more commonly noted in the elderly: the mechanism has not yet been determined.

The magnitude of autonomic tone can be assessed by the variability in the P-P interval. This is known as *heart rate variability*. When the PQ interval is relatively constant the R-R interval (usually measured during Holter analysis) can be used as a surrogate for the P-P interval. Henceforth, because heart rate variability programs assess the R-R interval rather than the true P-P interval, the term R-R interval will be used to indicate the actual P-P interval with the understanding that there is a constant relationship between the P wave and QRS complex. Beat-to-beat variability is certainly possible when other rhythms are present, such as atrial fibrillation; however, this will not reflect the sinus node variability. Three methods of heart rate variability are commonly used: geometric, time domain and frequency domain analysis.

Geometric heart rate variability analysis (Fig. 4.4) includes two- and three-dimensional tachograms of successive R-R intervals, a heart rate tachogram, Poincaré plots (Lorenz plots) of R-R intervals against R-R +1 intervals, and a R-R interval histogram. Tachograms in the dog have a distinctive pattern that reflects the sinus arrhythmia in this species. The patterns vary depending on the degree of parasympathetic tone. Dogs with prominent sinus arrhythmia tend to have a double banding representing the R-R intervals with a large reduction in the number of R-R intervals between these bands. This pattern in the normal dog suggests exit block from the sinus node as the probable mechanism for the generation of the sinus arrhythmia. The sinus node exit pathways of the dog have been extensively studied. The paucity of beats in this zone is also appreciated in the nonlinear Poincaré plots and the R-R interval histograms. The histogram does not represent a single Gaussian distribution, but instead has two or three seemingly distinct populations of R-R intervals. At faster heart rates, for example,

---

BOX 4.4.
NON-RESPIRATORY SINUS ARRHYTHMIA IN DOGS

HEART RATE: 60 -160 bpm.
INTERVAL R-R: variation in the sinus rhythm that is not associated with the phases of respiration.
WAVE P: present, sinus axis except in case of wandering pacemaker.
ATRIOVENTRICULAR CONDUCTION: present.

PQ INTERVAL: normal (60-130 ms) or with possible occurrence of first- or second-degree atrioventricular blocks during heart rate deceleration with the sinus arrhythmia the underlying rhythm.
QRS COMPLEX: normal (<70 ms), except in case of pre-existing intraventricular conduction disorders.
VENTRICULO-ATRIAL CONDUCTION: absent.
BLOCKED BEATS: none.

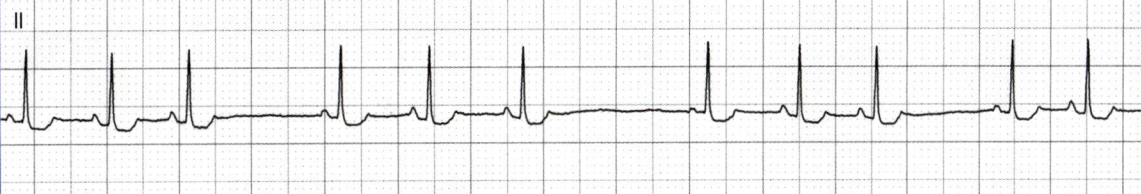

Dog, Beagle, male, 3 years.
Lead II - speed 25 mm/s - calibration 5 mm/1 mV.

Notes: non-respiratory sinus arrhythmia with a variable rate between 75 and 125 bpm. Note the P waves with sinus axis and irregular P-P intervals, with grouping of the QRS complexes in series of three. The QRS complexes and PQ intervals are normal.

in dogs with congestive heart failure, this pattern is absent. Some dogs do not have a distinct "zone of avoidance", but nonetheless fewer beats are present. Unlike the dog, the cat does not show such a pattern.

Time domain heart rate variability represents the variability of the R-R intervals and provides information with regards to the parasympathetic tone. Time domain analysis can be performed on selected intervals or for the entire 24 hours. A triangular index is included in some Holter analysis programs, but is not applicable in dogs because of the multi-distribution of R-R intervals in this species. The following are time domain parameters:
- SDNN – standard deviation of all R-R intervals (NN = normal P wave triggered R-R).
- SDANN – standard deviation of all five-minute R-R intervals.
- SDNN Index – mean of all five-minute R-R interval standard deviations.
- RMSSD – square root of the mean square of successive R-R interval differences.

Higher numbers of each of the above are indicative of greater variability and higher parasympathetic tone.

Frequency domain heart rate variability (Fig. 4.5) is the most complex to analyze. The power spectral density is obtained from the time series (R-R intervals) to determine how power (variance) varies with frequency. The nonparametric method known as fast Fourier transformation is perhaps the most commonly used method of analysis. Several frequency bands have been associated with autonomic tone, with the high frequency band reflecting parasympathetic tone. Although more commonly used to assess shorter-term heart rate variability, either in 5 minute increments or on the basis of 256 or 512 beats, 24-hour analyses can be done to determine ultra-low frequencies. These have been studied in the dog. It should be noted that although causes for the different bands have been proposed, there is considerable overlap and disagreement; therefore, firm conclusions cannot be drawn although high total power and greater density in the high frequency band is consistent with high vagal tone. The frequency bands most commonly considered are as follows:

- Total ≤0.4 Hz.
- Very low frequency ≤0.04 Hz.
- Low-frequency ≤0.04–0.15 Hz.
- High-frequency 0.15–0.4 Hz.

Waveform characteristics. The QRS-T waveforms in normal dogs and cats are similar to those of a sinus rhythm. However, just as with a sinus rhythm, the presence of abnormal QRS-T waveforms associated with conduction disturbances or coexisting arrhythmias does not preclude the existence of a sinus arrhythmia as the *underlying rhythm* because the sinus node function can still be normal. In contrast to the regular P wave morphology of a sinus rhythm, the P wave in sinus arrhythmia varies in morphology and amplitude in the dog. This variability most often tracks with the irregularity of the P-P intervals and is termed a *wandering pacemaker* (Figs. 4.1 and 4.2).

The cyclic variation characteristic of a wandering pacemaker is due to changes in the site of impulse origin within the sinus node and/or changes in the exit pathway from the sinus node. Due to the migration of the site where the sinus pulse originates and/or exits, the direction of the vector of atrial depolarization varies. These variations track with the changes in P-P intervals which track most commonly with the phases of respiration. In particular, during vagal predominance the inferior-posterior portion is initially activated and the impulse exits from the inferior pathway and descends along the posterior and middle internodal tract. This causes the P wave in leads II, III and aVF to have a lower amplitude with the P wave vector directed more towards lead I. During sympathetic dominance, however, the dominant pacemaker activity migrates to the level of the anterior-superior portion of the sinus node, the impulses exit from the superior pathway and then reach the atrioventricular node through the anterior internodal tract. This causes the P wave in leads II, III and aVF to have a greater amplitude with the P wave vector directed more towards leads II and aVF. In cases of pronounced respiratory sinus arrhythmia, the P waves that follow prolonged pauses can have a higher amplitude as a result of the increase in sympathetic tone secondary to a fall in blood pressure at the end of the pause.

Sinus arrhythmia

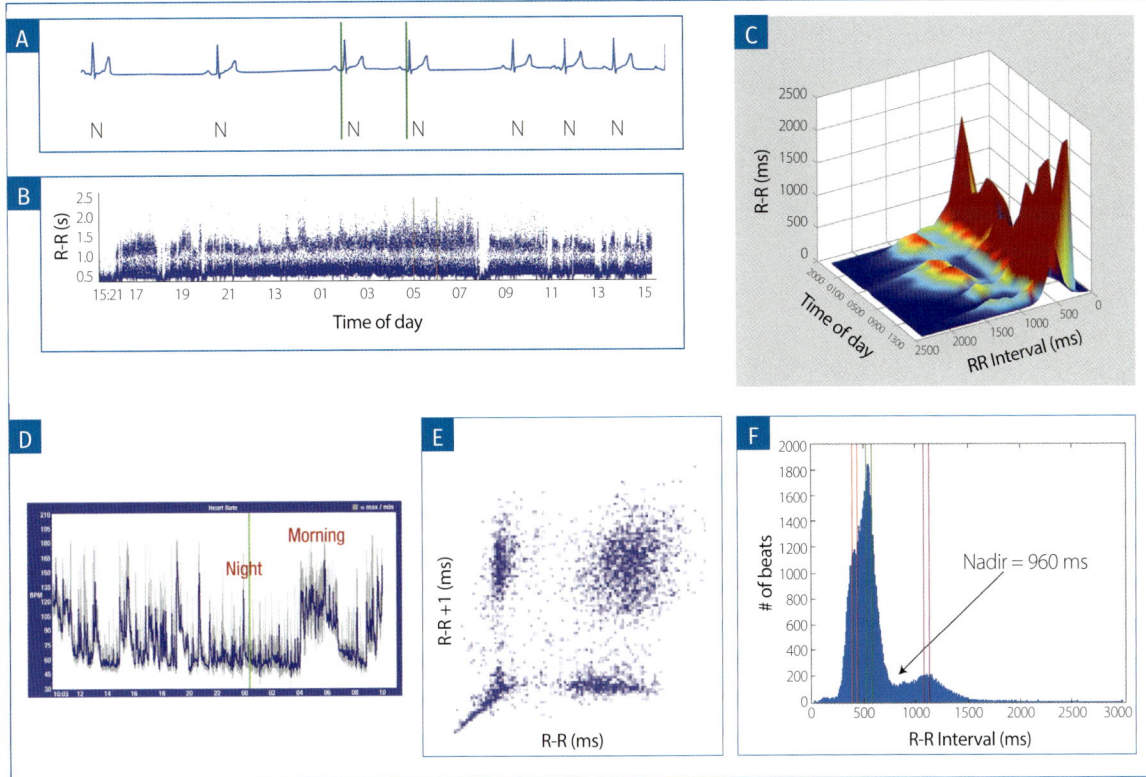

Figure 4.4. Representations of heart rate variability with geometric methods.
Each of these images is the result of an analysis of 24-hour Holter recordings from dogs.
A) Electrocardiogram showing the variability in the R-R interval during sleep in a normal Boxer.
B) Two-dimensional tachogram from a normal Boxer. The time of day is on the X-axis and the R-R interval (ms) is on the Y-axis. This two-dimensional representation of the R-R interval is a time series that is created when each interval is represented by a blue dot as they occur over time. Because a dog normally has more than 100,000 heart beats in a 24-hour period, such a compressed image results in similar intervals overlapping in the two-dimensional plot. A paucity of dots can be appreciated in the region of approximately 800-950 ms because of the low density of beats that occur at this approximate interval. In the compressed view this appears as a band of white/less blue. This area has been called the "zone of avoidance" of sinus beats. In this tachogram the R-R interval is seen to shorten at approximately 8 a.m. (08:00 hours), the time when the dog woke up. Other areas of faster heart rate can be appreciated as well. Longer R-R intervals occur during sleep. A two-dimensional tachogram does not fully represent the number of beats for a given R-R interval. However, tachograms created from much shorter time intervals can enable individual dots to be appreciated.
C) A three-dimensional tachogram from a normal Boxer gives a better representation of the beat density (number of beats at a particular time). Note that the density of R-R intervals is greatest between approximately 450 and 750 ms.
D) The heart rate tachogram is a time series representing the heart rate throughout the 24-hour period. The denser blue line represents a running average every 8 beats while the gray represents the minimum and maximum rate. Most dogs have slower heart rates during the night.
E) A Poincaré plot (Lorenz plot) represents the beat-to-beat variability of the R-R intervals in a given time period. For most Holter analysis systems if this geometric representation of heart rate variability is available, it is done for a selected hour. An R-R interval is plotted on the X-axis and the R-R interval is plotted on the Y axis. There is overlap such that the last R-R+1 becomes the R-R and is plotted against the following R-R interval (R-R+1). The beat-to-beat overlap continues throughout the plotting window. The dog has a unique pattern because of its inherently high vagal tone. There is a paucity of intervals in the center of the plot; this corresponds to the "zone of avoidance" seen in the tachogram. Variation in this region is common with different patterns.
F) A R-R interval histogram indicates the number of beats for a given R-R interval. A non-singular Gaussian distribution is appreciated.

Chapter 4. Normal sinus rhythms

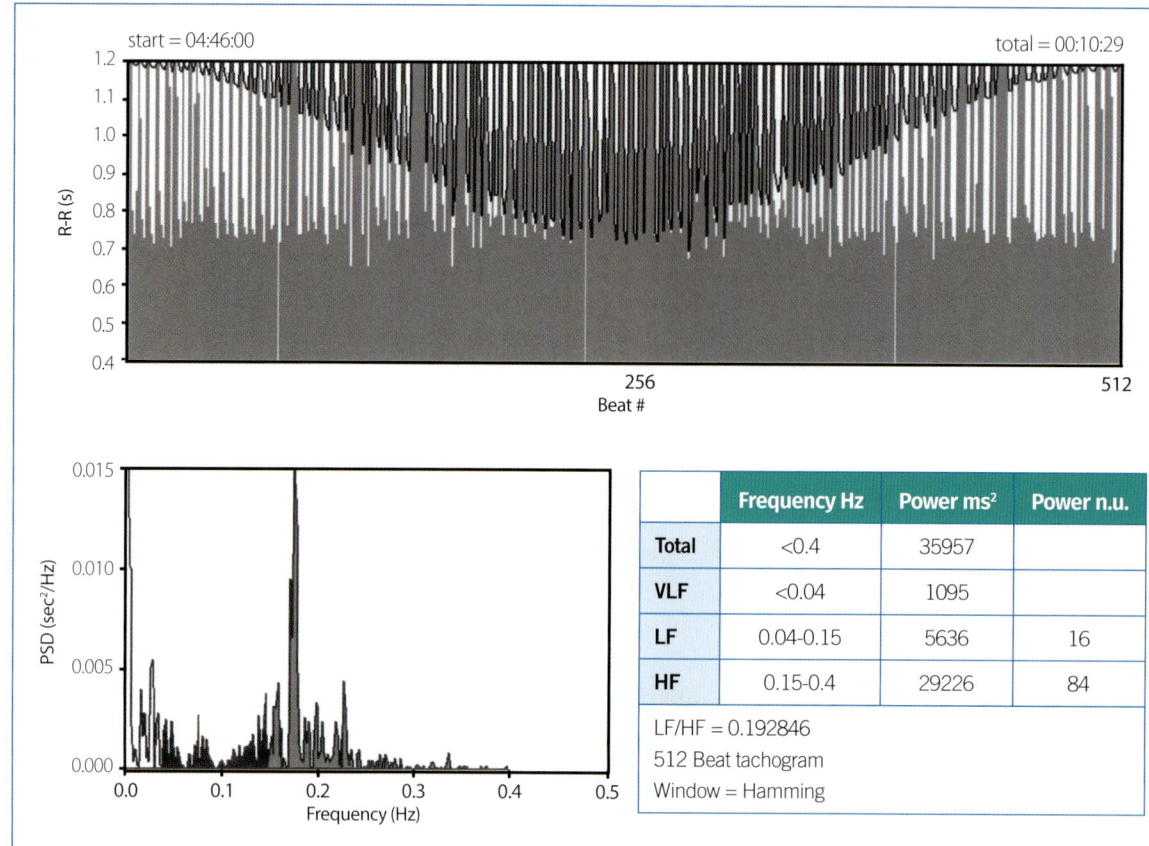

Figure 4.5. Frequency domain heart rate variability from a selected area on a 24-hour electrocardiographic recording. An example frequency domain shows the power density within certain ranges of frequency from very low to high frequency. When performing frequency domain analysis a time period (e.g. 5 minutes) or a number of beats (n = 512) is selected. Autonomic tone can be assessed based on the values at the different frequency levels. In this example the total power and frequency are high indicating a period of high vagal tone. Importantly, the indexed values show a high proportion in the high-frequency zone.

At times the wandering pacemaker seems to have a more extensive course of migration or exit to discharge the atrium. This has been termed a *sinus node-atrioventricular junction wandering pacemaker* (Fig. 4.2). With this type of wandering pacemaker the dominant pacemaker moves progressively from the sinus node to the pacemakers of the atrioventricular junction (during increases in parasympathetic tone). The P wave varies in polarity from positive to negative in lead II passing through intermediate forms, but always remaining positive, biphasic or isodiphasic in lead I. The P waves that result from impulses originating from the atrioventricular junction are negative and may actually have a shorter PQ interval.

With a wandering pacemaker the variation in P wave morphology makes it difficult to know how to perform measurements that are meaningful. In general, it should be assumed that the largest (greatest amplitude and greatest width) P wave should be within the normal limits (amplitude <0.4 mV, width <40 ms).

In the majority of normal dogs the PQ interval is constant and of normal duration. In some dogs (geriatric or those with very high vagal tone) the PQ interval may vary and increase as the P-P interval lengthens. This is because the parasympathetic tone affects atrioventricular node conduction at the same time that it affects sinus node rate.

Sinus rhythms with other arrhythmias

Identification of sinus P waves can be very important in the interpretation of arrhythmias. The following are examples:

Marching out P-P intervals - A frequent aid to understanding an arrhythmia is to recognize associations between P waves and QRS complexes. Moreover, interpretation of an electrocardiogram always involves determining regular and irregular rhythms. The fixed P-P interval is moved across the recording to find hidden P waves to understand their relationship to QRS complexes. This can be helpful in cases of sinus rhythm, but the irregularities of the P-P interval that are normally present in the dog because of sinus arrhythmia can make specific diagnoses more difficult. Some of the rules proposed for the interpretation of arrhythmias in humans may not apply to dogs, although they may have some application in the assessment of rhythm in the cat.

Atrioventricular dissociation - During ventricular tachycardia the sinus node usually continues to discharge, and, therefore, a sinus P wave may be seen without an associated QRS complex when capture of the ventricles is interrupted by the premature ventricular complex. At times the sinus P waves may be hidden within the QRS complex of the ventricular beat. Atrioventricular dissociation also occurs during third-degree atrioventricular heart block and sinus P waves may be seen between or within the escape complexes. In the case of focal junctional tachycardia, sinus P waves can synchronize with the Hisian rhythm (see p. 149).

Ventriculo-phasic sinus arrhythmia - This a rhythm characterized by the presence of variations of the P-P intervals induced by ventricular systole. This arrhythmia may occur with second- and third-degree atrioventricular blocks. In this type of arrhythmia, the variations of the P-P intervals depend on the effect of the mechanical systole which, during the ejection phase, stimulates the aortic and carotid baroreceptors. Activation of these receptors causes a vagal stimulation that begins about 600 ms after the QRS complex and lasts approximately 1 s. During this time, the parasympathetic system depresses sinus automaticity, with prolongation of the P-P interval following ventricular systole. Conversely, the P wave immediately following the QRS complex occurs prior to the increase in parasympathetic tone induced by systole. Therefore, P-P intervals which include a QRS complex are shorter than P-P intervals that follow a QRS complex (Fig. 4.6).

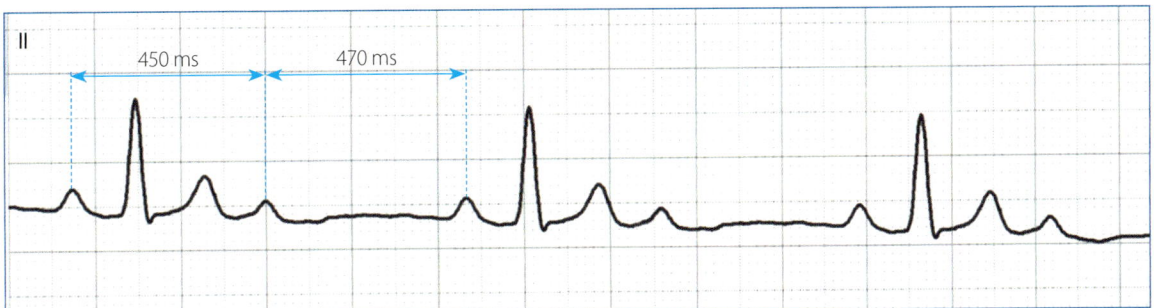

Figure 4.6. Ventriculo-phasic sinus arrhythmia during 2:1 second-degree atrioventricular block (Dog, Great Dane, male, 9 years. Lead II - speed 50 mm/s - calibration 10 mm/1 mV).
The dominant rhythm is sinus rhythm conducted with 2:1 second-degree atrioventricular block. Note the P-P intervals including a QRS complex are shorter (450 ms) than the P-P intervals not including a QRS complex (470 ms). These electrocardiographic findings are characteristic of ventriculo-phasic sinus arrhythmia (see text for explanations).

Suggested readings

1. Blacke RR, Shaw DJ, Culshaw GJ, et al. Poincaré plots as a measure of heart rate variability in healthy dogs. *J Vet Cardiol* 2018; 20:20-32.
2. Bollmann A, Hilbert S, John S, et al. Insights from preclinical ultra high-density electroanatomical sinus node mapping. *Europace* 2015; 17:489-494.
3. Chung EK. A reappraisal of ventriculophasic sinus arrhythmia. *Jpn Heart J* 1971; 12:401-404.
4. Fabry-Delaigue R, Duchene-Marullaz P, Lemaire P, Chambon M. Long-term observation of cardiac rhythm and automaticity in the dog after excision of the sinoatrial node. *J Electrocardiol* 1982; 15:209-219.
5. Furukawa Y, Takei M, Narita M, et al. Different sympathetic-parasympathetic interactions on sinus rate and atrioventricular conduction in dog hearts. *Eur J Pharmacol* 1997; 334:191-200.
6. Goldberg JM. Intra-SA-nodal pacemaker shifts induced by autonomic nerve stimulation in the dog. *Am J Physiol* 1975; 229:1116-1123.
7. Hamlin RL, Olsen I, Smith CR, et al. Clinical relevancy of heart rate in the dog. *J Am Vet Med Assoc* 1967; 151:60-63.
8. Hamlin RL, Smetzer DL, Smith CR. The electrocardiogram, phonocardiogram and derived ventricular activation process of domestic cats. *Am J Vet Res* 1960; 24:792-801.
9. Hamlin RL, Smith CR, Smetzer DL. Sinus arrhythmia in the dog. *Am J Physiol* 1966; 210:321-328.
10. Hanås S, Tidholm A, Egenvall A, et al. Twenty-four hour Holter monitoring of unsedated healthy cats in the home environment. *J Vet Cardiol* 2009; 11:17-22.
11. Hariman RJ, Hoffman BF, Naylor RE. Electrical activity from the sinus node region in conscious dogs. *Circ Res* 1980; 47:775-791.
12. Hezzell MJ, Humm K, Dennis SG, et al. Relationship between heart rate and age, bodyweight and breed in 10849 dogs. *J Small Anim Pract* 2013; 54:318-324.
13. Jackson BL1, Lehmkuhl LB2, Adin DB. Heart rate and arrhythmia frequency of normal cats compared to cats with asymptomatic hypertrophic cardiomyopathy. *J Vet Cardiol* 2014; 16:215-225.
14. Moise NS From cell to cageside: autonomic influences on cardiac rhythms in the dog. *J Small Anim Pract* 1998; 39:460-468.
15. Shykoff BE, Naqvi SS, Menon AS, et al. Respiratory sinus arrhythmia in dogs. Effects of phasic afferents and chemostimulation. *J Clin Invest* 1991; 87:1621-1627.
16. Wasmund SL, Pacchia CF, Page RL, et al. Mechanisms of sinus node cycle length changes during ventricular fibrillation. *Clin Auton Res* 2015; 25:399-406.
17. Yano K, Hayano M, Matsumoto Y. Sinus node function after selective elimination of sympathetic influences on the sinus node area of the dog. *Jpn Heart J* 1986; 27:71-81.
18. Yasuma F, Hayano J. Respiratory sinus arrhythmia: why does the heartbeat synchronize with respiratory rhythm? *Chest* 2004; 125:683-690.

CHAPTER 5

Chamber enlargement

In order to understand the electrocardiographic changes secondary to cardiac enlargement (chamber dilation or wall thickening), the model describing the heart as a dipole (see p. 21) and electrical currents (*wavefronts or forces*) of depolarization and repolarization as vectors is useful. Because the electrocardiogram is recorded from electrodes placed on the surface of the body, the deflections (or waveforms) that represent the summation of cardiac vectors are influenced by various factors, including the intensity of the electrical field generated by the cardiac dipole, the angle of intersection between the recording point and the axis of the vectors, the distance between the exploring electrode and the cardiac dipole, and the interaction of the electrical forces with the thoracic structures. It is also important to realize that the deflections and how they are displayed on the surface electrocardiogram are time-dependent such that delays in conduction time or concomitant depolarizations from different regions of the heart will be additive and affect the amplitude and morphology of the deflections. Considering the many factors that influence the electrocardiographic deflections, the electrocardiogram does not perform well for recognizing atrial and ventricular dilation or wall hypertrophy. The only structural changes of the heart detected by electrocardiography are those causing significant changes in direction and duration of the electrical current wavefront. Therefore, the sensitivity of the electrocardiogram for the detection of cardiac enlargement is low while the specificity is usually high.

Atrial enlargement

The P wave is the electrocardiographic representation of left and right atrial depolarization. Normally arising from the sinus node, the electrical wavefront of atrial depolarization travels first across the right atrial wall and then the left atrium. Although the summed vector corresponding to this depolarization wave is commonly represented in a two-dimensional image, the true atrial wave of depolarization propagates in a three-dimensional environment, and is more accurately described with at least three orthogonal leads. The resulting vector assumes a direction corresponding to the sequence of atrial activation, typically following a superior-to-inferior, anterior-to-posterior and right-to-left direction. The six-limb leads in the frontal plane are useful to describe the pattern of atrial depolarization. Normally the P wave has a positive deflection in the inferior leads (II, III and aVF), is positive, biphasic or isodiphasic in lead I and shows maximum negativity in aVR. Because the P wave is essentially always negative in aVR in normal dogs and cats, this lead can be used as a quick check to confirm the correct placement of the electrodes. However, measurements of the P wave amplitude and duration are usually performed using lead II. The duration of the P wave must be ≤40 ms in the dog (≤50 ms in giant breeds) and ≤35 ms in the cat, while the amplitude should be ≤0.4 mV in the dog and ≤0.2 mV in the cat. The ascending portion of the P wave is determined by right atrial depolarization and its descending portion by left atrial depolarization (Fig. 5.1A).

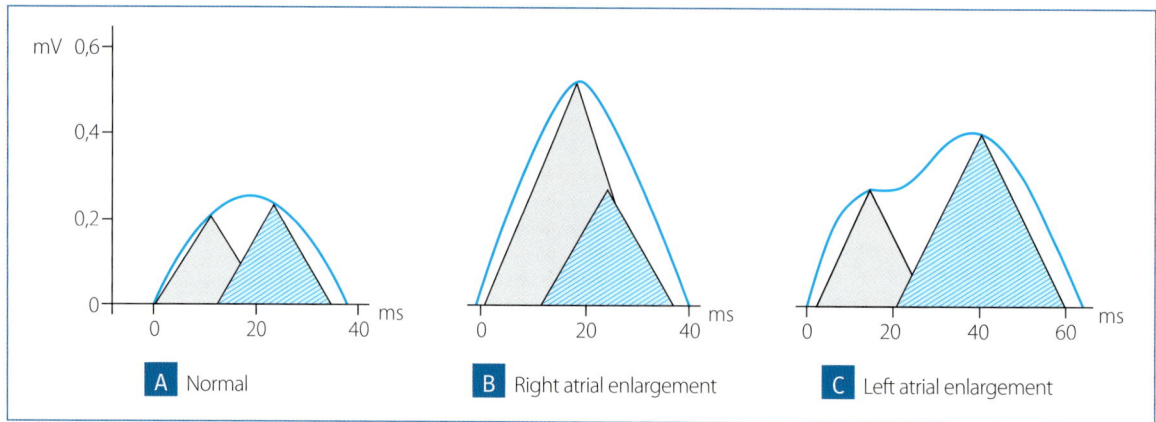

Figure 5.1. P wave components in lead II. A) In normal conditions, the ascending branch of the P wave is associated with activation of the right atrium (gray), and the descending branch with left atrial activation (blue). B) In the presence of right atrial enlargement, the component corresponding to right atrial activation has a larger magnitude and a prolonged duration, but it usually does not exceed the left atrial activation time. As a result, the P wave has increased amplitude and normal duration. C) In the presence of left atrial enlargement, the component of left atrial depolarization is delayed and its duration is increased. The P wave thus appears wider with a bifid (or bimodal) morphology.

The P wave amplitude is therefore more affected by the initial activation, attributable to the right atrial depolarization, while the P wave duration depends to a greater extent on the later activation of the left atrium. Importantly, however, marked right atrial enlargement can result in P wave prolongation. Overall, alterations in the P wave amplitude and duration are mostly the result of chamber dilation rather than wall thickening.

It is important to understand that in the dog the P wave morphology, particularly its amplitude, most often changes during respiratory sinus arrhythmia accompanying alterations in parasympathetic and sympathetic tone. The P wave amplitude in lead II is greater with shorter P-P intervals which are associated with higher sympathetic tone with inspiration; it is lower with longer P-P intervals which correspond to higher parasympathetic tone during expiration. However, if a sinus pause is prolonged because of a pronounced sinus arrhythmia the P wave after such a long pause may sometimes be taller in lead II. Indeed, a fairly long pause results in a drop in systemic blood pressure triggering activation of the baroreceptors and an increase in sympathetic tone. One effect of adrenergic stimulation is an increase in heart rate, but another effect is a shift of the exit pathway of the electrical impulse out of the sinus node. This exit pathway from the sinus node is more superior (closer to the cranial vena cava) and, therefore, the summed depolarization vector is directed in a more superior to inferior direction, in other words more towards the positive pole of lead II, increasing the amplitude of the P wave. It should also be mentioned that when dogs are given sympathomimetic or parasympatholytic drugs, the P wave amplitude increases. Additionally, the P wave amplitude will be greater if an electrocardiogram is recorded immediately after exercise. Conversely, with an increase in parasympathetic tone and a decrease in sympathetic tone the sinus node impulse shifts to an exit pathway from the sinus node that is more inferior. This results in a summed depolarization vector of the right and left atria that is more perpendicular to lead II, such that the amplitude of the P wave is decreased. With the changing P wave morphology (*wandering pacemaker*) and amplitude so commonly seen in the dog, which P wave should be measured? This question has not been answered.

Atrial repolarization (T_a wave; termed "T-sub-a") is represented by a deflection that is opposite in direction to the P wave but has a smaller amplitude. Atrial repolarization in the dog occurs within 140 ms after the onset of the P wave, and the interval from the onset of the P wave to the end of T_a is approximately 170 to 200 ms, although longer intervals have been reported during atrial pacing. T_a may, therefore, be seen within the PQ segment. The T_a wave is most evident when there is a delay in atrial repolarization due to a conduction disturbance or chamber enlargement; however, it may be seen in normal dogs depending upon the lead examined or the dog breed (e.g. it is commonly seen in Beagles). T_a waves may also be more evident with atrioventricular nodal block or during supraventricular tachycardias with varied atrioventricular conduction that result in P waves without QRS complexes (Fig. 5.2).

Right atrial enlargement

Right atrial enlargement is characterized by an increased amplitude of the P wave. The duration of right atrial depolarization may not be appreciated because it overlaps with left atrial depolarization. In extreme right atrial enlargement and conduction disturbances the P wave can be prolonged (Fig. 5.1B).

Right atrial enlargement is secondary to diseases that cause an increase in volume or pressure of the right atrial chamber (e.g. tricuspid regurgitation, atrial septal defect); or in cases of chronic airway and pulmonary diseases.

The diagnostic criteria for right atrial enlargement are: P waves with a sinus axis, peaked morphology and amplitude greater than 0.4 mV in dogs and greater than 0.2 mV in cats in lead II; T_a wave appearance identifiable as a depression of the PQ segment, the J point and the ST segment in the inferior leads (II, III and aVF) (Fig. 5.3). A P wave amplitude greater than 0.4 mV may be found in some breeds (e.g. Greyhound) in the absence of atrial enlargement.

Figure 5.2. Electrocardiographic representation of atrial repolarization (dashed blue line). Atrial repolarization, represented by a T_a wave on the electrocardiogram, is rarely visible because it has a small amplitude and is typically buried within the QRS complex.

Left atrial enlargement

Left atrial enlargement is likely to result in a prolongation of left atrial depolarization (*P mitrale*), which causes an increase in the width (duration) of the P wave (Fig. 5.1C).

Left atrial enlargement can develop because of pressure overload (e.g. mitral regurgitation, atrial septal defect in the presence of elevated right heart pressures, ventricular septal defects, patent ductus arteriosus).

The diagnostic criteria for left atrial enlargement are: P waves with a sinus axis and bifid (or bimodal) morphology in the inferior leads (II, III and aVF) and a duration greater than 40 ms in dogs (greater than

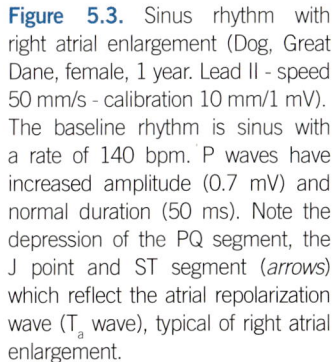

Figure 5.3. Sinus rhythm with right atrial enlargement (Dog, Great Dane, female, 1 year. Lead II - speed 50 mm/s - calibration 10 mm/1 mV). The baseline rhythm is sinus with a rate of 140 bpm. P waves have increased amplitude (0.7 mV) and normal duration (50 ms). Note the depression of the PQ segment, the J point and ST segment (*arrows*) which reflect the atrial repolarization wave (T_a wave), typical of right atrial enlargement.

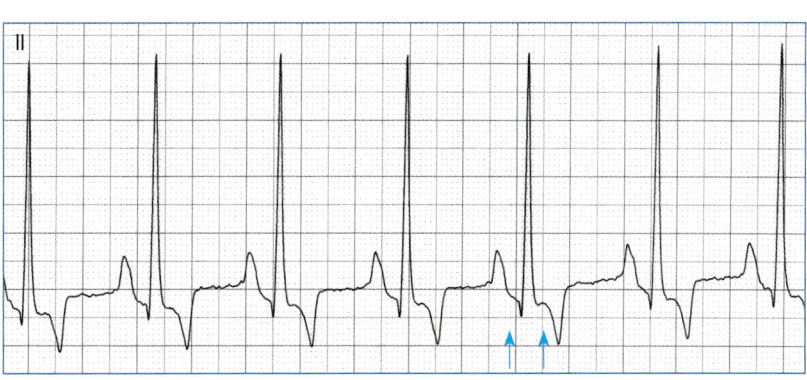

50 ms in giant breeds) and greater than 35 ms in cats (Figs. 5.1C and 5.4). A bifid P wave that is not prolonged should not be considered diagnostic of left atrial enlargement. It is important to re-emphasize that, although a markedly prolonged P wave duration is a specific marker of left atrial enlargement, its sensitivity remains low (many dogs with a markedly enlarged left atrium on an echocardiogram have a normal P wave duration on the electrocardiogram). Intra-atrial conduction delays caused by fibrosis, anoxia or myocarditis can cause bifid or bimodal P wave morphology without the coexistence of left atrial enlargement. Age is also a factor that affects P wave morphology, with duration being increased in older animals.

Biatrial enlargement

Biatrial enlargement, usually associated with chronic mitral and tricuspid valve disease, results in prolongation of left and right atrial depolarization.

The diagnostic criteria for biatrial enlargement are: P waves with a sinus axis, a duration greater than 40 ms in dogs (greater than 50 ms in giant breeds) and greater than 35 ms in cats, an amplitude greater than 0.4 mV in dogs and greater than 0.2 mV in cats and, often, with bifid morphology in the inferior leads (II, III and aVF) (Fig. 5.5).

Ventricular enlargement

The electrocardiogram cannot distinguish an increase in myocardial mass caused by an increase in ventricular wall thickness (concentric hypertrophy) from that caused by dilation (eccentric hypertrophy). Additional diagnostics (e.g. echocardiography) are required for this discrimination.

Right ventricular enlargement

Ventricular depolarization includes the propagation of the electrical wavefront in the interventricular septum, the right ventricle and the left ventricle, and can be represented by three vectors (see p. 43). In the presence of severe right ventricular enlargement, the initial vector of depolarization which corresponds to the interventricular septum is unchanged; the second vector is of greater magnitude than the third vector, and

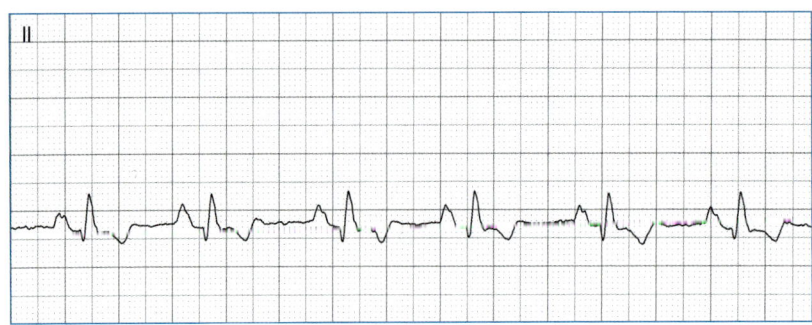

Figure 5.4. Sinus rhythm with left atrial enlargement (Dog, Doberman, male, 9 years. Lead II - speed 50 mm/s - calibration 10 mm/1 mV). The baseline rhythm is sinus with a rate of 120 bpm. P waves are increased in duration (60 ms) with a bifid (or bimodal) appearance, typical of left atrial enlargement.

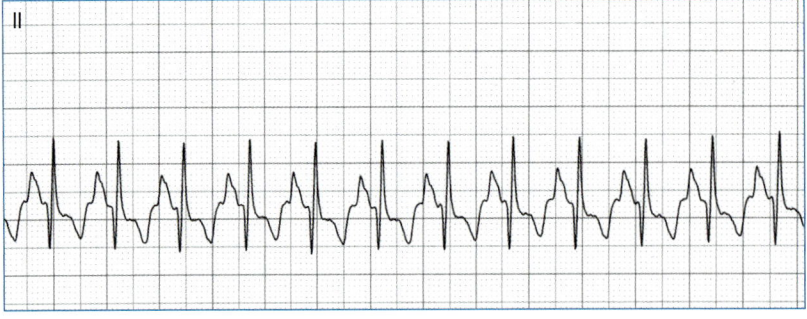

Figure 5.5. Sinus rhythm with biatrial enlargement (Dog, mixed breed, female, 1 year. Lead II - speed 50 mm/s - calibration 10 mm/1 mV).
The baseline rhythm is sinus tachycardia with a rate of 260 bpm. P waves have increased duration and amplitude (50 ms; 0.6 mV) and a bifid appearance, typical of biatrial enlargement.

oriented in an inferior-to-superior, left-to-right and posterior-to-anterior direction.

Electrocardiographic evidence of right ventricular enlargement can be identified with right-sided pressure or volume overload. Examples of conditions causing pressure overload include pulmonic stenosis, tetralogy of Fallot, right-to-left shunting patent ductus arteriosus, ventricular septal defect with Eisenmenger's syndrome, heartworm disease, pulmonary hypertension, and thromboembolism. An example of conditions causing volume overload is tricuspid regurgitation. Rarely, chronic lung disease or severe cardiomyopathy produce electrocardiographic evidence of right ventricular enlargement.

The electrocardiographic criteria of right ventricular enlargement in dogs are: normal QRS complex duration (<70 ms in dogs and <40 ms in cats), S waves in leads I (greater than 0.05 mV), II (greater than 0.35 mV), V_2 (greater than 0.80 mV) and V_4 (greater than 0.70 mV); Q waves in aVR (greater than 0.30 mV); an R/S ratio <0.87 in lead V_4; the algebraic sum of the QRS complex greater than −0.20 mV in lead I; and a positive T wave in lead I (greater than 0.25 mV). The mean electrical axis of the QRS complex in the frontal plane is shifted clockwise between +100 ° and −80 °, in the horizontal plane it is shifted clockwise between +105 ° and −31 °, and in the sagittal plane it is shifted clockwise between +91 ° and −12 °. Approximately 90 % to 95 % of electrocardiograms from dogs with right ventricular enlargement fulfill three or more of the above criteria. The rate of false positives is approximately 7 %. In approximately 80 % of dogs with severe right ventricular enlargement, there is a deep S wave in one of the precordial leads combined with a right axis deviation in the frontal plane (clockwise shift of the vector beyond +100 °). A deep S wave in leads II and aVF is only found in 40 % of dogs with severe right ventricular enlargement. Rarely, dogs with right ventricular enlargement have deep Q waves in leads I, II, III and aVF (Box 5.1).

The electrocardiographic criteria of right ventricular enlargement in cats are: normal QRS complex duration (≤40 ms); deep S waves in leads I, II, III, aVF, V_2 and V_4; and an axis deviation of the QRS complex in the frontal plane to the right (Box 5.2).

Left ventricular enlargement

The first (septal activation) and second (right ventricular activation) vectors are not affected by *left ventricular enlargement*. However, there is an increase in the magnitude of the third vector without a change in its orientation. The duration of ventricular depolarization is frequently increased but this cannot be distinguished from prolonged depolarization secondary to a left intraventricular conduction delay.

Electrocardiographic signs of left ventricular enlargement can be recognized with left-sided volume or pressure overload. Diseases leading to volume overload include chronic mitral valve disease, aortic insufficiency, patent ductus arteriosus with left-right shunt and an arteriovenous fistula. Diseases associated with left-sided pressure overload include sub-aortic stenosis or systemic hypertension. Finally, cardiomyopathies and systemic diseases leading to an increase in cardiac output (hyperthyroidism, chronic anemia) can create electrocardiographic signs of left ventricular enlargement.

The electrocardiographic features of left ventricular enlargement in dogs are not very sensitive and include: a minimal increase in the duration of the QRS complex (greater than 70 ms); an increase in R wave amplitude greater than 3 mV in leads II, aVF, V_2 and V_4; a R wave amplitude greater than 0.5 mV in lead I. Approximately 60 % of electrocardiograms from dogs with left ventricular enlargement fulfill two or more of the above-mentioned criteria. The rate of false positive results is approximately 7 % (electrocardiographic signs of left ventricular enlargement in the absence of structural changes). In approximately 10 % of dogs with left ventricular enlargement, the QRS complex displays a moderate left axis deviation. Other changes in the morphology of the QRS complex include notches and a decrease in the slope of the descending branch of the R wave (*slurring*), or prolonged R-peak time (also called intrinsicoid deflection). Deep negative T waves may be present. On occasion the ST segment is deviated in the opposite direction of the largest deflection of the QRS complex in leads I, II, III, aVF and V_{10} (Box 5.3).

The electrocardiographic criteria for left ventricular enlargement in cats include: an R wave in lead II greater than 0.9 mV; an R wave greater than 1 mV in leads V_2 and V_4; and a QRS complex with a duration greater than 40 ms (Box 5.4).

Chapter 5. Chamber enlargement

BOX 5.1.
RIGHT VENTRICULAR ENLARGEMENT IN DOGS

HEART RATE: depends on the sinus node firing rate.
R-R INTERVAL: depends on the regularity of the sinus node pacemaker.
P WAVE: present, sinus axis.
ATRIOVENTRICULAR CONDUCTION: present.
PQ INTERVAL: normal.

QRS COMPLEX: normal duration (≤70 ms); S waves in leads I (>0.05 mV), II (>0.35 mV), V_2 (>0.80 mV) and V_4 (>0.70 mV); Q waves in aVR (>0.30 mV); R/S ratio ≤0.87 in lead V_4; algebraic sum of QRS complex >−0.20 mV in lead I; mean electrical axis of the QRS complex in the frontal plane shifted clockwise between +100° and −80°.
VENTRICULO-ATRIAL CONDUCTION: absent.
BLOCKED BEATS: none.

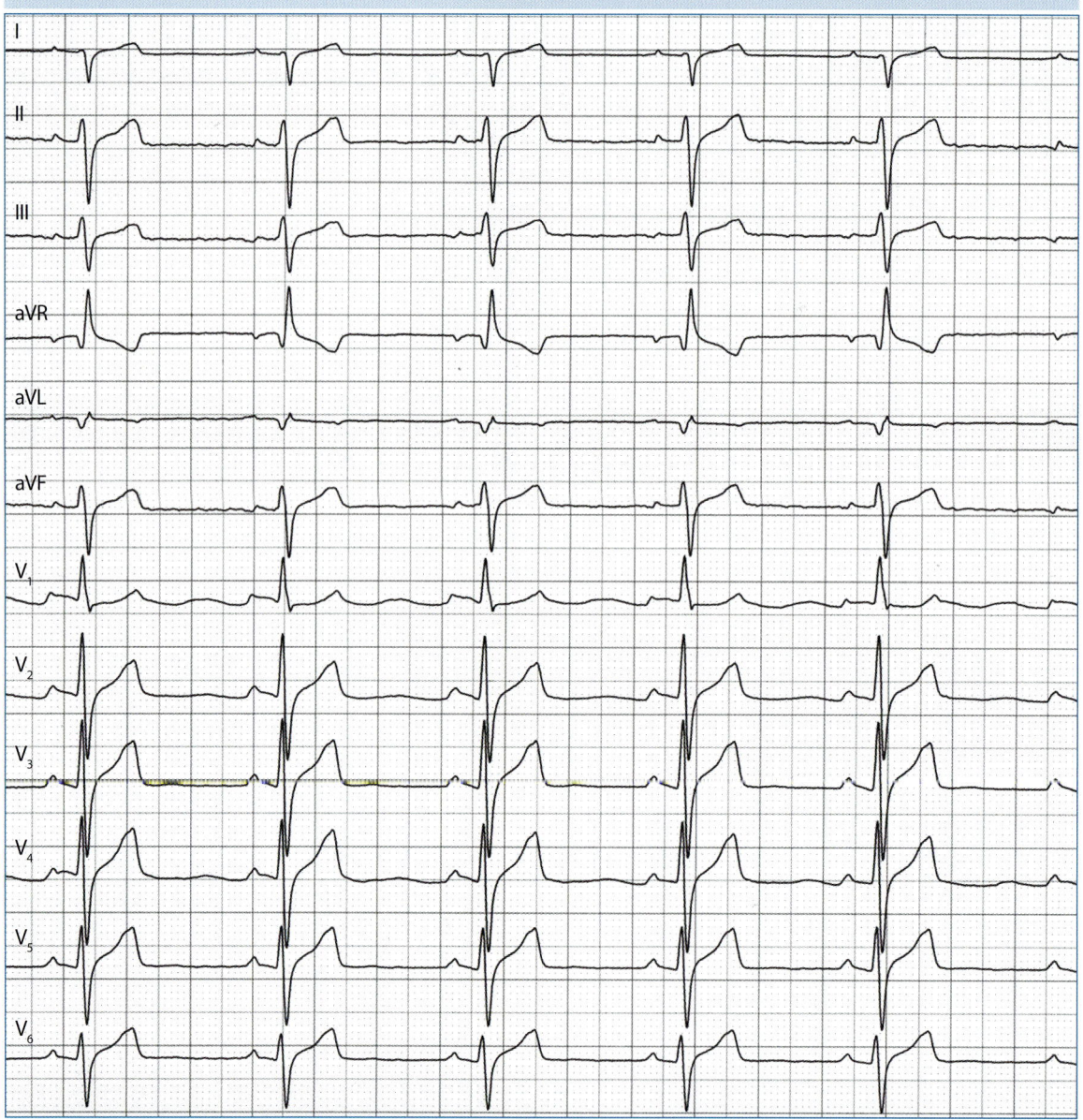

Dog, West Highland White Terrier, male, 3 years.
Twelve leads (I, II, III, aVR, aVL, aVF, V_1, V_2, V_3, V_4, V_5, V_6) - speed 50 mm/s - calibration 5 mm/1 mV.

Notes: sinus rhythm with a rate of 100 bpm and right ventricular enlargement. The QRS complex has a normal duration (60 ms) with deep S waves in the inferior leads (II, III, aVF) and a mean electrical axis in the frontal plane of −135°.

BOX 5.2.
RIGHT VENTRICULAR ENLARGEMENT IN CATS

HEART RATE: depends on the sinus node firing rate.
R-R INTERVAL: depends on the regularity of the sinus node pacemaker.
P WAVE: present, sinus axis.
ATRIOVENTRICULAR CONDUCTION: present.
PQ INTERVAL: normal.

QRS COMPLEX: normal duration (<40 ms); deep S waves in leads I, II, III, aVF, V_2 and V_4; mean electrical axis of the QRS complex in the frontal plane shifted clockwise between +160° and −80°.
VENTRICULO-ATRIAL CONDUCTION: absent.
BLOCKED BEATS: none.

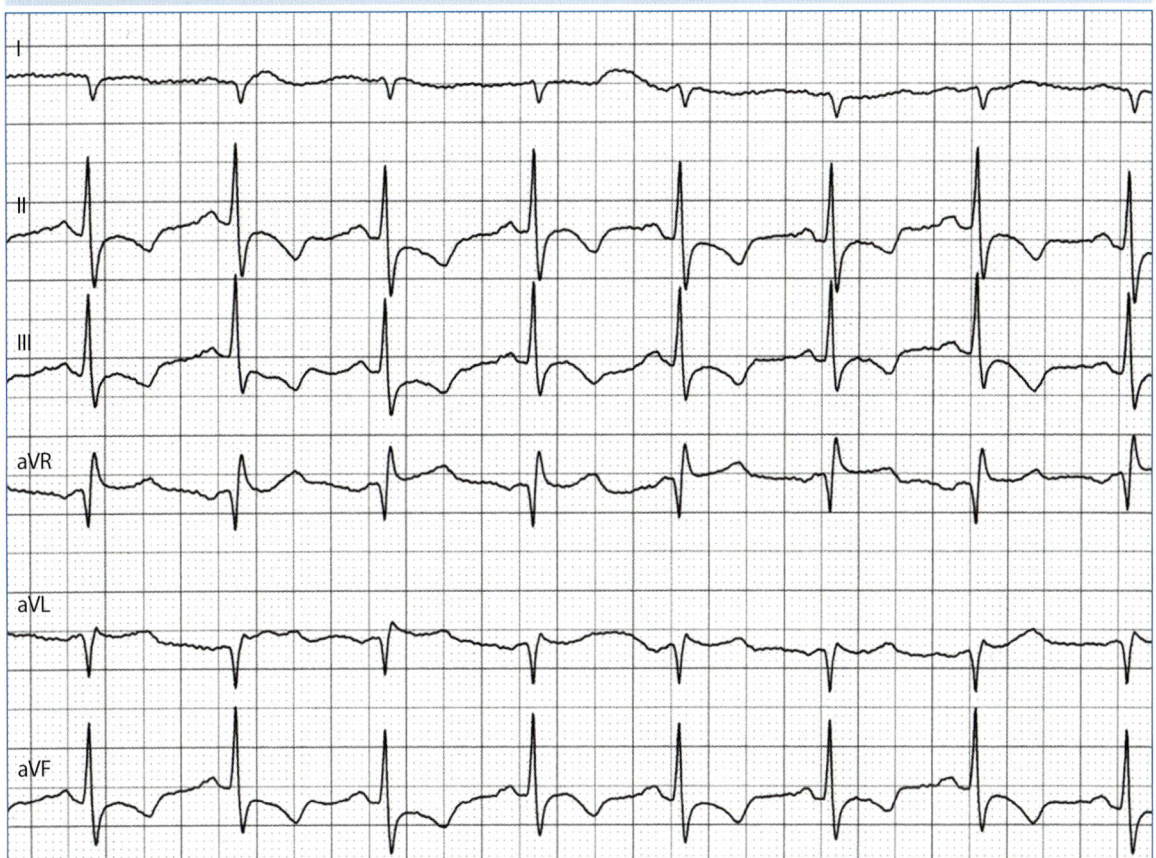

Cat, female, 13 years.
Six limb leads (I, II, III, aVR, aVL, aVF) - speed 50 mm/s - calibration 10 mm/1 mV.

Notes: sinus rhythm with a rate of 160 bpm with right ventricular enlargement. The QRS complex has a normal duration (40 ms) with deep S waves in the inferior leads (II, III, aVF) and a mean electrical axis in the frontal plane of +160°.

BOX 5.3.
LEFT VENTRICULAR ENLARGEMENT IN DOGS

HEART RATE: depends on the sinus node firing rate.
R-R INTERVAL: depends on the regularity of the sinus node pacemaker.
P WAVE: present, sinus axis.
ATRIOVENTRICULAR CONDUCTION: present.
PQ INTERVAL: normal.

QRS COMPLEX: increased duration (>70 ms); R waves in leads II, aVF, V_2 and V_4 >3 mV; R wave >0.5 mV in lead I; notching or slurring of the descending branch of the QRS complex. Delayed intrinsicoid deflection.
VENTRICULO-ATRIAL CONDUCTION: absent.
BLOCKED BEATS: none.

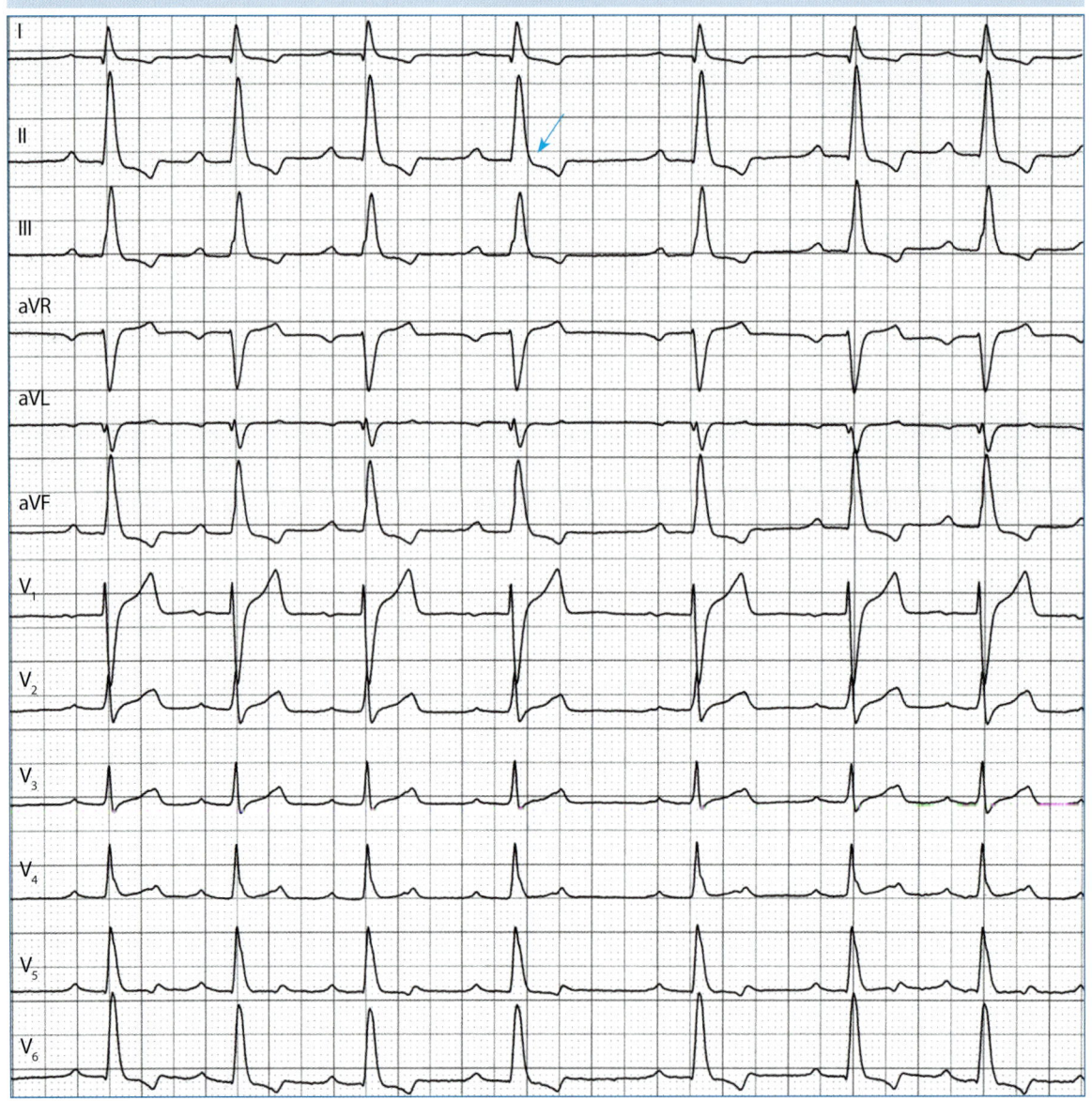

Dog, Jack Russell, male, 11 years.
Twelve leads (I, II, III, aVR, aVL, aVF, V_1, V_2, V_3, V_4, V_5, V_6) - speed 50 mm/s - calibration 5 mm/1 mV.

Notes: sinus rhythm with a rate of 140 bpm with left ventricular enlargement. The QRS complex has a normal morphology with an increased duration (75 ms) and mean electrical axis in the frontal plane of +66°. The slope of the descending portion of the R wave is decreased (slurring) (arrow).

Ventricular enlargement

BOX 5.4.
LEFT VENTRICULAR ENLARGEMENT IN CATS

HEART RATE: depends on the sinus node firing rate.
R-R INTERVAL: depends on the regularity of the sinus node pacemaker.
P WAVE: present, sinus axis.
ATRIOVENTRICULAR CONDUCTION: present.

PQ INTERVAL: normal.
QRS COMPLEX: increased duration (>40 ms); R wave >0.9 mV in lead II; R wave >1 mV in leads V_2 and V_4.
VENTRICULO-ATRIAL CONDUCTION: absent.
BLOCKED BEATS: none.

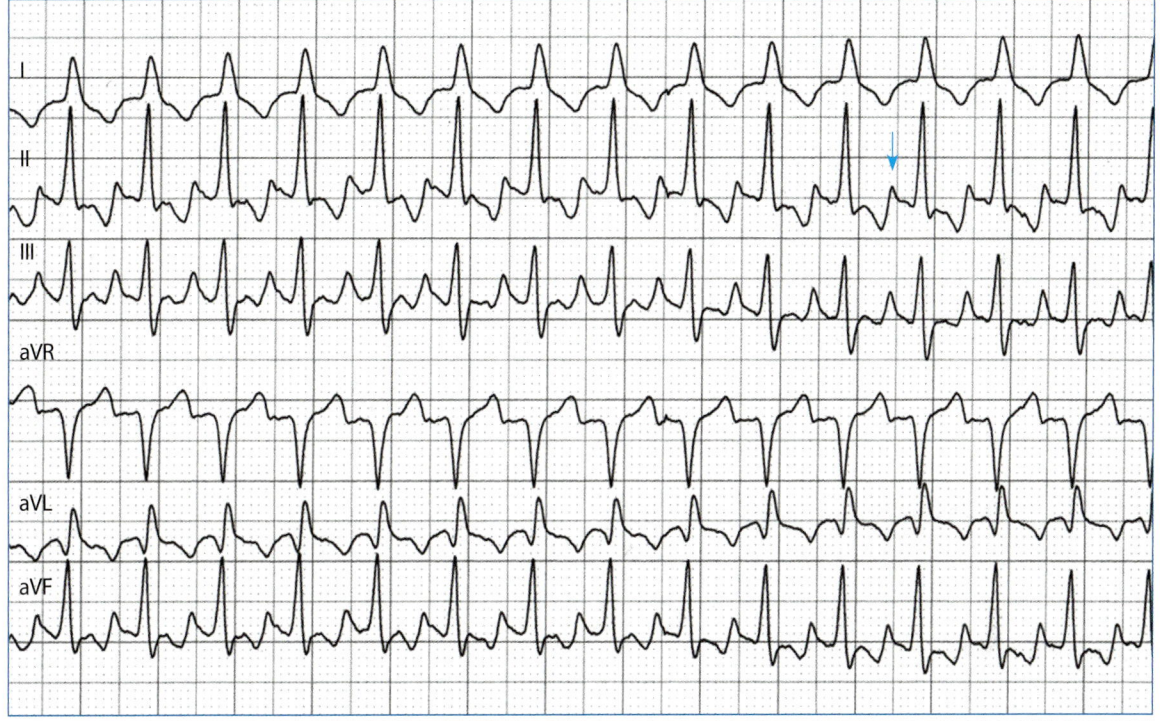

Cat, Persian, male, 9 years old.
Six limb leads (I, II, III, aVR, aVL, aVF) - speed 50 mm/s - calibration 10 mm/1 mV.

Notes: sinus tachycardia with a frequency of 300 bpm with left ventricular enlargement. The QRS complex has a normal morphology with increased duration and amplitude (50 ms; 1.2 mV) and the electrical axis is +70° in the frontal plane. Because of the high atrial rate, sinus P waves are inscribed in the preceding T wave (arrow).

Suggested readings

1. Boineau JP, Hill JD, Spach MS, et al. Basis of the electrocardiogram in right ventricular hypertrophy. Relationship between ventricular depolarization and body surface potentials in dogs with spontaneous RVH-contrasted with normal dogs. *Am Heart J* 1968; 76:605-627.
2. Brown FK, Brown WJ Jr, Ellison RG, et al. Electrocardiographic changes during development of right ventricular hypertrophy in the dog. *Am J Cardiol* 1968; 21:223-231.
3. Burwash IG, Morgan DE, Koilpillai CJ, et al. Sympathetic stimulation alters left ventricular relaxation and chamber size. *Am J Physiol* 1993; 264:R1-7.
4. Calvert CA, Losonsky JM, Brown J, et al. Comparison of radiographic and electrocardiographic abnormalities in canine heartworm disease. *Vet Radiol* 1986; 27:2-7.
5. Chen K. Reevaluation and revision of electrocardiographic criteria for the diagnosis of left ventricular hypertrophy in dogs. *J Chinese Vet Soc* 1988; 14:359-370.
6. Constable PD, Hinchcliff KW, Olson J, et al. Athletic heart syndrome in dogs competing in a long-distance sled race. *J Appl Physiol* 1994; 76:433-438.
7. Hamlin RL. Electrocardiographic detection of ventricular enlargement in the dog. *J Am Vet Med Assoc* 1968; 153:1461-1469.
8. Hill JD. Electrocardiographic diagnosis of right ventricular enlargement in dogs. *J Electrocardiol* 1971; 4:347-357.
9. Lombard CW, Spencer CP. Correlation of radiographic, echocardiographic, and electrocardiographic signs of left heart enlargement in dogs with mitral regurgitation. *Vet Radiol* 1985; 26:89-97.
10. Moise NS, Dietze AE, Mezza LE, et al. Echocardiography, electrocardiography, and radiography of cats with dilatation cardiomyopathy, hypertrophic cardiomyopathy, and hyperthyroidism. *Am J Vet Res* 1986; 47:1476-1486.
11. O'Grady M, DiFruscia R, Carley B, et al. Electrocardiographic evaluation of chamber enlargement. *Can Vet J* 1992; 33:195-200.
12. Perego M, Skert S, Santilli RA. Analysis of the atrial repolarization wave in dogs with third-degree atrioventricular block. *Am J Vet Res* 2014; 75:54-58.
13. Savarino P, Borgarelli M, Tarducci A, et al. Diagnostic performance of P wave duration in the identification of left atrial enlargement in dogs. *J Small Anim Pract* 2012; 53:267-272.
14. Scott CC, Leier CV, Kilman JW, et al. The effect of left atrial histology and dimension on P wave morphology. *J Electrocardiol* 1983; 16:363-366.
15. Stepien RL, Stepien RL, Hinchcliff KW, et al. Effect of endurance training on cardiac morphology in Alaskan sled dog. *J Appl Physiol* 1998; 85:1368-1375.
16. Rawlings CA, Lewis RE. Right ventricular enlargement in heartworm disease. *Am J Vet Res* 1977; 38:1801-1805.
17. Schober KE, Maerz I, Ludewig E, et al. Diagnostic accuracy of electrocardiography and thoracic radiography in the assessment of left atrial size in cats: comparison with transthoracic 2-dimensional echocardiography. *J Vet Intern Med* 2007; 21:709-718.
18. Trautvetter E, Detweiler DK, Bohn FK, et al. Evolution of the electrocardiogram in young dogs with congenital heart disease leading to right ventricular hypertrophy. *J Electrocardiol* 1981; 14:2752-2782.
19. Tsumoto S, Kawashima S, Iwasaki T. Unaltered size of right ventricular infarct in dogs with right ventricular hypertrophy induced by pressure overload. *Am J Physiol* 1995; 268:1781-1787.
20. Warman S, Perason G, Barrett E, et al. Dilatation of the right atrium in a dog with polymyositis and myocarditis. *J Small Anim Pract* 2008; 49:302-305.

Background to the diagnosis of arrhythmias

The diagnosis and treatment of cardiac arrhythmias is often complex and multifaceted. Background knowledge, observational skills, deductive reasoning, understanding consequences and appropriate diagnostics collectively contribute to unravelling the diagnosis and better managing the treatment. This chapter will highlight the following to improve the likelihood of an accurate diagnosis and treatment success:

- mechanisms underlying the initiation and perpetuation of arrhythmias (including the substrate and triggers),
- classification of arrhythmias (based on their site of origin, rate and patterning),
- haemodynamic consequences of arrhythmias (clinical signs, arrhythmic cardiomyopathy, sudden death),
- diagnostic tools for the identification of arrhythmias (short-term monitoring, event-triggered, long-term monitoring),
- finally, a stepwise approach to the interpretation of the electrocardiogram; this provides the opportunity to hypothesize on the mechanism of the arrhythmia, classify its origin better, recognize its systemic impact and decide whether further electrocardiographic diagnostic tools are required.

Mechanisms of arrhythmias

The arrhythmogenic mechanisms responsible for the initiation and perpetuation of tachycardias, conduction abnormalities and bradyarrhythmias are divided into abnormalities of (Table 6.1):
- impulse formation,
- impulse conduction, and
- impulse formation and conduction.

TABLE 6.1. Description of tachycardia type, arrhythmogenic mechanisms, site of origin of automatic focus, triggered activities and anatomical or functional reentry.

Tachycardia	Mechanism	Site
Sinus tachycardia	Enhanced normal automaticity	Sinus node
Focal atrial tachycardia	Abnormal automaticity Triggered activities	Atrial myocardium and tributary veins Atrial myocardium and tributary veins
Atrial flutter	Anatomical reentry	Right atrium
Atrial fibrillation	Functional reentry	Atrial myocardium and tributary veins
Atrioventricular reciprocating tachycardias	Anatomical reentry	Atrial and ventricular myocardium, AV node and Purkinje system and accessory pathway
Focal and non-paroxysmal junctional tachycardia	Enhanced normal automaticity	Atrioventricular node and His bundle
Accelerated idioventricular rhythm	Enhanced normal automaticity	Purkinje fibers
Monomorphic ventricular tachycardia	Anatomical reentry	Ventricular myocardium and/or arteries
Polymorphic ventricular tachycardia	Triggered activities	Ventricular myocardium or Purkinje fibers

It must be emphasized that it is usually not possible to characterize the electrophysiological substrate of arrhythmias precisely from analysis of the surface electrocardiogram. Importantly, an arrhythmia can be initiated by one mechanism and perpetuated by a different one. Rhythm patterns on a 24-hour Holter recording and data from intracardiac mapping studies can provide additional clues to further elucidate the mechanism causing the arrhythmia.

Abnormalities of impulse formation: automaticity and triggered activity

Normal and abnormal automaticity

Automaticity is the ability of a myocyte to generate an action potential spontaneously. In cells that have the property of automaticity, the membrane potential progressively depolarizes during the diastolic interval (phase 4 of the action potential) until the threshold potential is reached leading to the initiation of an action potential (phase 0). Normal automaticity is a characteristic of the pacemaker cells of the sinus node, the atrioventricular junction, and cells of the His-Purkinje system.

Disorders of impulse formation include:
- depression of normal automaticity,
- enhanced normal automaticity,
- abnormal automaticity, and
- triggered activity.

Depression of normal automaticity

Under normal conditions, the depolarization rate of the sinus P cells is usually faster than that of all other pacemaker cells within the atrioventricular junction and the His-Purkinje system, and for this reason it is called the "dominant pacemaker" of the heart. The faster rate of the sinus node inhibits the depolarization of other atrial pacemaker cells and with normal conduction through the atrioventricular node for depolarization of the ventricle, the ventricular pacemaker cells are suppressed. The suppression of the subsidiary pacemakers is known as *overdrive suppression* (see p. 15). In brief, overdrive suppression of subsidiary pacemaker cells is caused by hyperpolarization (more negative resting membrane potential). A cell is driven to this more negative potential because of enhanced activity of the sodium-potassium exchange pump. This pump is enhanced because, with faster rates, more sodium enters the cell. However, once activated the exchange pump creates a net positive loss from the cell as more sodium is moved out of the cell than potassium enters. Consequently, the latent pacemaker must depolarize further to reach the threshold for activation. With normal automaticity of the sinus node, the rate of spontaneous depolarization is strongly influenced by autonomic tone. In the presence of autonomic blockade, the inherent sinus node discharge rate of the dog is 90 to 100 bpm. During periods of high vagal tone, sinus rate can typically decrease to 30 or 40 bpm, and it can reach 250 bpm in response to adrenergic stimulation. The rate of sinus node depolarization that corresponds to a normal sinus rhythm on the electrocardiogram of awake dogs in the hospital environment is not usually lower than 60 bpm. The upper limit of what is considered normal depends on the underlying demeanor of the dog or cat and the current stress of the situation. Additionally, it depends on age. Under the circumstances of having an electrocardiogram performed in hospital, the dog will most often still have a sinus arrhythmia detected because of the strong influence of the parasympathetic system in the animal. Consequently, the majority of dogs under examination will have heart rates <140 bpm. However, when dealing with a nervous, anxious or fractious dog the sinus rate will be faster and there will be sinus rhythm or sinus tachycardia. For cats examined in hospital, quite often the heart rate ranges between 160 to 220 bpm. In dogs, the normal automaticity of the atrioventricular junction results in a heart rate of 40 to 60 bpm. The rate of depolarization of the Purkinje fibers is approximately 30 bpm.

Depression of normal automaticity results in a decrease of the discharge rate of the automatic focus or in a total interruption of its automatic activity. Depression of sinus node automaticity results in sinus bradycardia or sinus arrest. Whenever the rate of the sinus node is below the rate of depolarization of the subsidiary pacemakers, these latter can initiate an escape beat or an escape rhythm.

Depression of normal automaticity can occur secondary to autonomic dysfunction (increase in parasympathetic tone or decrease in sympathetic tone), metabolic disorders (electrolyte abnormalities, such as hyperkalemia, hypothyroidism or hypothermia), ischemia (interruption of blood supply via the sinus node artery), fibrosis within the sinus node and around its exit pathways, or ion channel dysfunction.

Enhanced normal automaticity

Enhanced normal automaticity is an increase in the discharge rate of pacemaker cells. This mechanism can be associated with an increase in the slope of phase 4, a change of the resting transmembrane potential towards less negative values, or by a shift of the threshold potential towards more negative values (Fig. 1.11).

Under normal conditions the sinus node is the dominant pacemaker, but occasionally the subsidiary pacemaker rate can exceed the sinus rate. The ionic mechanisms responsible for enhanced normal automaticity in the sinus node and atrioventricular junction include an increase in the magnitude of the "funny" current (I_f), a decrease in outward potassium currents (I_K) at the end of phase 3, and an increase in calcium current (I_{CaL}) usually as a result of adrenergic stimulation. Hypoxemia and hypokalemia also promote enhanced normal automaticity by inhibiting the Na+/K+ pump, which results in a less negative diastolic membrane potential.

Enhanced normal automaticity is the mechanism of sinus tachycardia (Boxes 8.1 and 8.2) and of non-paroxysmal junctional tachycardia (Box 8.4).

Abnormal automaticity or depolarization-induced automaticity

Abnormal automaticity is observed in working atrial and ventricular myocytes that normally do not depolarize spontaneously. Myocytes can acquire the property of automaticity if their resting membrane potential shifts to less negative values (from −70/90 mV to −40/60 mV) and approaches the threshold potential. This effect is frequently observed as a result of ischemia and reperfusion (hyperkalemia, low intracellular pH, high adrenergic tone). The rate of depolarization is directly related to the resting membrane potential value. The less negative the membrane potential, the faster the rate. Abnormal automaticity is usually not stopped by overdrive suppression. Abnormal automaticity is also a feature of Purkinje fibers when their membrane potential changes to less negative values (approximately −60 mV), for example with myocardial ischemia.

Abnormal automaticity is the cause of some focal atrial and multiform ventricular tachycardias. A tachycardia with a phase of rate acceleration ("warm-up") at its onset and rate deceleration ("cool-down") before it terminates is likely automatic in origin (Fig. 8.11). When the arrhythmia originates from a single focus, the morphology of the P' waves of automatic atrial tachycardias usually remains identical from initiation to return to the sinus rhythm. In addition, automatic supraventricular tachycardias can persist even during atrioventricular block. Accelerated idioventricular rhythms, depending on their site of origin, can be due to enhanced normal or abnormal automaticity. However, available clinical tools do not enable identification of the ion channel alteration responsible for this electrophysiological disorder.

Triggered activity

Triggered activity corresponds to membrane potential oscillations, called after-depolarizations, following the onset of an action potential. Based on their timing relative to the phases of the action potential, after-depolarizations are classified as:
- early after-depolarization (EAD), and
- delayed after-depolarization (DAD).

After-depolarizations cause arrhythmias when the membrane potential oscillations reach the threshold potential and initiate an action potential. Triggered activity can result in a single premature beat or an arrhythmia that persists for a variable number of beats.

Early after-depolarization

Early after-depolarizations have been studied experimentally in canine mid-myocardial cells and Purkinje fibers (see studies by C. Antzelevitch). The mid-myocardial cells of the dog are more likely than the endocardial or epicardial cells to develop early after-depolarizations because of a lower concentration of the ion channel I_{Ks}. The potassium ion channels are responsible for repolarization and bringing the membrane potential back to its resting level. If the balance between inward and outward currents is not maintained there will be a propensity to early after-depolarizations. A reduced concentration or blockade of potassium channels (potassium channel blocking drugs such as sotalol block I_{Kr}) can potentiate this type of triggered activity. In addition to a reduction of repolarizing currents, early after-depolarizations may develop as a consequence of increased availability of calcium current (I_{CaL}), an increase in the sodium-calcium exchange current because of greater intracellular calcium or up-regulation of the exchanger such as can occur with catecholamines. Each of these mechanisms alone or in combinations can push the cell to depolarization. Differences exist with regards to the sensitivity of the Purkinje fibers and ventricular mid-myocardial cells of the dog to intracellular calcium levels. Experimentally, drugs such as ryanodine can abolish early after-depolarizations in canine mid-myocardial cells, but not in Purkinje fibers. Some of these data may have application in dogs and drug responsiveness of identified arrhythmias. Importantly, although classically considered a bradycardia associated mechanism for arrhythmias, early after-depolarizations can be induced with certain beta and alpha-adrenergic agonists when combined with vagal stimulation. Early after-depolarizations can develop during phase 2 of the action potential (Fig. 6.1) when the transmembrane potential is around –30 mV, or phase 3, when the transmembrane potential is approximately –60 mV.

Clinically the factors predisposing to the development of early after-depolarizations include bradycardia, hypothermia, myocardial stretch, hypoxia and acidosis. Prolongation of the action potential can also be induced by drugs that block repolarizing K+ currents, such as quinidine, procainamide, bretylium and sotalol. Early after-depolarization-induced arrhythmias include *torsade de pointes* and polymorphic ventricular tachycardia. Early after-depolarizations from the Purkinje fibers of the left ventricle have been shown to be the mechanism inciting arrhythmia onset in the inherited form of ventricular arrhythmias in German Shepherd dogs (Figs. 10.14 and 10.15). Although these dogs have arrhythmias initiated by early after-depolarizations most frequently with slower heart rates and longer R-R intervals as the classic set up for this mechanism, younger and more severely affected dogs may have non-sustained runs of polymorphic ventricular tachycardia with varying sinus rates and conditions (Figs. 6.2 and 6.3). In some cases, early after-depolarizations only serve as the trigger of an arrhythmia that is then perpetuated by a different electrophysiological mechanism, such as reentry.

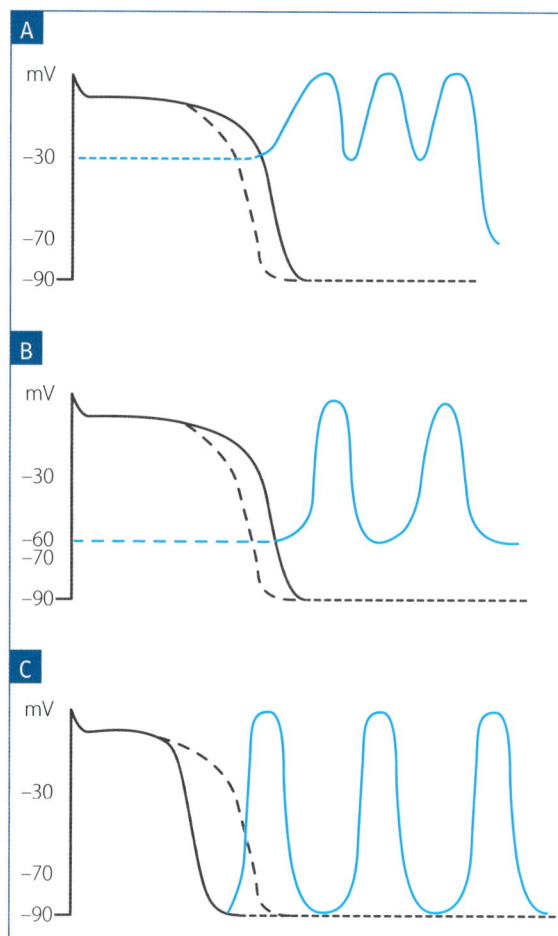

Figure 6.1. Triggered activity. Early after-depolarization (EAD) occurring during phase 2 of the action potential (plateau early after-potentials) (A) or during phase 3 (phase 3 early after-depolarizations) (B). Delayed after-depolarization (DAD) secondary to depolarizing currents occurring after complete repolarization (phase 4). Tachycardia, which is associated with a shortening of action potential duration, promotes delayed after-depolarization by increasing intracellular calcium (C). Whenever membrane oscillations of early or delayed after depolarization reach threshold, they trigger an action potential, which appears on the surface electrocardiogram as an ectopic complex.

Delayed after-depolarization

Delayed after-depolarizations are depolarizing currents that arise during phase 4 of the action potential. They occur when intracellular Ca^{2+} overload results in activation of the Na^+/Ca^{2+} exchanger and a net influx of Na^+. The long-lasting calcium current (I_{CaL}) does not contribute to delayed after-depolarizations (Fig. 6.1).

Predisposing factors to delayed after-depolarizations include high levels of circulating catecholamines, myocardial reperfusion, hypokalemia, hypomagnesemia, hypercalcemia, and digitalis toxicity.

Arrhythmias induced by delayed after-depolarizations include atrial tachycardias secondary to digitalis toxicity, focal junctional tachycardia and ventricular tachycardia associated with reperfusion injuries. Arrhythmias secondary to delayed after-depolarization can be triggered by sinus tachycardia and rapid pacing.

Abnormalities of impulse conduction

Conduction is the ability of the heart muscle to propagate an electrical stimulus from cell to cell.

Conduction blocks

Depression of electrical impulse conduction is called *block*. A block can be a delay of conduction or a complete interruption of electrical impulse propagation. Blocks can be divided into physiological and pathological, partial (or incomplete) and complete, and finally anatomical and functional.

A *physiological* block is an interruption of impulse propagation in a given structure because the cycle length of the electrical stimulus is shorter than the time it takes for this structure to recover from its refractory period. Examples of physiological block are aberrant intraventricular conduction (see p. 286) and second-degree atrioventricular block during rapid supraventricular tachycardias, for example atrial flutter. Physiological atrioventricular

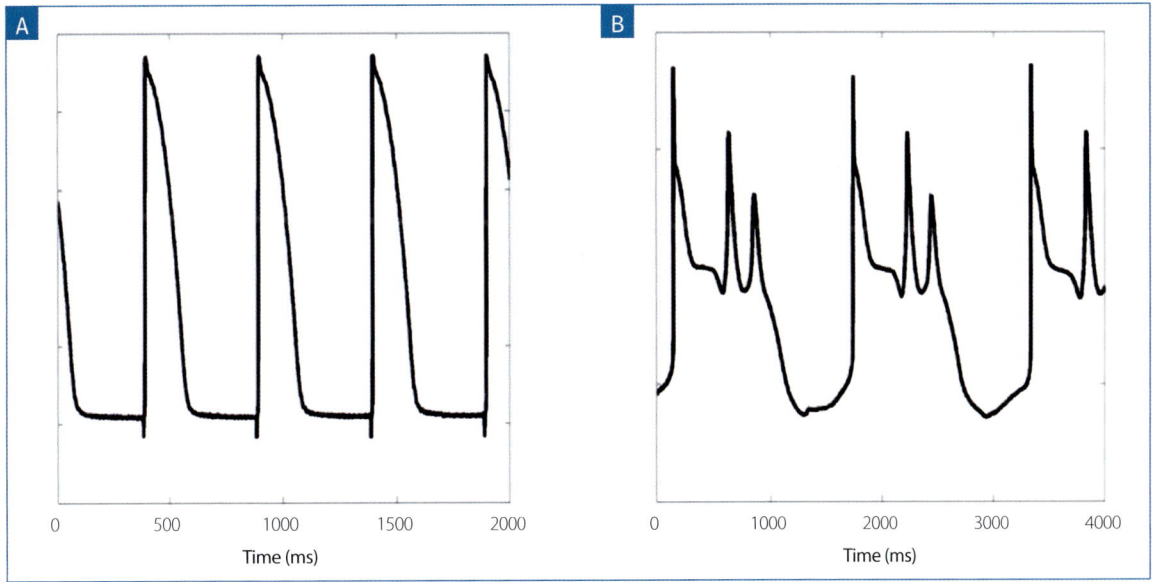

Figure 6.2. Early after-depolarizations. Action potential recorded from a Purkinje fiber without early after-depolarizations (A). Spontaneous early after-depolarizations occurring during phase 3 of the action potential recorded from a Purkinje fiber of the left ventricle from a German Shepherd puppy afflicted with inherited ventricular arrhythmias and at risk of sudden death (B).

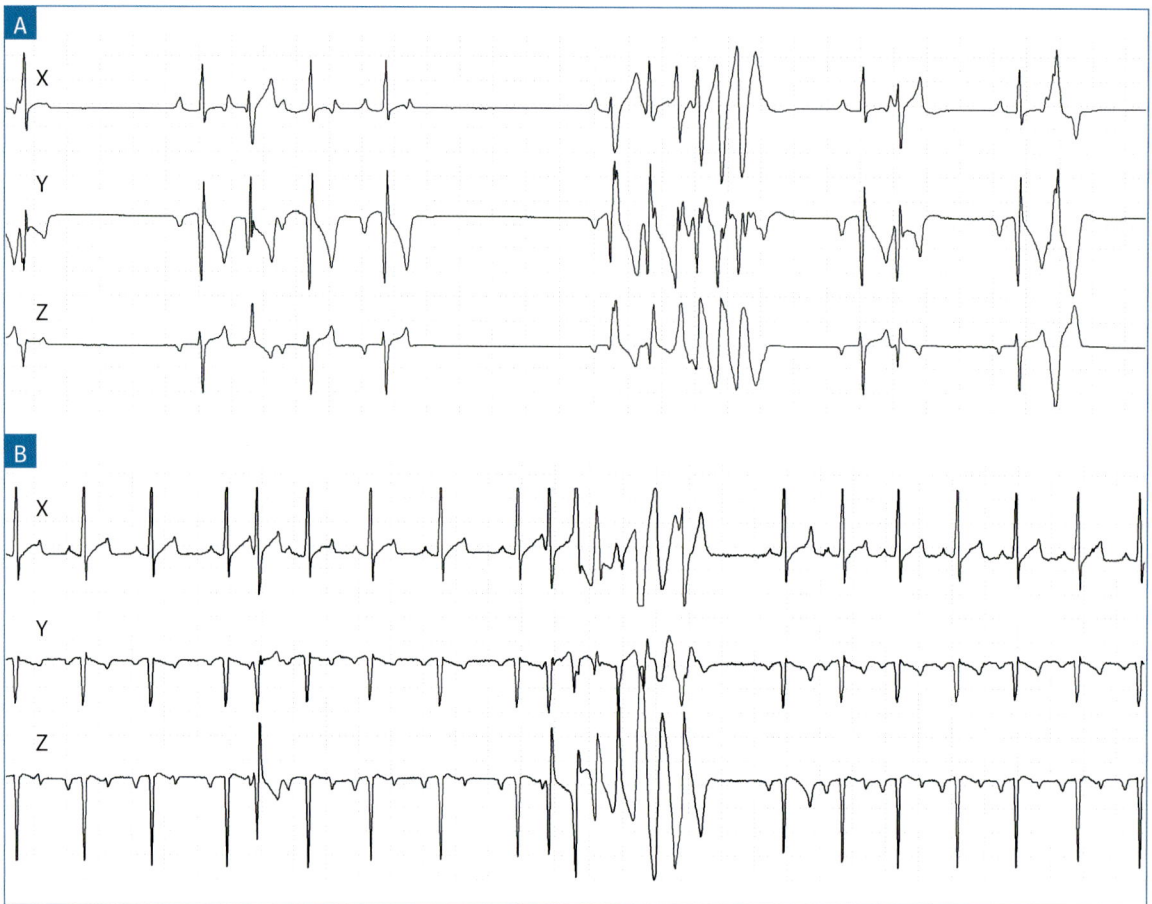

Figure 6.3. Polymorphic nonsustained ventricular arrhythmias in German Shepherd dogs. Although early after-depolarizations are classically thought of as a bradycardia associated mechanism for arrhythmias, they can also occur without pauses or bradycardia. Frequently, nonsustained runs of polymorphic ventricular tachycardia initiated by early after-depolarizations occur during sleep or rest following exercise with the associated slower heart rates. In frame (A) a sleeping 6-month-old German Shepherd dog is seen to have a ventricular escape beat followed by polymorphic ventricular tachycardia. Frame (B) shows that the dog also developed the arrhythmia while awake.

block in the presence of rapid atrial activity protects the ventricles from an excessive ventricular response rate that would compromise hemodynamics.

A *pathological* block is an unexpected interruption of impulse conduction in a segment of the conduction system. Pathological blocks can be anatomical or functional. For example, anoxia or cell degeneration lead to a decrease in myocardial metabolism and accumulation of intracellular Ca^{2+} and Na^+. This change then results in a constant state of depolarization with progressive decrease in conduction velocity until complete block.

A *partial* or *incomplete* block is characterized by a localized slowing of conduction velocity.

A *complete* block is a complete interruption of impulse propagation. When the block affects intraventricular conduction, it is described as complete when the duration of the QRS complex on the surface electrocardiogram exceeds 80 ms in the dog and 40 ms in the cat.

An *anatomical* block is caused by a lesion of the specialized conduction system, the atrial or the ventricular working myocardium.

A *functional* block, also called rate-dependent, occurs when an electrical impulse reaches an area of myocardium during its refractory period. Functional blocks are commonly associated with a rapid heart rate (tachycardia-dependent block or phase 3 block) when electrical impulses are completely or partially blocked in myocytes that have not fully recovered from the previous action potential. Functional block is also associated with bradycardia (bradycardia-dependent block or phase 4 block), which is thought to be secondary to a decrease in cell excitability during long diastolic intervals.

It is well-established that conduction is more rapid when it occurs along the longitudinal axis rather than along the transverse axis of cardiac muscle fibers. These are the anisotropic properties of conduction in the heart. Typically, in the normal heart the anisotropic ratio of conduction velocity between the long and transverse axes of fiber orientation is approximately 2:1. In the healthy myocardium, cell-to-cell conduction occurs predominantly in the longitudinal axis of the myocytes, and is reduced in the transverse direction explaining this ratio of conduction, which is known as *uniform anisotropic conduction*. A particular type of functional block corresponds to *non-uniform anisotropic conduction*. Non-uniform anisotropic conduction is present when transverse conduction of electrical impulses is markedly decreased in some areas of the myocardium, causing a greater differential between longitudinal and transverse conduction. As a result, impulse propagation through the myocardium follows an irregular course, described as zig-zag conduction between areas of block.

Reentry

In the normal heart, a wavefront of depolarization is initiated in the sinus node and is followed by sequential activation of cardiac myocytes. Once all the cells are in a refractory state the electrical impulse dies out.

However, when an area of myocardium that is still refractory cannot be initially activated by the electrical wavefront (*unidirectional block*), it can serve as a pathway for the electrical wavefront to re-excite the heart as long as it has regained excitability before full depolarization of the rest of the myocardial tissue. This phenomenon is called reentry. If the electrical impulse persists within the *reentrant circuit*, it becomes the substrate of a tachyarrhythmia.

Several factors are necessary for reentry:
- a circuit,
- a unidirectional block in a branch of the circuit,
- slow conduction velocity in a branch of the circuit,
- an appropriate cycle length, and
- a trigger.

The *circuit* is the path followed by the electrical impulse during a reentry. It can be present in any part of the heart and can include the atrial myocardium, the ventricular myocardium, the atrioventricular node, the Purkinje network and atrioventricular accessory pathways. The size and shape of the reentrant circuit is determined by the conduction velocity and refractory period of the myocytes.

The circuit has two branches, which can be called α and β (Fig. 6.4). By convention, branch α conducts impulses in the antegrade direction, and branch β conducts in a retrograde direction. The branches of the circuit are separated by an anatomical or functional central area of block (non-conducting tissue), which constrains impulses within the circuit.

If the two branches of the circuit have the same conduction velocity and refractory period, impulses proceed along the two separate routes, and then gather distal to the area of block in a single wavefront (Fig. 6.4A). Conversely, if the refractory period of one of the branches of the circuit is prolonged, an impulse that propagates down one branch may be unable to travel in the other branch that is still refractory. If it remains refractory after the impulse has reached the extremity of the first branch, distal to the area of block, reentry is not possible (Fig. 6.4B). However, if the branch with the longest refractory period had time to recover from refractoriness because of slow conduction within the first branch of the circuit, the impulse can conduct retrogradely. At this point, the impulse stops or re-excites the antegrade branch of the circuit (Fig. 6.4C). If the reentrant phenomenon is limited to a single heartbeat, it is called an *echo beat*, but if it is sustained over time it gives rise to a reciprocating (or reentrant) tachycardia.

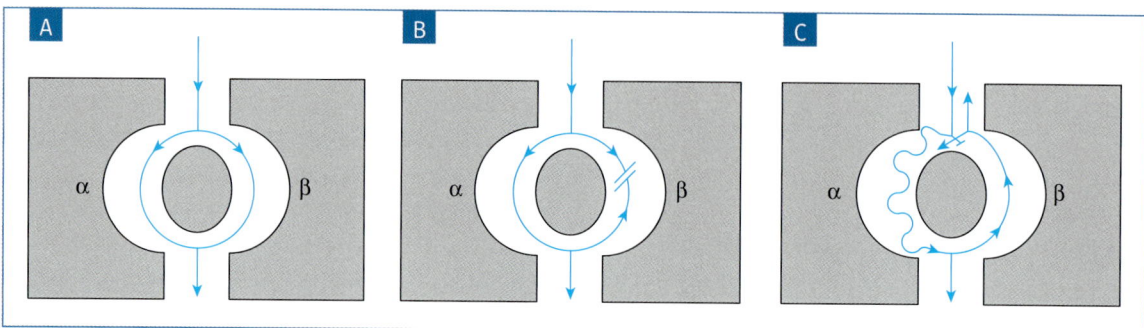

Figure 6.4. The concept of reentry. Electrical impulse propagation around an area of block and conditions for the formation of a reentry. See text for explanations.

The maintenance of reciprocating arrhythmias and electrical impulse direction inside the reentrant circuit depend on conduction velocity and refractory periods within the circuit. The size of the circuit must be equal to or exceed the cycle length of the reentry. Cycle length is the product of conduction velocity and refractory period.

Premature atrial or ventricular ectopic beats and abrupt changes in the sinus rhythm cycle length can serve as triggers for reentrant arrhythmias.

Reentry is likely the most common mechanism of tachyarrhythmias; however, this has not been proven for many atrial and ventricular arrhythmias in dogs. Reentrant arrhythmias include atrial flutter, some forms of atrial fibrillation, atrioventricular nodal reciprocating tachycardia (in humans, but currently not identified in dogs), atrioventricular reciprocating tachycardias, and certain forms of ventricular tachycardia associated with ischemia and myocardial fibrosis.

Types of reentry

Reentry can be divided into anatomical or functional (Fig. 6.5). *Anatomical* or *classic* reentry is characterized by an electrical circuit that is defined by anatomical structures. It, therefore, has a stable path, location and size. An example of anatomical circuit is represented by orthodromic atrioventricular reciprocating tachycardias. This circuit consists of the His-Purkinje system as the antegrade branch (atrium to ventricle), and an atrioventricular accessory pathway as the retrograde branch. The atria and the ventricles close the circuit proximally and distally, respectively. *Functional* reentries are characterized by a circuit that develops around a central core formed by refractory tissue. For this reason, functional reentries do not remain at a precise anatomical location and the circular movement can vary in size and path in relation to the electrophysiological characteristics of the area that sustains the reentry. Atrial fibrillation is an example of functional reentrant arrhythmia.

There are differences between anatomical and functional reentries related to the presence of an *excitable gap* and the factors that influence heart rate. An excitable gap is a segment of excitable tissue between the "head" and the "tail" of the reentrant wavefront. There is an excitable gap when the circuit is longer than the cycle length of the reentry. Excitable gaps are typical of anatomical reentries, although they can be found with some types of functional reentries (Fig. 6.5). In a predetermined anatomically circuit, the rate depends on the length of the circuit and the conduction velocity of the impulse within the circuit. Conversely, the rate of a functional reentry only depends on the refractory period of the excitable tissue; when the refractory period of the tissue is shorter, impulses can travel faster.

Six classical models of reentry circuit have been described: the ring, leading circle, figure of eight, spiral wave or rotor, reflection and phase 2 reentry. The ring

Abnormalities of impulse conduction

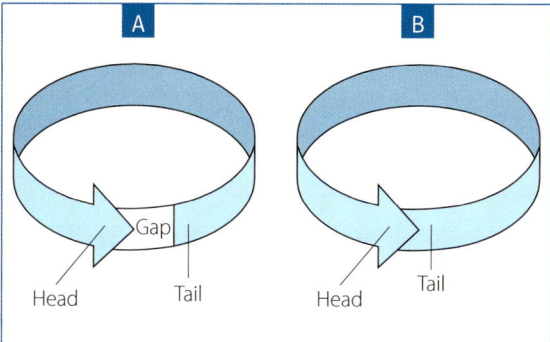

Figure 6.5. Wavefront during typical anatomical (A) and functional reentry (B). The anatomical reentry is characterized by a separation (*gap*), represented by the white area, between the head and the tail of the reentrant circuit, which corresponds to excitable tissue (*excitable gap*). An excitable gap is present when the wavelength (conduction velocity × refractory period) of the reentry is smaller than the length of the anatomical circuit. An excitable *gap* is not usually present in a functional reentry circuit; therefore, as soon as the myocytes in the circuit recover excitability, they are immediately re-activated by the wavefront of depolarization.

model is based on an anatomical obstacle, while the others are functional reentries.

The *ring model* is the simplest form of anatomical reentry. In this type of circuit, the impulse travels along the perimeter of cardiac structures that serve as "obstacles". These barriers can be represented by normal anatomical structures or be an area of fibrosis. The characteristic of the ring reentry is to be anchored to a specific anatomical structure. The most common clinical forms of this type of reentry include atrioventricular reciprocating tachycardias (Boxes 8.7 and 8.8), typical and atypical atrial flutter (Boxes 8.11- 8.13), atrioventricular nodal reciprocating tachycardia and most sustained monomorphic ventricular tachycardia (Box 10.3) with structural heart disease (Fig. 6.6A).

The *leading circle model* applies to functional reentries that are represented by a reentrant wavefront circling around the same fixed functionally refractory core. The central core is maintained in a refractory state by constant electrical activations originating from the reentrant circuit. The size of the circuit is determined by the refractory period of the tissue. There is no excitable gap between the head and the tail of the reentry. As soon as a portion of the circuit recovers from its refractory state, it is re-activated again by the electrical wavefront. The smaller the circuit, the faster the tachycardia. This model may apply to some forms of atrial fibrillation (Fig. 6.6B).

The *figure-of-eight* reentry corresponds to two reentrant circuit that share a common central pathway. Electrical impulses travel in opposite directions in the two circuits (clockwise and counterclockwise). The common portion of the circuits is usually an area of slow conduction (Fig. 6.6C).

The *spiral wave* model is the two-dimensional representation of the leading circle concept. In this model, the reentrant wavefronts have the appearance of a spiral (or rotor) rotating within the myocardium around a core. Spiral waves can be initiated by transient changes in myocardial properties and are not anchored to one specific site. The main rotor, sometimes referred to as "mother wave" can be the source of less stable rotors called "daughter waves". This model applies to some forms of atrial fibrillation (Figs. 6.6D and 6.6E).

Reflection refers to a form of reentry in which the electrical impulse travels antegradely and then retrogradely in a linear segment of tissue (for example a Purkinje fiber) that contains an area of depressed conduction. Initially, the impulse travels parallel to the area of depressed conduction, which has not yet recovered from its prolonged refractory period (unidirectional block). By the time the impulse reaches the level of the distal end of the area of depressed conduction, the tissue is again excitable and able to conduct the impulse retrogradely (Fig. 6.6F).

Phase 2 reentry is an arrhythmogenic mechanism that develops at a transmural level, because of the difference in the duration of action potentials between the epicardial, mid-myocardial (M-cells) and endocardial layers. Alteration in inward or outward currents can amplify the heterogeneity of action potential duration between layers of myocardium and promote reentry.

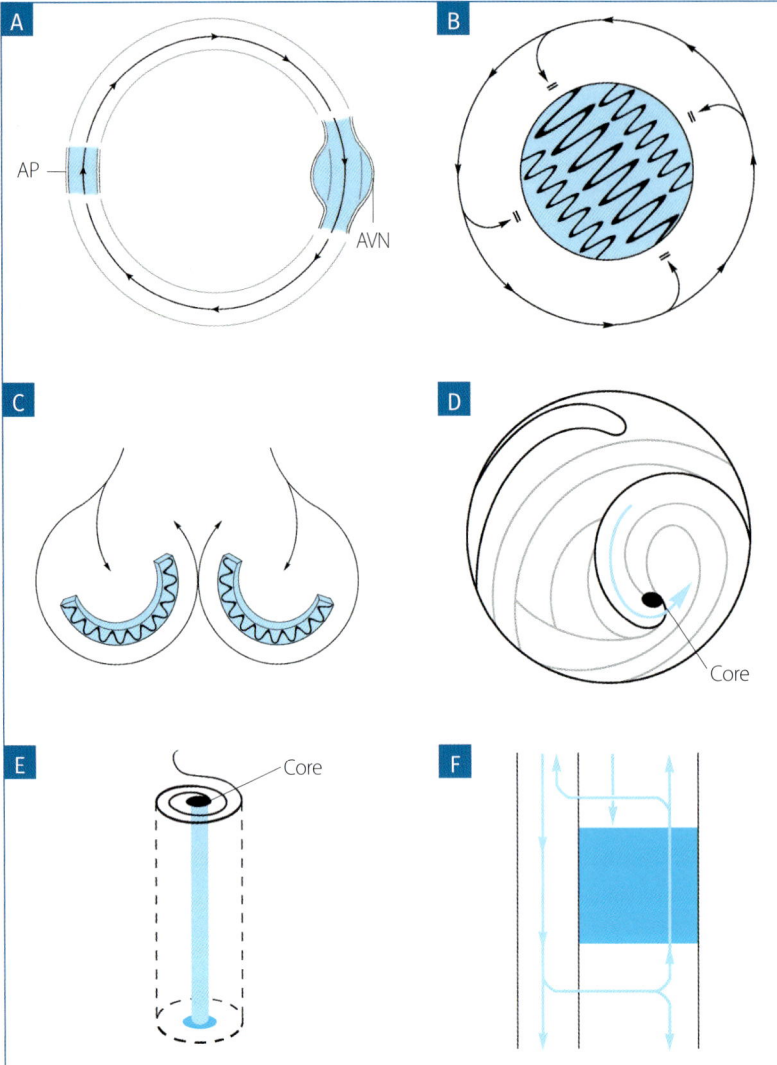

Figure 6.6. Types of reentry: A) Ring model (circle movement reentry) during atrioventricular reciprocating tachycardia mediated by an accessory pathway. The reentrant circuit includes the atrial and ventricular myocardium, the atrioventricular junction and the accessory pathway; B) leading circle model which describes the mechanism of functional reentry. The membrane potential of the cells of the central region is passively influenced by the reentrant circuit and maintained above threshold potential, which prevents it from depolarizing (electrotonic influence); C) figure-of-eight reentry is formed by two reentrant loops that travel around a functional line of block (in blue) in opposite direction (clockwise and counterclockwise), and share a portion of the circuit between the areas of block; D) spiral wave model, which corresponds to a two-dimensional representation of the leading circle model. The spiral wave circles around its refractory core; E) scroll wave corresponding to a three-dimensional representation of the spiral wave. The core is called the filament; F) reflection is a form of reentry occurring in a single linear portion of myocardium that includes one area of depressed conduction (blue). An impulse first travels parallel to the area of depressed conduction, and then is able to travel retrogradely through it once it has recovered from refractoriness. *AVN*: atrioventricular node; *AP*: accessory pathway.

Classification of arrhythmias

The classification of arrhythmias described in this book (Table 6.2) has been adapted for veterinary patients from consensus guidelines published for the diagnosis and treatment of rhythm disorders in humans.

The term bradycardia or bradyarrhythmia defines a ventricular rate below 60 bpm in dogs, and 140 bpm in cats. However, it must be remembered that with the advent of 24-hour electrocardiographic monitoring it is well-established that healthy dogs can have heart rates lower than 60 bpm while sleeping and cats can have heart rates below 140 bpm. This group of arrhythmias includes disorders of sinus node automaticity (sinus bradycardia, sinus arrest, sinus standstill), sino-atrial and atrioventricular conduction disturbances, atrial standstill and sino-ventricular rhythm.

The term tachycardia or tachyarrhythmia describes a cardiac rhythm with four or more consecutive beats occurring at a rate above that expected for a normal dog or cat under the given circumstances. The precise definition for a tachycardia must be left open for the clinical situation. For example, a sleeping dog with a heart rate of 150 bpm is likely abnormal, although a dog in a veterinary hospital could easily have a heart rate of 150 bpm. This of course is also true for the cat. In both species, the sinus rates can vary dramatically depending on autonomic influences.

Tachycardias are classified as supraventricular or ventricular based on their anatomical substrate (Table 6.3). A *supraventricular* tachycardia is dependent on at least one supraventricular anatomical structure to persist over time. These supraventricular structures include the sinus node, the atrial myocardium, the atrial portion of the atrioventricular junction, the coronary sinus, the pulmonary veins, the venae cavae, the ligament of Marshall and the Marshall vein. Atrioventricular reciprocating tachycardias are dependent not only on supraventricular structures (atrial myocardium, atrioventricular node) but also on the ventricular myocardium.

Supraventricular tachyarrhythmias that only use the atrioventricular junction as their anatomical substrate are called infra-atrial supraventricular tachycardias. This group includes atrioventricular nodal reciprocating tachycardia, focal junctional tachycardia, non-paroxysmal junctional tachycardia, and reciprocating nodo-ventricular tachycardia mediated by nodo-ventricular or nodo-fascicular fibers (also referred to as *Mahaim fibers*).

Ventricular tachycardias originate from ventricular anatomical structures including the walls of the ventricles, the intraventricular specialized conduction system, the Purkinje fibers, the left and right outflow tracts, the aortic root and the initial segment of the pulmonary artery (Table 6.3).

The anatomical substrate of tachyarrhythmias is usually determined from their electrocardiographic

TABLE 6.2. Classification of rhythm disorders in dogs and cats

Rhythm disturbances		Bradycardia and conduction disturbances	Ectopic beats and rhythms
Supraventricular	**Ventricular**		

■ Sinus tachycardia
■ Atrioventricular nodal reciprocating tachycardia
■ Focal junctional tachycardia
■ Non-paroxysmal junctional tachycardia
■ Atrioventricular reciprocating tachycardias
  ■ Orthodromic atrioventricular reciprocating tachycardia
  ■ Permanent junctional reciprocating tachycardia
  ■ Antidromic atrioventricular reciprocating tachycardia
■ Focal atrial tachycardia
■ Multifocal atrial tachycardia or chaotic atrial rhythm
■ Macroreentrant atrial tachycardia
  ■ Cavo-tricuspid isthmus dependent atrial flutter
  ■ Cavo-tricuspid isthmus non dependent atrial flutter
■ Atrial fibrillation
	■ Idioventricular rhythm
	■ Accelerated idioventricular rhythm
	■ Monomorphic ventricular tachycardia
	  ■ Nonsustained
	  ■ Repetitive
	  ■ Sustained
	  ■ Incessant
	  ■ Ventricular flutter
	■ Polymorphic ventricular tachycardia
	■ Torsade de pointes
	■ Bidirectional ventricular tachycardia
	■ Ventricular fibrillation
		■ Sinus bradycardia
		■ Sinus arrest
		■ Sinus standstill
		■ Atrial standstill
		■ Sino-ventricular rhythm
		■ Asystole or ventricular arrest
		■ Pulseless electrical activity or electromechanical dissociation
		■ Intra-atrial conduction delay or block
		■ Sino-atrial block
		■ Atrioventricular block
		  ■ First-degree
		  ■ Second-degree
		    ■ Wenckebach
		    ■ Möbitz
		    ■ Fixed 2:1
		    ■ Advanced
		  ■ Third-degree
		  ■ Paroxysmal
		■ Intraventricular blocks
		  ■ Monofascicular
		  ■ Bifascicular
		  ■ Trifascicular
			■ Supraventricular ectopic beats and rhythms
			  ■ Atrial ectopic beats
			  ■ Atrial ectopic rhythm
			  ■ Junctional ectopic beats
			  ■ Junctional ectopic rhythm
			  ■ Atrial parasystole
			  ■ Dissociation or unilateral atrial rhythm
			■ Ventricular ectopic beats and rhythms
			  ■ Ventricular ectopic beats
			  ■ Idioventricular rhythm
			  ■ Ventricular parasystole

TABLE 6.3. Classification of tachycardias based on the anatomical substrate

Tachycardia	Anatomical substrate
Supraventricular tachycardias	
Atrioventricular nodal reciprocating tachycardia	Slow and rapid atrioventricular nodal pathway ± perinodal atrial myocardium ± coronary sinus
Atrioventricular reciprocating tachycardia mediated by accessory pathway	Atrial myocardium, atrioventricular node, His bundle, bundle branches and fascicles, ventricular myocardium, accessory pathway
Focal atrial tachycardia	Atrial myocardium, coronary sinus, pulmonary vein, caval veins, sinus node and sino-atrial junction
Atrial flutter	Atrial myocardium and coronary sinus
Atrial fibrillation	Atrial myocardium, coronary sinus, pulmonary veins and caval veins
Focal and non-paroxysmal junctional tachycardia	Atrioventricular node and the His bundle
Ventricular tachycardias	
Monomorphic ventricular tachycardia	Ventricular myocardium, left and right ventricular outflow tract, pulmonary artery, aortic sinuses of Valsalva
Polymorphic ventricular tachycardia	Ventricular myocardium
Torsade de pointes	Ventricular myocardium
Ventricular fibrillation	Ventricular myocardium and the Purkinje fibers

characteristics. Other electrocardiographic parameters used to describe tachyarrhythmias include their duration and the regularity of the ventricular rhythm (R-R intervals).

The duration of the QRS complex is used to classify tachycardias as narrow QRS complex tachycardias (<70 ms in dogs and <40 ms in cats) and wide QRS complex tachycardias (>70 ms in dogs and >40 ms in cats). Typically, narrow QRS complex tachycardias are supraventricular in origin, and wide QRS complex tachycardias are ventricular in origin. However, intraventricular conduction delays (bundle branch blocks, rate-related *aberrancy*) can give supraventricular tachycardias the appearance of wide QRS complex arrhythmias.

Ventricular tachycardia is described as monomorphic when all QRS complexes have the same morphology, pleomorphic if there is more than one QRS morphology during a run of tachycardia but the QRS complexes are not continuously changing; and finally, a ventricular tachycardia is said to be polymorphic, when the QRS complex morphology varies on a beat-to-beat basis. A bidirectional ventricular tachycardia is characterized by alternating QRS morphology, characterized by a 180-degree shift of the electrical axis between consecutive QRS complexes.

The regularity of the R-R intervals is another electrocardiographic criterion useful for the classification of tachycardias. A tachycardia is defined as regular when the R-R intervals are constant, and it is called irregular if the R-R intervals vary. A particular type of irregularity, occurring at the initiation and termination of certain tachyarrhythmias, corresponds to the "*warm-up*" and "*cool-down*" phases of the tachycardia. During the "warm-up" phase at the time of the onset of the arrhythmia, the R-R intervals progressively shorten due to the increase in the discharge rate of an ectopic focus. Conversely, during the "cool-down" phase, a progressive increase in R-R intervals precedes termination of the tachycardia.

Depending on their mode of initiation, termination, and duration tachyarrhythmias can be classified as (Table 6.4):
- *non-sustained*, when they last less than 30 s,
- *sustained*, when they last more than 30 s or if they require medical intervention because of hemodynamic collapse within the initial 30 s,
- *incessant* (or *permanent*), when they last for more than 12 hours including brief periods of sinus rhythm. The terms incessant or permanent are therefore misnomers because the tachyarrhythmia is necessarily continuous,

- *repetitive*, when frequent episodes of non-sustained tachycardia are interrupted by short periods of sinus rhythm, and
- *paroxysmal*, when their initiation and termination is abrupt.

Hemodynamic consequences of arrhythmias

The hemodynamic consequences of cardiac arrhythmias can cause adverse clinical signs and potentially deterioration leading to death. For any given arrhythmia, the hemodynamic effects often vary between patients because of the complexity of the interplay of multiple factors (age, underlying cardiac or systemic disease, integrity of cardiovascular reflexes, influence of autonomic nervous system, etc.). Medications that alter myocardial function, enhance or suppress the parasympathetic or sympathetic system, or induce sedation/anesthesia can influence the hemodynamic response to arrhythmias. Myocardial function is likely the most important determinant of tolerance to an arrhythmia. Specific characteristics of an arrhythmia that are usually associated with a more negative impact on blood pressure and perfusion include:
- rate and duration of tachycardia,
- coupling interval of premature complexes,
- rate and duration of bradycardia,
- abruptness of rate variation,
- sequence of activation of the ventricles, and
- temporal relationship between atrial and ventricular activation.

Tissue perfusion is the ultimate function of the cardiovascular system. Systemic arterial blood pressure varies in the dog because of sinus arrhythmia (Fig. 6.7A). Moreover, the determinants of cardiac function are complex. For example, an increase in heart rate will decrease diastolic filling time which could potentially decrease stroke volume because of decreased preload and decreased myocardial stretch (Frank-Starling law). However, the effect varies with the speed and degree of changes in heart rate. Importantly, to counteract the potential for a decrease in stroke volume associated with the shorter diastolic period, the cardiac contractility increases with an increase in heart rate, a phenomenon known as the *Bowditch effect* (or *Treppe or Staircase effect*), which was first described by Henry Bowditch in 1871. One explanation for this phenomenon is that at higher heart rates Na^+/K^+-ATPase is unable to keep up with the influx of sodium. The higher intracellular sodium means that more sodium is available to be exchanged for Ca^{2+} via the Na^+/Ca^{2+} exchanger; this mechanism results in the accumulation of intracellular calcium which has a positive inotropic effect. This positive inotropic effect increases the stroke volume with an increase in blood pressure. Commonly this occurs in dogs when the heart rate increases with sinus arrhythmia (Fig. 6.7A). It should be emphasized that this response is present in the normal heart, whereas in contrast, a diseased heart is not capable of increasing contractility with increased rate. Furthermore, the Bowditch effect has an upper rate limit because at high rates the opposite effect occurs. This upper rate limit varies with age, medications and underlying disease. Having an adequate heart rate can be critical to maintaining an adequate blood pressure in and of itself. This is particularly evident when animals are anesthetized (Fig. 6.7B).

Although arrhythmias may have negative hemodynamic effects, when ectopic beats or rhythms exist but at rates similar to the underlying sinus rhythm, the disturbance of blood pressure and perfusion may be minimal.

TABLE 6.4. Classification of cardiac arrhythmias based on anatomical, electrocardiographic and clinical criteria

Anatomical criteria	Electrocardiographic criteria	Clinical criteria
Site of origin	**QRS duration**	**Mode of presentation**
Supraventricular	Narrow	Paroxysmal
Ventricular	Wide	Permanent or incessant
	Morphology	Repetitive
	Monomorphic	
	Bidirectional	**Duration**
	Polymorphic	Sustained (>30 s)
	Cycle length	Non sustained
	Irregular	
	Regular	
	Warm up/cool down	

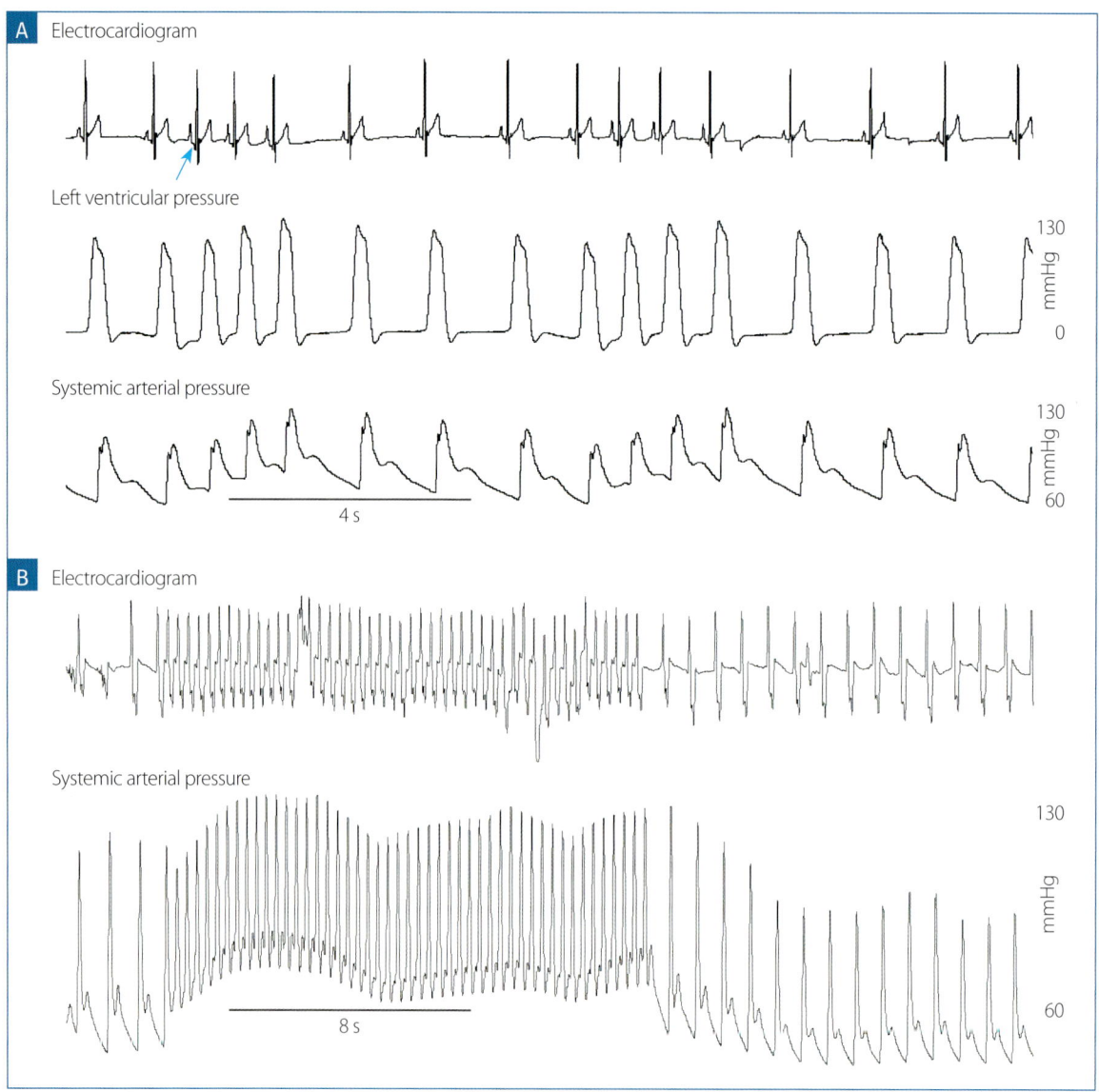

Figure 6.7. Electrocardiogram and pressure recordings from an anesthetized dog with a sinus arrhythmia and a dog undergoing a pacemaker implantation. These recordings illustrate the effect of changes in heart rate on blood pressure.
A) During sinus arrhythmia changes in the autonomic input to the sinus node result in changes in the left ventricular and systemic arterial pressures as the heart rate increases and decreases. With vagal withdrawal, the sinus rate increases and so does the intraventricular and systemic pressures. Note on the electrocardiogram that the P wave is taller with the shorter P-P interval, which is typical of the wandering pacemaker in the dog. Additionally note the more prominent T_a wave of the taller P waves (arrow). The systolic and diastolic pressures decrease with the slower heart rate in part because of increased parasympathetic tone causing vasodilation. Note also that the pulse pressure (pulse width) is greater (larger difference between systolic and diastolic pressure) when the R-R intervals are longer. Consequently, the femoral pulse may feel stronger. The gradual increase in left ventricular pressure that is causing the increase in systemic arterial pressure at the faster heart rate is likely the phenomenon known as the Bowditch effect, also known as the Treppe effect or staircase effect. See text for details of the mechanism.
B) The Bowditch effect is evident in this recording of an anesthetized dog undergoing pacemaker implantation. Initially, the pacing rate was 70 bpm. The rate was increased to 180 bpm with an increase in the systemic arterial pressure. After approximately 5 s the systemic arterial pressure stabilized at a slightly lower level with variation due to mechanical ventilation. When the pacing rate was reduced to 75 bpm the blood pressure decreased and then stabilized.

It is also important to realize the complexity and relationships between cardiac rhythm and blood pressure in disease states (Fig. 6.8). Detection of these rhythms by physical examination may be difficult because pulse deficits may not be found. This is in contrast to premature complexes (also termed extrasystoles or extrasystolic beats) that have a *short coupling interval* (the coupling interval is the time between two beats) (Figs. 6.9 and 6.10).

With an extrasystolic beat the stroke volume is reduced and the ryanodine receptors responsible for the release of calcium are refractory to activation. Thus, premature beats are typically associated with a weak cardiac contraction. The shorter the coupling interval, the weaker the contraction. However, these beats are typically followed by a stronger contraction with the subsequent beat through a mechanism known as *post-extrasystolic potentiation*. It should be emphasized that the

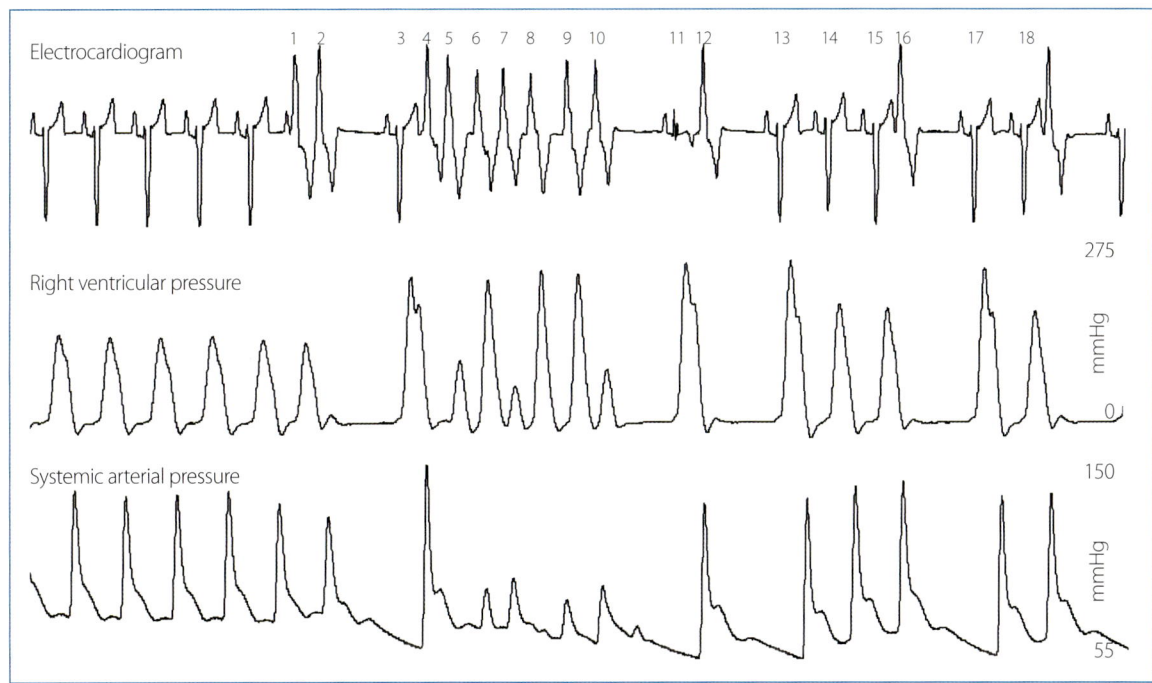

Figure 6.8. Electrocardiogram, right ventricular pressure recording and systemic arterial pressure in a dog with severe pulmonic stenosis. These tracings demonstrate the complexity associated with the rhythm, timing, and disease state. The beat identified as 1 is a premature ventricular complex preceded coincidentally by a P wave albeit with a short PQ interval. Because the interval is similar to the sinus rhythm (note that this dog has very deep negative deflections in lead II because of severe right ventricular hypertrophy) and there may be some atrial contribution to the ventricular filling, the blood pressure generated is similar to that of sinus beats. Closely coupled ventricular premature complex 2 generates a barely detectable pressure difference in the right ventricle and no systemic arterial pressure. However, the post-extrasystolic beat 3 results in a marked increase in right ventricular pressure as well as in the systemic arterial pressure. The left ventricular pressures are not presented, but would have likely generated a greater intraventricular pressure. The severity of the condition in this particular dog adds complexity, as it is likely that it has super-systemic right ventricular pressures that could have a varied influence on the left ventricle. A short non-sustained run of ventricular tachycardia with a variable R-R interval is identified with beats 4-10. Note the variable ventricular pressure generated. In this disease state the higher right ventricular pressure does not translate into a high systemic arterial pressure with this rhythm. Beat 11 is a fusion beat with a post-extrasystolic potentiation and pressure that is followed by 12 a premature ventricular complex that does not generate a ventricular pressure nor systemic pressure. Note that sinus beat 13 generates a similar pressure as 11 while the two sinus beats that follow 13-14 have a similar ventricular pressure, but yet appear to have a Bowditch (staircase) effect on systemic blood pressure. The premature beat 16 does not generate a pressure, but does result in post-extrasystolic potentiation of the right ventricular pressure. Note that the post-extrasystolic potentiation identified in the right ventricular profile of beats 3, 13 and 17 is similar; however, the systemic arterial pressure profile is different. This is because of the electrophysiological and hemodynamic effects that precede these beats.

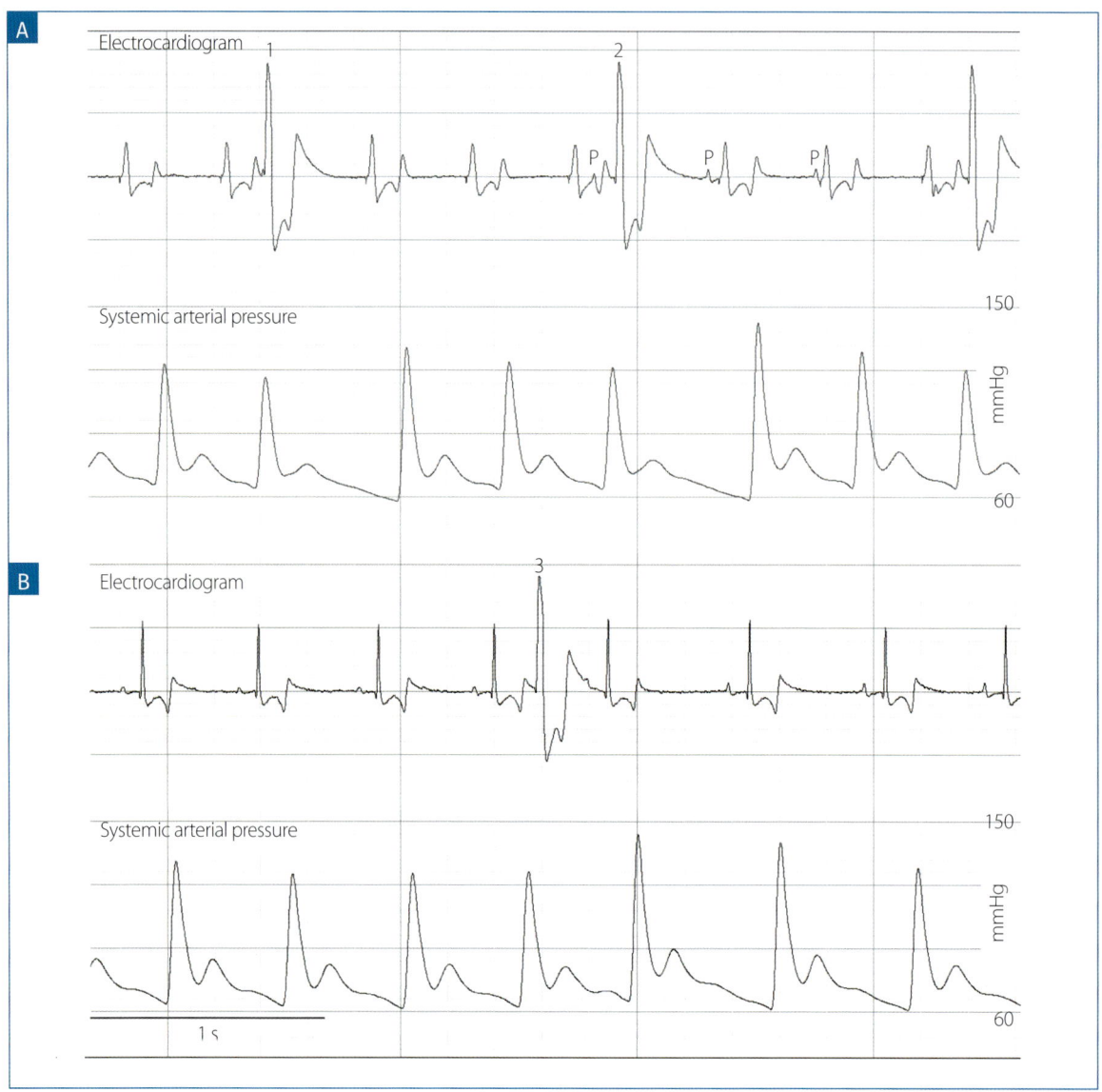

Figure 6.9. Electrocardiogram and systemic arterial pressure recorded from a dog during pacemaker implantation for sinus node dysfunction.
(A) During ventricular pacing premature ventricular complexes occurred which resulted in post-extrasystolic potentiation. Note the increased systemic arterial pressure associated with the premature ventricular complex 1. The premature ventricular complex did not generate a systemic pressure but the next paced beat produced a higher systolic pressure and a lower diastolic pressure (wider pulse pressure). The second premature ventricular complex 2, which is followed by another paced beat that coincidentally is preceded by a P wave, generates an even greater systolic pressure. A likely and perhaps even more important reason for beat 2 to generate an even greater post-extrasystolic potentiated beat is the more closely coupled beat that follows.
(B) During a period of sinus rhythm a premature ventricular complexes 3 is interpolated between two sinus beats without a longer period of diastole. Regardless, post-extrasystolic potentiation is identified (see text for mechanism). This type of hemodynamic consequence, however, may not occur in animals with obstructive hypertrophic cardiomyopathy. In this situation premature complexes result in a decrease in the systemic arterial pressure that follows the next sinus beat. This is caused by the increased inotropic effect resulting in an increase in left ventricular outflow tract obstruction. In humans this phenomenon is called the Brockenbrough-Braunwald-Morrow sign. The decrease in pressure occurs for a single beat.

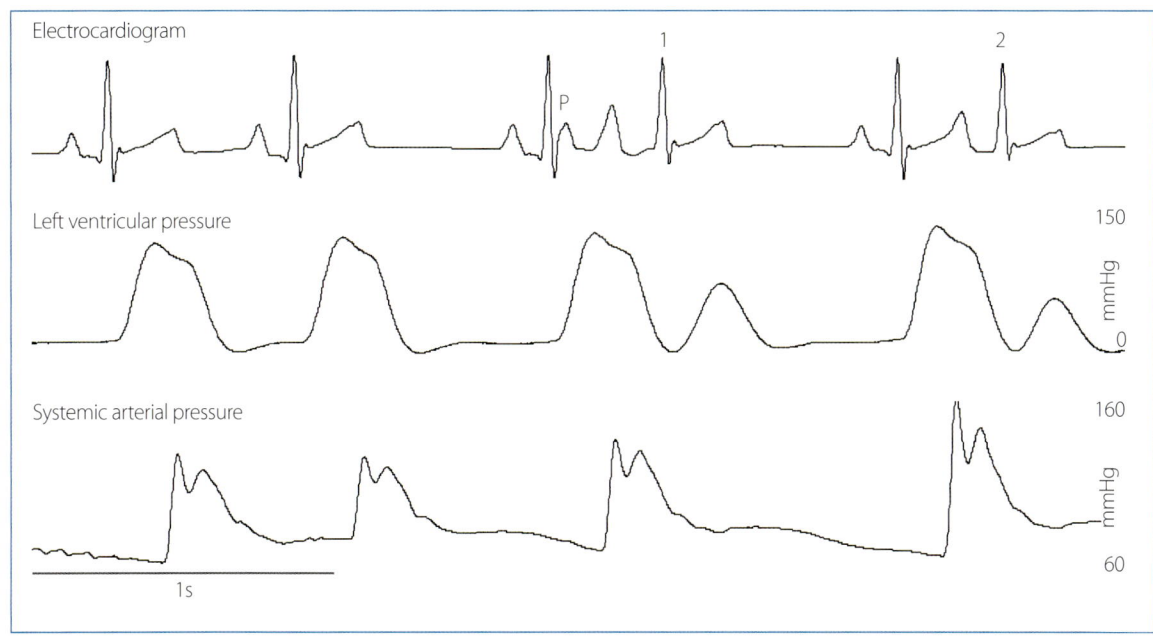

Figure 6.10. Electrocardiogram, left ventricular pressure and systemic arterial pressure recording from a dog. Two premature atrial complexes are identified. A P wave (P) can be identified during the ST segment of the preceding sinus beat before the ventricular complex identified as 1. Although the PQ interval is long, it is likely associated with this complex. A P wave for beat 2 is not seen. The premature atrial complexes do generate pressures within the left ventricle and post-extrasystolic potentiation is illustrated in the systemic arterial pressure of 1. Although an overshoot exists in this recording, the change in pressure can be appreciated.

pressure generated in the ventricle may not necessarily correlate with the systemic pressure depending on multiple factors (e.g. outflow tract obstruction, compliance of the arterial system, extrasystolic interval). Previously the post-extrasystolic potentiation was explained in part by the Frank-Starling mechanism, as the pause following a premature beat increases filling time. The recovery of contractile strength occurs with an increased extrasystolic interval (known as *mechanical restitution*); however, the increased pressure generated is minimal. Numerous studies have instead shown that the increased force of contraction of the beat following an extrasystole is independent of loading conditions and related to the *force-frequency* and *force-interval* relationships. With a premature beat that has a short coupling interval the refractory ryanodine receptors result in a smaller calcium transient. This results in less negative feedback to sarcolemmal calcium influx which increases cytosolic calcium resulting in a sarcoplasmic reticulum loaded with calcium (caused by SERCA 2a). The ryanodine receptors then recover during the time before the post-extrasystolic beat, which permits increased calcium released from the sarcoplasmic reticulum. This increased calcium is then available to bind to troponin C and cause a stronger contraction.

In the evaluation of tachycardia it is also important to ascertain whether the hemodynamic effects such as hypotension are the result of an excessively rapid rate or if the rapid rate is in response to hypotension. Moreover, an increase in heart rate in response to hypotension must be differentiated from a primary cardiac arrhythmia (Figs. 6.11 and 6.12). Differentiation of a supraventricular tachycardia during the initial examination is not always straightforward when the history is unknown or hemodynamic monitoring has not been instituted. Additionally, it is important to realize that the presence of an electrical depolarization of the ventricles does not necessarily result in an effective ventricular contraction (Fig. 6.8).

Figure 6.11. A semi-continuous electrocardiogram and systemic blood pressure recording from a dog undergoing occlusion of a patent ductus arteriosus. These recordings demonstrate several important relationships between hemodynamics and the electrocardiogram including the P wave location relative to the T wave, atrioventricular nodal conduction fatigue and the effect of ST segment changes on the P and T waves.

(A) A sinus rhythm with a heart rate of 108 bpm is recorded with a blood pressure that shows a wide pulse pressure (large difference between systolic and diastolic pressure) because of diastolic runoff due to the patent ductus arteriosus. The downward directed bracket labeled with an "A" indicates the PR interval (no Q wave identified in this lead). This interval is used to compare to the PR interval in frame C.

(B) Time: 5 min 17 s after frame A. During the passage of a transesophageal echocardiographic probe the dog developed a sinus tachycardia. Note the drop in blood pressure. Is this drop due to the tachycardia or is it a stimulus for the tachycardia? Note that the P and T wave overlap. The bracket directed upward encompasses the QT interval. The bracket directed downward indicates the PR interval that was measured in frame E at the same heart rate. These intervals are compared to those at the same heart rate in frame E.

(C) Time: 5 min 39 s after frame A. The reason that the dog developed a sinus tachycardia was unknown, but the rate continued to increase with a continued drop in blood pressure. The P wave is now seen in the ST segment such that the P wave precedes the T wave. The bracket directed upward encompasses the QT interval and helps to differentiate the P and T wave. The downward directed bracket is the PR interval measured in frame A. Here with the faster sinus rate, the PR interval has increased and falls outside of this bracketed interval. Atrioventricular nodal conduction has, therefore, slowed during this sinus tachycardia. The ability of the atrioventricular node to conduct is influenced by recovery, facilitation and fatigue. Wenckebach periodicity occurs when inadequate recovery of atrioventricular nodal conduction occurs with shorter P-P intervals that leads to atrioventricular block. In this case, the protracted rapid rate results in nodal "fatigue" with a prolonged atrioventricular conduction time and consequently, a prolonged PR interval. Importantly, atrioventricular nodal conduction is complex and is very sensitive to autonomic influences as well as the impact of rate. For an additional comparison examine frame E.

(D) Time: 7 min 14 s after frame A. The blood pressure has plummeted and a rapid heart rate continues. Likely, ST segment depression exists because of poor myocardial perfusion and is indicated by the down-directed arrow preceding the P wave. A larger negative deflection follows the P wave and is likely a T_a wave that is more exaggerated probably because of coexisting atrial myocardial hypoxia. Boluses of intravenous fluids were begun and anesthetic gas stopped.

(E) Time: 10 min 13 s after frame A. Note that although the heart rate of 219 bpm is the same as that in frame B, the extended period of time with rapid sinus tachycardia has resulted in atrioventricular nodal conduction fatigue as shown by the longer PR interval here in frame E. Compare the down-directed brackets

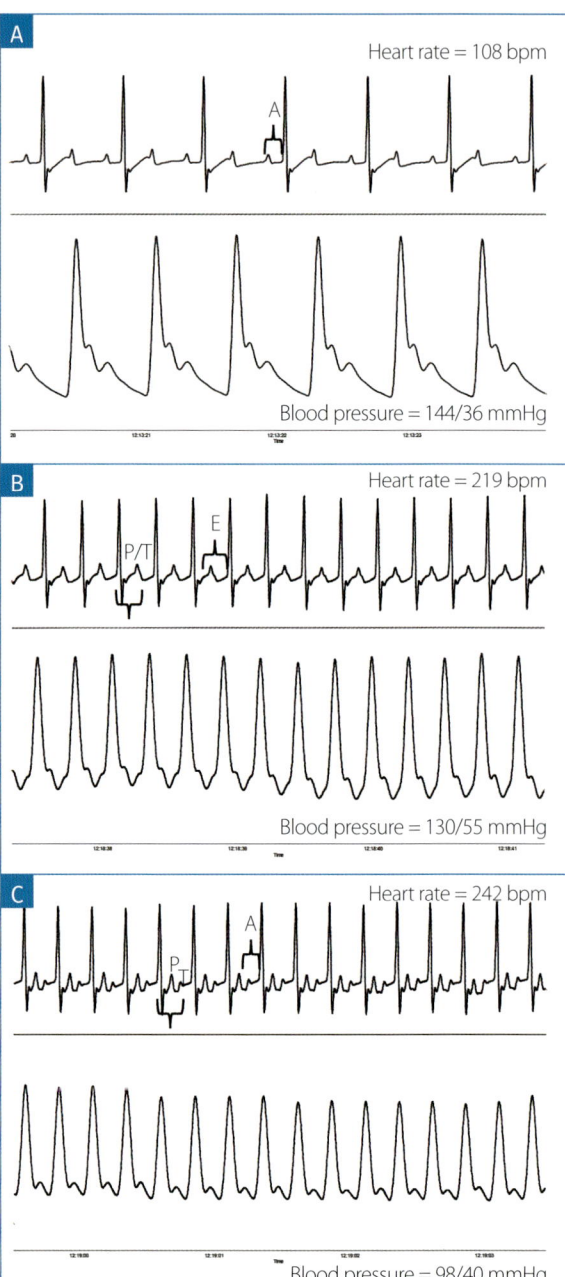

of B and E. The comparison of frame B with frame E illustrates the point that the complexity of conduction can result in a different electrocardiogram waveform pattern in the same patient, although the heart rate is the same. It should be noted that young dogs are very capable of having sinus tachycardia with rates above 250 bpm.

(F) Time: 11 min 8 s after frame A. The dog began to respond to treatment with a slowing of the heart rate, increase in blood pressure and less ST segment depression.

Hemodynamic consequences of arrhythmias | 111

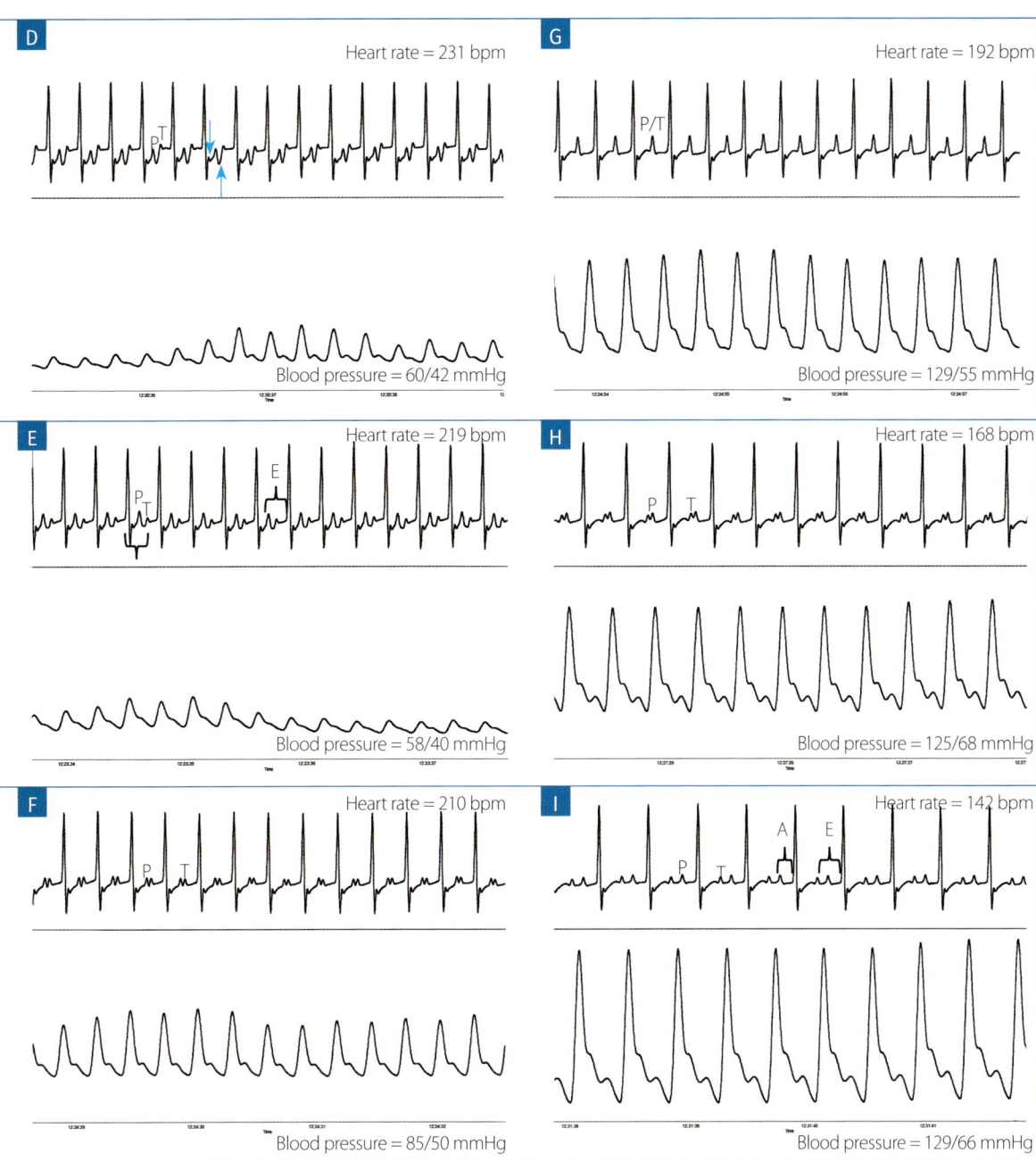

(G) Time: 11 min 27 s after frame A. The heart rate continued to decrease and the blood pressure to increase. Note with the shorter P-P interval the P and T overlap.

(H) Time: 13 min 56 s after frame A. The heart rate has slowed and the blood pressure has increased. Atrioventricular conduction time is normalizing. The balance of rate and conduction permits the P wave to follow the T wave.

(I) Time: 19 min 9 s after frame A. The sinus rate continued to slow back to normal and 15 minutes later returned to within 10 % of the initial rate. In this frame, with a rate of 142 bpm, the P and T waves have a normal time relationship. The bracket labeled A is the PR interval identified in frame A and for comparison the bracket labeled E is the PR interval identified in frame E. They are shown together here to illustrate the effect of heart rate and PR interval. The procedure was completed with successful ductal occlusion and the dog recovered uneventfully. The exact mechanism for the hypotension and sinus tachycardia were not determined.

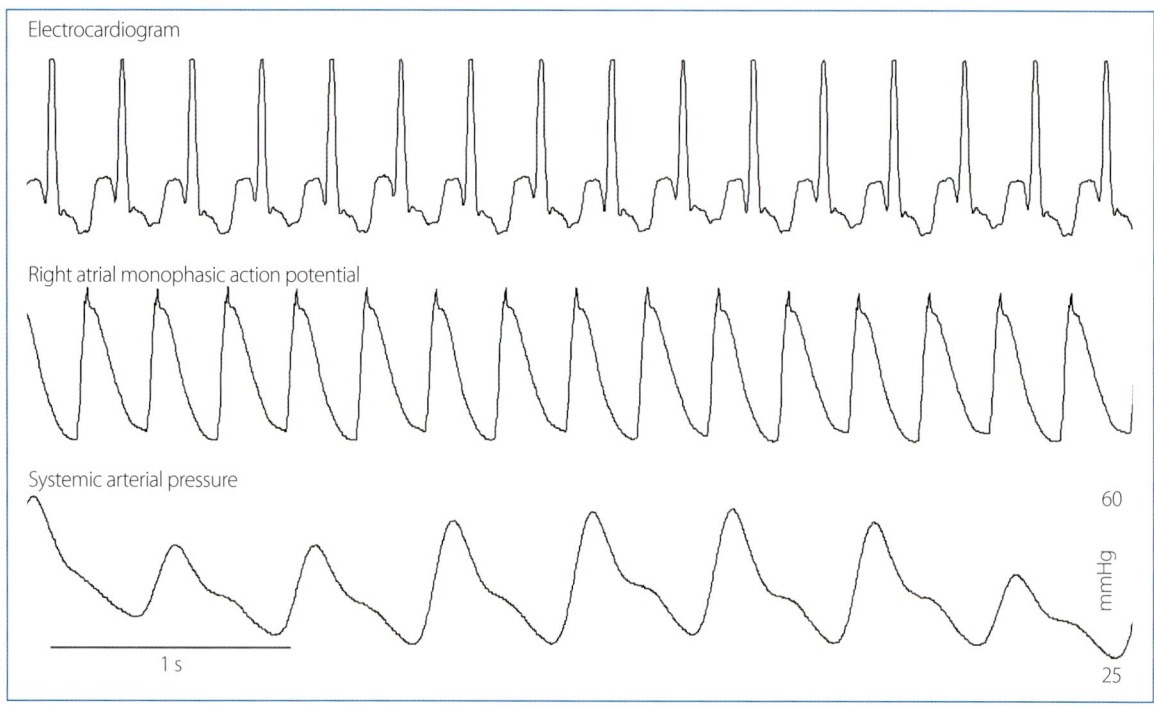

Figure 6.12. Electrocardiogram, intracardiac right atrial monophasic action potential and systemic arterial pressure in a dog with rapid atrial and ventricular rates. Atrioventricular conduction is 1:1; however; pulsus alternans occurs when the left ventricular systolic pressure is less than the aortic pressure on alternate beats so that the aortic valve does not open with halving of the pulse rate. The pressures are very low. On a physical examination such a relationship between heart sounds and pulse must be differentiated from a bigeminal rhythm. In addition to supraventricular tachycardias, pulsus alternans can occur with severe myocardial disease.

The duration of an arrhythmia has a major role in the hemodynamic consequences and associated clinical signs. Paroxysmal and rapid tachycardias (Fig. 6.13) can lead to an acute reduction in cardiac output and blood pressure, and result in weakness and syncope. Although incessant tachycardias may be well-tolerated, they lead to structural and functional cardiac changes over time, dominated by ventricular systolic dysfunction. The term tachycardiomyopathy, or arrhythmia-induced cardiomyopathy is used to describe the cardiac remodeling secondary to arrhythmias. The main characteristic of arrhythmia-induced cardiomyopathy is that it is partially or completely reversible once the arrhythmia is controlled. Tachycardiomyopathy is the result of an increase in myocardial oxygen demand, neurohormonal system activation, an alteration of calcium metabolism, myocyte elongation and extracellular matrix remodeling.

Slowing of the ventricular rate below the normal range is associated with an increase in each stroke volume because of a longer filling time, but it is usually not sufficient to compensate for the reduction in heart rate, which results in a decrease in cardiac output (stroke volume per minute). The reduction in ventricular rate is also responsible for an increase in mean right atrial pressure and alteration of caval blood flow into the atrium. The reduction in cardiac output triggers compensatory systems (adrenergic system, renin angiotensin aldosterone system and vasopressin) to maintain systemic perfusion. Over time, the increase in circulating volume combined with the elevation in atrial pressure can lead to bradycardia-induced cardiomyopathy and heart failure. Importantly, abrupt slowing of heart rate such as can occur with sinus node dysfunction will lead to acute drops in blood pressure (Fig. 6.14).

Under normal conditions, the temporal relationship between atrial systole and ventricular systole (*atrioventricular synchrony*) is important to optimize ventricular filling (Fig. 6.15) at the end of diastole, especially during

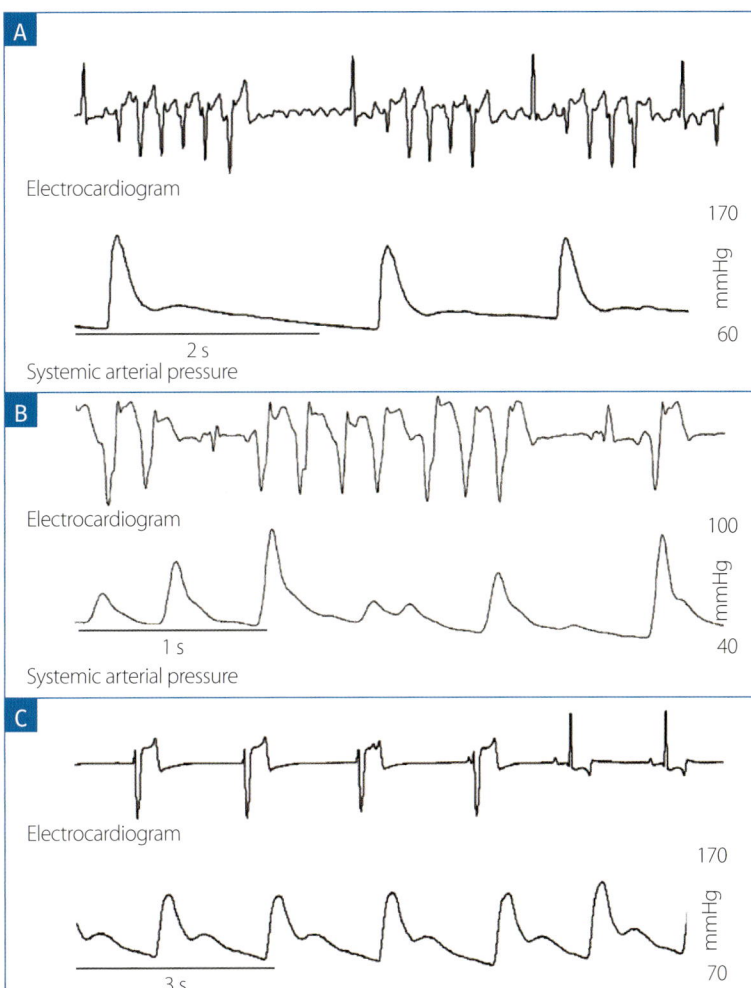

Figure 6.13. Electrocardiograms and systemic arterial pressure recordings from three dogs with ventricular rhythms.
(A) Recording from a young German Shepherd dog with atrial fibrillation and nonsustained ventricular tachycardia. The nonsustained runs of ventricular tachycardia failed to generate a measurable systemic blood pressure.
(B) Recording from a dog with severe pulmonic stenosis undergoing a balloon valvuloplasty which developed non-sustained runs of ventricular tachycardia that generated variable systemic pressures. Note the long delay between electrocardiographic beat identification and blood pressure deflection in this dog.
(C) Recording from a dog with sinus node dysfunction during pacemaker implantation. An idioventricular rhythm of 48 bpm generated a systemic pressure similar to that of sinus beats.

periods of elevated heart rate. Variations of the temporal relationship between the atrial and ventricular contraction secondary to PQ interval prolongation, atrioventricular dissociation or ventriculo-atrial retrograde conduction can result in a decrease in cardiac output, valvular insufficiency and elevated atrial pressure. When atrial contraction is not followed by a ventricular contraction (as in second- or third-degree atrioventricular heart block) the ventricular pressures increase and can exceed those of the right and left atrium resulting in diastolic regurgitation (Fig. 6.16).

In the presence of atrioventricular dissociation and ventriculo-atrial conduction, atrial and ventricular contraction can occur simultaneously. Atrial contraction against closed atrioventricular valves results in retrograde flow into the venae cavae (the "canon" a wave on examination of the jugular pulse) and pulmonary veins, and an increase in intra-atrial pressures (Fig. 6.17). The ultimate example of atrioventricular dissociation occurs during ventricular fibrillation during which the sinus node can continue to fire even in the face of the devastating ventricular rhythm (Fig. 6.18).

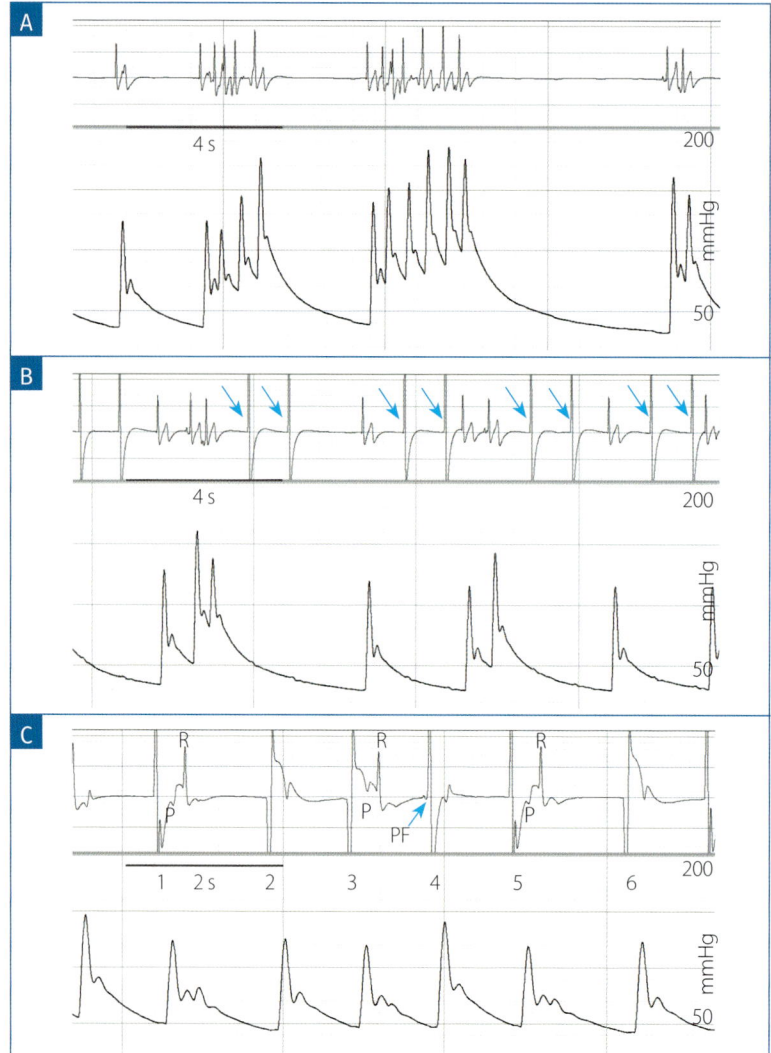

Figure 6.14. Electrocardiographic and systemic arterial pressure recordings from a dog with sinus node dysfunction undergoing permanent pacemaker implantation. Transcutaneous pacing was required due to excessively long pauses triggered by tachycardia. This figure illustrates the profound effects of sinus pauses on the systemic blood pressure and consequently perfusion. It also illustrates the importance of always paying attention not only to the electrical activity identified on the electrocardiogram, but also evidence of electromechanical association regardless of the arrhythmia or situation.
(A) During periods of sinus arrest the systemic blood pressure drops. Very late sinus and junctional complexes interrupt the sinus pauses.
(B) The sinus pauses became progressively longer and transcutaneous pacing was started. The arrows indicate the artifact during pacing. Note, however, that the capture was not occurring and no systemic pressure was generated. It is very important when monitoring the electrocardiogram during such pacing (or during any arrhythmia) to know that there is an electromechanical relationship. Large pacing artifacts from transcutaneous pacing can be confused with ventricular capture.
(C) Complexes 1 and 5 are successfully captured transcutaneous beats. A retrograde P wave (P) is identified that then results in an antegrade atrioventricular conduction and a narrow QRS complex (R). Beats 2, 3 and 6 begin with a negative deflection followed by a wide positive deflection. The pacing lead rather than the transcutaneous patches initiates these beats. The arrow indicates a pseudo-fusion (PF) complex. This is a pseudo-fusion because a sinus complex is hidden within the pacing artifact and the pacing artifact does not result in the capture. At this time the pacing lead was being secured. Retrograde P waves are common in dogs with sinus node dysfunction that are paced. These may be singular negative P waves that are blocked, or they may conduct antegrade down the atrioventricular node resulting in a QRS complex.

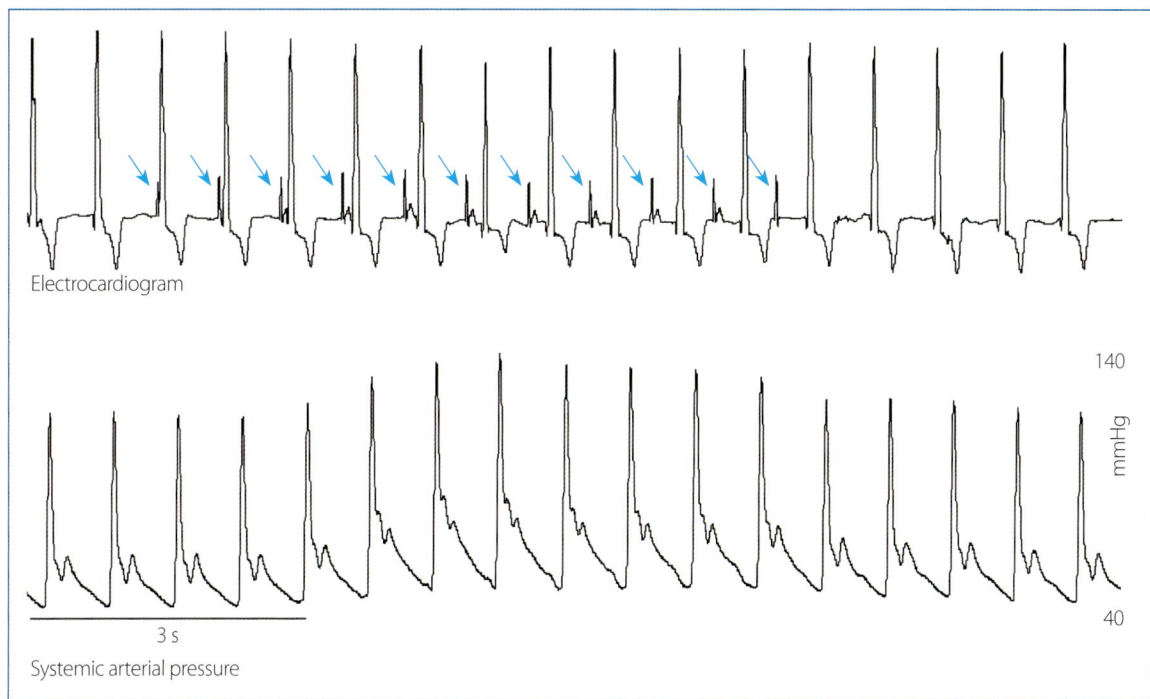

Figure 6.15. Electrocardiogram and systemic arterial pressure recorded from a dog with sinus node dysfunction undergoing pacemaker implantation with the lead in the atrium. This image illustrates the importance of atrioventricular synchrony and the effect that the PQ interval, and therefore, atrial systole has on stroke volume. The underlying rhythm is ventricular. Arrows indicate pacing artifact spike. It cannot be determined if the two initial spikes generate a P wave; however, the following pacing attempts result in a P wave. The pacing spikes are occurring at a constant interval. A very gradual and minimal slowing of the ventricular rate results in a change in the paced PQ interval. The change in this interval results in gradual augmentation of the ventricular filling and preload that then increases the systemic arterial pressure. When the PQ interval becomes too long (second to last P wave) or it does not capture (last P wave) the systemic pressure decreases.

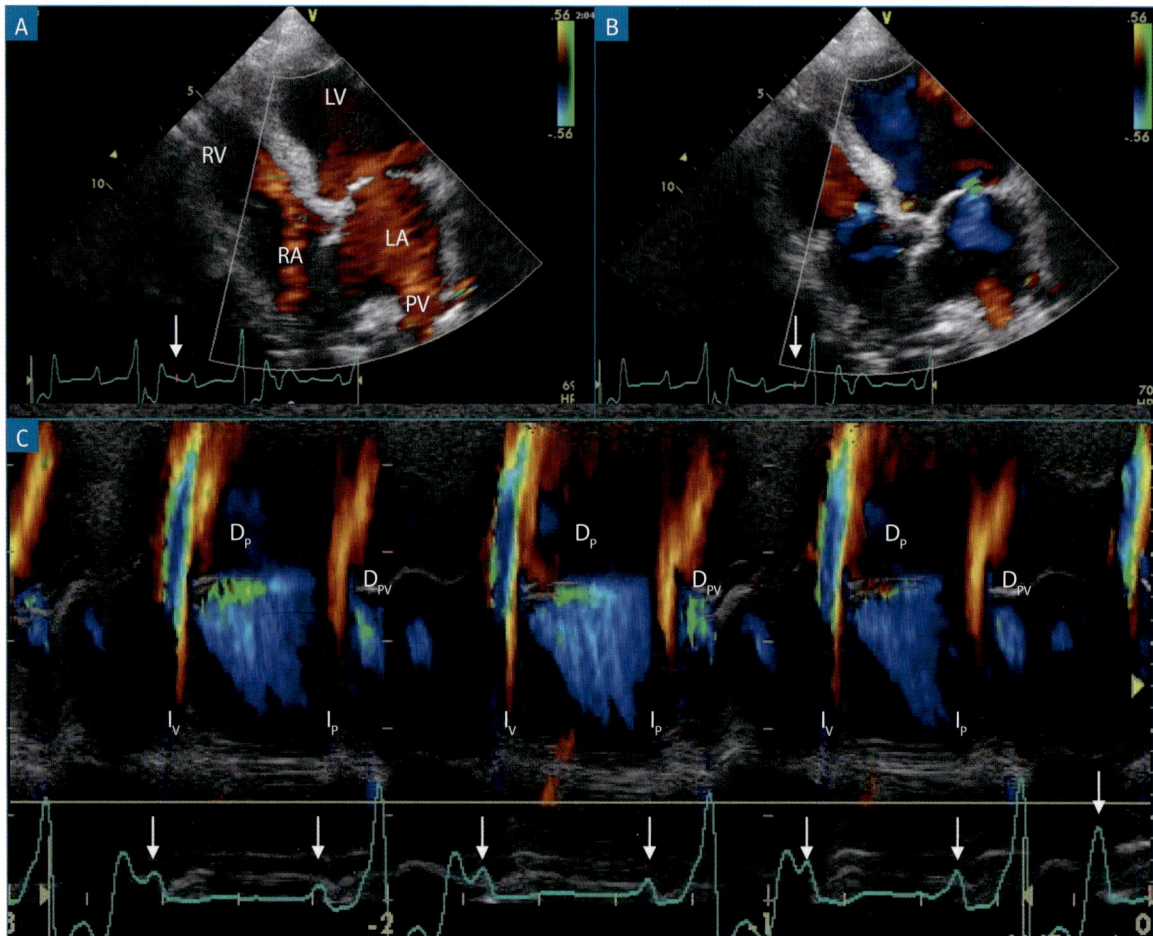

Figure 6.16. Two-dimensional and M-mode color flow Doppler echocardiographic examinations illustrating the hemodynamic consequences of third-degree atrioventricular nodal block.
(A) Inflow from the venae cavae to the right atrium/ventricle (RA, RV) and from the pulmonary veins (PV) to the left atrium/ventricle (LA, LV) occurs because the normal early diastolic pressure gradient favors flow from the atria into the ventricles. This flow occurs at the end of ventricular systole that was initiated by a ventricular escape complex (arrow). The color flow Doppler map codes the direction of flow towards the transducer (from atria to ventricles) as red (A).
(B) Diastolic atrioventricular valvular regurgitation is identified after the P wave of third-degree atrioventricular block (arrow). The color flow Doppler map codes the direction of flow away from the transducer (from both right and left ventricles to the atria) as blue.
(C) The color flow M-mode echocardiogram directed through the center of the mitral valve illustrates the effect of timing, pressure gradients and flow. The arrows on the electrocardiogram indicate P waves. The duration of diastolic regurgitation was dependent on whether it was interrupted by the ventricular systole caused by a ventricular escape complex. Following the end of ventricular systole, blood flow into the ventricles (early diastolic filling) is identified as an aliased red signal (I_V). Following atrial systole, blood flow into the ventricles is identified as a low velocity red signal (I_P). Following the completion of early diastolic flow and atrial systole, pressures increase in the ventricles such that they exceed atrial pressures resulting in a reversal of flow. This reversed pressure gradient results in backward flow (diastolic regurgitation across the atrioventricular valves) and is identified as a low velocity blue color. The duration of diastolic regurgitation is longer during P-P intervals (D_P) and shorter when a ventricular escape complex occurs between two P-P intervals (D_{PV}).

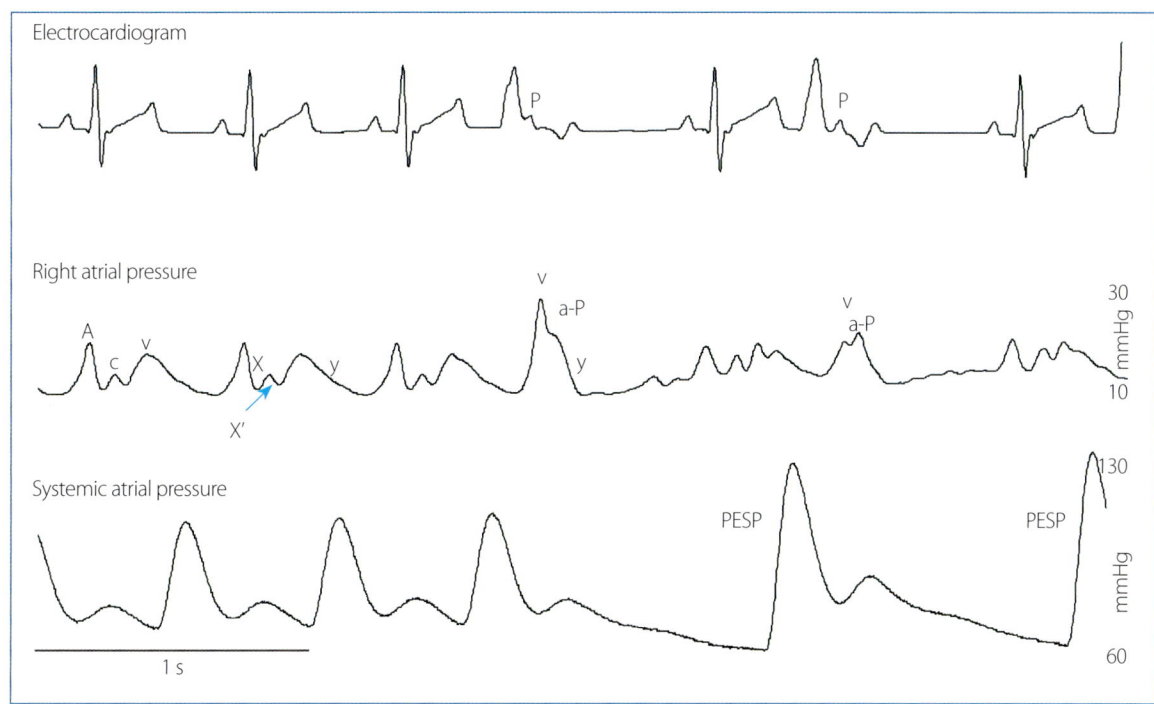

Figure 6.17. Electrocardiogram, right atrial pressure and systemic arterial pressure in a dog with pulmonic stenosis and right heart failure. The electrocardiogram shows a sinus rhythm with two premature ventricular complexes. The indicated P waves occur at the time of the ventricular contraction when the atrioventricular valves are closed. This is atrioventricular dissociation, which occurs with ventricular arrhythmias and third-degree atrioventricular heart block. In the right atrial pressure tracing the components of the pressure waveforms are identified and correlate with the electrocardiographic events. The intra-atrial pressures are elevated because of right heart failure. Atrial contraction (a), which occurs after the P wave, is followed by a positive deflection due to isovolumic contraction of the ventricle (c) and ventricular contraction (v) occurs after the QRS complex. It should be noted that the "c" wave is not always apparent as it is dependent on heart rate and PQ/PR interval. The downward deflections occur after the atrial contraction (x), after isovolumic contraction (x') (arrow) and after ventricular contraction (y). A premature ventricular complex is seen on the electrocardiogram which is followed on the right atrial pressure recording as a large V and in addition the atrial contraction corresponding to the disassociated P wave results in a large positive deflection. A sinus beat follows which in the systemic arterial pressure recording shows a post-extra-systolic potentiated pressure (PESP). This potentiation is the result of more sodium and calcium ions entering the myocardial cell than can be handled by the sodium pump and the mechanisms for calcium exit. This is known as the force-frequency relationship. In the second premature ventricular complex the timing of the ventricular and atrial contraction result in modification of the waveform. The reason for the altered right atrial pressure associated with the sinus beat between the two ventricular complexes is not readily apparent.

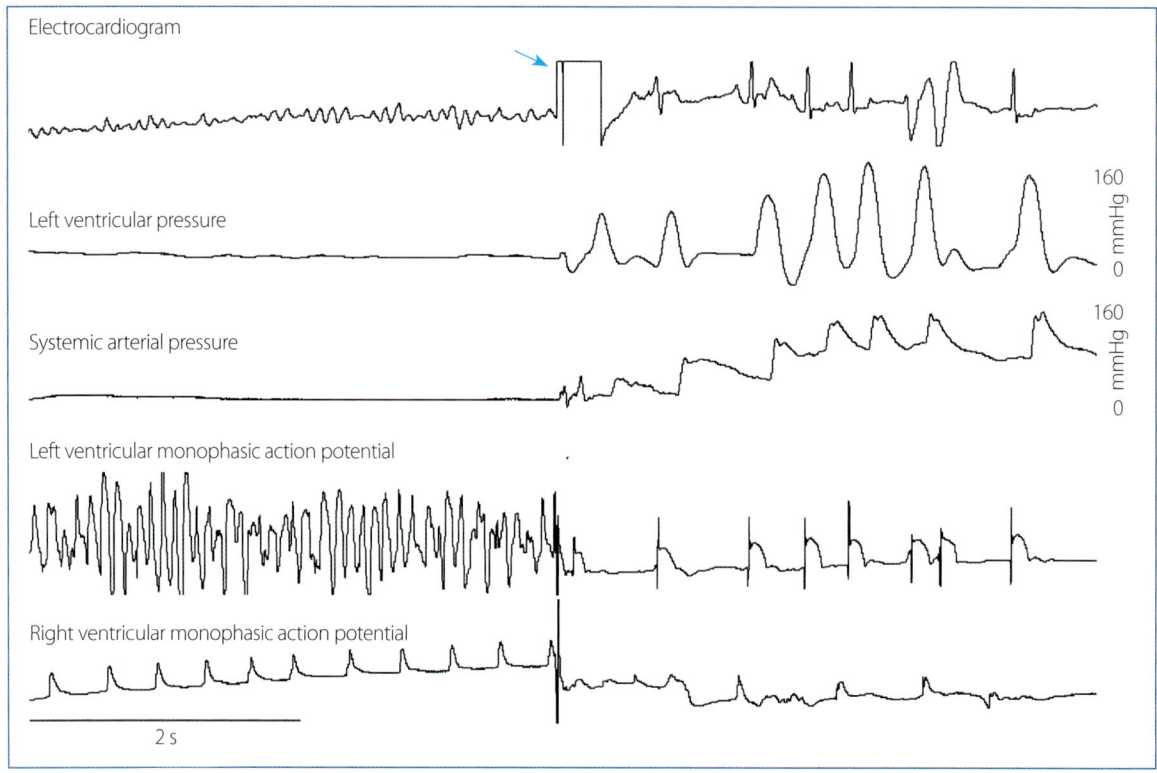

Figure 6.18. Electrocardiogram, left ventricular and systemic arterial pressures, left ventricular and right atrial monophasic action potential intracardiac recordings from a dog in ventricular fibrillation. The electrocardiogram shows the typical undulations of ventricular fibrillation. Without effective ventricular contractions, no ventricular or systemic pressures are generated for perfusion. The intracardiac recording from the left ventricular endocardium shows ventricular fibrillation while the intracardiac recording from the right atrial endocardium continues to show atrial depolarization because sinus rhythm coexists with the ventricular fibrillation. The arrow indicates the point when a shock of 150 J was delivered and the heart was successfully defibrillated. The electrocardiogram shows sinus beats and a ventricular couplet. Note that the first ventricular complex following the sinus beat has a long coupling interval and generates an effective blood pressure while the second ventricular complex that has a short coupling interval is ineffective in generating a systemic pressure. Note the return of an organized action potential in the left ventricular monophasic action potential recording.

During atrial fibrillation the variation in the ventricular response rate results in irregular R-R intervals with associated variation in the systemic blood pressure and perfusion (Fig. 6.19). On a beat-to-beat basis the rhythm is irregular; however, long-term monitoring shows prominent effects of the autonomic nervous system. The ventricular response rate can increase dramatically with sympathetic tone. Dogs that do not have extremely high ventricular response rates have slowing during the sleep hours an effect that becomes more prominent with successful treatment to decrease atrioventricular conduction. The development of atrial fibrillation can profoundly cause decompensation and congestive heart failure in myocardial disease or atrioventricular valve degeneration.

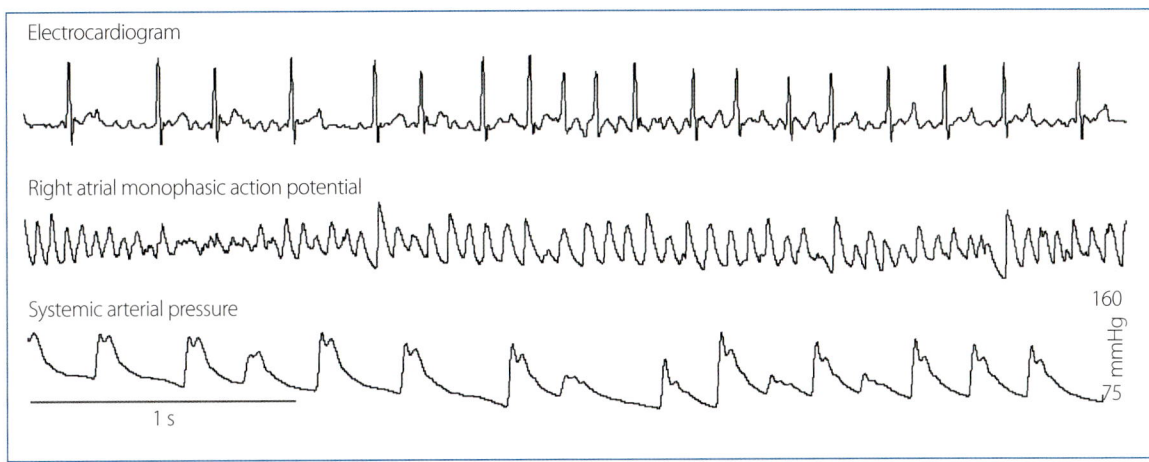

Figure 6.19. Electrocardiogram, intracardiac right atrial monophasic action potential and systemic arterial pressure in a dog with functional atrial fibrillation triggered by sedation with opioids and catheter movement. The recording from the endocardial surface of the right atrium shows the action potential variation during this type of atrial fibrillation which varies from fractionated to a more organized waveform. The ventricular response rate is seen to increase when the depolarizations in the atria become slower and more organized. The latter phenomenon results in less concealed conduction in the atrioventricular node with the consequence of a faster ventricular rate. With the higher heart rate the systemic arterial pressure is seen to decrease. Additionally, variability in the systemic pressure is identified.

Arrhythmia-related clinical signs

Dogs with bradyarrhythmias (third-degree atrioventricular block or persistent atrial standstill) develop right-sided congestive heart failure after a period of a few weeks to a few months. Clinical signs include ascites, less commonly pleural effusion and cachexia. Syncope is caused by transient cerebral hypoperfusion during periods of asystole that last at least 8 seconds.

Supraventricular and ventricular tachycardias cause signs of weakness and syncope, usually during periods of activity. Acute signs are more common with paroxysmal tachycardias, especially in animals with pre-existing systolic dysfunction. In general, supraventricular tachycardias are better tolerated than ventricular tachycardias, which are more frequently associated with syncope, and on occasion cardiogenic shock.

Both incessant supraventricular and ventricular tachycardias with high ventricular rate can result in tachycardiomyopathy (or arrhythmia-induced cardiomyopathy), a form of myocardial dysfunction that mimics dilated cardiomyopathy and leads to congestive heart failure. The features of tachycardiomyopathy include a decrease in ejection fraction, increases in left ventricular end-diastolic and end-systolic volumes and an increase in the pulmonary capillary wedge pressure. Tachycardiomyopathy is partially or completely reversible if the arrhythmia can be controlled. In dogs, experimental pacing studies suggest that a sustained ventricular rate of 220 bpm for several weeks consistently results in ventricular dysfunction.

Diagnosis of arrhythmias

In the past, 3-min electrocardiograms recorded on grid paper were the standard. Now with the advent of electronic electrocardiograms and the capability of recording 6 and 12-lead electrocardiograms for 5 to 60 minutes at a time, a more thorough evaluation is possible. With longer recording times there is the opportunity for changes in rhythm to give clues to the diagnosis. Table 6.5 provides a summary of evaluations or questions to assist in the diagnosis of arrhythmias.

TABLE 6.5. Step-by-step approach to the electrocardiographic evaluation of arrythmias

1. Technique.
a. Assess recording for sweep speed and calibration.
b. Assess recording for filtering (changes in filtering can alter amplitude measurements).
c. Assess recording for artifact.

2. Assess ventricular complexes (QRS complex).
a. Determine rate of ventricular complexes (normal rate, tachycardia, bradycardia).
b. Determine if all ventricular complexes look the same (different origin or different conduction).
c. Classify ventricular complex morphology as within normal duration and amplitude and classify ventricular complexes as narrow or wide (differentiation of ventricular versus supraventricular origin).
d. Determine if ventricular rhythm is regular or irregular.
e. Determine if irregular rhythm present with normal rate, tachycardia or bradycardia.
f. Are there individual/single premature complexes (short R-R interval usually <400 ms).
g. If premature complexes present, determine if their QRS complex morphology is narrow (normal duration, amplitude) or wide.

3. Assess atrial complexes (P waves, F waves, f waves, absent atrial complexes).
a. Identify P waves.
b. Determine the rate of atrial complexes.
c. Determine if rate of atrial complexes equals rate of ventricular complexes.
d. Determine relationship of P waves with ventricular complex.
   i. Associated.
   ii. Not associated.
e. Evaluate P wave morphology as it relates to P-P interval.
f. Evaluate P wave morphology across all leads.
g. If no P waves identified, are there flutter waves, fibrillation waves or no atrial activity.
h. Is atrial rhythm regular or irregular.

4. Assess relationship between atrial and ventricular complexes.
a. Are there P waves without QRS complexes (determination of atrioventricular nodal block or atrial tachycardia with physiologic block).
b. Restatement of (a): are P waves associated with ventricular complexes (each QRS has a P wave).
   i. Are there more P waves than QRS complexes (physiologic or pathologic atrioventricular nodal block with ventricular escape rhythm).
   ii. Are there more QRS complexes than P waves (ventricular tachycardia with atrioventricular dissociation identified, can also be junctional in origin).
c. Determine PQ interval (prolongation or preexcitation).
d. Determine if PQ interval is consistent (determination of first-degree atrioventricular block, intermittent conduction across accessory pathway, variation in atrioventricular conduction associated with autonomic tone).
e. Are there F waves with irregular ventricular rhythm (determination of atrial flutter).
f. Baseline undulations of f waves with irregular ventricular rhythm (determination of atrial fibrillation).

5. Determine underlying rhythm over which premature complexes or pauses identified.
a. Sinus rhythm or sinus arrhythmia.
b. Atrial fibrillation.
c. Atrial flutter.
d. Atrial standstill.

6. Assess patterns.
a. Are there pauses of the atrial and ventricular rhythm determination of sinus pauses usually >2 s for in-hospital ECG, usually <500 pauses >2 s on 24-hour Holter normal).
b. Are pauses interrupted by a late sinus beat, atrial escape beat, junctional escape beat or ventricular escape beat.
c. Are there multiple P waves in a row without associated ventricular/QRS complex but ventricular complexes present at slow rate (atrioventricular block with junctional or ventricular escape rhythm).
d. Are there patterns of ventricular or atrial premature beats present (bigeminy, trigeminy, quadrigeminy).
e. Are there patterns of multiple ventricular or atrial ectopic beats present (couplets, triplets, nonsustained tachycardia, sustained tachycardia).
f. Are there changes in QRS morphology associated with an increase or decrease in heart rate (rate-dependent intraventricular blocks)
g. Are there particular patterns associated with the occurrence of premature complexes (following long short R-R intervals, occurrence with excitement, occurrence with slow or fast heart rate, constant/variable coupling interval).
h. Determine if morphologies are constantly changing, have a pattern, or remain constant.

7. Assess P-QRS-T complex across all electrocardiographic leads.

a. P wave amplitude and morphology changes in the dog due to wandering pacemaker. P wave amplitude and morphology in the cat are much more consistent.

b. Measurement of the P wave in the dog is problematic because it changes due to the wandering pacemaker. Be aware that with faster heart rates and anticholinergics, the P waves will be taller in lead II.

c. Verify normal QRS wave vectors of depolarization (normal dogs and cats have negative QRS wave in lead aVR). If not normal, investigate criteria for conduction block or ventricular hypertrophy.

d. Verify normal P wave vector of depolarization (normal dogs and cats have positive P waves in lead II and negative P waves in aVR). If P waves do not have normal vector first verify positioning of leads, if correct, then evaluate for ectopic focus.

e. Some breeds of dog and some cats have low amplitude P waves in frontal plane, check precordial leads for P wave. If P waves not identified, evaluate for arrhythmia.

f. Verify proportions of T wave to QRS complex (usually abnormal in the dog is a large amplitude T wave, be aware that cats can have a T wave larger than the QRS complex in the frontal plane). If T wave tall, symmetrical and spiked, check for hyperkalemia.

g. In assessing for origin of arrhythmias review QRS morphology across frontal plane and precordial leads.

8. Assessment of difficult rhythm disorders.

a. With a difficult rhythm, record over several minutes to see if rhythm changes occur so as to identify clues to the arrhythmia.

b. Try maneuvers to change the rhythm and assist in diagnosis such as vagal maneuvers, exercise, or excitement.

c. Drug intervention to assist in diagnosis can be used.

d. If precordial leads are not recorded, record as they may be of assistance.

e. If a rhythm disorder is suspected but not identified during routine electrocardiography, use longer-term monitoring such as 24-hour Holter recordings.

Several other techniques have been developed to obtain longer recordings of the cardiac rhythm: 24-hour Holter systems, external event recorders, and more recently implantable loop recorders.

However, none of these recording devices provide detailed information on the exact location of arrhythmogenic substrates or the electrophysiological mechanism of arrhythmias. These limitations have led to the development of electrophysiological mapping, which consists in recording the intra-cardiac electrical activity via catheters precisely positioned in the cardiac chambers under fluoroscopic guidance.

Holter monitoring

In 1949, Dr. Norman Holter designed a system to record a continuous electrocardiogram for 24 hours. Although the term "24-hour ambulatory electrocardiographic monitoring" is used, most commonly veterinary clinicians use the term "Holter monitoring". Holter monitoring is indicated in the assessment of syncope (transient loss of consciousness), near-syncope (partial transient loss of consciousness), collapse, arrhythmias (bradycardias and tachycardias), effect of anti-arrhythmic treatment, pacemaker malfunction, or screening for cardiomyopathies. Certainly, other means of rhythm assessment outside of the hospital environment are of value in the appraisal of cardiac rate and rhythm. These include implantable loop recorders and event recorders. However, Holter monitoring (which can have extended monitoring times as well) provides a great deal of information that may not be obtained from other modalities.

This diagnostic evaluation can be performed in dogs and cats and is becoming even more plausible as technology advances with smaller recording devices. A variety of recording systems have been developed that either have wires connected to patches or wireless small stick-on patches that are then connected to the recording device. The latter may not give adequate differentiation between leads without a great deal of signal amplification, which can potentially increase artifacts. When using the wired electrode patches, they may be positioned to provide an orthogonal bipolar system X, Y and Z to record the electrocardiogram in three anatomical planes (frontal, sagittal and horizontal) or alternatively the precordial leads V_1, V_2, V_3 and V_5 can be used to record the electrocardiogram in the horizontal plane. The recording device is most often secured within the pouch of a wearable "Holter vest" that is designed for dogs and cats. The ideal situation is to have this recording made while the dog is in the home environment. After recording the electrocardiogram, the digitized data is downloaded for software analysis. Although the analysis algorithms have improved, all still demand careful editing for proper beat annotation (identification).

When interpreting the results of Holter analysis the following features are examined:
- heart rate,
- heart rate variability,
- frequency and timing of the arrhythmias, and
- triggers for the arrhythmias.

The evaluation of heart rate entails the examination of numerous parameters. Average heart rate is simply one of the initial parameters assessed. It is vitally important to understand and know for a given Holter analysis system what this average heart rate means. Is this based on the sinus rhythm? Is this based on the total heartbeats regardless of beat identification? Some systems are able to provide both. Hourly average heart rate can be assessed from the hourly table provided by most analysis programs. Such tables often give the minimum and maximum heart rate for any given hour as well. Again, it is vital to know if this heart rate is sinus or total R-R intervals. A heart rate tachogram provides a graphic display of geometric heart rate variability over the 24 hours. It must be determined for any given analysis program how the average heart rate is being calculated and displayed on this graph. Some use a rolling average of 8 beats with a display of the minimum and maximum heart rate shown as bars and others use the standard deviation of the average heart rate. From this graph the heart rate distribution at certain points during the day may be correlated with the diary that is kept by the owner. The majority of dogs have a sleep cycle that is most consistently seen with a slower heart rate between midnight and 7 a.m. Of course, this will vary depending upon household activities. It is also very common for some of the fastest heart rates to occur during the application or removal of the Holter monitor.

Quite often associated with the heart rate tachogram there is a graph indicating the timing and duration of pauses. The definition of a pause can be selected, but usually within a prescribed range. Some prefer to set this definition of a pause as greater than 2 s and others greater than 3 s. It is vitally important to recognize that if a pause is indicated in the narrative or graphic presentation this area needs to be visualized on the full disclosure adequately. Quite often pauses occur with an interruption by an escape beat and repeated pauses. Therefore, if an individual relies totally on the narrative report without investigating the existence of secondary pauses, they will not be identified and recognized as potential problems. Quite often the minimum and maximum heart rates are over emphasized as it must be remembered that these are singular points in time. A more important parameter to assess is the amount of time that a dog spends with a heart rate less than 50 bpm or above 120 bpm. These two parameters can be adjusted but in general, such assessment gives a perspective of the overall clustering of heart rate. In general the majority of dogs spend greater than 80 % of their day with a heart rate between these two values. Most dogs spend less than 1 hour with a heart rate less than 50 bpm and less than 3 hours with a heart rate greater than 120 bpm.

Heart rate variability can be determined from the R-R intervals recorded during the 24-hour Holter. Such assessment can be done for all or part of the recording. Geometric, time domain, and frequency domain can be used. It is important to remember that when heart rate variability is considered it is in the context of what the sinus node is doing; however, the P-P interval is not what is being assessed. Consequently, if heart rate variability is to be used accurately only sinus beats should be used for the calculations of the various parameters studied. Although heart rate variability is primarily considered in the assessment of the autonomic system and its effect on the sinus node, importantly, geometric heart rate variability serves a very valuable role in understanding rhythm disorders with specific patterns developing with certain types of arrhythmias.

Geometric heart rate variability involves the use of graphs and other visual means in the assessment of R-R intervals. These graphs include heart rate tachogram, sinus interval histogram, ventricular interval histogram, supraventricular interval histogram, R-R interval 24 hour tachogram, hourly R-R interval tachogram, and Poincaré plots. It should be noted that the R-R interval tachogram is a linear two-dimensional representation over time that appears as a compressed image. In the standard 24-hour R-R interval tachogram, repeated intervals overlay each other because of the compression, and therefore the appreciation of beat density is lost. This can be regained by the use of three-dimensional R-R interval tachograms which incorporate a histogram with the tachogram. The Poincaré plot is also a two-dimensional geometric representation of the heart rate variability; however, it is a nonlinear representation of the beat-to-beat intervals. A Poincaré plot is created by plotting a given R-R interval on the X-axis against the next R-R interval on the Y-axis (R-R interval +1). Importantly, the next interval that serves as the location on the X-axis overlaps by one and is the previous R-R interval +1. Thus, the graph is R-R interval versus R-R interval +1. In the Holter analysis packages these are often represented by the hour but if a particular algorithm permits a specific time interval to be assessed this may provide information as desired. Additionally, a full 24-hour image of the Poincaré plot can be obtained; however, the beat density is so great that valuable information is difficult to obtain. Importantly the still images cannot portray the exact dynamics in play. To assist in this, animated Poincaré plots can be used.

Time domain heart rate variability includes: (1) SDNN: standard deviation of all NN intervals, (2) SDANN: standard deviation of all 5-min NN interval means, (3) SDNN Index: mean of all 5-min NN interval standard deviations, and (4) RMSSD: square root of the mean squared successive NN interval differences. The triangular index is available in many software packages; however, this is likely not a usable parameter as it is determined from the total number of beat intervals divided by the height of the histogram. Because the distribution of beats in the dog represented by the histogram does not have a single bell-shaped curve but is skewed or has several semi-bell-shaped curves, it may not be accurate. Time domain heart rate variability can be determined over the entire 24-hour period or by selecting time periods of interest during a designated period.

Frequency domain heart rate variability is usually determined over shorter periods of time, although longer periods may also be considered so long as there is stability. For short-term frequency domain assessment period is usually chosen as a 5-min interval, 256 beats or 512 beats. Additionally, different filtering methods are selected (e.g. Hamming, Hanning windows). With frequency domain heart rate variability the values are reported as the power spectral density (s^2/Hz) on the Y-axis with frequency (Hz) on the X-axis. The power in ms^2 as the total <0.4 Hz, very low frequency <0.04 Hz, low frequency <0.04-0.15 Hz, and high-frequency <0.15-0.4 Hz. Additionally, the low-frequency/high-frequency ratio is reported, and importantly the indexed power is given in units of n.u.

Geometric heart rate variability has provided insight with regards to the unique patterning of the sinus beating in the dog. The dog does not have the same type of pattern as humans, cats, or horses. The canine beat distribution is unique with a bifurcating pattern associated with high vagal tone. In the dog the Poincaré plot shows this distribution as short-short intervals during the times that a sinus rhythm associated with a faster heart rate is present. This is during times of higher sympathetic tone and lower parasympathetic tone. This appears on the plot as points that cluster together, forming a fuzzy bar of points along the line of identity. Usually, at approximately 700 ms there is a triangular cluster of points that then projects to bars (arms) representing short-long intervals and long-short intervals. These represent the time of high parasympathetic tone in the dog (Fig 6.20). This bifurcated pattern is recognized on the R-R interval tachogram as a region of decreased density. It appears as a paucity of beat intervals (zone of avoidance) between approximately 700 and 1200 ms. Several different patterns are present on the Poincaré plot in normal dogs. Likely, depending on the balance of parasympathetic and sympathetic tone beats along the arms will cluster more or less and a cloud of R-R intervals representing long-long intervals is seen below the line identity. Geometric heart rate variability can be of value not only in the assessment of normal and abnormal sinus node function, but can give evidence to the type of arrhythmia that is present. For example, atrial fibrillation has a distinctive pattern, as do 2:1 and 3:1 atrioventricular nodal heart blocks, atrial flutter, couplets, or abrupt changes in rhythm such as cardioversion.

124 | Chapter 6. Background to the diagnosis of arrhythmias

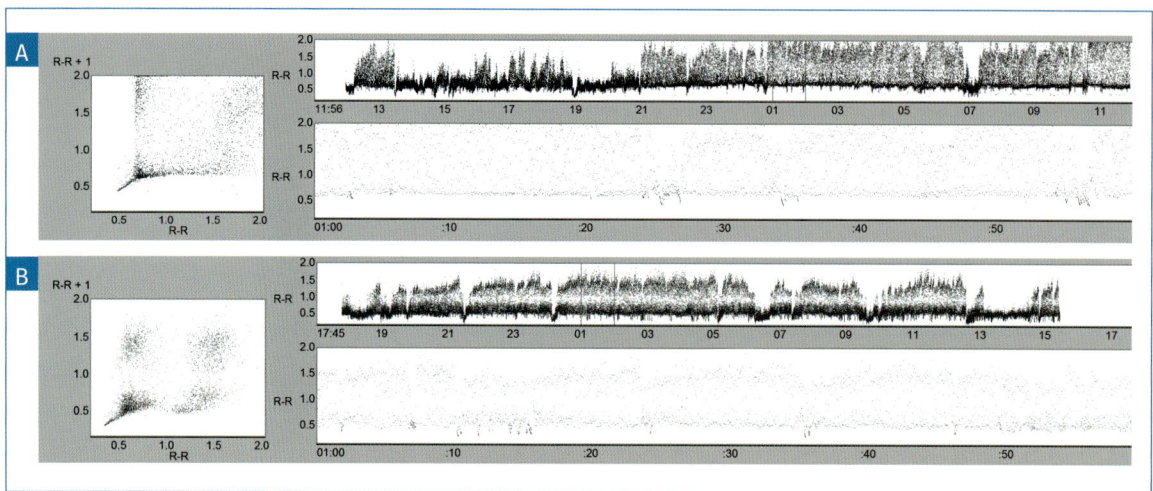

Figure 6.20. Holter recording from a Doberman and Boxer showing a 24-hour tachogram for each dog and a selected 1-hour Poincaré plot.
(A) The beat-to-beat intervals along the line of identity between approximately 500 and 600 ms represents beats with a more constant interval that occur during higher sympathetic tone. In this Doberman at approximately 650 ms the beat-to-beat intervals diverge into "arms" because of increased parasympathetic input. A low density cloud of long-long intervals is seen. The tachogram shows the beat density spread for 24 hours and during the hour represented in the Poincaré plot.
(B) The beat-to-beat intervals for the Boxer show a different clustering associated with sympathetic and parasympathetic tone. The tachogram also shows a different beat clustering.

Of course one of the primary reasons for performing 24-hour Holter monitoring is to assess the presence and severity of arrhythmias. Each of the above assessments are made, but to diagnose the specific arrhythmia, the actual beats are examined. Examination of the P-QRS-T complexes is essential and can be done from looking at selected report strips, full disclosure at a speed that permits adequate assessment of coupling intervals and short strips whereby the intervals between beats are indicated. It is not possible to fully appreciate the results of a Holter recording by simply looking at a very compressed image of a full disclosure. This is particularly true if one is trying to assess the response to treatment of arrhythmias. In addition to knowing the frequency and complexity of arrhythmias, the distribution or triggers of these arrhythmias can lend important information that may have an impact on the type of treatment that is given. For example, do the ventricular arrhythmias occur more with excitement or more during the evening during sleep? The type of patterning over many beats may give evidence of particular mechanism for the arrhythmia. This may be additionally assisted by the study of animated Poincaré plots. It is also important to realize that some dogs may not have a large ventricular load, but do have dangerous ventricular tachycardia. Careful evaluation of beat-to-beat patterning before the pause is also important. For example evidence of a neurocardiogenic reflex would be a tachycardia followed by gradual slowing and then excessively long pauses.

As a general statement, if a dog has sufficient cardiac arrhythmias (supraventricular or ventricular) to demand the institution of treatment that dog should have a baseline 24-hour Holter recording and follow-up recordings. If this type of monitoring is not done, then the response to medication will not be known. It is impossible to make a full and accurate appraisal based on a short electrocardiogram performed in the clinic. It is also important to realize and accept that in general the majority of dogs can tolerate a 24-hour period to obtain a baseline recording before antiarrhythmic medication is instituted. If a baseline recording is not obtained, it is impossible to determine whether the medication is having an antiarrhythmic or a proarrhythmic effect or no effect at all. Of course, there are circumstances in which a baseline recording is not in the best interest of the patient, but these are the exception. In general, an 85 % reduction in the frequency of an arrhythmia with treatment is necessary in order to be sure that the effect is not just day-to-day variability.

Holter analysis packages commonly include graphs for QT plotting and assessment. In addition, they often offer one of several QT correction formulas to use in the assessment of the QT interval. Such formulas have been established to be flawed and of limited value in the assessment of canine heart rate and QT relationships. The relationship of the QT to R-R interval is non-linear. Some formulas over-correct while others under-correct at varying heart rates. Moreover, there is a QT hysteresis that occurs in its relationship to the R-R interval. Development of methods to relate the QT interval to heart rate are an ongoing struggle. One procedure used in the analysis of 24-hour ambulatory electrocardiographic recordings evaluates the stability of beat-to-beat QT interval with respect to the TQ interval (electrical diastole). This is called QT/TQ restitution. Restitution is the ability of the heart to recover from one beat to the next. During very rapid heart rates the TQ interval can approach zero (e.g. ventricular tachycardia). The QT/TQ ratio provides an assessment of the relationship of the electrical systolic period to the electrical diastolic period. Restitution curves of this relationship have been associated with transition from ventricular tachycardia to ventricular fibrillation based on the steepness of the restitution relationship. The steeper the slope (>1) the more likely it is that instability exists. The longer the QT interval relative to this TQ interval the more likely it is for fibrillation to occur.

Some miscellaneous comments with regards to evaluation of the Holter recording are warranted. Dogs change their body position often when wearing the monitor and this will result in dramatic alterations and changes in the P-QRS-T complex. Such changes must be understood and not misdiagnosed as a problem. Most often these changes are accompanied by motion artifacts. Variability in the frequency of arrhythmias can occur with no medical intervention and this is why very strict criteria must be used to be sure that a drug has an antiarrhythmic effect or to blame a drug for a pro-arrhythmic effect. Moreover, with the analysis of many recordings in dogs it can be realized that the normal young adult dog has virtually no arrhythmias. Additionally, arbitrary numbers to define a dog as affected or not affected during screening based on some limit of premature complexes could be problematic. Additional studies are required to learn what are true normal values. For example, an evaluation of geriatric dogs and their heart rate patterns and frequency of arrhythmias is needed. Treatment effects of medications demand study.

Event recorders

An event recorder is a device that can monitor the heart rhythm for up to 7 days using the wearable version, and for up to 36 months with implantable loop recorders. This diagnostic tool is indicated in animals that experience rare clinical signs that could be attributed to an arrhythmia, whenever standard tests (3 to 5-min electrocardiogram, a 24-hour Holter monitor and an echocardiogram) have failed to identify a cause.

External event recorders record the electrocardiogram from a pair of electrodes that are secured to the skin on the thorax. Implantable event recorders have the size of a USB flash drive and can be placed subcutaneously on the left hemithorax at the level of the heart.

Event recorders continuously record the electrocardiogram and a 5 to 10-min segment of the tracing is saved for later review. The device can be programmed to automatically save a portion of the electrocardiogram if the heart rate falls outside a pre-defined range. The save function can also be triggered manually if the pet owner witnesses an episode of weakness or syncope (Figs. 6.21 and 6.22). Event recorders reveal the cause of syncope in up to 85 % of the cases, usually if the recording is triggered manually.

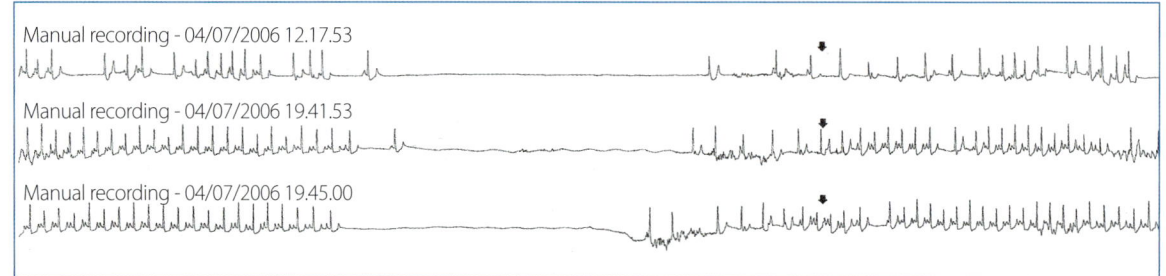

Figure 6.21. Recordings obtained with an external event recorder in a dog with arrhythmic syncope secondary to sinus node dysfunction (Dog, German Dachshund, female, 10 years. Each tracing is 30 s in duration - calibration 5 mm/1 mV).
Note in the three tracings the presence of episodes of supraventricular tachycardia followed by sinus arrest lasting 8.9, 7.7 and 8.3 s, respectively. Arrows indicate the time when the owner witnessed an episode of syncope and triggered the recording. The device was designed to save the electrocardiogram a few seconds before and after manual activation.

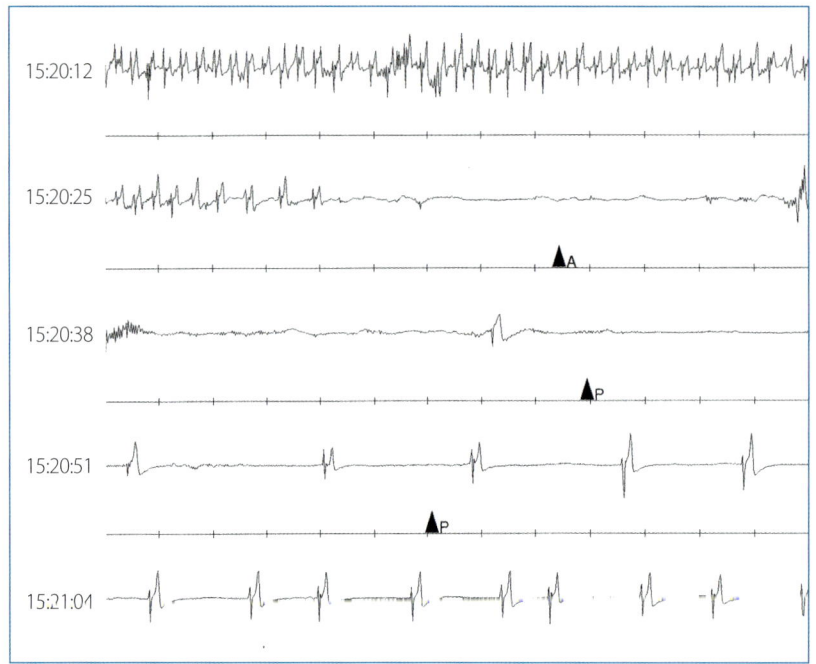

Figure 6.22. Recording obtained with an implantable loop recorder in a dog with suspected reflex syncope (Dog, English Bulldog, male, 2 years - speed 12.5 mm/s - calibration 6.3 mm/1 mV).
The first tracing shows a sinus tachycardia with a mean heart rate of 173 bpm, followed by a sinus arrest lasting 17.6 s and interrupted by an ventricular escape rhythm, first with a discharge rate of 10 bpm. The ventricular rhythm gradually increases to 80 bpm. The triangle followed by the letter A indicates the automatic activation of the device, based on pre-programmed parameters for the detection of bradycardia. The black triangles followed by the letter P indicate when the owner manually activated the device during the syncopal event.

Electrophysiology study

Although electrophysiological studies in veterinary medicine are currently limited to a few institutions worldwide, knowing the diagnostic and therapeutic indications will assist in optimal care of dogs with arrhythmias. It should be noted that historically electrophysiological studies in the research arena were conducted in dogs, thus valuable data are available in the literature. This methodology is limited to dogs of adequate size and is not possible, at present, in the cat. As a deeper understanding of clinical arrhythmias in the dog develops and as methods advance to make procedures more technically feasible and affordable the use of such studies will become more common. In human medicine contact catheter directed cardiac mapping has been supplanted in many cases by noncontact three-dimensional reconstruction of the electrical activity of the heart. The latter has broadened the diagnostic and therapeutic abilities for the treatment of arrhythmias; however, extensive training is required to master the use of this equipment and interpret the

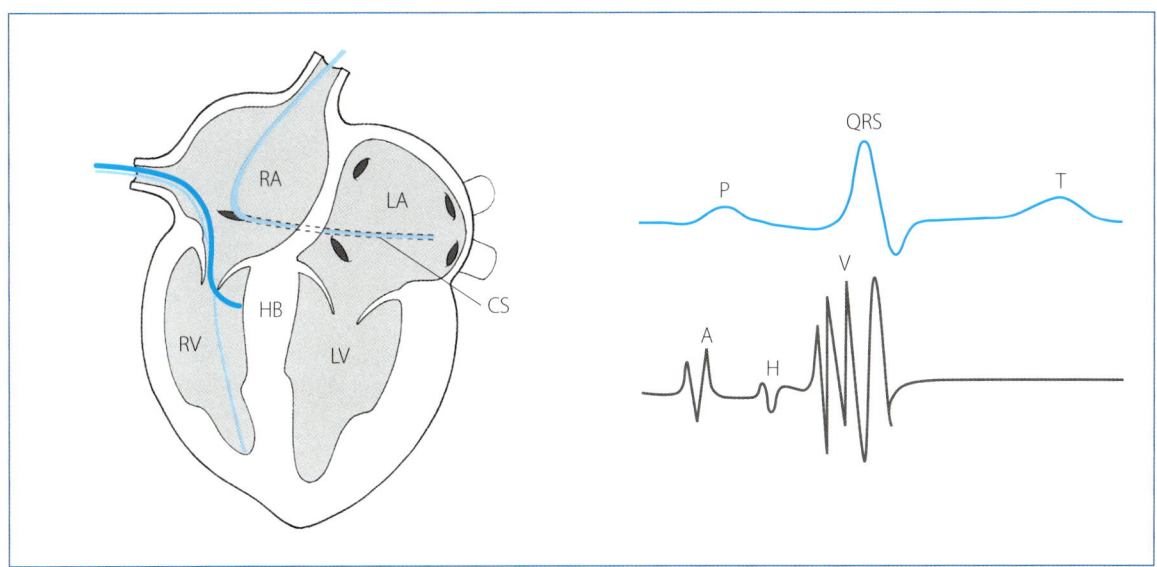

Figure 6.23. Schematic representation of the position of the catheters during an electrophysiological study. A decapolar catheter is inserted into the coronary sinus, a quadripolar catheter enters the right atrium via the caudal vena cava and is placed at the atrioventricular junction where a His electrogram can be recorded. The position of the His catheter identifies the apex of the triangle of Koch (the position of the atrioventricular node). A third catheter is positioned in the apex of the right ventricle. This catheter is also used to map the atrial chamber. On the right side of the figure, a representation of the surface electrocardiogram in lead II and its corresponding intracardiac electrograms. An A (atrial) wave corresponds to the P wave, a H (His) electrogram indicates the activation of the atrioventricular junction, and a V (ventricular wave) corresponds to the QRS complex on the surface electrocardiogram. *CS*: coronary sinus; *RA*: right atrium; *LA*: left atrium; *HB*: His bundle; *RV*: right ventricle; *LV*: left ventricle.

information yielded. Furthermore, at present, the size of the catheters limits the use to larger dogs. The reasons for performing an electrophysiological study in a dog include the diagnosis and treatment of:
- focal atrial tachycardias,
- accessory pathways,
- atrial flutter,
- atrial fibrillation with high ventricular response rate refractory to medical treatment, and
- selected reentrant ventricular tachycardias.

Perhaps the diagnosis and treatment with radiofrequency ablation of an accessory pathway causing relentless atrioventricular reentrant tachycardia in a young dog (commonly Labrador Retrievers) is one of the most rewarding uses of an electrophysiological study in the dog. Additionally, recent advances have discovered that in some large and giant breed dogs with "lone" atrial fibrillation after cardioversion an underlying focal atrial tachycardia arising from the pulmonary veins is the underlying mechanism that triggers the arrhythmia. Ablation of this tissue eliminates the substrate for the arrhythmia. In some situations medical treatment to control an excessively high ventricular response rate during atrial fibrillation is inadequate or the dog cannot tolerate the medication. Under these circumstances ablation of the atrioventricular node to cause third-degree atrioventricular block with an implantation of a permanent pacemaker serves as an alternative to medical treatment.

Contact catheter-based electrophysiological studies are based on the recording of intracardiac electrical activity (electrograms) and pacing techniques to identify the substrate (*intracardiac mapping*) and mechanism of arrhythmias. In dogs, such studies require general anesthesia. Several intracardiac catheters are inserted from the jugular and femoral veins into the cardiac chambers to study the right heart. Direct recordings of the left cardiac chambers require a transeptal puncture of the inter-atrial septum. A standard electrophysiological study requires a decapolar (10 electrodes) catheter positioned inside the great cardiac vein, a quadripolar catheter maintained against the membranous interventricular septum and an ablation catheter that is successively directed in the apex of the right ventricle, the right atrium and around the tricuspid valve annulus. The decapolar catheter placed in the great cardiac vein records the left atrial electrograms from its distal electrodes, and its most proximal electrodes record electrical activity at the level of the coronary sinus ostium on the floor of the right atrium. It is useful to differentiate right-sided from left-sided arrhythmias (Fig. 6.23). The quadripolar catheter, also called the His catheter, is critical as it indicates the position of the atrioventricular node, which could be accidentally damaged during a radiofrequency procedure. Radiofrequency catheter ablation is a therapeutic procedure used to eliminate the arrhythmia substrate. Specifically, the radiofrequency current is converted into heat, causing targeted coagulation necrosis of the myocardial tissue, which is then replaced by fibrous tissue. The ablation catheter is also used to record electrical activity and stimulate the right ventricle, the different regions of the right atrium and the tricuspid valve annulus.

Suggested readings

1. Abbott JA. Heart rate and heart rate variability of healthy cats in home and hospital environments. *J Feline Med Surg* 2005; 7:195-202.
2. Akhtar M, Tchou PJ, Jazayeri M. Mechanisms of clinical tachycardias. *Am J Cardiol* 1988; 61:9-19.
3. Antzelevitch C, Bernstein MJ, Feldman HN, et al. Parasystole, reentry, and tachycardia: a canine preparation of cardiac arrhythmias occurring across inexcitable segments of tissue. *Circulation* 1983; 68:1101-1115.
4. Bailey JC, Anderson GJ, Pippenger D, et al. Reentry within the isolated canine bundle of His. Possible mechanism for reciprocal rhythm. *Am J Cardiol* 1973; 32:808-813.
5. Bardy GH, Ungerleider RM, Smith WM, et al. A mechanism of torsades de pointes in a canine model. *Circulation* 1983; 67:52-59.
6. Bethge KP. Classification of arrhythmias. *J Cardiovasc Pharmacol* 1991; 17:13-19.
7. Blomstrom-Lundqvist C, Scheinman MM, Aliot EM, et al. ACC/AHA/ESC guidelines for the management of patients with supraventricular arrhythmias–executive summary. A report of the American College of Cardiology/American Heart Association Task Force on Practice Guidelines and the European Society of Cardiology Committee for Practice Guidelines (writing committee to develop guidelines for the management of patients with supraventricular arrhythmias) developed in collaboration with NASPE-Heart Rhythm Society. *J Am Coll Cardiol* 2003; 42:1493-1531.
8. Bright JM, Cali JV. Clinical usefulness of cardiac event recording in dogs and cats examined because of syncope, episodic collapse, or intermittent weakness: 60 cases (1997-1999). *J Am Vet Med Assoc* 2000; 216:1110-1114.
9. Brignole M, Alboni P, Benditt DG, et al. Guidelines on management (diagnosis and treatment) of syncope-Update 2004. *Eur Heart J* 2004; 25:2054-2072.
10. Calvert CA, Jacobs G, Pickus CW, et al. Result of ambulatory electrocardiography in overtly healthy Doberman Pinscher with echocardiographic abnormalities. *J Am Vet Med Assoc* 2000; 217:1328-1332.
11. Calvert CA, Wall M. Effect of severity of myocardial failure on heart rate variability in Doberman Pinscher with and without echocardiographic evidence of dilated cardiomyopathy. *Am J Vet Res* 2000; 61:506-511.
12. Castellanos A, Myerburg RJ. The electrophysiologic manifestations of abnormal automatic activity arising in depolarized foci. *Circulation* 1983; 67:9-10.
13. Childers RW. Supernormality: recent developments. *Pacing Clin Electrophysiol* 1984; 7:1115-1120.
14. Cranefield PF. Action potentials, afterpotentials, and arrhythmias. *Circ Res* 1977; 41:415-423.
15. Davis MJ, Gore RW, Determinants of cardiac function: simulation of a dynamic cardiac pump for physiology instruction. *Adv Physiol Educ* 2001; 25:13-35.
16. El-Sherif N, Gomes JA, Restivo M, et al. Late potentials and arrhythmogenesis. *Pacing Clin Electrophysiol* 1985; 8:440-462.
17. Ferasin L. Recurrent syncope associated with paroxysmal supraventricular tachycardia in a Devon Rex cat diagnosed by implantable loop recorder. *J Feline Med Surg* 2009; 11:149-152.
18. Glass L, Guevara MR, Shrier A. Universal bifurcations and the classification of cardiac arrhythmias. *Ann N Y Acad Sci* 1987; 504:168-178.
19. Goldreyer BN, Kastor JA, Kershbaum KL. The hemodynamic effects of induced supraventricular tachycardia in man. *Circulation* 1976; 54:783-789.
20. Gopinathannair R, Etheridge SP, Marchilinski FE. Arrhythmia-induced cardiomyopathies: mechanisms, recognition, and management. *J Am Coll Cardiol* 2015; 66:1714-1728.

Suggested readings

21. Guimond C, LeBlanc RA, Pelletier B, et al. Supernormal conduction and atrial echo beats in the dog. *Eur Heart J* 1981; 2:499-507.
22. Gussak I, Antzelevitch C. Cardiac repolarization bridging basic and clinical sciences. Edited by Humana Press 2003.
23. Hanås S, Tidholm A, Egenvall A, et al. Twenty-four hour Holter monitoring of unsedated healthy cats in the home environment. *J Vet Cardiol* 2009; 11:17-22.
24. Hilwig RW. Cardiac arrhythmias in the dog: detection and treatment. *J Am Vet Med Assoc* 1976; 169:789-798.
25. Hirose M, Laurita KR. Calcium-mediated triggered activity is an underlying cellular mechanism of ectopy originating from the pulmonary vein in dogs. *Am J Physiol Heart Circ Physio* 2007; 292:1861-1867.
26. Hocini M, Loh P, Ho SY, et al. Anisotropic conduction in the triangle of Koch of mammalian hearts: electrophysiologic and anatomic correlations. *J Am Coll Cardiol* 1998; 1:629-636.
27. Hoffman BF, Rosen MR. Cellular mechanisms for cardiac arrhythmias. *Circ Res* 1981; 49:1-15.
28. James R, Summerfield N, Loureiro J, et al. Implantable loop recorders: a viable diagnostic tool in veterinary medicine. *J Small Anim Pract* 2008; 49:564-570.
29. Janssen PML. Myocardial contraction-relaxation coupling. *Am J Physiol Heart Circ Physiol* 2010; 299:H1741-1749.
30. Lau EW. Infra-atrial supraventricular tachycardias: mechanism, diagnosis and management. *Pacing Clin Electrophys* 2008; 31:490-498.
31. MacKie BA, Stepien RL, Kellihan HB. Retrospective analysis of an implantable loop recorder for evaluation of syncope, collapse, or intermittent weakness in 23 dogs (2004-2008). *J Vet Cardiol* 2010; 12:25-33.
32. Miller RH, Lehmkulh LB, Bonagura JD, et al. Retrospective analysis of the clinical utility of ambulatory electrocadiographic (Holter) recordings in syncopal dogs: 44 cases (1991-1995). *J Vet Intern Med* 1999; 13:111-122.
33. Moe GK, Antzelevitch C. Reflection as a mechanism of reentrant cardiac arrhythmias. *Physiol Bohemoslov* 1987; 36:243-253.
34. Moe GK, Jalife J. Reentry and ectopic mechanisms in the genesis of arrhythmias. *Arch Inst Cardiol Mex* 1977; 47:206-211.
35. Moe GK, Jalife J, Antzelevitch C. Models of parasystole and reentry in isolated Purkinje fibers. *Mayo Clin Proc* 1982; 57:14-19.
36. Nattel S. Pulmonary vein cellular electrophysiology and atrial fibrillation: does basic research help us understand clinical pulmonary-vein arrhythmogenesis? *Heart Rhythm* 2005; 2:1346.
37. Rosen MR. The relationship of delayed afterdepolarizations to arrhythmias in the intact heart. *Pacing Clin Electrophysiol* 1983; 6:1151-1156.
38. Samet P. Haemodynamic sequelae of cardiac arrhythmias. *Circulation* 1973; 47:399-407.
39. Santilli RA, Ferasin L, Voghera SG, et al. Use of implantable loop recorder (Reveal) to evaluate the cause of unexplained syncope in dogs. *J Am Med Assoc* 2010; 236:78-82.
40. Sasyniuk BI, Mendez C. A mechanism for reentry in canine ventricular tissue. *Circ Res* 1971; 28:3-15.
41. Scherf D. Remarks on the nomenclature of cardiac arrhythmias. *Prog Cardiovasc Dis* 1970; 13:1-25.
42. Sprenkeler DJ, Vos MA. Post-extrasystolic Potentiation: Link between Ca^{2+} Homeostasis and Heart Failure? *Arrhythm Electrophysiol Rev* 2016; 5: 20–26.
43. Tse G. Mechanisms of cardiac arrhythmias. *J Arrhythmia* 2016; 32:75-81.
44. Ware WA. Twenty-four ambulatory electrocardiography in normal cats. *J Vet Intern Med* 1999; 13:175-180.
45. Willis R, McLeod K, Cusack J, et al. Use of an implantable loop recorder to investigate syncope in a cat. *J Small Anim Pract* 2003; 44:181-183.
46. Wit AL, Cranefield PF. Triggered and automatic activity in the canine coronary sinus. *Circ Res* 1977; 41:434-445.

CHAPTER 7

Supraventricular beats and rhythms

The terms supraventricular ectopic beats and rhythms refer to rhythm disorders originating from structures other than the sinus node, including the atrial myocardium, the atrioventricular node, the coronary sinus, the pulmonary veins, the venae cavae and the ligament or vein of Marshall. Supraventricular ectopic beats and rhythms may occur in the presence or absence of cardiac disease, or be secondary to systemic diseases. Their arrhythmogenic mechanisms include enhanced automaticity, triggered activity and anatomical or functional reentry.

Supraventricular arrhythmias can be subdivided into atrial ectopic beats/rhythms and junctional ectopic beats/rhythms, depending on whether they originate in the atrium or the atrioventricular region, respectively.

Ectopic atrial beats and rhythms

An *atrial ectopic beat* is a spontaneous depolarization originating from the working atrial myocardium or from the venous structures connected to the atria. An atrial ectopic beat is defined as *premature* (atrial premature beat, atrial premature contraction) if it occurs earlier than the expected impulse from the underlying rhythm. Conversely, it is called an atrial escape beat when it occurs after a pause of the basic rhythm (usually sinus rhythm) (see p. 136). When more than three atrial ectopic beats occur sequentially, they are called *atrial rhythm*.

An atrial rhythm with a firing rate below the sinus discharge rate is called atrial escape rhythm, while an atrial rhythm with a firing rate greater than 180 bpm in dogs and 220 bpm in cats is called atrial tachycardia.

There are many diseases associated with atrial premature beats, including atrial enlargement secondary to mitral and tricuspid insufficiency, cardiomyopathy, myocarditis, advanced stages of pulmonary hypertension and congenital heart diseases. Tumors infiltrating or compressing the atrial myocardium, such as chemodectoma, hemangiosarcoma and lymphosarcoma, can induce atrial premature beats. Extracardiac factors that can contribute to atrial premature beats include toxemia, uremia, digitalis toxicity, anesthetic drugs and vagal hyperactivity.

In some cases, atrial premature beats originate from venous structures in the absence of structural cardiac diseases (for example: ectopic beats from the pulmonary veins triggering atrial fibrillation).

Atrial escape beats usually occur during a reduction in the discharge rate of the dominant sinus pacemaker.

To identify the site of origin of an atrial ectopic beat, it is necessary to evaluate the morphology and the electrical axis of the ectopic P wave (P') recorded in the frontal plane from the unipolar and bipolar limb leads (I, II, III, aVR, aVL and aVF). The P' wave axis determined in the horizontal plane from the precordial leads (V_1-V_6) is not useful for this purpose in dogs and cats.

In general, the more distant the depolarization wavefront is from the sinus node, the more pronounced are the alterations of the morphology and axis of the P' wave.

Atrial ectopies originating from the roof of the atria propagate in a superior-to-inferior direction, and those arising from the floor of the atria propagate along an inferior-to-superior axis (Fig. 7.1). Right atrial ectopic beats have a leftward axis direction, and left atrial ectopies have a rightward axis direction.

Chapter 7. Supraventricular beats and rhythms

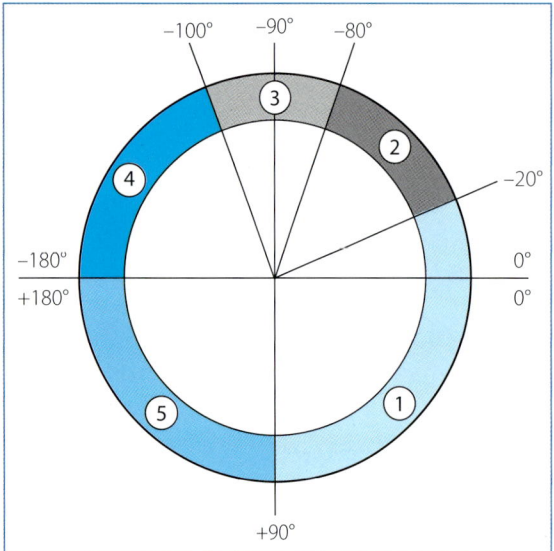

Figure 7.1. Direction of the vector of atrial depolarization in the frontal plane for sinus beats, supraventricular ectopic beats and junctional ectopic beats. Sector 1 indicates the electrical axis for the sinus P wave or an ectopic P' wave originating from the upper right atrium; sector 2 corresponds to the electrical axis of a lower right atrial ectopic P' wave; sector 3 corresponds to the electrical axis of a junctional P' wave; sector 4 corresponds to the electrical axis of a lower left atrial ectopic P' wave; sector 5 corresponds to the electrical axis of an upper left atrial ectopic P' wave.

Therefore, depending on their origin, atrial ectopic beats and rhythms can be classified as:
- right upper atrial,
- right lower atrial,
- left upper atrial, and
- left lower atrial.

Right upper atrial beats and rhythms

Ectopic beats and rhythms originating from the lateral and superior region of the right atrium (*crista terminalis*, right auricle, cranial vena cava, right pulmonary veins) have the following electrocardiographic characteristics:
- positive P' wave in the inferior leads (II, III and aVF); positive, biphasic or isodiphasic in lead I and maximum negativity in lead aVR. The mean electrical axis of the P' wave on the frontal plane is directed superior-to-inferior and ranges from −20° to +90°,
- normal P'Q interval, and
- normal QRS complex duration (≤70 ms in dogs and ≤40 ms in cats) and morphology, as the ventricular depolarization follows the normal conduction pathways (atrioventricular node and His-Purkinje system). The QRS complex may, however, be wide in the presence of intraventricular conduction disturbances, or intraventricular aberrant conduction (Fig. 7.2).

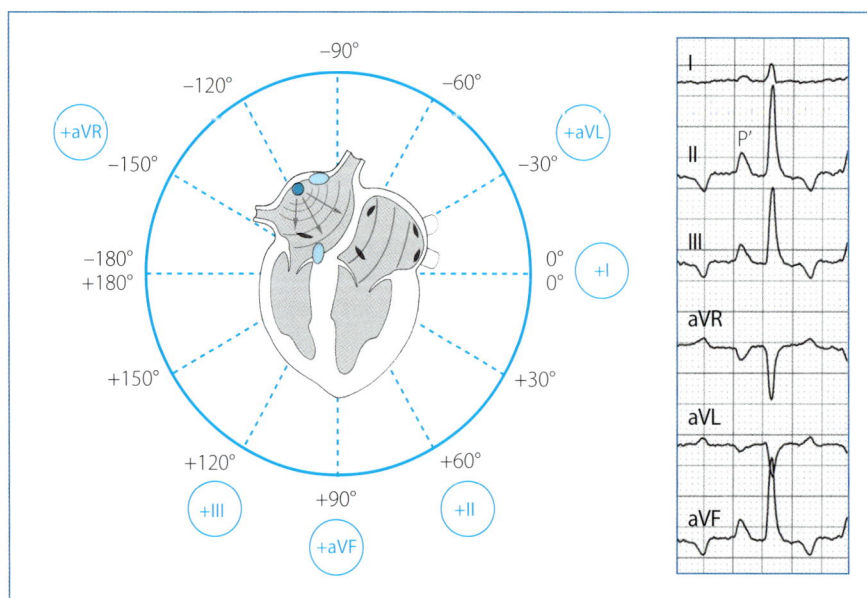

Figure 7.2. Upper right atrial ectopic beat. Ectopic atrial depolarization morphology in the six limb leads. In this example, the P' wave axis is +74° - speed 50 mm/s - calibration 10 mm/1 mV. See text for explanations.

Atrial ectopies originating from the right atrial roof cannot always be distinguished from normal sinus beats as both have an axis of −20 ° to +90 °.

Right lower atrial beats and rhythms

Ectopic beats and rhythms originating from the inferomedial region (inter-atrial septum) and posteromedial (ostium of the coronary sinus) right atrium have the following electrocardiographic characteristics:
- negative P' wave in the inferior leads (II, III, and aVF); positive P' in leads I, aVL and aVR. The mean electrical axis of the P' wave in the frontal plane is directed inferior-to-superior and ranges from −20 ° to −80 °; the P' wave duration can be increased, particularly for ectopic beats arising from the posterior area of the right atrium,
- prolonged P'Q interval when ectopies arise from the coronary sinus ostium, and normal P'Q interval for ectopies that arise from the inter-atrial septum, and
- normal QRS complex except in the presence of structural or functional intraventricular conduction abnormalities (Fig. 7.3).

Left upper atrial beats and rhythms

Ectopic beats and rhythms originating from the upper region of the left atrium (left pulmonary veins, left auricle) show the following electrocardiographic characteristics:
- positive P' wave in the inferior leads (II, III and aVF); negative or isodiphasic P' wave in lead I and maximum negativity in aVL. The mean electrical axis of the P' wave on the frontal plane is directed superior-to-inferior and ranges between +90 ° and +180 °,
- normal P'Q interval, and
- normal QRS complex except in the presence of a structural or functional intraventricular conduction abnormalities (Fig. 7.4).

Left lower atrial beats and rhythms

Ectopic beats and rhythms originating from the inferolateral region (ligament or vein of Marshall, coronary sinus ostium, great cardiac veins and mitral annulus) have the following electrocardiographic characteristics:
- negative P' wave in the inferior leads (I, II, III and aVF), positive P' wave in aVR. The mean electrical axis of the P' wave in the frontal plane is directed inferior-to-superior and ranges from −100 ° to −180 °,
- normal P'Q interval, and
- normal QRS complex except in the presence of structural or functional intraventricular conduction abnormalities (Fig. 7.5).

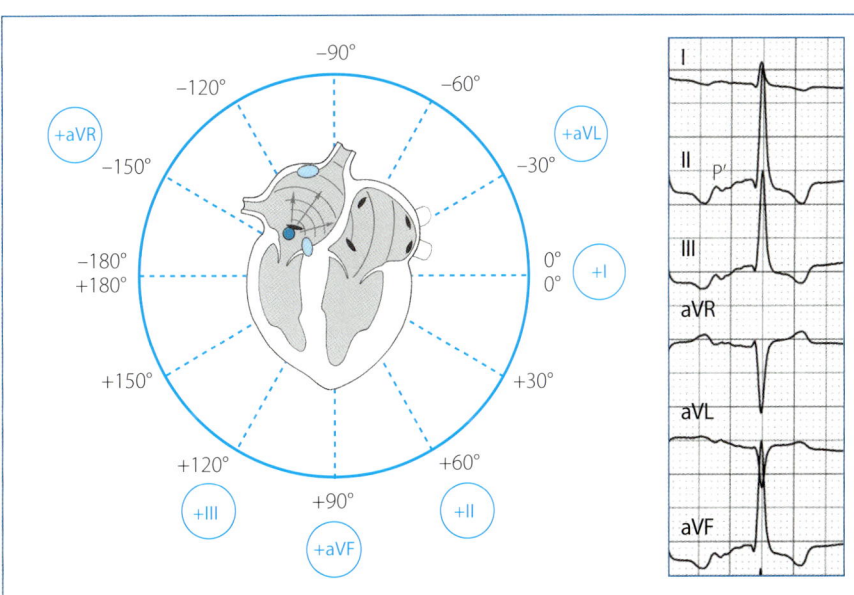

Figure 7.3. Lower right atrial ectopic beat. Ectopic atrial depolarization morphology in the six limb leads. In this example, the P' wave axis is −72 °. Note that the PQ interval is prolonged at 180 ms - speed 50 mm/s - calibration 5 mm/1 mV. See text for explanations.

A wavefront coming from the sinus node (P wave) may, occasionally fuse with a second wavefront originating from an ectopic site (P' wave). In this case, the atrial myocardial mass is partially depolarized by the electric impulse arising from the sinus node and partially by the electric impulse of ectopic origin. This phenomenon is more frequent when the rate of the atrial ectopic beats is similar (isorhythmic) to the sinus node rate. On the electrocardiogram, the *atrial fusion beats* (P" waves) have an intermediate morphology between the sinus P wave and the ectopic P' wave. Depending on the degree of fusion, the P" wave morphology and polarity vary.

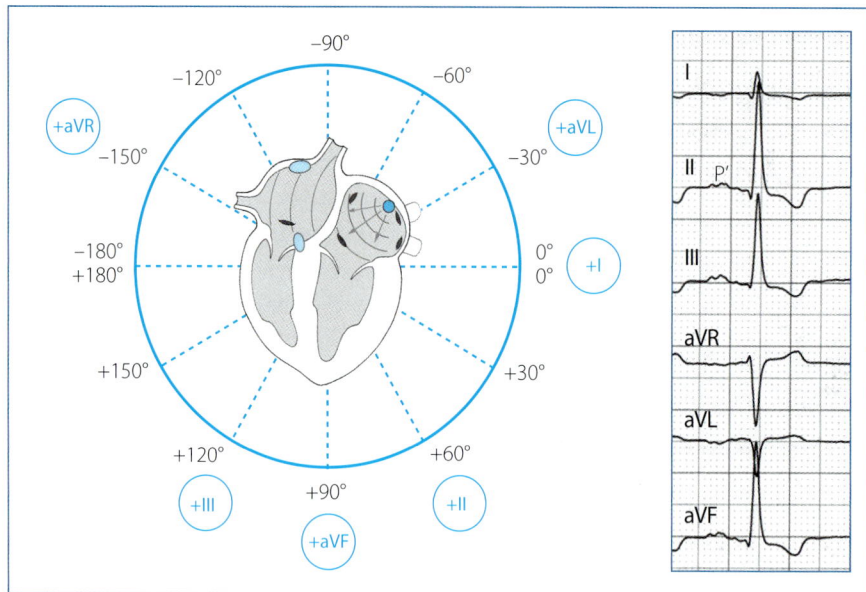

Figure 7.4. Upper left atrial ectopic beat. Ectopic atrial depolarization morphology in the six limb leads. In this example, the P' wave axis +163 ° - speed 50 mm/s - calibration 5 mm/1 mV. See text for explanations.

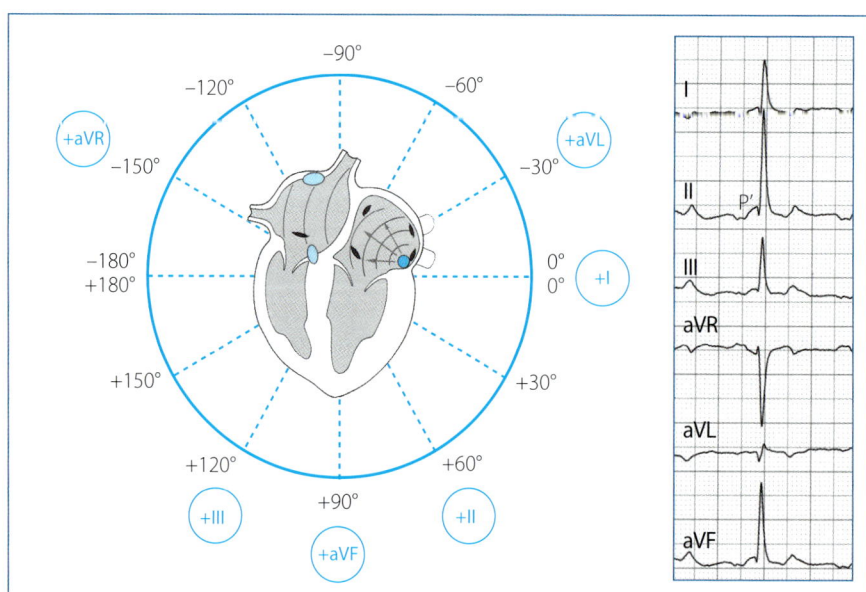

Figure 7.5. Lower left atrial ectopic beat. Ectopic atrial depolarization morphology in the six limb leads. In this example, the P' wave axis is equal to −123 ° - speed 50 mm/s - calibration 10 mm/1 mV. See text for explanations.

Junctional ectopic beats and rhythms

An impulse that originates from the atrioventricular junction is defined as a *junctional ectopic beat*.

The junctional region is the normal conduction pathway between the atria and ventricles, and it can be divided into three segments: the atrionodal (AN) area, the nodo-Hisian (NH) area and the His bundle. All share the property of automatic activity, and therefore have the ability to serve as subsidiary pacemakers.

A junctional ectopic beat is called premature when it occurs earlier than the expected impulse of the underlying rhythm. Whenever a junctional ectopic beat occurs at the end of a pause, it is defined as a junctional *escape beat*. A *junctional rhythm* corresponds to more than three consecutive junctional ectopic beats with a rate of 60 to 100 bpm in dogs; it is called a *junctional escape rhythm* if the rate is close to 60 bpm. The term *junctional tachycardia* is used when the rate is above 100 bpm.

A junctional escape rhythm occurs when the rate of the sinus rhythm decreases below the inherent rate of the junctional pacemaker cells, when the sinus node stops firing (sinus arrest), or in the presence of an impulse exit block from the sinus node (sino-atrial block).

During a junctional rhythm, atrial activation occurs in a retrograde direction, that is, depolarization propagates in an inferior-to-superior direction. In addition, because the impulse originates in the atrioventricular region (positioned anteriorly at the base of the inter-atrial septum), it simultaneously activates both atria. In electrophysiology this is described as *concentric retrograde atrial activation* (Figs. 7.1 and 7.6A). Concentric retrograde atrial activation must be differentiated from *eccentric retrograde atrial activation*, which describes an inferior-to-superior depolarization of the atria from a site other than the junctional region (see p. 17). Eccentric retrograde atrial activation is observed with inferior atrial rhythms and focal atrial tachycardias, and during atrioventricular reciprocating tachycardias (Figs. 7.1 and 7.6B).

During a junctional rhythm, the retrograde P' wave can be seen slightly before or after the QRS complex, or it may not be visible if it is superimposed on the QRS complex. The position of the P' wave relative to the QRS complex depends not only on the site of origin of the impulse within the junctional region (AN, NH or His), but also the pathway traveled and the conduction velocity of the electrical impulse in the antegrade and retrograde directions. For example, a different temporal relationship is observed between the P' wave and the QRS complex, according to whether the electrical impulse travels retrogradely along the fast or slow pathway of the atrioventricular node. It is not, therefore, recommended

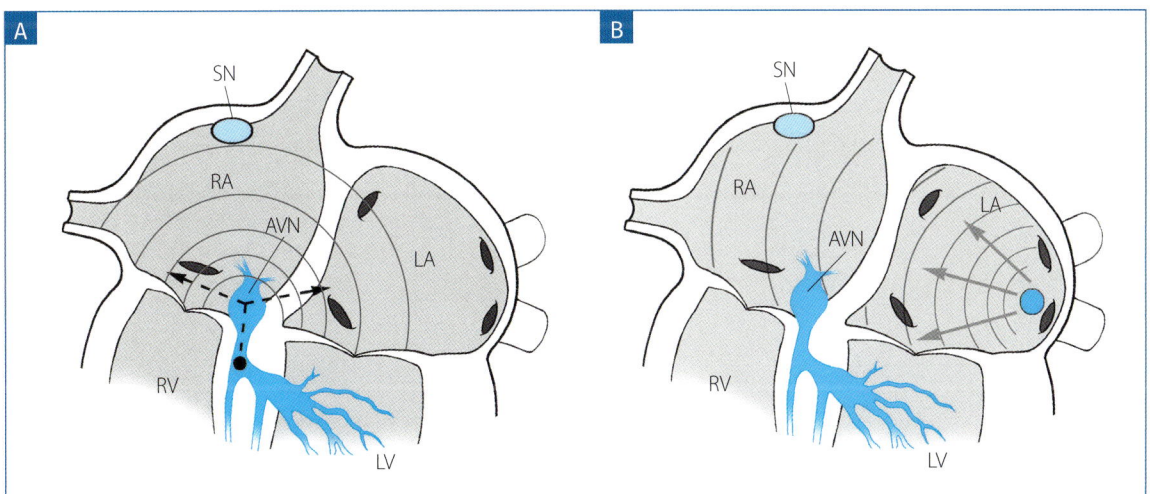

Figure 7.6. Concentric (A) and eccentric (B) retrograde atrial activation. See text for explanations. *RA*: right atrium; *LA*: left atrium; *SN*: sinus node; *AVN*: atrioventricular node; *RV*: right ventricle; *LV*: left ventricle.

classifying junctional rhythms as superior, mid- or inferior rhythms based on the position of the retrograde P' wave relative to the QRS complex.

When the atrial activation precedes the activation of the ventricles (because the ectopic focus is in the superior region of the junction and/or the impulse

BOX 7.1.
JUNCTIONAL RHYTHM WITH P' WAVE PRECEEDING THE QRS COMPLEX IN THE DOG

HEART RATE: 60-100 bpm; the rhythm is defined as a junctional escape rhythm if the rate is between 40 and 60 bpm.
R-R INTERVAL: regular.
P'WAVE: present, with concentric atrial retroactivation (axis between −80° and −100°).

ATRIOVENTRICULAR CONDUCTION: present.
P'Q INTERVAL: reduced compared to sinus rhythm.
QRS COMPLEX: normal (≤70 ms) except if preexisting intra-ventricular conduction disorders.
VENTRICULO-ATRIAL CONDUCTION: absent.
BLOCKED BEATS: none.

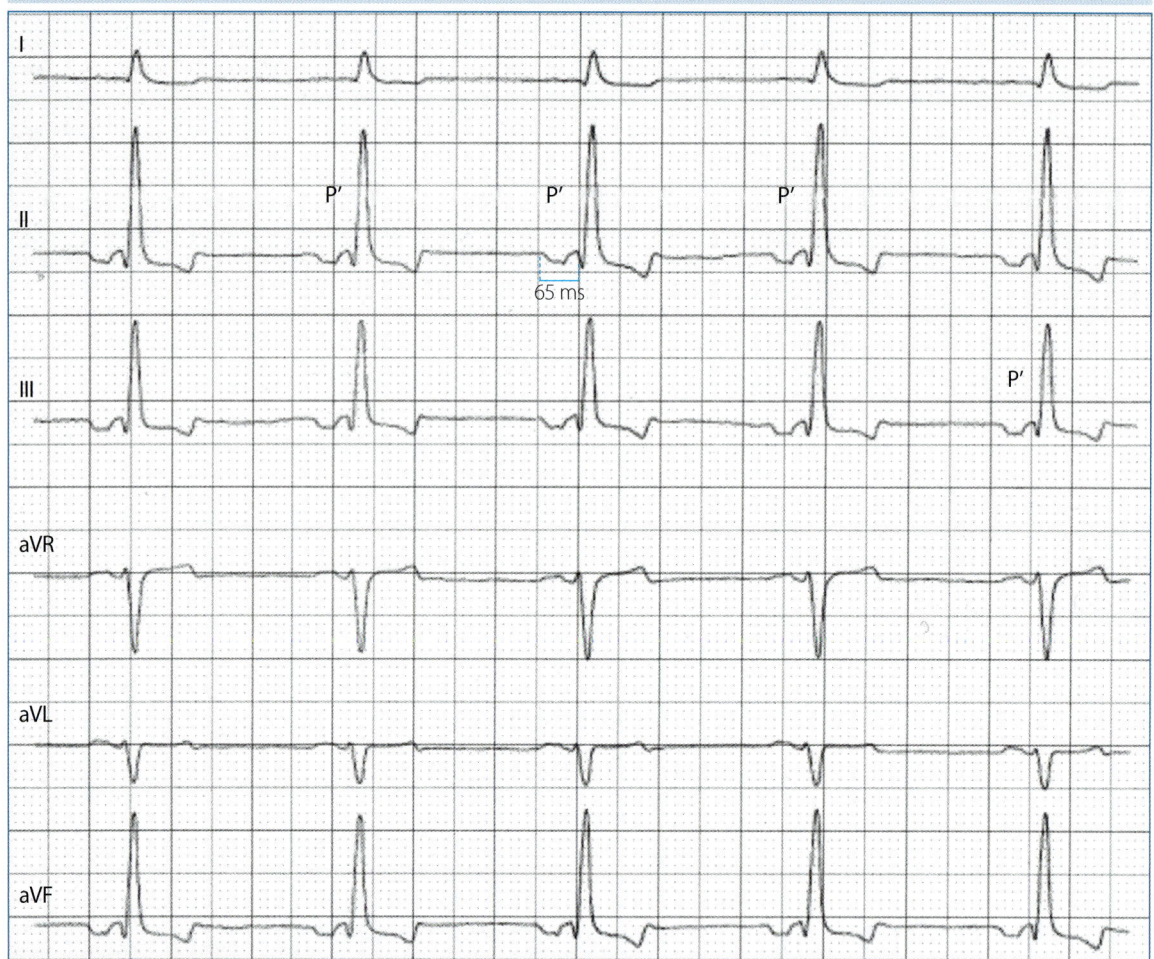

Dog, Greyhound, female, 4 years.
Six limb leads (I, II, III, aVR, aVL, aVF) - speed 50 mm/s - calibration 10 mm/1 mV.

Junctional rhythm with a heart rate of 100 bpm; the P' waves precede the QRS complexes, are negative in the inferior leads (II, III and aVF) and have the same amplitude in aVR and aVL (axis −90°). The P'Q interval is slightly shorter than normal (65 ms) and the amplitude and duration of the QRS complex are normal.

Junctional ectopic beats and rhythms

travels faster retrogradely than antegradely), the P' wave precedes the QRS complex, and the P'Q interval is usually shorter than the PQ interval from the sinus beats (Box 7.1).

If the P'Q interval is similar or longer than the PQ interval of the sinus beats, it is consistent with a junctional rhythm with intra-atrial or atrioventricular conduction delay; another possibility is an ectopic atrial rhythm. When the atrial and ventricular activation are simultaneous, the P' wave is not visible because it is superimposed on the QRS complex (Box 7.2).

When atrial depolarization follows ventricular activation, P' waves can be identified in the initial portion of the ST segment, and typically form pseudo-S waves in the inferior leads (II, III and aVF). P' waves resulting from a junctional rhythm typically have a mean electrical axis ranging from −80° to −100° in the frontal plane and the amplitude of the P' wave is the same in aVR and aVL (Box 7.3).

BOX 7.2.

JUNCTIONAL RHYTHM WITH P' WAVE SUPERIMPOSED ON THE QRS COMPLEX IN THE DOG

HEART RATE: 60-100 bpm; the rhythm is defined as a junctional escape rhythm if the rate is between 40 and 60 bpm.
R-R INTERVAL: regular.
P' WAVE: not visible.
ATRIOVENTRICULAR CONDUCTION: not evaluable.

P'Q INTERVAL: not evaluable.
QRS COMPLEX: normal (≤70 ms) except if preexisting intraventricular conduction disorders.
VENTRICULO-ATRIAL CONDUCTION: absent.
BLOCKED BEATS: none.

Dog, Labrador Retriever, Male, 6 years.
Six limbs leads (I, II, III, aVR, aVL, aVF) - speed 50 mm/s - calibration 5 mm/1 mV

Junctional rhythm with a heart rate of 100 bpm. The P' waves are superimposed on the QRS complex and are not, therefore, visible. The QRS complexes are normal, R-R intervals are regular.

Chapter 7. Supraventricular beats and rhythms

BOX 7.3.
JUNCTIONAL RHYTHM WITH P' WAVE FOLLOWING THE QRS COMPLEX IN THE DOG

HEART RATE: 60-100 bpm; the rhythm is defined as a junctional escape rhythm if the rate is between 40 and 60 bpm.
R-R INTERVAL: regular.
P' WAVE: present, with concentric atrial retro-activation (axis between –80 ° and –100 °).

ATRIOVENTRICULAR CONDUCTION: absent.
P'Q INTERVAL: absent.
QRS COMPLEX: normal (≤70 ms) except if preexisting intra-ventricular conduction disorders.
VENRICULO-ATRIAL CONDUCTION: present (1:1).
BLOCKED BEATS: none.

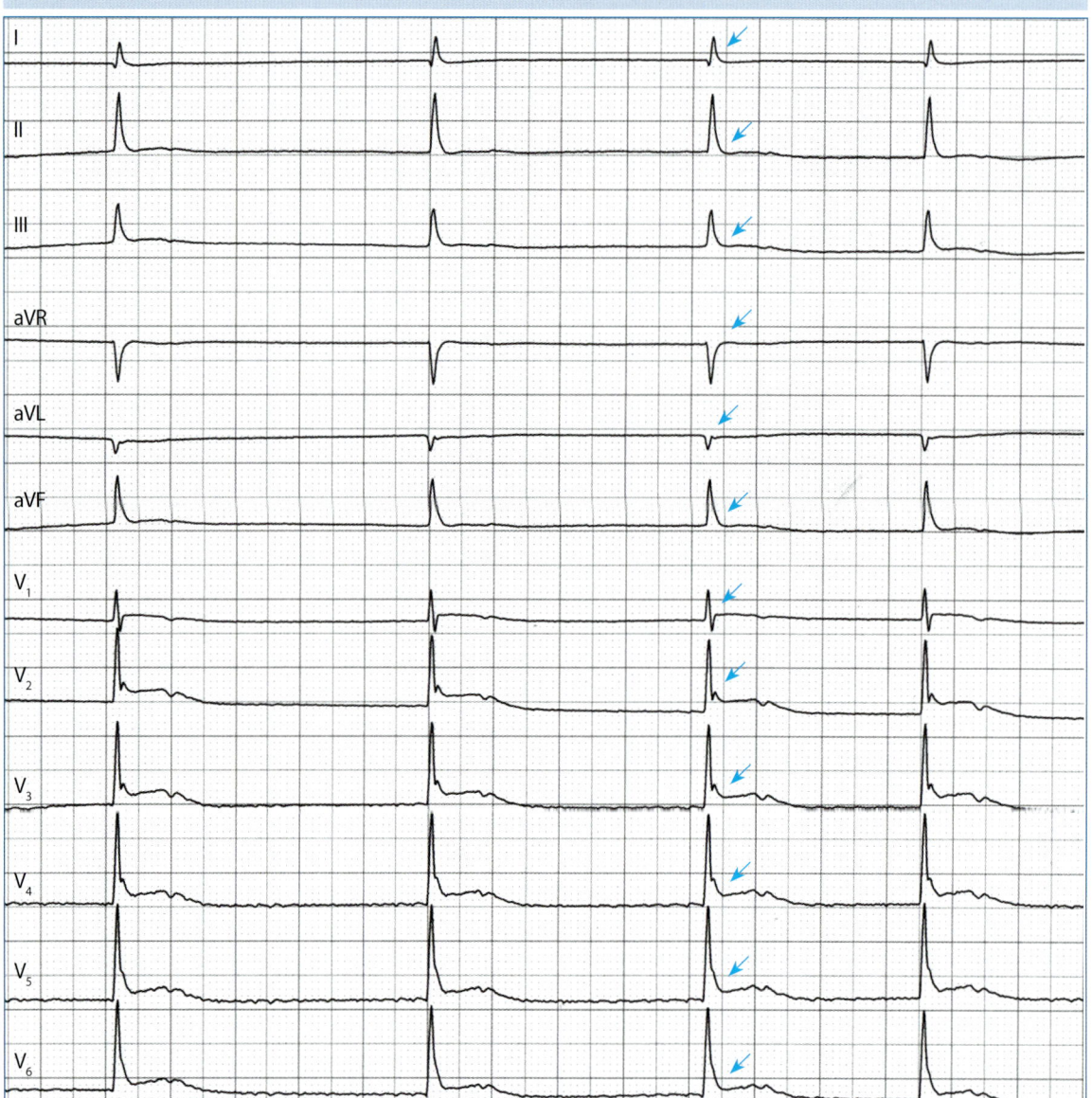

Dog, West Highland White Terrier, female, 13 years.
Twelve leads (I, II, III, aVR, aVL, aVF, V$_1$, V$_2$, V$_3$, V$_4$, V$_5$, V$_6$) - speed 50 mm/s - calibration 5 mm/1 mV.

Junctional rhythm with a heart rate of 70 bpm during third-degree sino-atrial block or sinus standstill. Note the absence of sinus P waves and the presence of narrow QRS complexes (50 ms) of junctional origin. There is 1:1 ventriculo-atrial conduction, characterized by the presence of P' waves in the first portion of the ST segment (arrows); this is particularly evident in V$_2$, V$_3$ and V$_4$. The P' wave is negative in inferior leads (II, III and aVF) and is of equal amplitude in aVR and aVL (axis –90 °).

During a junctional rhythm, the ventricles are activated in the antegrade direction along the normal His-Purkinje system. The duration and morphology of the QRS complex are, therefore, usually normal, unless preexisting disorders of intraventricular conduction are present.

Patterns of ectopic supraventricular beats

Once complexes have been identified on the surface electrocardiogram as supraventricular (atrial or junctional) ectopies based on the electrical axis of the P' waves, they should be classified as premature or escape beats. This is done by comparing the length of the sinus P-P intervals and the P-P' interval (*coupling interval*) (Figs. 7.7 and 7.8). If the P-P' interval is shorter than the sinus P-P interval, the supraventricular ectopy is called *premature*; alternatively, if the P-P' interval is greater than the longest sinus P-P interval, the supraventricular ectopy is an *escape beat*.

When a premature atrial ectopic beat originates from the atrial myocardium, the P' wave tends to be superimposed on the T wave of the previous beat (Figs. 7.9 and 7.10). P' waves resulting from ectopies originating from the tributary veins (cranial and caudal vena cava, great cardiac vein and pulmonary veins) typically occur within the ST segment of the previous beat (Fig. 7.11).

Premature supraventricular beats are frequently followed by a pause. The pause is called *compensatory* if the sum of the P-P' and P'-P intervals is equal to twice the sinus P-P interval (Fig. 7.7). The presence of a compensatory post-extrasystolic pause indicates that the depolarization wavefront originating from the ectopic focus does not depolarize the sinus node and does not, therefore, interfere with its next pacing cycle. Conversely, the post-extrasystolic pause is called *non-compensatory* when the sum of the P-P' and P'-P intervals is less than twice the sinus P-P interval, which indicates that the ectopic atrial beat depolarizes the sinus node and resets its pacing cycle.

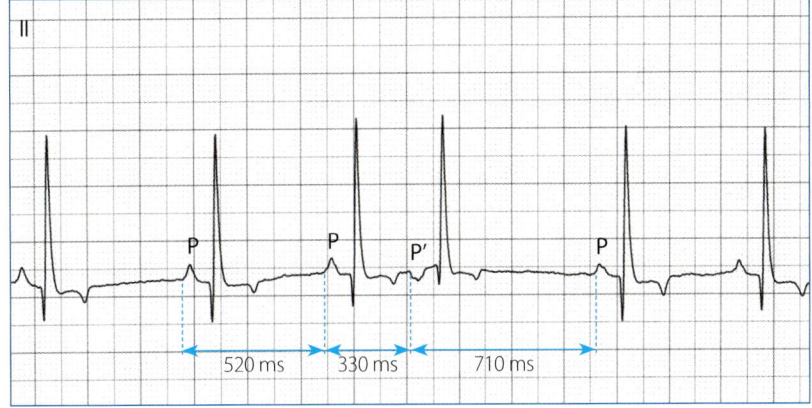

Figure 7.7. Premature atrial beat followed by a compensatory pause (Dog, Poodle, female, 14 years. Lead II - speed 50 mm/s - calibration 10 mm/1 mV). The cycle length of the sinus rhythm (P-P) is 520 ms. The P-P' interval is 330 ms; the atrial ectopic beat is defined as premature since the P-P' interval is shorter than the P-P interval between two sinus beats. Following the premature atrial beat, there is a compensatory post-extrasystolic pause, because the sum of the P-P' and P'-P intervals (1040 ms) is twice the duration of the P-P interval (520 ms).

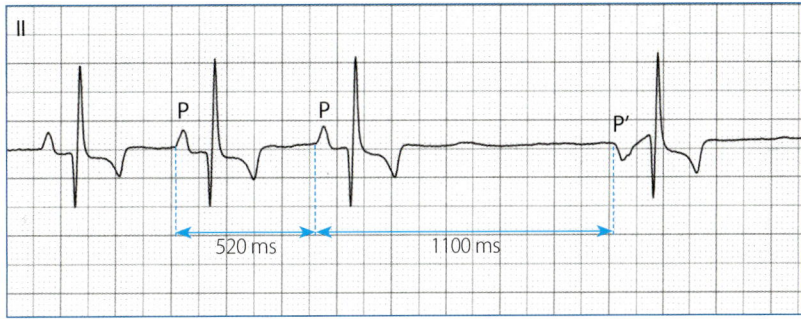

Figure 7.8. Escape atrial beat (Dog, Labrador Retriever, male, 4 years. Lead II - speed 50 mm/s - calibration 10 mm/1 mV). The cycle length of the sinus rhythm (P-P) is 520 ms. The P-P' interval is 1100 ms; the ectopic beat is defined as an escape beat because the P-P' interval is longer than the P-P interval between two sinus beats.

The post-extrasystolic pause is defined as *overcompensatory* if the sum of the P-P' and P'-P intervals is longer than twice the sinus P-P interval. This type of pause is related to an interruption of the sinus node pacemaker activity in response to atrial depolarization from the premature beat. This observation can raise the suspicion of sinus node dysfunction.

It is, however, important to note that the presence of pronounced sinus arrhythmia in the dog, which results in a highly variable sinus P-P interval on the electrocardiogram, complicates the distinction between compensatory, non-compensatory and overcompensatory post-extrasystolic pauses and these rules can often be applied only in cats, in which regular sinus rhythm is usually present.

If a supraventricular premature beat does not to interfere with the sinus rhythm, it is called *interpolated*. In this case, the ectopic beat is not followed by a post-extrasystolic pause, and the sinus P-P interval remains constant.

Premature ectopic beats can be isolated or display allorhythmic patterns, including bigeminy, trigeminy, quadrigeminy, couplets and triplets. *Atrial bigeminy* corresponds to one sinus beat alternating with one atrial ectopic beat (Fig. 7.9); *atrial trigeminy* is two sinus beats alternating with an atrial ectopic beat; *atrial quadrigeminy* is three sinus beats alternating with an atrial ectopic beat. Two consecutive premature atrial ectopic beats are called an *atrial couplet* (Fig. 7.10), three consecutive atrial ectopic beats form an *atrial triplet*. When the number of consecutive atrial ectopic beats exceeds three, the term atrial rhythm or tachycardia is used depending on the heart rate.

Relationship between atrial and ventricular activation

The P'Q interval of an atrial premature beat is influenced by its prematurity and the duration of the refractory period of the atrioventricular nodal region. The earlier the supraventricular ectopy, the greater the likelihood that the impulse will be slowed down (prolonged P'Q) or blocked in the atrioventricular node (decremental conduction of the atrioventricular node). The P'Q interval is prolonged if the atrial impulse enters the atrioventricular junction during a state of relative refractoriness. When the P'Q interval is equal to or shorter than the sinus PQ interval, it suggests that the origin of the ectopic beat is

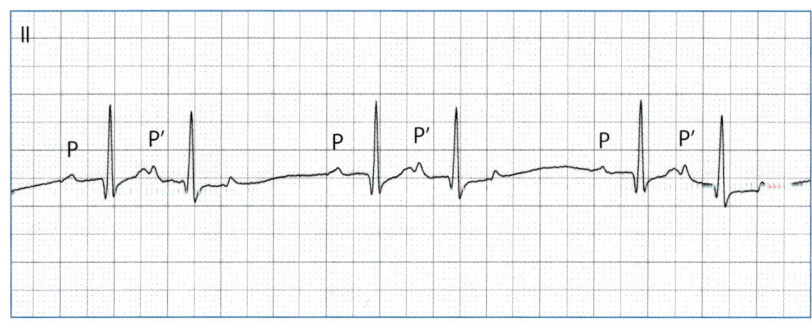

Figure 7.9. Atrial bigeminy (Dog, Great Dane, female, 1 year. Lead II- speed 50 mm/s - calibration 10 mm/1 mV). Sinus beats (P) alternate with premature atrial beats (P'). The P' waves have a superior-to-inferior axis and occur on the descending limb of the previous T wave.

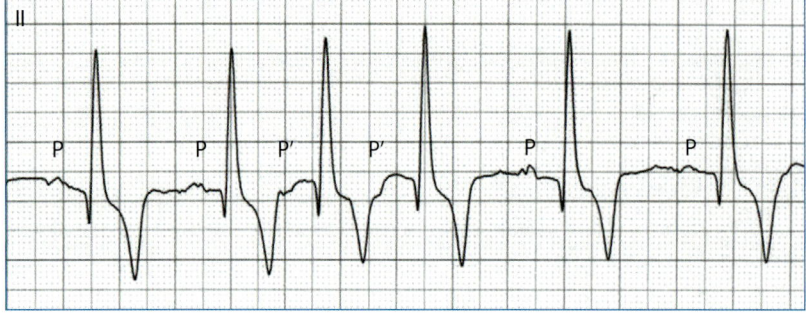

Figure 7.10. Atrial couplet (Dog, German Shepherd, female, 11 years. Lead II - speed 50 mm/s - calibration 10 mm/1 mV). The first two and the last two beats are sinus in origin (P). The third and the fourth beats are premature atrial ectopic beats (P') that form a couplet.

close to the atrioventricular node. If a premature atrial impulse reaches the atrioventricular junction during its refractory period, its conduction to the ventricles is not possible (*blocked P' wave*) (Fig. 7.11), resulting in an apparent second-degree atrioventricular block.

The QRS complex resulting from an atrial premature beat usually has normal morphology and duration. However, if the ectopic beat reaches one of the two ventricular bundle branches in a refractory state, it is conducted aberrantly, and the QRS that follows the P' wave displays a bundle branch block morphology on the electrocardiogram.

Atrial parasystole

Atrial parasystole is a particular type of ectopic atrial rhythm characterized by the presence of an atrial focus that has the property of enhanced normal or abnormal automaticity, or triggered activities and is protected from the electrical influences of the surrounding myocardial tissue (*entrance block*). As a result, the parasystolic focus depolarizes spontaneously and regularly without being reset by the underlying sinus depolarizations (*classic parasystole*). As the atrial myocardium can be alternatively depolarized by the sinus node or the parasystolic focus, it is not uncommon that the atrial tissue is in a refractory state when the parasystolic focus discharges. In some cases, the entrance block is not complete and therefore the dominant sinus activity can still interact with the parasystolic focus and alter its firing rate (*modulated parasystole*).

On the electrocardiogram, atrial parasystole is characterized by ectopic P' waves and interectopic P'-P' intervals that are multiples of a common denominator (Fig. 7.12). The amplitude and duration of the P' waves depend on the location of the parasystolic focus. It should be noted that with a parasystolic rhythm fusion beats and inconsistent coupling intervals of the ectopic beat and the sinus beat exist. These electrocardiographic features of the parasystolic rhythm are likely more prevalent because they are easier to confirm with ventricular parasystolic rhythms; the electrocardiogram with a suspected atrial parasystolic rhythm should be carefully examined for these characteristics. Importantly, long recordings may be required to have sufficient data for examination.

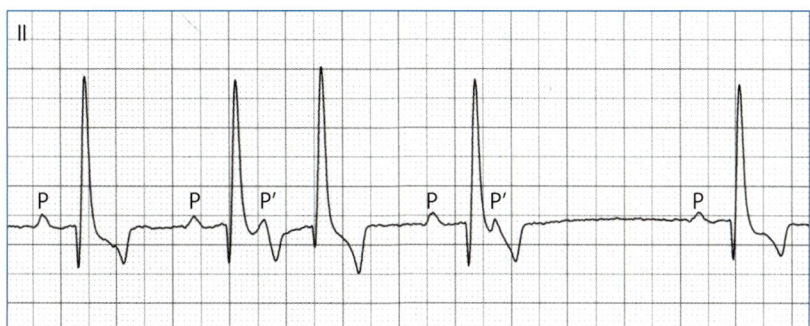

Figure 7.11. Blocked premature atrial beat (Dog, German Shepherd, female, 8 years. Lead II - speed 50 mm/s - calibration 10 mm/1 mV). The first, second, fourth and fifth beats are sinus beats (P). The third beat is a premature atrial beat (P') likely arising from a venous structure (pulmonary vein) since the atrial depolarization occurs in the ST segment of the previous beat. The P'Q interval is prolonged which reflects delayed conduction (*decremental conduction*) in the atrioventricular node in response the prematurity of the atrial ectopic beat. A P' wave is also visible in the ST segment of the fourth beat. It has the same axis and prematurity as the previous ectopic beat but is blocked in the atrioventricular node.

Chapter 7. Supraventricular beats and rhythms

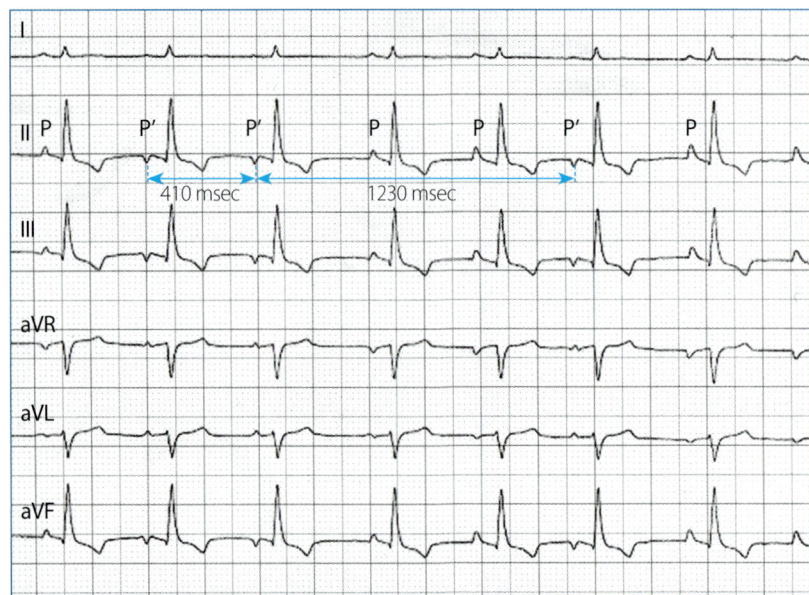

Figure 7.12. Atrial parasystole (Dog, mongrel, female, 12 years. Six-lead electrocardiogram -speed 50 mm/s - calibration 5 mm/1 mV). Note the presence of P waves with a sinus axis (P) and ectopic P' waves coming from the lower right atrium. The P-P' interval is variable. The first P'-P' is 410 ms and the second is 1,230 ms, which is exactly three times the shortest P'-P' interval (410 ms) which corresponds to the common denominator. This is consistent with atrial parasystole.

Atrial dissociation

The term *atrial dissociation* or *unilateral atrial rhythm* is used to describe the simultaneous presence of two independent atrial rhythms that do not interfere with each other. Typically, one of the two rhythms is the sinus rhythm, although cases of atrial dissociation in which the rhythm was a tachycardia or atrial flutter have been described. The other rhythm (*unilateral atrial rhythm*) is confined to one portion of the atrial myocardium, due to complete failure of electrical impulse transmission between the two atria (inter-atrial block) or within a portion and the rest of one atrium (intra-atrial block). The electrical impulse originating from the unilateral ectopic atrial rhythm usually does not propagates to the ventricles.

Atrial dissociation can be observed in human patients with severe congestive heart failure and is generally considered a negative prognostic factor. In dogs, there are only a few clinical reports and none of these cases have been confirmed by intracardiac electrophysiological study.

Atrial dissociation must be differentiated from *pseudo-atrial dissociation* secondary to artifacts. These artifacts can be a loss of contact of the electrodes or rhythmic movements of the animal. In cats, it has been shown that diaphragmatic activity induced by stimulation of the phrenic nerve can generate on the surface electrocardiogram deflections similar to a P wave that is positive in the inferior leads. When pseudo-atrial dissociation is caused by respiratory artifacts, the P' waves disappear during periods of apnea.

Electrocardiographically, atrial dissociation is characterized by sinus P waves that are normally conducted to

Atrial dissociation

BOX 7.4.
ATRIAL DISSOCIATION OR ECTOPIC ATRIAL UNILATERAL RHYTHM IN THE DOG

HEART RATE: depends on the firing rate of the sinus node.
R-R INTERVAL: depends on regular discharge of the sinus node.
P WAVE: normal sinus P waves and smaller ectopic P' waves with a slightly irregular interectopic interval (P'-P').

ATRIOVENTRICULAR CONDUCTION: only for sinus P waves; absent for P' waves.
PQ INTERVAL: normal.
QRS COMPLEX: normal.
VENTRICULO-ATRIAL CONDUCTION: absent.
BLOCKED BEATS: all P' waves.

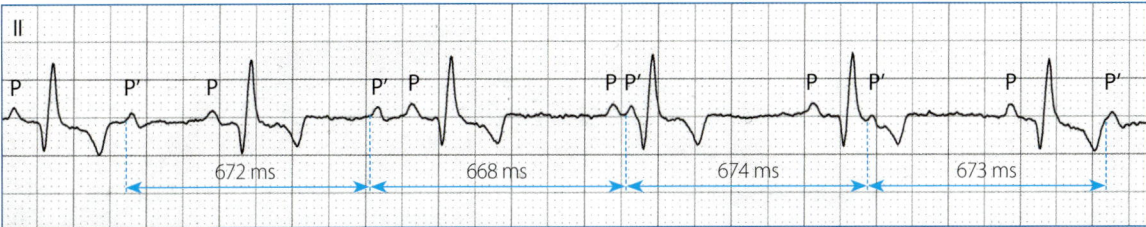

Dog, Afghan Greyhound, male, 11 years. Lead II - speed 50 mm/s - calibration 5 mm/1 mV.

Atrial dissociation or ectopic atrial unilateral rhythm. Note the coexistence of normally conducted sinus P waves and P' ectopic waves not conducted to the ventricles with a cycle length (P'-P') of 670 ms. P' waves have a shorter duration and lower amplitude than the sinus P wave. The P' waves do not disrupt the P-P and R-R sinus intervals.

the ventricles, and P' waves of different morphology and reduced amplitude and duration compared to the sinus P waves because the tissue depolarized is limited to one atrium or a small part of it. Those P' waves must not be associated with breathing, muscle movements or other factors that could induce artifacts. Ectopic P' waves have no effects on the sinus P-P and R-R intervals, they are never conducted to the ventricles, and therefore they are never followed by a QRS complex. P" waves with different morphology and prolonged duration can be observed when the ectopic P' wave is superimposed on the sinus P wave. This waveform should not be confused with a fusion of the two wavefronts since the ectopic atrial rhythm never reaches the contralateral atrial myocardium.

Assessment of the P'-P' interval is important to distinguish atrial dissociation from atrial parasystole and blocked premature atrial ectopic beats. In the presence of atrial dissociation, the interectopic P'-P' interval is not perfectly regular. In the case of atrial parasystole, the impulses that arise from a protected atrial focus can be conducted to the myocardium of both atria and ventricles as long as they reach the atrial myocardium in an excitable state. In addition, the interectopic P'-P' intervals vary but are multiples of a common denominator. Non-conducted atrial premature beats usually have a fixed coupling interval between the sinus P wave and the ectopic P' wave (P-P') (Box 7.4).

Suggested readings

1. Alella A, Granata L, Losano G. Dynamics of cardiac arrhythmias. Auricular extrasystoles. *Boll Soc Ital Biol Sper* 1966; 42:984-985.
2. Chen JH, Lien WP, Chen JJ, et al. Automaticity of the SN and A-V junctional tissue before and after chemical denervation in the dog. *Chest* 1989; 95:653-657.
3. Chung BKY, Walsh TJ, Massie E. A review of atrial dissociation, with illustrative cases and critical discussion. *Am J Med Sciences* 1965; 49:472-477.
4. Clapp S, Driscoll DJ, Mitrani I, et al. Comparative effects of age and sedation on sinus node automaticity and atrioventricular conduction. *Dev Pharmacol Ther* 1981; 2:180-187.
5. Eliska O, Eliskova M. Morphology of the region of the coronary sinus in respect to coronary sinus rhythm. *Int J Cardiol* 1990; 29-141-153.
6. Jones SB, Euler DE, Hardie E, et al. Comparison of SA nodal and subsidiary atrial pacemaker function and location in the dog. *Am J Physiol* 1978; 234:471-476.
7. Jones SB, Euler DE, Randall WC, et al. Atrial ectopic foci in the canine heart: hierarchy of pacemaker automaticity. *Am J Physiol* 1980; 238:788-793.
8. Kovacevic A, Sastravaha A. Clinically silent atrial dissociation in a dog. *J Vet Cardiol* 2007; 9:135-137.
9. Li YH, Lo HM, Lin JL, et al. Atrial dissociation after atrial compartment operation for chronic atrial fibrillation in mitral valve disease. *Pacing Clin Electrophysiol* 1998; 21:756-759.
10. Moore EN, Jomain SL, Stuckey JH, et al. Studies on ectopic atrial rhythms in dogs. *Am J Cardiol* 1967; 19:676-685.
11. Neely BH, Urthaler F, Hageman GR. Differences in the determinants overdrive suppression between sinus rhythm and slow atrioventricular junctional rhythm. *Circ Res* 1985; 57:182-191.
12. Oreto G, Luzza F, Satullo G, et al. Sinus modulation of atrial parasystole. *Am J Cardiol* 1986; 58:107-109.
13. Ramos A, Gelband H, Flinn CJ, et al. Benign nature of atrial dissociation in pediatric patients. *Pediatr Cardiol* 1983; 4:13.
14. Scollan K, Bulmer BJ, Heaney AM. Electrocardiographic and echocardiographic evidence of atrial dissociation. *J Vet Cardiol* 2008; 10:53-55.
15. Scott ME, Finnegan OC. Atrial dissociation. *Br Heart J* 1975; 37:539-542.
16. Szekely A, Zamolyi K, Harsanyi A, et al. Atrial dissociation. A case of unilateral slow atrial rhythm. *J Electrocardiol* 1988; 21:106-110.
17. Tan AY, Zhou S, Jung BC, et al. Ectopic atrial arrhythmias arising from canine thoracic veins during in vivo stellate ganglia stimulation. *Am J Physiol Heart Circ Physiol* 2008; 295:691-698.
18. Tse WW. Effect of epinephrine on automaticity of the canine atrioventricular node. *Am J Physiol* 1975; 229:34-37.
19. Waldo AL, Vitikainen KJ, Hoffman BF. The sequence of retrograde atrial activation in the canine heart: correlation with positive and negative retrograde P waves. *Circ Res* 1975; 37:156-163.
20. Woehlck HJ, Vicenzi MN, Bajic J, et al. Anesthetics and automaticity of dominant and latent pacemakers in chronically instrumented dogs. IV. Dysrhythmias after sinoatrial node excision. *Anesthesiology* 1995; 82:1447-1455.
21. Zipes DP, Dejoseph RL. Dissimilar atrial rhythms in man and dog. *Am J Cardiol* 1973; 32:618-628.
22. Zucker IH, Gilmore JP. Left atrial receptor discharge during atrial arrhythmias in the dog. *Circ Res* 1973; 33:672-677.

CHAPTER 8

Supraventricular tachycardias

The term supraventricular tachycardia is applied to a group of arrhythmias whose substrate includes at least one supraventricular anatomical structure. These supraventricular structures are the atrial myocardium, the atrioventricular node, the coronary sinus, the pulmonary veins, the venae cavae and the ligament or vein of Marshall. Atrioventricular reciprocating tachycardias include not only a supraventricular structure but also atrioventricular accessory pathways and the ventricular myocardium as part of their reentrant circuit.

Supraventricular tachycardias typically have rates above 180 bpm in adult dogs, and 220 bpm in puppies and cats. Ventricular activation usually occurs through the intraventricular conduction system, which results in a QRS complex of normal duration (<70 ms in dogs and <40 ms in cats) on the electrocardiogram. For this reason, supraventricular tachycardias are also called "narrow" QRS complex tachycardias. The duration of the QRS complex is a useful tool to differentiate supraventricular tachycardias from ventricular ("wide" QRS complex) tachycardias (QRS complex greater than 70 ms in dogs, and greater than 40 ms in cats). However, intraventricular conduction delays and antegrade conduction of supraventricular impulses along an accessory pathway can alter the morphology and duration of the QRS complex, and make the distinction between supraventricular tachycardias and ventricular tachycardias challenging.

Although *atrial fibrillation* does not always manifest itself as a tachycardia, it is included with the other types of supraventricular tachycardias in this book. The following supraventricular rhythms are described in this chapter:
- sinus tachycardia,
- atrioventricular nodal reciprocating tachycardia,
- focal junctional and non-paroxysmal junctional tachycardia,
- tachycardias mediated by atrioventricular accessory pathways,
- focal atrial tachycardia,
- multifocal atrial tachycardia,
- macroreentrant atrial tachycardia (atrial flutter), and
- atrial fibrillation.

Sinus tachycardia

Sinus tachycardia is characterized by an increase in the firing rate of the sinus node above 180 bpm in adult dogs, and 220 bpm in puppies and cats, in response to physiological or pathological stimuli. The maximum heart rate that can be reached during sinus tachycardia has not been clearly defined, but rates of 240 to 250 bpm are not uncommon in adult dogs during periods of excitement or exercise.

The possible electrophysiological mechanisms for sinus tachycardia include:
- enhanced normal automaticity of sinus pacemaker cells,
- a change in the origin of the site of atrial depolarization, which moves superiorly within the sinus node, and
- the presence of a reentrant microcircuit located within the sinus node, the atrial tissue surrounding the sinus node or the region of the *crista terminalis*.

Whenever sinus tachycardia results from enhanced normal automaticity, it is described as *physiological sinus tachycardia*. It is triggered by an increase in sympathetic tone associated with a decrease in parasympathetic tone.

This physiological sinus tachycardia can be the result of a response to physiological events. Some examples of these events include: exercise, excitement and fear. A physiological sinus tachycardia can also occur as a response to pathological conditions, for example, disease states that are associated with an increased metabolic demand or low cardiac output. Specific examples include blood loss, shock, cardiac tamponade and severe anemia. Sinus tachycardia can also result from the administration of drugs (anticholinergics, catecholamines, β-agonists).

Physiological sinus tachycardia should be distinguished from *inappropriate sinus tachycardia*, which is a persistent increase in heart rate in the absence of an apparent cause. Although inappropriate sinus tachycardia is a well described phenomenon in people, it has as yet to be proven in dogs and cats. However, electrocardiograms recorded from dogs with sinus node dysfunction have characteristics that may be compatible with the diagnosis of inappropriate sinus tachycardia rather than atrial tachycardia. One possible mechanism includes *reentrant sinus tachycardia*, which is caused by a reentrant circuit in the region of the sinus node and is responsible for paroxysmal and non-sustained episodes of tachycardia.

The electrocardiogram during sinus tachycardia is characterized by a sinus rate greater than 180 bpm in adult dogs, and 220 bpm in puppies and cats, and P waves with a sinus axis, i.e. from −20 ° to +90 ° in the dog and from ±0 ° to + 90 ° in the cat. It should be noted that the amplitude of the P wave in the dog is often greater during sinus tachycardia than during a normal sinus rate. The PQ interval is usually between 60-130 ms in dogs, and 50-90 ms in cats. On occasion when electrocardiograms or Holter monitoring is performed on puppies during sinus tachycardia a sudden second-degree heart block occurs with a single non-conducted P wave. This is not a sign of an abnormality. Whenever the tachycardia is very rapid, or when first-degree atrioventricular block is present during tachycardia, the P waves may be superimposed on the previous T wave and be difficult to detect. QRS complexes usually have a normal morphology and duration unless functional or preexisting intraventricular conduction disturbances are present. The onset and termination of physiological sinus tachycardia is gradual (warm-up and cool-down periods), which is typical of normal enhanced automaticity (Boxes 8.1 and 8.2). It is important to recognize in clinical practice but, particularly when the recording speed/sweep speed of the electrocardiogram is inappropriately fast, this warm-up and cool-down may be difficult to appreciate. An accurate determination of these periods requires that the speed under such conditions should be a minimum of 50 mm/s, but the phenomenon may actually be better appreciated at 100 mm/s. Moreover, young dogs and cats can increase their heart rate extremely quickly so that again, appreciation of the warm-up is more difficult. Often the cool-down may be more apparent. Another clinical concept to note is that when examining a patient who has physiologic sinus tachycardia in response to a pathological condition the rapid heart rate is sustained and it is, therefore, difficult to identify the warm-up and cool-down. This can make it difficult to know with certainty whether sinus tachycardia is the correct diagnosis. This problem may be resolved through diligent determination of the triggering pathological condition (e.g. cardiac tamponade) to determine that in fact the likely diagnosis is sinus tachycardia.

Atrioventricular nodal reciprocating tachycardia

Atrioventricular nodal reciprocating tachycardia develops along an anatomical reentry circuit that includes the atrioventricular node and the surrounding atrial tissue. This circuit is formed by two anatomically and functionally distinct pathways, a fast and a slow pathway (*longitudinal dissociation*) in the right atrium (see p. 16). In most cases, the fast pathway is located anteriorly near the apex of Koch's triangle, while the slow pathway extends inferoposteriorly from the compact area of the atrioventricular node to the tricuspid ring near the ostium of the coronary sinus.

Atrioventricular nodal reciprocating tachycardia begins when a premature beat reaches the fast pathway during its refractory period and is conducted in an antegrade direction along the slow pathway. Because of the

Atrioventricular nodal reciprocating tachycardia | 147

BOX 8.1.
PHYSIOLOGICAL SINUS TACHYCARDIA IN THE DOG

HEART RATE: >180 bpm in adult dogs, >220 bpm in puppies.
R-R INTERVAL: regular.
P WAVE: present, sinus axis (between –20 ° and +90 °).
ATRIOVENTRICULAR CONDUCTION: present.
PQ INTERVAL: usually normal.
QRS COMPLEX: narrow (≤70 ms) unless preexisting intraventricular conduction abnormalities.
VENTRICULO-ATRIAL CONDUCTION: absent.
BLOCKED BEATS: usually none.
INITIATION AND TERMINATION MODALITY: gradual (warm-up and cool-down).

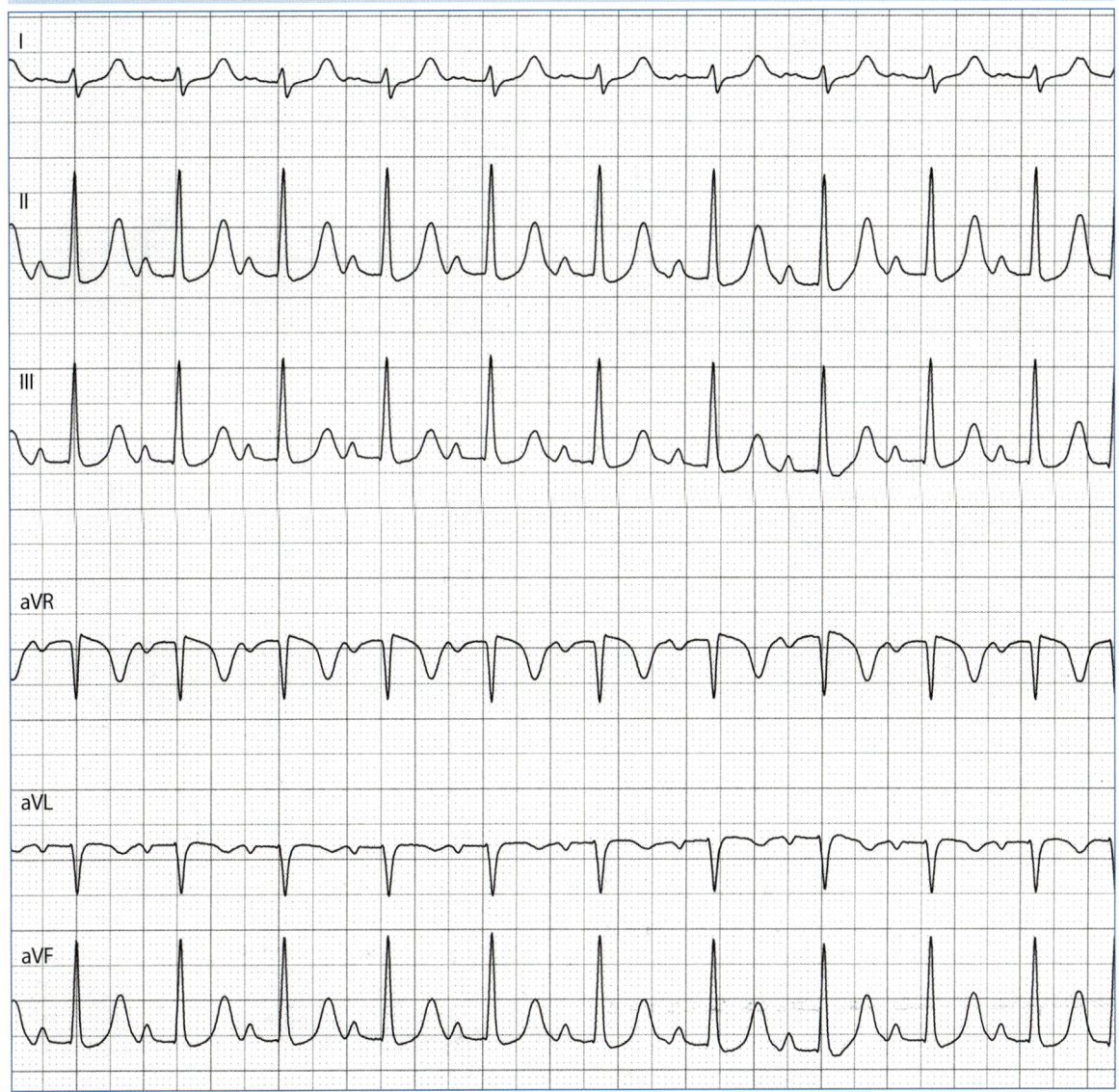

Dog, Pekingese, male, 16 years.
Six limb leads (I, II, III, aVR, aVL, aVF) - speed 50 mm/s - calibration 10 mm/1 mV.

Notes: sinus tachycardia with a rate of 220 bpm, characterized by P waves with a sinus axis (+75°), normal PQ intervals and QRS complexes.

Chapter 8. Supraventricular tachycardias

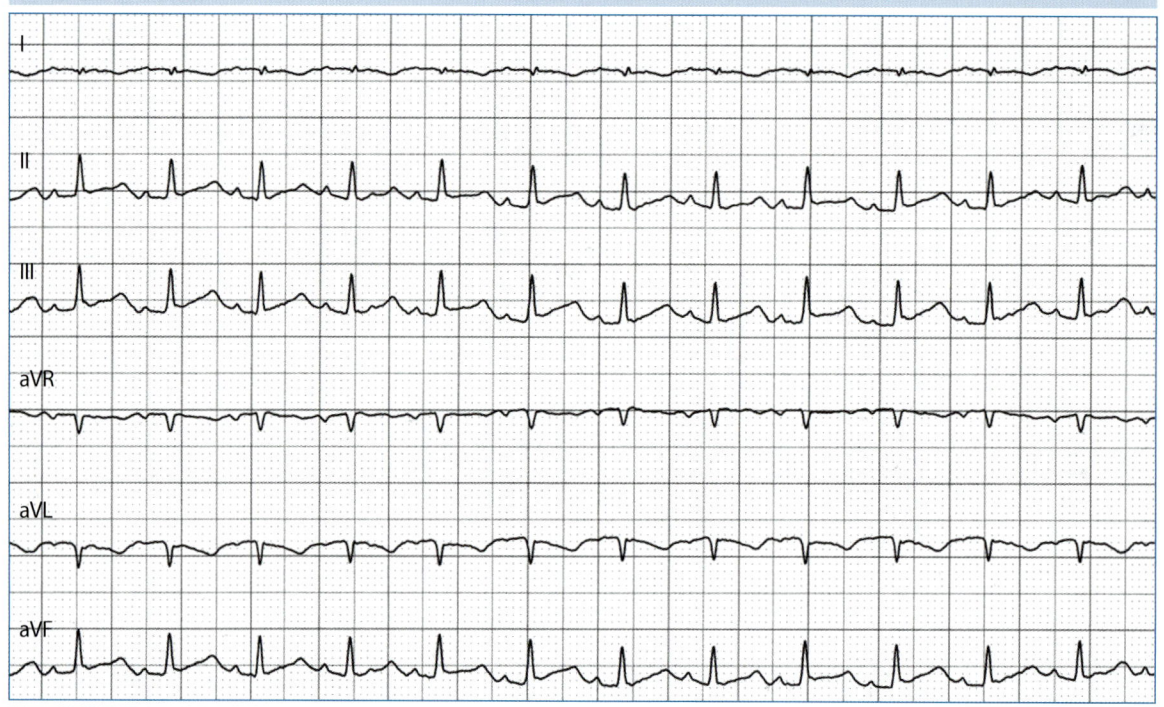

BOX 8.2.
PHYSIOLOGICAL SINUS TACHYCARDIA IN THE CAT

HEART RATE: >220 bpm.
R-R INTERVAL: regular.
P WAVE: present, sinus axis (between +0° and +90°).
ATRIOVENTRICULAR CONDUCTION: present.
PQ INTERVAL: normal.

QRS COMPLEX: narrow (≤40 ms), unless preexisting intraventricular conduction abnormalities.
VENTRICULO-ATRIAL CONDUCTION: absent.
BLOCKED BEATS: usually none.
INITIATION AND TERMINATION MODALITY: gradual (warm-up and cool-down).

Cat, Domestic Short Hair, male, 14 years.
Six limb leads (I, II, III, aVR, aVL, aVF) - speed 50 mm/s - calibration 10 mm/1 mV.

Notes: sinus tachycardia with a rate of 250 bpm, characterized by P waves with a sinus axis (+60°), normal PQ intervals and QRS complexes.

slower conduction velocity, the impulse reaches the distal portion of the atrioventricular node after the fast pathway has recovered from its refractory period. It is therefore able to conduct retrogradely (in a ventriculo-atrial direction) to the atrium. When a single impulse conducts retrogradely, it results in an *echo beat* (Fig. 8.1).

Various form of atrioventricular nodal reciprocating tachycardias are recognized in people depending on the direction of the electrical impulse as it travels along the fast pathway and the slow pathway. There is a common form, also referred to as *slow-fast*, an uncommon form, or *fast-slow*, and finally intermediate forms, such as the *slow-slow form* of *tachycardia*. In the common form, the impulse travels down to the ventricles along the slow pathway and travels back to the atria through the fast pathway; in the uncommon form it goes down to the ventricles along the fast pathway and goes back to the atria along the slow pathway, and in the intermediate forms, the impulse uses pathways characterized by slow conduction properties in both directions.

Importantly, atrioventricular nodal reciprocating tachycardia has not been documented to occur spontaneously in the dog. It is only after surgical dissection of the right atrium that isolates the right atrium from the atrioventricular node that this tachyarrhythmia has been induced in the experimental dog. However, dual atrioventricular nodal pathways have been confirmed with anatomical studies of the dog heart and spontaneous echo beats are documented in the dog. The fact this tachyarrhythmia has not been clinically identified in the dog, as well as the difficulty in inducing this arrhythmia experimentally, led researchers in the 1990s to hypothesize that the dog was unable to sustain this arrhythmia. It was hypothesized that the atrium of the dog was unable to maintain the atrioventricular nodal reciprocating tachycardia because of an anatomical "brake" in the anterior atrial septum and this was a factor that differed from people. Moreover, it was suggested that the internodal and atrionodal conduction pathways contribute to the maintenance of the reentrant circuit.

Focal junctional tachycardia and non-paroxysmal junctional tachycardia

The term junctional tachycardia defines a supraventricular arrhythmia that originates from the area of the atrioventricular junction. The origin of this rhythm is not in the compact node itself as this region lacks automaticity. Junctional rhythms when studied electrophysiologically do have a His deflection and studies in the dog showed that His bundle rhythms have a P wave, which usually follows the QRS complex, but with an origin in the upper region of the junctional area the P wave usually precedes or is buried within the QRS complex.

Two types of junctional tachycardia have been described:
- focal junctional tachycardia, and
- non-paroxysmal junctional tachycardia.

Focal junctional tachycardia

Focal junctional tachycardia results from enhanced automaticity or triggered activity in the junctional area, proximal to the apex of Koch's triangle and posterior to the distal atrioventricular bundle and the compact atrioventricular node.

This type of tachycardia is reported in people during childhood in its congenital or postoperative form. In the dog, it is more common in young Labradors and its manifestation as an incessant rhythm can worsen preexisting heart failure.

The electrocardiographic characteristics of focal junctional tachycardia are (Fig. 8.2):
- a mostly regular ventricular rate between 100 and 160 bpm,
- presence of isorhythmic (indicating similar rates) atrioventricular dissociation, and
- periods of retrograde (ventriculo-atrial) conduction with a 1:1 ratio.

Isorhythmic atrioventricular dissociation describes the concomitant presence of two rhythms, one sinus and the other one junctional or ventricular in origin that have similar discharge rates. The sinus rhythm depolarizes the atria in the antegrade direction; the junctional or ventricular ectopic rhythm depolarizes the ventricles. Electrocardiographically isorhythmic atrioventricular dissociation is characterized by sinus P waves that are not associated with the QRS complex, although they remain in close proximity to the QRS complex. The P-P and R-R intervals are similar and there are slight variations

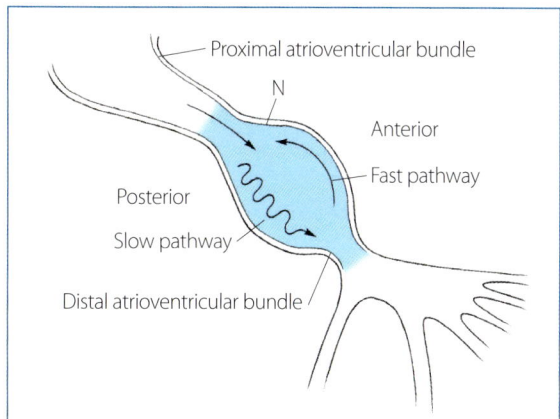

Figure 8.1. Longitudinal dissociation in the atrioventricular node of the dog. The figure shows the intranodal circuit formed by the slow pathway and the fast pathway. When the electric impulse travels once through the circuit formed by the two pathways it gives rise to an echo beat; if it travels several times sequentially, it initiates an atrioventricular nodal reciprocating tachycardia. *N*: compact atrioventricular node.

of the PQ intervals. As a result of small variations of the discharge rate of one of the two foci, the P waves may approach or overlap the QRS complexes (Fig. 8.2B). When the two independent rhythms maintain the same rate for short or relatively long periods, it is described as isorhythmic atrioventricular dissociation with *accrochage or synchronization*.

Type I and type II isorhythmic atrioventricular dissociation with synchronization have been described. Type I is characterized by a continuous fluctuation of the distance between the sinus P wave and the QRS complex which originates in the junctional region. Throughout the electrocardiogram, the P wave approaches and then gradually moves away from the QRS complex resulting in a periodic variation of PQ and QP intervals (Fig. 8.2B). The P wave never moves through the ST segment toward the subsequent QRS complex because the sinus rhythm and the junctional rhythm have approximately the same rate. Type I synchronization is attributed to cyclic variations of arterial blood pressure. Whenever the P wave moves closer to the QRS complex until the two waveforms overlap, the decreased contribution of atrial contraction to ventricular filling leads to a small drop in blood pressure, which stimulates the arterial baroreceptors. As a result, sympathetic tone is activated and leads to a shortening of the P-P intervals on the electrocardiogram, which corresponds to an increase in sinus node discharge rate. Finally, when the PQ interval returns back to physiological values, blood pressure increases, sinus node discharge rate slows down and the P waves migrate again toward the QRS complexes (Fig. 8-2B). Type II synchronization is characterized by a fixed relationship between P waves and QRS complexes (Fig. 8.2C). Different mechanisms have been proposed to explain isorhythmic atrioventricular dissociation with type II synchronization. The most popular concept is that the mechanical stimulus from the pulsation of the sinus node artery can have a synchronizing effect on the sinus node, atrioventricular node or ventricular conduction system cells.

Retrograde (ventriculo-atrial) activation occurs when the discharge rate of the junctional pacemaker exceeds the sinus rate and suppresses the sinus node pacemaker by an impulse depolarizing the atrial myocardium retrogradely, a mechanism known as *overdrive suppression* (see p. 15). The atrial retrograde activation arising from the junctional region is called concentric and the ratio of ventriculo-atrial conduction is 1:1 (Fig. 8.2D and Fig. 8.3).

In summary, focal junctional tachycardia has a mean heart rate in the dog of 100-160 bpm, and its onset is

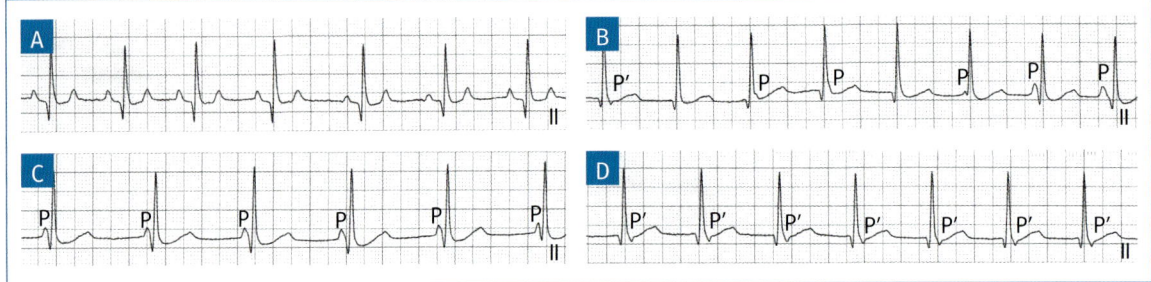

Figure 8.2. Electrocardiographic features of focal junctional tachycardia and the relationship between P waves, P' waves and QRS complexes (Dog, Labrador, male, 2 years. Lead II - speed 50 mm/s - amplitude 10 mm/1 mV).
A) Sinus rhythm.
B) Focal junctional tachycardia with isorhythmic atrioventricular dissociation and type I synchronization. Note the first beat characterized by 1:1 ventriculo-atrial conduction with a P' wave inscribed in the initial part of the ST segment appearing as a pseudo-S wave (Fig. 8-2D). Starting from the third beat, in response to the baroreceptor reflex, the sinus P wave is initially inscribed into the descending limb of the R wave, before moving to the left of the QRS complex back to its original position.
C) Focal junctional tachycardia with isorhythmic atrioventricular dissociation and type II synchronization. Note the constant relationship between the QRS complex and the dissociated sinus P wave.
D) Focal junctional tachycardia with a 1:1 ventriculo-atrial conduction ratio. Note the P' waves characteristic of concentric ventriculo-atrial conduction inscribed in the initial part of the ST segment appearing as pseudo-S waves. To appreciate the P' wave the complex during tachycardia must be compared with the ST segment of the sinus beat (Fig. 8-2A).

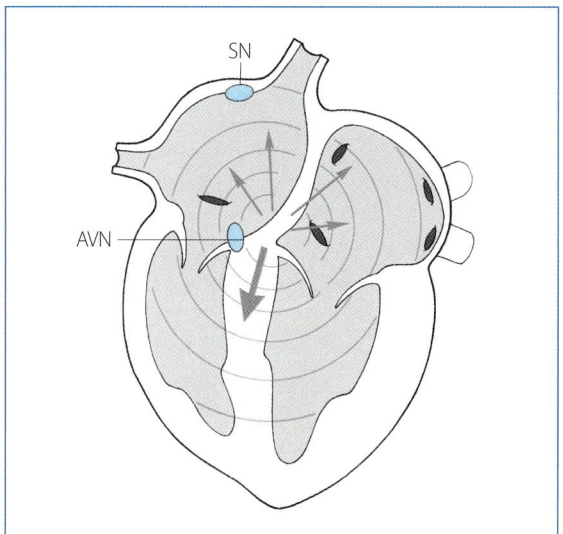

Figure 8.3. Concomitant activation of the atria in a retrograde direction and of the ventricles in an antegrade direction from a junctional focus. *AVN*: atrioventricular node; *SN*: sinus node.

gradual. Most of the time, focal junctional tachycardia displays isorhythmic atrioventricular dissociation, characterized by P waves with a sinus axis dissociated from the narrow QRS complexes (≤70 ms in dogs and ≤40 ms in cats) that originate in the junctional region. During isorhythmic atrioventricular dissociation, the PQ interval is variable and some P waves overlap with the QRS complexes; type I or type II synchronization is sometimes present. If the junctional pacemaker reaches a discharge rate above the sinus node, concentric retrograde atrial conduction occurs with a 1:1 ratio. When retrograde P' waves follow the QRS complexes, they appear in the initial portion of the ST segment as pseudo S-waves in the inferior leads (II, III and aVF) and a positive polarity with similar amplitude in aVR and aVL. The mean electric axis of these P' waves in the frontal plane is between −80 ° and −100 ° (Fig. 8.3 and Box 8.3). This rhythm should be differentiated from non-paroxysmal junctional tachycardia, which usually has a slower rate and does not display atrioventricular dissociation.

Non-paroxysmal junctional tachycardia

Non-paroxysmal junctional tachycardia which is also known as *accelerated atrioventricular junctional rhythm* is caused by enhanced normal automaticity of a proximal junctional pacemaker or triggered activity. The term non-paroxysmal indicates that the rhythm does not have a sudden onset or a sudden offset. The retrograde atrial activation occurs from the junction and precedes ventricular activation with a shorter than normal atrioventricular conduction time. Ventricular depolarization is usually normal along the intraventricular conduction system.

The electrocardiographic features of non-paroxysmal junctional tachycardia include a ventricular rate between 60 and 130 bpm, constant atrioventricular association with a 1:1 conduction ratio, although rarely, Wenckebach-type (Mobitz I) second-degree atrioventricular block can occur. P' waves precede narrow QRS complexes (<70 ms in dogs and <40 ms in cats) and their electrical axis is between −80 ° and −100 ° (concentric retrograde activation). The P'Q interval is shorter than the sinus PQ interval. Finally, and a key feature that explains the term non-paroxysmal, this tachycardia has a gradual onset and termination (Box 8.4).

Atrioventricular tachycardias mediated by accessory pathways

Atrioventricular accessory pathways consist of congenital muscular bundles, also called Kent bundles, which remain after the formation of the cardiac fibrous skeleton. Under normal conditions, the fibrous skeleton, which serves as the supporting structure for the atrioventricular and semilunar valves, electrically insulates the atria from the ventricles, preventing the transmission of atrial impulses to the ventricles except through the atrioventricular bundle. The accessory pathways penetrate the fibrous skeleton, thus creating a direct connection between the atria and the ventricles, and form a second conduction pathway in addition to the atrioventricular node. In dogs, accessory pathways can be isolated or multiple and are located, in most cases, around the tricuspid valve annulus.

Chapter 8. Supraventricular tachycardias

BOX 8.3.
FOCAL JUNCTIONAL TACHYCARDIA IN THE DOG

HEART RATE: 100-160 bpm.
R-R INTERVAL: regular.
P WAVE: present, sinus axis (between −20 ° and +90 °) during isorhythmic atrioventricular dissociation, otherwise P' waves with inferior-to-superior concentric axis (between −80 ° and −100 °) during 1:1 ventriculo-atrial retrograde conduction.
ATRIOVENTRICULAR CONDUCTION: absent.
PQ INTERVAL: variable.

QRS COMPLEX: narrow (≤70 ms) unless preexisting intraventricular conduction abnormalities.
VENTRICULO-ATRIAL CONDUCTION: occasionally present with 1:1 ratio.
BLOCKED BEATS: P waves during isorhythmic atrioventricular dissociation.
INITIATION AND TERMINATION MODALITY: gradual (warm-up and cool-down).

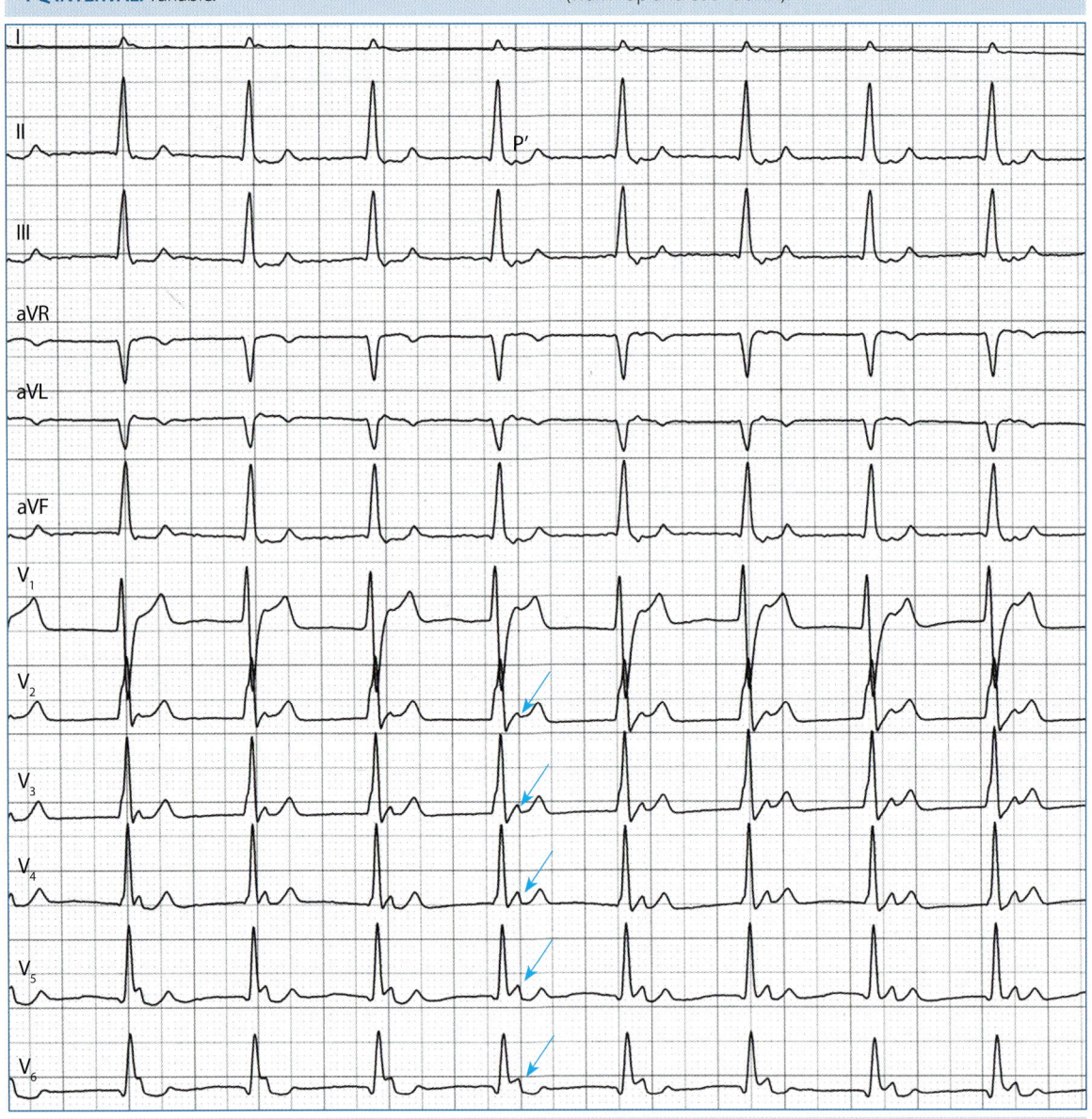

Dog, Labrador Retriever, Male, 2 years.
Twelve leads (I, II, III, aVR, aVL, aVF, V₁, V₂, V₃, V₄, V₅, V₆) - speed 50 mm/s - calibration 10 mm/1 mV.

BOX 8.4.
NON-PAROXYSMAL JUNCTIONAL TACHYCARDIA IN THE DOG

HEART RATE: 60-130 bpm.
R-R INTERVAL: regular.
P'WAVE: present, inferior-to-superior concentric axis (between −80° and −100°).
ATRIOVENTRICULAR CONDUCTION: present.
P'Q INTERVAL: shorter than the sinus PQ interval.

QRS COMPLEX: narrow (≤70 ms) unless preexisting intraventricular conduction abnormalities.
VENTRICULO-ATRIAL CONDUCTION: absent.
BLOCKED BEATS: rarely, Wenckebach type (Mobitz I) second-degree atrioventricular block.
INITIATION AND TERMINATION MODALITY: gradual (warm-up and cool-down).

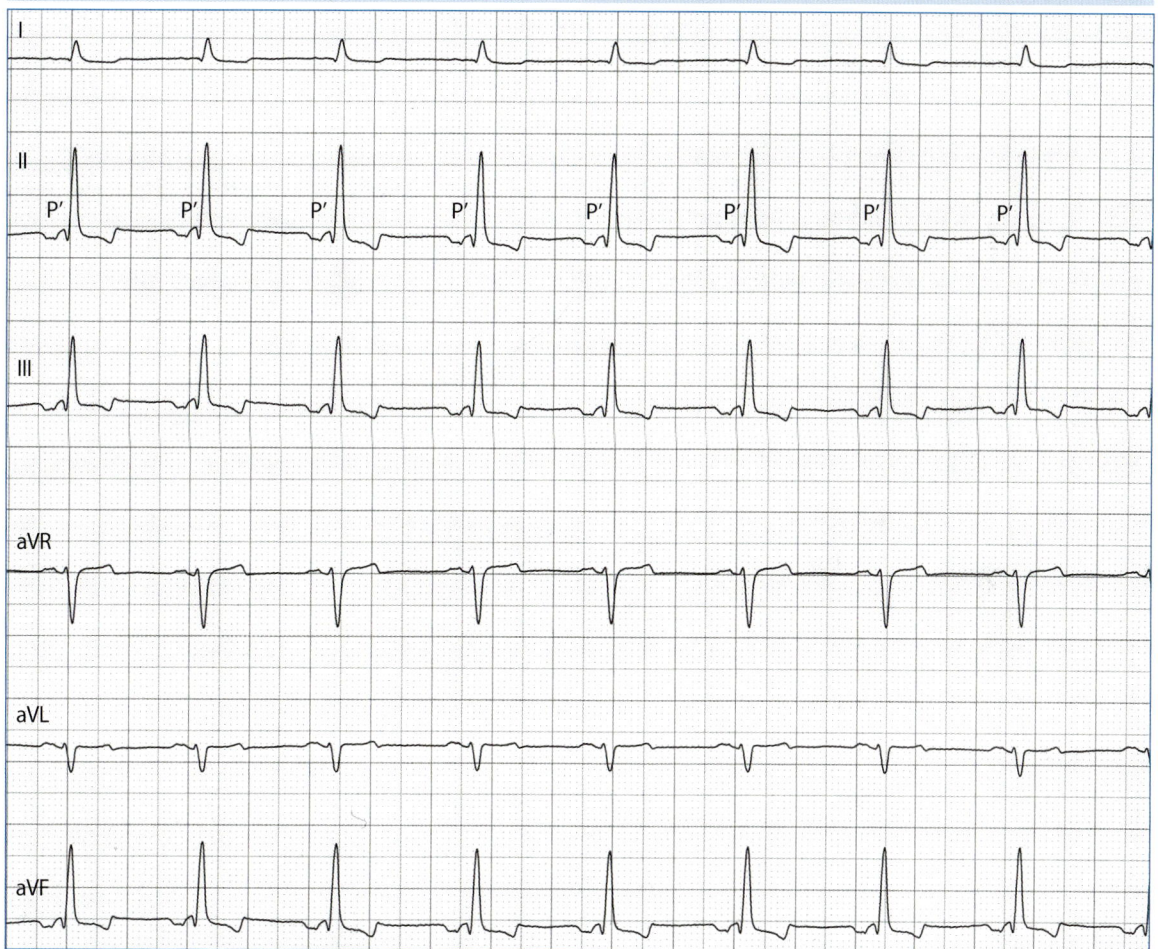

Dog, Greyhound, female, 4 years.
Six limb leads (I, II, III, aVR, aVL, aVF) -speed 50 mm/s - calibration 5 mm/1 mV.

Note: non-paroxysmal junctional tachycardia with a discharge rate of 130 bpm. P' waves with an inferior-to-superior concentric axis (−90°), P'Q interval duration of 70 ms, narrow QRS complexes with a duration of 55 ms and 1:1 atrioventricular conduction.

Notes: focal junctional tachycardia with a rate of 160 bpm. There is concentric 1:1 retrograde conduction with P' waves with an inferior-to-superior axis (from −90°) following the QRS complexes (arrows). Therefore the P' wave is negative in leads II, III and aVF. A small positive deflection is seen following the negative P' wave; however, this returns to the ST segment and could represent the T_a wave. The P' waves are more obvious in leads V_2 to V_6 (arrows). As these deflections are lined up with the P'in the limb leads the negative deflection in the latter is better appreciated.

Based on their anatomical site, they are classified into: left and right postero-septal; left and right posterior; left and right lateral; left and right anterior; antero-septal and mid-septal (Fig. 8.4). The conduction of electrical impulses along accessory pathways can be bi-directional (i.e. atrioventricular and ventriculo-atrial direction), unidirectional in the antegrade (atrioventricular) direction or unidirectional in the retrograde (ventriculo-atrial) direction. In dogs, conduction along accessory pathways is bidirectional in one-third of cases, and is retrograde in two-thirds of cases.

When antegrade conduction along an accessory pathway is possible, sinus impulses are simultaneously conducted to the ventricles through both the atrioventricular node and the atrioventricular accessory pathway. The electrocardiographic feature of this type of conduction is called *ventricular pre-excitation*. Retrograde conduction along the accessory pathway is critical for the formation of the anatomical reentrant macro-circuit that is the substrate for atrioventricular orthodromic reciprocating tachycardia and permanent junctional reciprocating tachycardia.

In dogs, arrhythmias associated with the presence of accessory pathways are orthodromic atrioventricular reciprocating tachycardia, permanent junctional reciprocating tachycardia and pre-excited atrial fibrillation.

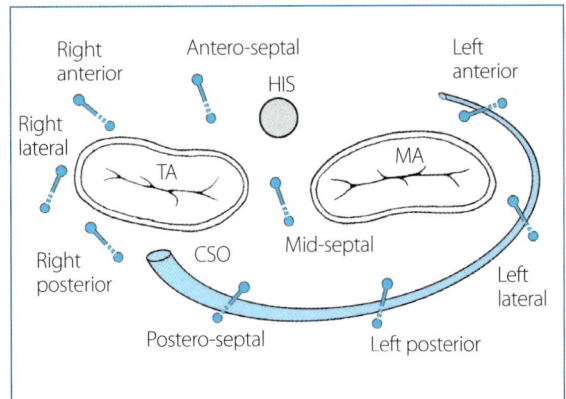

Figure 8.4. Anatomic distribution of atrioventricular accessory pathways in dogs around the mitral and tricuspid annuli. *TA*: tricuspid annulus; *MA*: mitral annulus; *CSO*: coronary sinus ostium; *HIS*: His bundle.

Ventricular pre-excitation

The term ventricular pre-excitation refers to the activation of a portion of the ventricular myocardium sooner than if the impulse only conducted along the normal atrioventricular conduction pathways (Fig. 8.5). It requires a supraventricular impulse to conduct faster through the accessory pathway than it conducts along the atrioventricular node. Usually, conduction through accessory

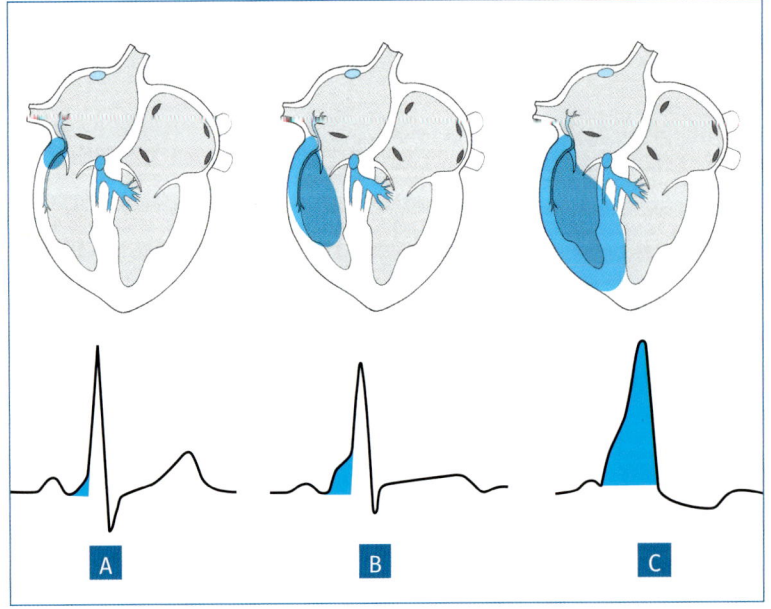

Figure 8.5. Activation of the ventricular myocardium along an atrioventricular accessory pathway with antegrade conduction. The atrial wavefront reaches the ventricles prematurely through the accessory pathway and later along the normal nodo-Hisian system. Depending on the relationship between the time of impulse conduction along the accessory pathway and the normal nodo-Hisian conduction, it results in different degrees of pre-excitation of the ventricular myocardium. From A to C a progressive prolongation of the atrioventricular conduction time results in a greater degree of ventricular pre-excitation (blue color). The degree of ventricular pre-excitation is characterized electrocardiographically by a progressive shortening of the PQ interval and with a progressive alteration of the morphology of the QRS complex and the T wave; ventricular depolarization is prolonged and the delta wave is more apparent.

pathways follows an all-or-none rule, that is either a supraventricular impulse conducts without delay or it blocks. It is different from the conduction through atrioventricular node that can be prolonged when the supraventricular rate increases, a property known as decremental conduction. In other words, when the rate of the impulses arriving at the atrioventricular node becomes increasingly rapid, the conduction through the atrioventricular node becomes slower. Retrograde conduction with decremental characteristic along an accessory pathway has been demonstrated on a few occasions in dogs.

Ventricular pre-excitation is described as *overt* when antegrade conduction along the accessory pathway is present, and it is called *non-manifest* when the sign of conduction along the accessory pathway (that is, a short PQ interval) is absent on the electrocardiogram. There are three mechanisms that can explain a normal PQ interval during pre-excitation: the presence of intra-atrial conduction delay that prolongs the initial portion of the PQ interval; a long distance between the atrial insertion of the accessory pathway and the sinus node; finally, slow conduction along the accessory pathway. Non-manifest pre-excitation must be distinguished from concealed ventricular pre-excitation, which corresponds to an accessory pathway that only conducts in a retrograde direction. Ventricular pre-excitation is described as *intermittent* when it alternates with periods of sinus rhythm with normal PQ intervals.

Accessory pathways are more commonly found in young (usually less than 2 years) Labrador Retrievers and Boxers. These dogs usually have a history of exercise intolerance, episodic weakness or congestive heart failure secondary to arrhythmia-induced cardiomyopathy. In some dogs, the accessory pathways are associated with other congenital cardiac defects, including tricuspid dysplasia, pulmonary valve stenosis and atrial septal defects. In cats, accessory pathways have more commonly been reported in American Shorthairs with hypertrophic cardiomyopathy.

The main electrocardiographic characteristics of a sinus rhythm with overt pre-excitation include:
- a short PQ interval,
- a delta wave,
- a wide QRS complex, and
- alterations of ventricular repolarization.

Short PQ interval

The PQ interval is short if it lasts less than 60 ms in dogs and 50 ms in cats. A short PQ interval reflects the reduction in conduction time between atria and ventricles associated with the propagation of the electric impulse through an accessory pathway. Indeed, conduction in an accessory pathway is typically faster than conduction along the normal atrioventricular conduction pathways. The degree of pre-excitation may vary depending on the location of the accessory pathway.

The degree of PQ interval shortening depends on:
- the conduction time through the accessory pathways and its antegrade refractory period,
- the antegrade conduction time through the atrioventricular node and its refractory period,
- the influence of the autonomic nervous system on the atrioventricular node,
- the distance between the atrial insertion site of the accessory pathway and the normal conduction system; for example, left-sided accessory pathways may only result in minor degrees of ventricular pre-excitation and a normal PQ interval (Fig. 8.5, Boxes 8.5 and 8.6) because of the increased distance between the atrial insertion of the accessory pathway and the sinus node. In contrast, right-sided accessory pathways will have a greater degree of ventricular pre-excitation,
- the intra-atrial conduction time, and
- the refractory period of the atrial myocardium.

Wide QRS complex and delta wave

In the presence of ventricular pre-excitation the QRS complex represents a fusion beat between the depolarization wavefront coming from the accessory pathway and the wavefront coming from the atrioventricular node and conduction along the intraventricular conduction system. Typically, the initial activation of the ventricles originates from the point of insertion of the accessory pathway to the ventricular myocardium. Since the atrioventricular accessory pathway conducts faster than the atrioventricular node, it allows early initiation of ventricular depolarization. This early depolarization of a portion of the ventricular myocardium appears on the surface electrocardiogram as an alteration of the initial portion of the QRS complex, called *delta wave* (δ).

The delta wave is followed by a Q, R or S wave from which it is sometimes separated by a notch. The portion of the ventricles activated by the accessory pathway is variable and depends on the location of its ventricular insertion, as well as the conduction times and refractory periods of the accessory pathway and the nodo-Hisian system. The extent of ventricular mass that is pre-excited depends, then, on the relationship between the activation time through the bundle of Kent and the activation time through the normal atrioventricular system. These time intervals represent the *total activation time*. The earlier the activation through the accessory pathway, the greater the pre-excited ventricular mass, and the more evident are the electrocardiographic signs of ventricular pre-excitation (Fig. 8.5).

Therefore, in addition to PQ interval shortening, electrocardiographic characteristics of ventricular pre-excitation include the presence of a δ wave and a QRS complex with bizarre morphology and increased duration (greater than 70 ms in dogs and greater than 40 ms in cats) (Boxes 8. 5 and 8.6). These electrocardiographic features must be distinguished from:
- late (or diastolic) ventricular ectopic beats with a P wave that is dissociated from it but occurs just before the wide QRS complex, giving the appearance of a short PQ interval,
- atrial or junctional ectopic rhythm with a short PQ interval and a pre-existing bundle branch block that result in a wide QRS complex, and
- *splintering* of the QRS complex. Splintered QRS complexes have an rR ', Rr', RR' or rr' pattern. *Splintering* of the QRS complex can be induced by alterations in ventricular depolarization secondary to fibrosis, accessory pathways, ischemia or apoptosis within the conduction system or ventricular myocardium. The presence of a splintered QRS complex associated with electrocardiographic signs of right atrial enlargement suggests the diagnosis of tricuspid dysplasia (Fig. 8.6).

Alterations of the ST segment and T wave

Whenever depolarization of the ventricles uses an accessory pathway, their repolarization is also altered, which appears on electrocardiogram as ST segment displacement and asymmetric T waves that have opposite polarity to that of the delta wave (Boxes 8.5 and 8.6).

Orthodromic atrioventricular reciprocating tachycardia

Orthodromic atrioventricular reciprocating tachycardia is the most common arrhythmia resulting from the presence of an accessory pathway in dogs and cats. The tachycardia uses an anatomical macro-reentrant circuit formed by the accessory pathway and the atrioventricular node connected superiorly by the atrial myocardium and inferiorly by the ventricular myocardium. The electrical impulse travels in an antegrade (from atrium to ventricle) direction along the atrioventricular node, and a retrograde (from ventricle to atrium) direction along the accessory pathway (Fig. 8.7).

Orthodromic atrioventricular reciprocating tachycardias depend on accessory pathways that can at least conduct impulses retrogradely, although some are able to conduct impulses in both directions. The initiation of the tachycardia is sudden. First an ectopic premature atrial depolarization is blocked in the anterograde direction in the accessory pathway and is conducted to the ventricles

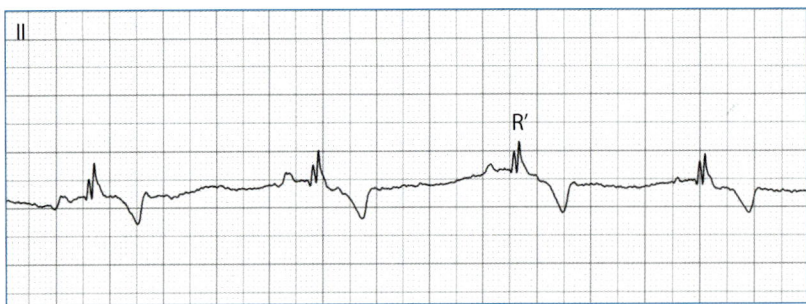

Figure 8.6. Sinus rhythm with *splintering* of the QRS complex (Dog, Giant Schnauzer, male, 8 years. Lead II - speed 50 mm/s - calibration 20 mm/1 mV).
The dominant rhythm is a sinus rhythm. The QRS complexes have a rR' morphology. The second positive wave (R ') does not intersect the isoelectric line. This type of QRS complex is said to be splintered.

Atrioventricular tachycardias mediated by accessory pathways | 157

BOX 8.5.
VENTRICULAR PRE-EXCITATION IN THE DOG

HEART RATE: dependent on the firing rate of the sinus node.
R-R INTERVAL: dependent on the regularity of the sinus rhythm.
P WAVE: present, sinus axis (between −20 ° and +90 °).
ATRIOVENTRICULAR CONDUCTION: present.

PQ INTERVAL: short (≤60 ms).
QRS COMPLEX: wide (>70 ms), with the presence of an initial delta wave. The T wave and delta wave have opposite polarities.
VENTRICULO-ATRIAL CONDUCTION: absent.
BLOCKED BEATS: none.

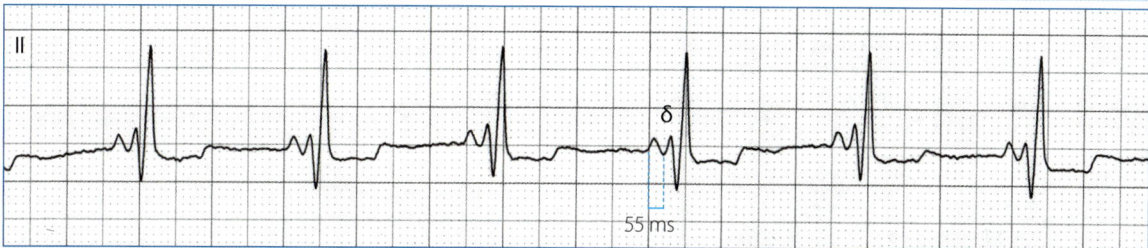

Dog, Labrador, male, 2 years.
Lead II - speed 50 mm/s - calibration 10 mm/1 mV.

Notes: ventricular pre-excitation. Normal sinus rhythm with a rate of 140 bpm, short PQ interval (55 ms), wide QRS complexes (80 ms) with the presence of an initial delta wave (δ).

BOX 8.6.
VENTRICULAR PRE-EXCITATION IN THE CAT

HEART RATE: dependent on the firing rate of the sinus node.
R-R INTERVAL: dependent on the regularity of the sinus rhythm.
P WAVE: present, sinus axis (between +0 ° and 90 °).
ATRIOVENTRICULAR CONDUCTION: present.
PQ INTERVAL: short (≤50 ms).

QRS COMPLEX: wide (>40 ms), with the presence of an initial delta wave. The T wave and delta wave have opposite polarities.
VENTRICULO-ATRIAL CONDUCTION: absent.
BLOCKED BEATS: none.

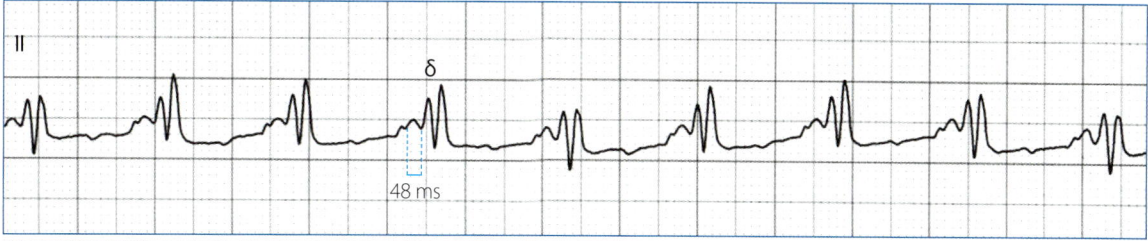

Cat, Domestic Short Hair, male, 2 years.
Lead II - speed 50 mm/s - calibration 10 mm/1 mV.

Notes: ventricular pre-excitation. Normal sinus rhythm with a rate of 180 bpm, short PQ interval (48 ms), wide QRS complexes (70 ms) with the presence of an initial delta wave (δ).

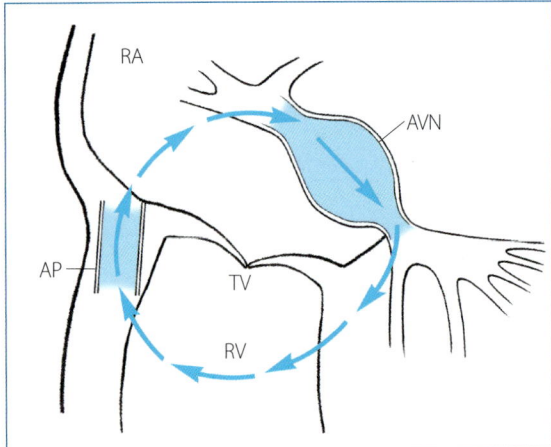

Figure 8.7. Orthodromic atrioventricular reciprocating tachycardia circuit. The electrical impulse is conducted antegradely (atrioventricular direction) along the atrioventricular node and retrogradely (ventriculo-atrial direction) along the accessory pathway. *RA*: right atrium; *AVN*: atrioventricular node; *AP*: accessory pathway; *TV*: tricuspid valve; *RV*: right ventricle.

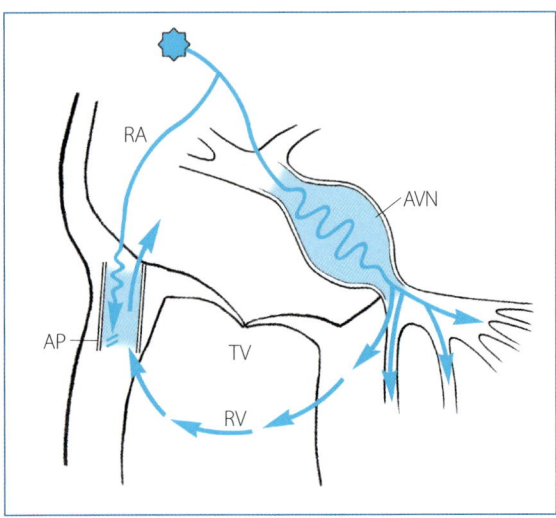

Figure 8.8. Initiation of orthodromic atrioventricular reciprocating tachycardia by an atrial premature beat. See text for explanations. *RA*: right atrium; *AVN*: atrioventricular node; *AP*: accessory pathway; *TV*: tricuspid valve; *RV*: right ventricle.

through the atrioventricular node. Then, the electrical impulse reaches the ventricular myocardium at the ventricular insertion site of the accessory pathway, finds it in an excitable state, and is conducted retrogradely back to the atria. After propagating to the entire atrial myocardium, the electrical impulse travels again through the atrioventricular node and repeats the reentrant circuit (Fig. 8.8). Premature ventricular ectopic beats can also initiate orthodromic atrioventricular reciprocating tachycardias whenever they are blocked retrogradely in the atrioventricular node but conduct along the accessory pathway, activate the atria and return to the ventricles along the normal conduction system, which initiates the cycle of tachycardia. Orthodromic atrioventricular reciprocating tachycardia can also start secondary to a critical variation of sinus node cycle length and therefore of atrial and ventricular refractoriness without any supraventricular or ventricular ectopic trigger.

During orthodromic atrioventricular reciprocating tachycardia, the retrograde activation of the atrial myocardium is called *eccentric*, because it starts at the atrial insertion of the pathway, usually located away from the atrioventricular node. The electrical activation of the two atria is, therefore, sequential (see p. 17).

The tachycardia terminates suddenly. This can result spontaneously from a block in the antegrade direction along the atrioventricular node or retrogradely along the accessory pathway. The tachycardia may also be terminated by a premature atrial or premature ventricular beat which enters the reentrant circuit. In clinical practice, orthodromic atrioventricular reciprocating tachycardia can be stopped with a precordial chest-thump that mechanically induces a ventricular ectopy, which interferes with the perpetuation of the reentrant circuit (Fig. 8.9).

Electrocardiographic characteristics of orthodromic atrioventricular reciprocating tachycardias include:
- narrow QRS complexes (≤70 ms in dogs and ≤40 ms in cats) with a ventricular rate between 190 and 300 bpm in dogs and usually above 300 bpm in cats,
- regular R-R intervals,
- QRS complex electrical alternans,
- 1:1 ventriculo-atrial conduction, usually eccentric,
- P' wave with variable axis in the frontal plane depending on the insertion site of the accessory pathway, but always with an inferior-to-superior direction, and
- short R-P' intervals.

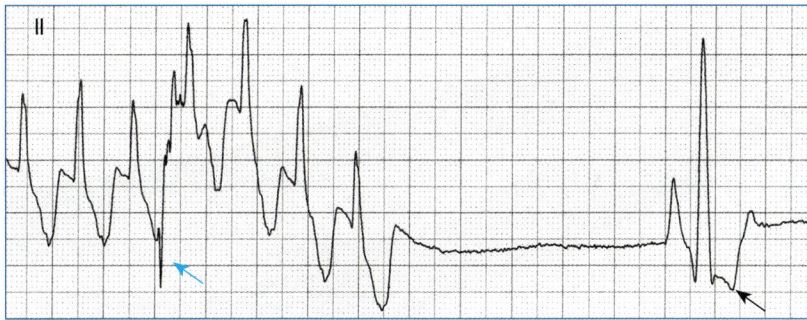

Figure 8.9. Orthodromic atrioventricular reciprocating tachycardia interrupted by a chest thump (Dog, Labrador, male, 9 months. Lead II - speed 50 mm/s - calibration 20 mm/1 mV).
The first three beats are an orthodromic atrioventricular reciprocating tachycardia. The mechanical extrastimulus induced by the chest thump (blue arrow) interrupts the tachycardia after four beats. Subsequently, a pause is interrupted by a sinus complex with evidence of a negative P' wave in the ST segment (black arrow) demonstrating the presence of retrograde atrial conduction along the accessory pathway not followed by a ventricular depolarization (antegrade atrioventricular block).

The QRS complexes usually have normal duration and morphology because ventricular activation occurs along the His-Purkinje system. In some cases, QRS complexes can be wide because of a rate-dependent intraventricular conduction disturbance or a pre-existing anatomical bundle branch block. R-R intervals are perfectly regular. However, in rare cases of orthodromic atrioventricular reciprocating tachycardia, there is *alternation in cycle length*, a R-R interval variation of at least 20 ms (see p. 291). This may be caused by the simultaneous presence of multiple accessory pathways with different conduction times or by the alternation of conduction through the fast and slow atrioventricular nodal pathways. Orthodromic atrioventricular reciprocating tachycardia is often characterized by *electrical alternans*, a beat-to-beat variation in R wave amplitude ≥0.1 mV in at least one lead. It is a reliable diagnostic tool to recognize orthodromic atrioventricular reciprocating tachycardia, although this electrocardiographic feature can also be seen in other supraventricular tachycardias (see p. 181). Electrical alternans may be due to beat-to-beat oscillation of the relative refractory period of the His-Purkinje system and of the diastolic interval following a sudden increase of the heart rate above a critical value. Orthodromic atrioventricular reciprocating tachycardias are characterized by P' waves after the QRS complexes with a 1:1 ventriculo-atrial conduction ratio. The P' waves can be found in the ST segment or, rarely in the ascending branch of the T wave (see p. 181).

Given the predominance of right atrioventricular accessory pathways in the dog, the retrograde atrial activation is eccentric with an electrical axis in the frontal plane that is directed inferior-to-superior toward lead aVR, which corresponds to negative P' waves in leads II, III and aVF and positive P' waves in leads I, aVL and aVR (Box 8.7).

During orthodromic atrioventricular reciprocating tachycardia, the RP' interval (from the beginning of the QRS complex to the onset of the P' wave) is defined as short, because it is less than 50 % of the R-R interval that includes it. This is the result of the retrograde conduction of the electrical impulse along the accessory pathway, which usually has a rapid conduction velocity. The length of the P'R interval reflects the atrioventricular conduction time during tachycardia. It is more than 50 % of the R-R interval that includes it, because the electrical impulse coming from the atria undergoes the typical conduction delay of the atrioventricular node. In dogs, the RP'/P'R ratio is usually ≤ 0.7 during orthodromic atrioventricular reciprocating tachycardia.

Permanent junctional reciprocating tachycardia

Permanent junctional reciprocating tachycardia as described by Coumel is a form of atrioventricular reciprocating tachycardia in which the antegrade limb of the circuit is the atrioventricular node and the retrograde limb is a right postero-septal accessory pathway with unidirectional retrograde conduction (*concealed pathway*), which

Chapter 8. Supraventricular tachycardias

BOX 8.7.
ORTHODROMIC ATRIOVENTRICULAR RECIPROCATING TACHYCARDIA IN THE DOG

HEART RATE: 190-300 bpm.
R-R INTERVAL: regular.
P' WAVE: present, retrograde conduction, usually negative in inferior leads and positive in aVR and aVL.
ATRIOVENTRICULAR CONDUCTION: present (1:1).
P'R INTERVAL: greater than the R-P'.
QRS COMPLEX: narrow (≤70 ms) unless concomitant functional or anatomical disorders of intraventricular conduction. Often visible electrical alternans.
VENTRICULO-ATRIAL CONDUCTION: present. 1:1 along the accessory pathway.
R-P' INTERVAL: short, less than 50 % of the R-R interval that includes P'. RP'/P'R ratio ≤0.7.
BLOCKED BEATS: none.
INITIATION AND TERMINATION MODALITY: sudden.

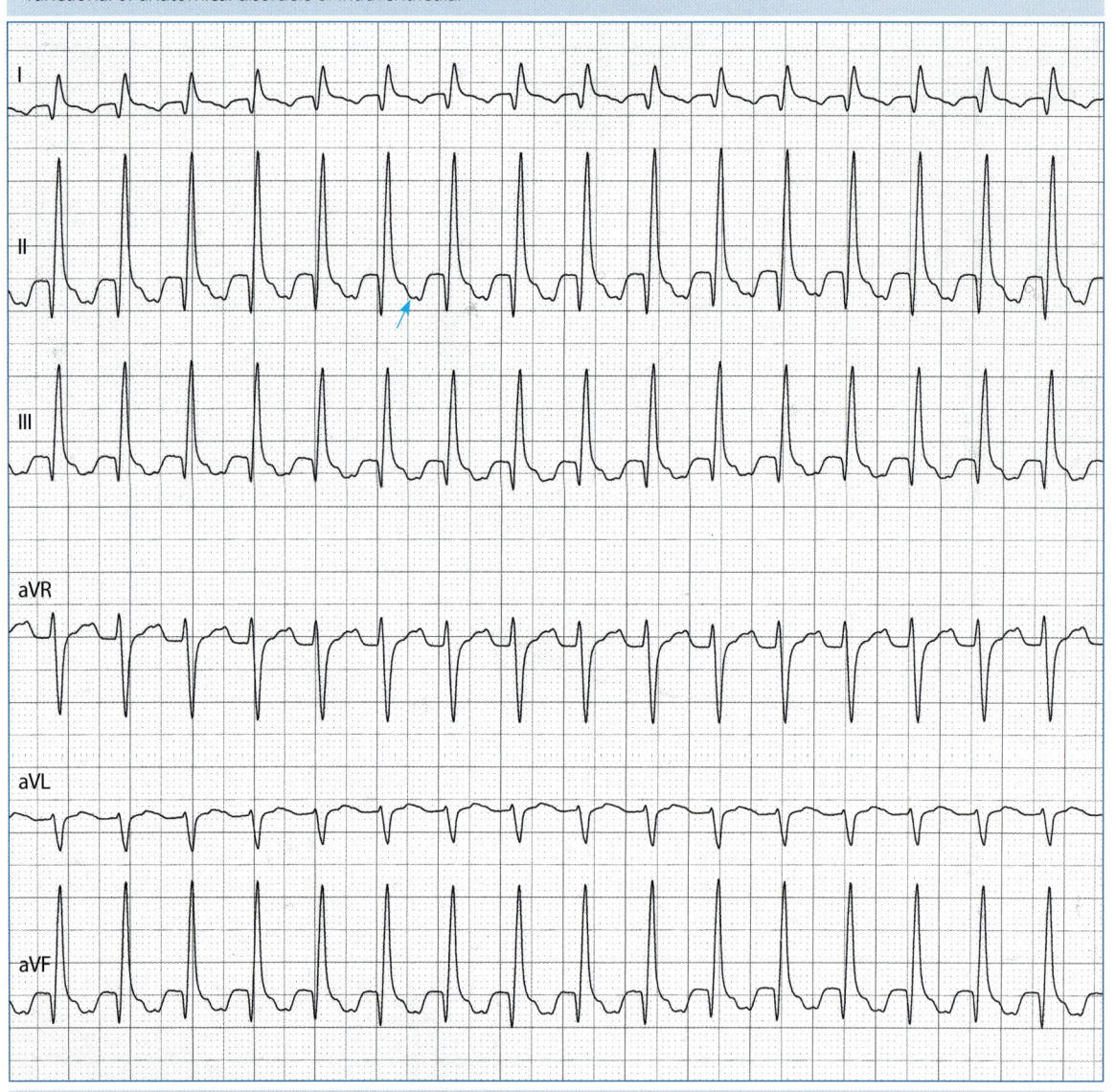

Dog, Boxer, male, 1 year.
Six limb leads (I, II, III, aVR, aVL, aVF) - speed 50 mm/s - calibration 5 mm/1 mV.

Notes: orthodromic atrioventricular reciprocating tachycardia with a ventricular rate of 300 bpm. QRS complexes are evident with normal morphology and duration (55 ms); regular R-R intervals (200 ms); P' waves (arrow) visible in the initial portion of the ST segment with a RP'/ P'R ratio of 0.5.

also has decremental properties. Permanent junctional reciprocating tachycardia is, as its name suggests, usually permanent, and begins with critical changes in the sinus cycle length. It can lead to severe cases of arrhythmia-induced cardiomyopathy.

Electrocardiographic characteristics of permanent junctional reciprocating tachycardia include (Box 8.8):
- narrow QRS complexes (≤70 ms in dogs) with a ventricular rate ranging from 230 to 250 bpm in dogs,
- regular R-R intervals with cycle length irregularity due to variation of the ventriculo-atrial conduction along the accessory pathway with decremental retrograde conduction,
- presence of electrical alternans of the QRS complex,
- 1:1 ventriculo-atrial conduction; always eccentric,
- a P' wave with an inferior-to-superior direction, with negative P' waves in leads II, III and aVF and an axis on the frontal plane directed towards avR and aVL, and
- a long and variable RP' interval with a RP'/P'R greater than 0.7.

Antidromic atrioventricular reciprocating tachycardia

Antidromic atrioventricular reciprocating tachycardias use the same anatomical circuit as orthodromic tachycardias, but the electrical impulse travels in the opposite direction. The ventricles are, therefore, activated by the accessory pathway in the antegrade direction and then the impulse returns to the atria retrogradely along the atrioventricular node. As a result, the tachycardia displays wide QRS complexes (greater than 70 ms in dogs and greater than 40 ms in cats) and regular R-R intervals that need to be differentiated from ventricular tachycardia and other supraventricular tachycardias conducted with aberrancy (see p. 231). During the tachycardia retrograde atrial activation is concentric, with P' waves inscribed within the QRS complex. This type of tachycardia has not yet been described in dogs and cats.

Pre-excited tachycardias

In the presence of an accessory pathway with a short antegrade refractory period, different types of supraventricular tachycardias can be conducted to the ventricles along the pathway. Because the refractory period of this structure is very short, it is possible that a large number of atrial depolarizations reach the ventricles, resulting in a very fast ventricular response rate. Indeed, unlike the atrioventricular node, the accessory pathway does not play the role of a "filter". In this situation, supraventricular tachycardias are described as *pre-excited* and are characterized by wide QRS complexes, a fast ventricular rate and usually regular R-R intervals. The QRS complexes can be fully pre-excited or show various degrees of fusion with the electrical wavefront traveling simultaneously through the atrioventricular node and partially depolarizing the ventricles. So far, atrial fibrillation intermittently conducted to the ventricles along an accessory pathway is the only pre-excited supraventricular tachycardia that has been described in dogs (Fig. 8.10).

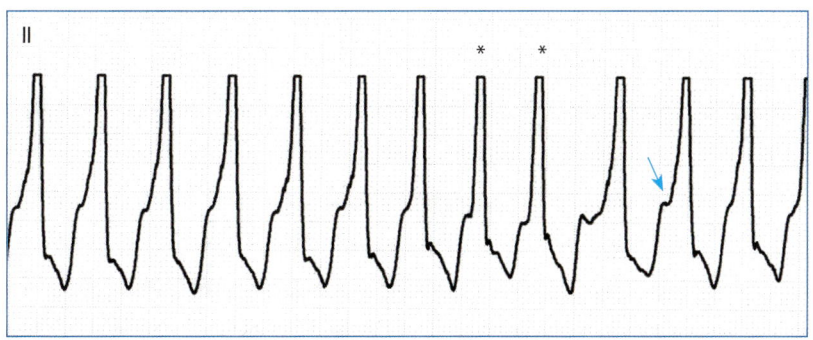

Figure 8.10. Pre-excited atrial fibrillation (Dog, Golden Retriever, male, 2 years. Lead II - speed 50 mm/s - calibration 10 mm/1 mV). Most QRS complexes correspond to the maximum degree of ventricular pre-excitation and increased duration (85 ms). The eighth and ninth beats (*) have a shorter duration (60 ms) than the other QRS complexes, because of different degrees of pre-excitation. The wide QRS complexes are characterized by a notch on the ascending branch of the R wave, called the delta wave (arrow), and the R-R intervals are irregular.

Chapter 8. Supraventricular tachycardias

BOX 8.8.
PERMANENT JUNCTIONAL RECIPROCATING TACHYCARDIA IN THE DOG

HEART RATE: 230-250 bpm.
R-R INTERVAL: regular, rarely irregular.
P' WAVE: present, retro-conducted, usually negative in inferior leads and positive in aVR and aVL.
ATRIOVENTRICULAR CONDUCTION: present (1:1).
P'R INTERVAL: shorter than the R-P'.
QRS COMPLEX: present (≤70 ms) unless concomitant functional or anatomical disorders of intraventricular conduction. Often visible electrical alternans.
VENTRICULO-ATRIAL CONDUCTION: present. 1:1 along the accessory pathway.
R-P' INTERVAL: long, more than 50 % of the R-R interval that includes P'. RP'/P'R ratio >0.7. On occasion variable if decremental conduction along the accessory pathway.
BLOCKED BEATS: none.
INITIATION AND TERMINATION MODALITY: sudden.

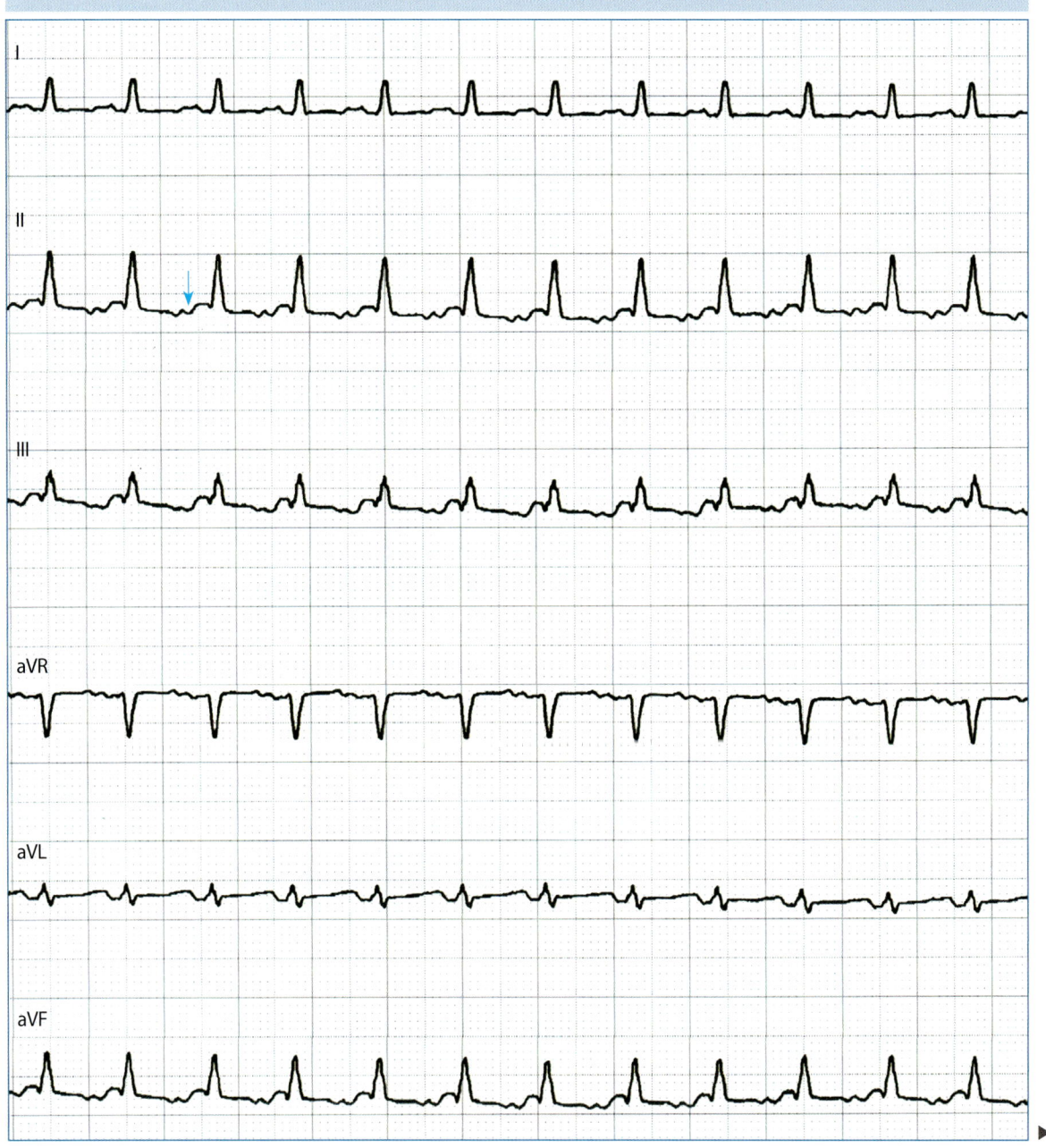

Focal atrial tachycardia

Focal atrial tachycardias originate from ectopic foci in the atria or the veins directly connected to the atria. The sinus node and the atrioventricular node are not involved in the initiation or maintenance of these tachyarrhythmias.

The foci are located in close proximity to well-defined anatomical landmarks, including the *crista terminalis*, the inter-atrial septum, the right and left auricles, the triangle of Koch, the tricuspid and mitral annulus, the cranial and caudal venae cavae, the pulmonary veins, the coronary sinus, and the vein or ligament of Marshall.

The arrhythmogenic mechanisms of focal atrial tachycardias include enhanced abnormal automaticity, triggered activity and micro-reentry. It is rarely possible to determine the mechanism of the arrhythmias from the electrocardiogram.

Atrial tachycardia can occur in the absence of structural cardiac disease or be associated with various cardiac and systemic diseases, including atrial enlargement, myocarditis, congenital or acquired heart disease, cardiac tumors, overdose of antiarrhythmics (for example digoxin toxicity), hyperthyroidism, general anesthesia or hypokalemia.

The electrocardiographic characteristics of focal atrial tachycardias include:
- narrow QRS complexes (≤70 ms in dogs and ≤40 ms in cats) with a ventricular rate between 210 and 330 bpm in dogs,
- regular R-R intervals with the possibility of periods of irregularities (*cycle length irregularity*),
- a long R-P' interval,
- possible presence of Wenckebach-type (Mobitz I) second-degree atrioventricular block, and
- P' waves with a variable axis in the frontal plane depending on the site of the ectopic focus, but in most cases with a superior-to-inferior direction.

The QRS complexes are usually narrow (≤70 ms in dogs and ≤40 ms in cats), except in the presence of functional or anatomical disorders of intraventricular conduction.

R-R intervals are generally regular in sustained forms of focal atrial tachycardias, but can be irregular due to variations in the rate of discharge of the ectopic focus; furthermore, during non-sustained focal atrial tachycardias R-R intervals tend to shorten after the initiation of the tachycardia and increase before the termination of the tachycardia ("warm up" and "cool down" phenomena). A characteristic of many focal atrial tachycardias is *irregularity of the cycle length*, defined as a variation of R-R intervals of at least 20 ms caused by changes in the firing rate of an automatic ectopic focus, the presence of atrioventricular nodal block and the variable conduction of electrical impulses along the fast or slow pathway of the atrioventricular node.

The location of the ectopic focus determines the axis of the P' waves. P' waves with a superior-to-inferior axis (positive P' waves in leads II, III and aVF) are more common in dogs. Generally, during focal atrial tachycardia, the P' wave precedes the QRS complex with a normal P'Q interval. If the ectopic focus discharges at a high rate, the P' wave can overlap with the T wave of the previous beat, which gives a typical shape referred to as the "camel sign" in the inferior leads (see p. 183).

Although there is no ventriculo-atrial conduction of impulses during focal atrial tachycardias, the ratio of the RP' and the P'R intervals is used to differentiate them from other forms of supraventricular tachycardias. Focal atrial tachycardias belong to the group of supraventricular tachycardias with a long RP' interval, and the RP'/P'R ratio is usually greater than 0.7 (Box 8.9).

English Bulldog, male, 5 years.
Six limb leads (I, II, III, aVR, aVL, aVF) - speed 50 mm/s - calibration 5 mm/1 mV.

Notes: permanent junctional reciprocating tachycardia with a ventricular rate of 230 bpm, normal QRS complexes with a duration of 60 ms; regular R-R intervals (260 ms); P' waves (arrow) following the T of the previous QRS complex with an inferior-to-superior axis (–45 °) and a RP'/ P'R ratio of 1.16.

Chapter 8. Supraventricular tachycardias

BOX 8.9.
FOCAL ATRIAL TACHYCARDIA IN THE DOG

HEART RATE: 210-330 bpm.
R-R INTERVAL: regular, with periods of irregularity
P' WAVE: present, usually with a superior-to-inferior axis.
ATRIOVENTRICULAR CONDUCTION: present (1:1) or possible existence of Wenckebach type (Mobitz I) second-degree atrioventricular block.
P'R INTERVAL: shorter than RP'.
QRS COMPLEX: narrow (≤70 ms) unless concomitant functional or anatomical disorders of intraventricular conduction.
VENTRICULO-ATRIAL CONDUCTION: absent.
R-P' INTERVAL: long, more than 50 % the R-R interval that includes P'. RP'/P'R ratio >0.7.
BLOCKED BEATS: yes, from time to time with Wenckebach type second-degree atrioventricular block.
INITIATION TERMINATION MODALITY: sudden in reentrant or triggered forms, gradual in automatic forms.

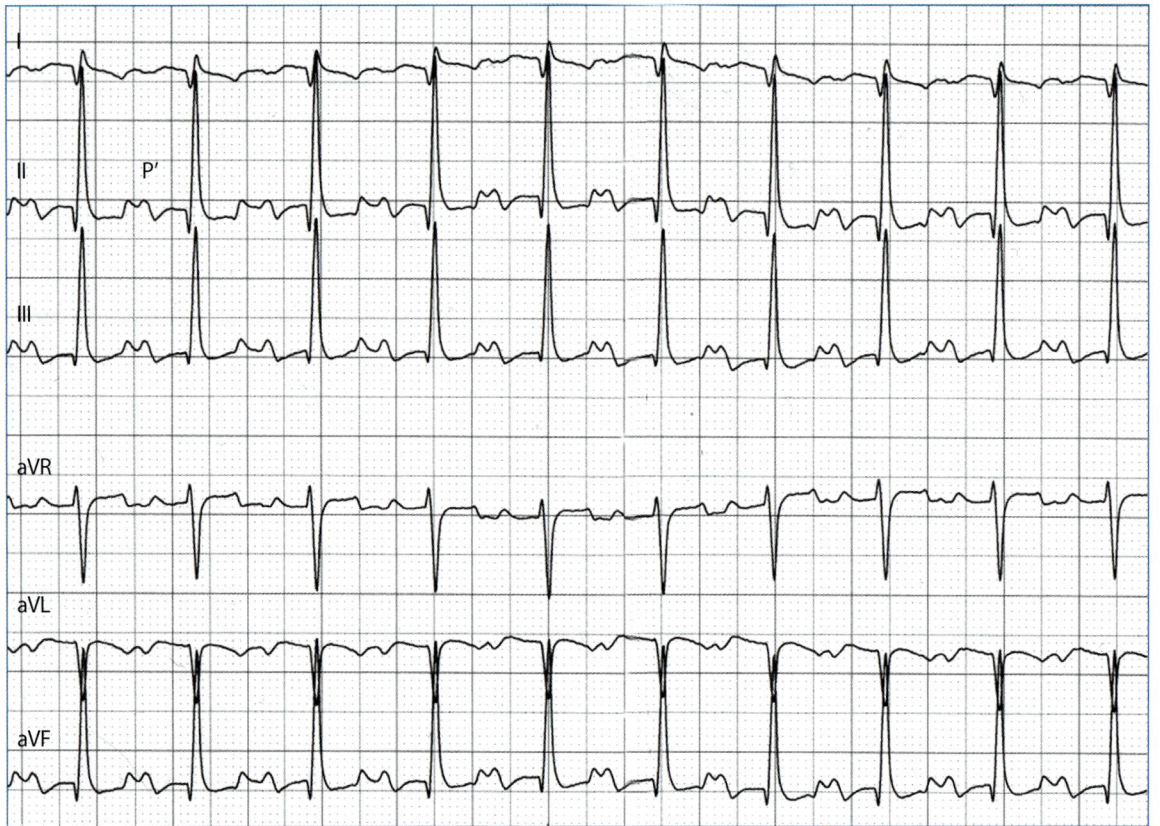

Dog, Rottweiler, female, 7 months.
Six limb leads (I, II, III, aVR, aVL, aVF) - speed 50 mm/s - calibration 10 mm/1 mV.

Notes: focal atrial tachycardia with a firing rate of 210 bpm originating from the left atrial roof. Note the presence of positive P' waves with a superior-to-inferior axis and negative polarity in leads I and aVL. The RP'/P'R ratio is 1.14. Note that the T_a wave that follows the P' wave is a negative deflection when the P' wave is positive, but is a positive deflection when the P' wave is negative.

In addition, focal atrial tachycardias can be further classified as:
- self-limiting atrial tachycardia,
- sustained paroxysmal atrial tachycardia,
- incessant atrial tachycardia,
- paroxysmal atrial tachycardia with atrioventricular block, and
- pulmonary vein atrial tachycardia.

Self limiting atrial tachycardia
This form of focal atrial tachycardia, characterized by the presence of runs of approximately 6 to 12 beats is usually considered benign and often accompanies chronic mitral valvular disease and chronic obstructive pulmonary diseases (Fig. 8.11).

Paroxysmal sustained atrial tachycardia
Paroxysmal sustained atrial tachycardia is a rhythm disturbance lasting 30 s or more, with a sudden onset and termination. It is usually associated with heart disease, including congenital heart defects, acquired valvular defects, myocarditis and cardiomyopathy. In many cases, there are multiple foci that initiate the tachycardia. The probable arrhythmogenic mechanisms for this type of tachycardia include micro-reentry and triggered activity.

Incessant atrial tachycardia
This type of tachycardia lasts more than 12 hours per day; it is rare and is usually associated with myocardial diseases. The incessant nature of this tachycardia can lead to arrhythmia-induced cardiomyopathy.

Paroxysmal atrial tachycardia with block
Paroxysmal atrial tachycardia with block is typically secondary to digitalis toxicity, which, by its negative dromotropic effect, induces second-degree atrioventricular block (Fig. 8.12).

Pulmonary vein atrial tachycardia
The atrial myocardium extends into the walls of the pulmonary veins, forming sleeves with a complex myofiber arrangement and anisotropic conduction that promotes reentry and ectopic focus activity. Spontaneous action potentials (automaticity) and early-afterdepolarizations (triggered activity) have been recorded from myocytes in isolated pulmonary vein preparations. Arrhythmogenicity is more pronounced in the right and left superior pulmonary veins. During tachycardia, the pulmonary vein firing rate is very rapid and the firing can occur as single beats or rapid (cycle length of 150-180 ms) and irregular bursts (Fig. 8.13). High temperature and circulating

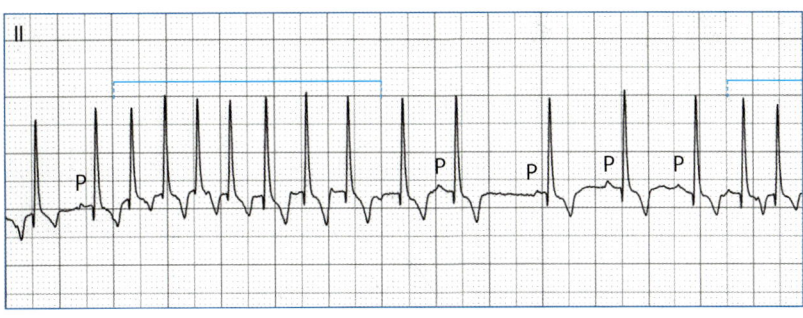

Figure 8.11. Self-limiting atrial tachycardia (Dog, mongrel, male, 13 years. Lead II - speed 25 mm/s - calibration 5 mm/1 mV).
The tracing shows some sinus beats (P) interspersed with runs of self-limiting atrial tachycardia (square) with irregular R-R intervals, characteristic of the warm-up and cool-down periods at the beginning and end of the tachycardia.

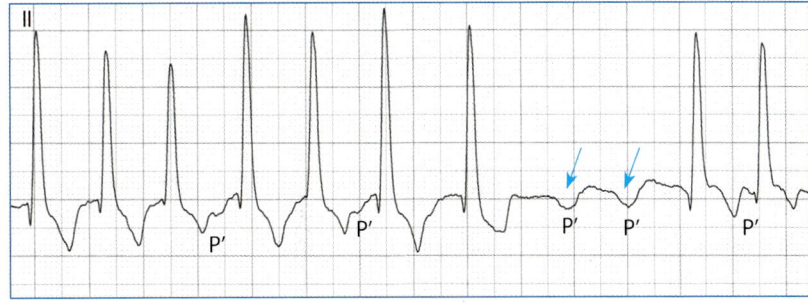

Figure 8.12. Paroxysmal atrial tachycardia with block (Dog, English Setter, male, 8 years. Lead II - speed 50 mm/s - calibration 10 mm/1 mV).
The tracing shows an atrial tachycardia followed, after the first seven beats, by a block with a 3:1 atrioventricular conduction ratio. Note the ectopic P' waves not conducted (*arrows*) followed by the return of atrial tachycardia with a 1:1 conduction ratio.

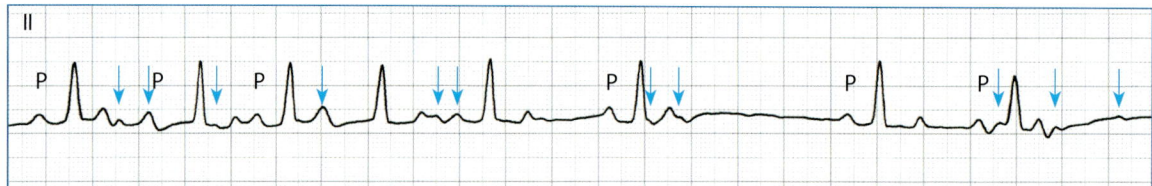

Figure 8.13. Pulmonary vein firing. (Dog, Irish Wolfhound, male, 5 year. Lead II - speed 50 mm/s - calibration 10 mm/1 mV). The tracing shows a sinus rhythm (P waves) interrupted by frequent atrial ectopies occurring as isolated impulses or organized in bursts and an atrial rate from 400 to 550 bpm. The second, fourth and the fifth ectopies are conducted to the ventricles, with prolonged atrioventricular conduction time. Note that the second sinus P wave is concomitant to the venous ectopy.

catecholamines promote pulmonary vein firing, while acetylcholine and phenylephrine reduce pulmonary vein activity. The effective refractory period of the cells in the proximal portion (close to the ostium) of the pulmonary veins is shorter than in the distal region, and for this reason vein ectopies are commonly concealed. In that case, no ectopic P' waves can be seen on the surface electrocardiogram. In humans, pulmonary vein firing is considered an important trigger for atrial fibrillation. It likely contributes to its induction and maintenance. Ectopic foci with the wall of the superior vena cava are also involved in the induction of atrial fibrillation.

Pulmonary vein firing is characterized by the presence of single identical P' waves usually in the ST segment of the previous beat (Fig. 7.11), or by a burst of P' waves with variable morphology and a superior-to inferior axis in the frontal plane (positive in leads II, III and aVF) and negative in leads I and aVL. The atrial rate is variable but very rapid and the impulse is usually conducted to the ventricles with high atrioventricular conduction ratios (from 4:1 to 6:1).

Multifocal atrial tachycardia

Multifocal atrial tachycardia also called *atrial chaotic rhythm* is characterized by irregular and continuously changing atrial activation, due to the presence of several atrial ectopic foci that are alternately activated.

The arrhythmogenic mechanism of multifocal atrial tachycardia is triggered activity by delayed after-depolarizations promoted by β-adrenergic stimulation. This arrhythmia is generally associated with severe atrial disease secondary to acute cardiac or pulmonary disease, digitalis toxicity, metabolic or electrolyte disorders.

The electrocardiographic characteristics of multifocal atrial tachycardia include a ventricular rate greater than 180 bpm in dogs and narrow QRS complexes (≤70 ms in dogs) unless an anatomical or functional intraventricular conduction block is present. R-R intervals are irregular. There are at least three different ectopic P' waves, at least three P'Q intervals of different duration, and segments of isoelectric line interposed between the P' waves (Box 8.10). During multifocal atrial tachycardia, normal sinus beats should not be present, while Wenckebach-type (Mobitz I) second-degree atrioventricular block is common. This type of tachycardia often degenerates into atrial fibrillation.

Macro-reentrant atrial tachycardia (atrial flutter)

The term *macro-reentrant atrial tachycardia* refers to a particular type of supraventricular tachycardia that is perpetuated by large anatomical or functional circuits in the right atrium or left atrium. This is in contrast to a micro-reentrant atrial tachycardia which involves a very small area of myocardium. In clinical circles this type of arrhythmia is still often referred to as *atrial flutter*. When reading the literature concerning types of atrial flutter/macro-reentrant atrial tachycardia even as late as the early 2000s the various classifications can be confusing. It is important to realize that the classification and naming of this group of rhythms have evolved as understanding of the mechanism of this arrhythmia has developed. Numerous types of macro-reentrant atrial tachycardia/atrial flutter are described in people, and many of these rhythms, which are uncommon in humans, do not occur in the dog. Previously, Wells classified atrial

Macro-reentrant atrial tachycardia (atrial flutter)

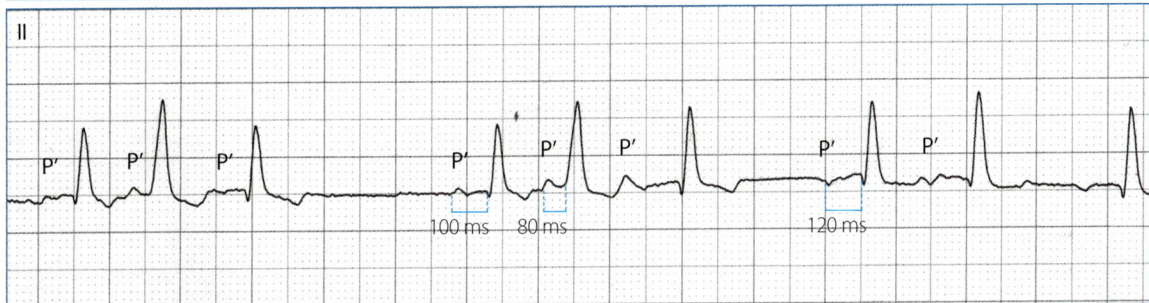

BOX 8.10
MULTIFOCAL ATRIAL TACHYCARDIA IN THE DOG

HEART RATE: greater than 180 bpm in adult dogs.
R-R INTERVAL: irregular.
P'WAVE: present; at least three P' waves from different foci.
ATRIOVENTRICULAR CONDUCTION: present (1:1) or with possible evidence of Wenckebach type second-degree atrioventricular block.
P'Q INTERVAL: at least three intervals of different durations.

QRS COMPLEX: narrow (≤70 ms) unless concomitant functional or anatomical disorders of intraventricular conduction.
VENTRICULO-ATRIAL CONDUCTION: absent.
BLOCKED BEATS: present, occasionally with Wenckebach type second-degree atrioventricular block.
INITIATION AND TERMINATION MODALITY: incessant character.

Dog, German Shepherd, male, 10 years old.
Lead II - speed 50 mm/s - calibration 10 mm/1 mV.

Notes: multifocal atrial tachycardia with a discharge rate between 180 and 220 bpm; evident narrow QRS complexes (60 ms) with irregular R-R intervals, at least three P' waves with three different morphologies and axes; P'Q intervals of different durations. Isoelectric line visible between the P' waves and the T waves.

---

flutter as type I (anatomical substrate) or type II (electrophysiologically functional substrate). An anatomical substrate means that there is an area of slowed conduction that is structurally present enabling the macro-reentrant circuit, whereas functional reentry indicates that there is no structural component but that the area of slowed conduction is caused by electrophysiological alterations (e.g. dispersion of refractoriness due to heightened vagal tone). Recently, the classification has been based on electrophysiological mechanisms and the anatomical substrate for the arrhythmia, and, therefore, the names reflect this categorization. In 2001 Saoudi, et al. opened the discussion to a reevaluation of the understanding of atrial flutter while the further clarification of Page, et al. in 2016 is summarized below as it pertains to the dog.

Basically there are three types of macro-reentrant atrial tachycardias/atrial flutters that are based on the location of the macro-reentrant circuit and the electrophysiological mechanisms (anatomical reentry and functional reentry):

- typical or cavotricuspid isthmus-dependent atrial flutter (two types),
- atypical or non-cavotricuspid isthmus-dependent atrial flutter, and
- other types of atypical atrial flutter (including functional reentry).

Cavotricuspid isthmus-dependent atrial flutter

A band of conductive tissue that is located between the caudal vena cava and the tricuspid valve is called the cavotricuspid isthmus. This portion of the right atrium is the vital component of the macro-reentrant anatomical circuit of the most common types of atrial flutter in this anatomical structure and is the basis for most cases of atrial flutter in both people and dogs. According to Wells' original classification these were known as type I atrial flutter. So far, in dogs typical and reverse typical atrial flutters have been confirmed by intracardiac electrophysiological studies.

Typical or cavotricuspid isthmus-dependent atrial flutter

Atrial flutter is a tachycardia characterized by an organized atrial rhythm, with an average atrial rate in dogs greater than 300 bpm; the most common form of atrial flutter is cavotricuspid isthmus-dependent atrial flutter (Fig. 8.14). The cavotricuspid isthmus is characterized by an area of slow conduction located in the inferior right atrium, between the emergence of the caudal vena cava, the Eustachian ridge and the annulus of the tricuspid valve. The remaining part of the circuit is composed of a ring of muscle that comprises the inter-atrial septum and the anterior wall of the right atrium joined superiorly at the roof of the right atrium. Depending on the direction of the wavefront around the tricuspid valve annulus, two forms of cavotricuspid-dependent atrial flutter are recognized: (1) the typical form in which atrial activation along the reentrant circuit is counterclockwise, and (2) the reverse typical form in which the activation is clockwise. The use of the word "typical" has been used to indicate that these two types of atrial flutter use the same structural location of slowed conduction for the reentrant loop, but that they revolve in two different directions. The perspective for the definition of counterclockwise versus clockwise is based on viewing the atrial circuit from the ventricular side of the atrioventricular valve annulus.

Atrial flutter can be found in the absence of structural cardiac disease or be associated with cardiac diseases that cause atrial enlargement, such as mitral insufficiency, arrhythmogenic cardiomyopathy, myocarditis, atrial septal defect and tricuspid valve dysplasia. Atrial flutter may degenerate into atrial fibrillation, and similarly atrial fibrillation can rearrange into atrial flutter.

The *typical cavotricuspid isthmus-dependent atrial flutter* (Fig. 8.15A, Box 8.11) appears on the electrocardiogram with regular and identical flutter waves (F waves) that have a characteristic "sawtooth" appearance in the inferior leads (II, III and aVF). The atrial rate ranges between 300 and 450 bpm in dogs. F waves are formed by a succession of: 1) a slow descending segment; 2) a rapid negative deflection; 3) an equally rapid rise, followed by; 4) a small positive cusp which surmounts the first slow descending portion of the next cycle (Fig. 8.15A). These variations in the polarity of the F waves represent the changes of impulse direction within the macro-reentrant circuit, and depolarization of

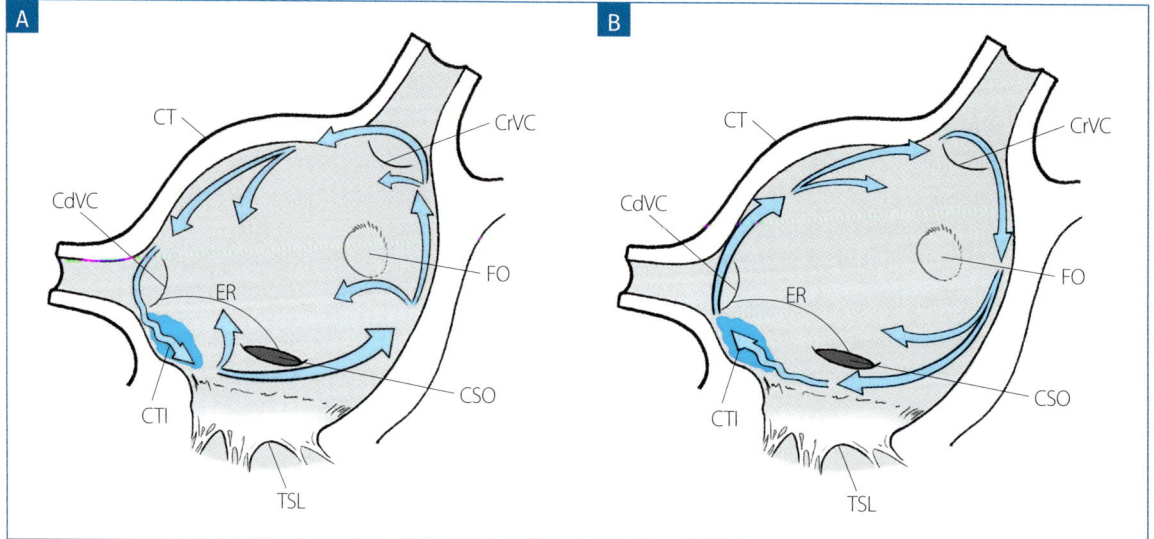

Figure 8.14. Right atrial circuit forming the substrate for cavo-tricuspid isthmus-dependent atrial flutter. Depending on the direction of the electrical impulse around the tricuspid valve annulus, two types of flutter are recognized: when the impulse circulates counterclockwise the atrial flutter is called typical (A), and when the impulse circulates clockwise the atrial flutter is called reverse typical (B). *CrVC*: cranial vena cava; *CdVC*: caudal vena cava; *CSO*: coronary sinus ostium; *ER*: Eustachian ridge; *CT*: crista terminalis; *FO*: fossa ovalis; *TSL*: tricuspid valve septal leaflet. The posterior region represented by the light blue area is the cavo-tricuspid or Cosio isthmus (*CTI*).

the right and left atria. The negative cusp of the F wave is induced by the inferior-to-superior activation of the inter-atrial septum. F waves are best visualized in leads II, III, aVF and V_1 since, in most cases, atrial activation occurs along the inferior-to-superior axis, i.e. the vector moves away from lead aVF. It should be mentioned that the deflections in atrial flutter can be difficult to define. This difficulty can arise from the historical identification of the flutter waves with a capital F over the positive deflection in lead II and the other inferior leads. However, the F waves during counterclockwise typical cavotricuspid isthmus-dependent atrial flutter are described as "negative" in these leads. With this most common type of atrial flutter it should be realized that the flutter waves are actually both negative and positive deflections that are continuously present as the loop of macro-reentry is constantly circling around the right atrium with conduction to the left atrium. The initial portion of F waves is usually negative in the inferior leads (II, III and aVF) and negative in V_1.

The *reverse typical cavotricuspid isthmus-dependent atrial flutter* (Fig. 8.15B, Box 8.12) has a positive deflection that is seen in the inferior leads (II, III and aVF) due to the superior-to-inferior activation of the inter-atrial septum, and a rounded appearance in V_1. In some cases, the isoelectric line can be interposed between the F waves. It has been suggested that this is due to the presence of an area of very slow conduction or possibly the summed vectors of the atrial depolarization that result from this reentrant path of activation.

The regularity of the F-F intervals is a characteristic that differentiates atrial flutter from fibrillation.

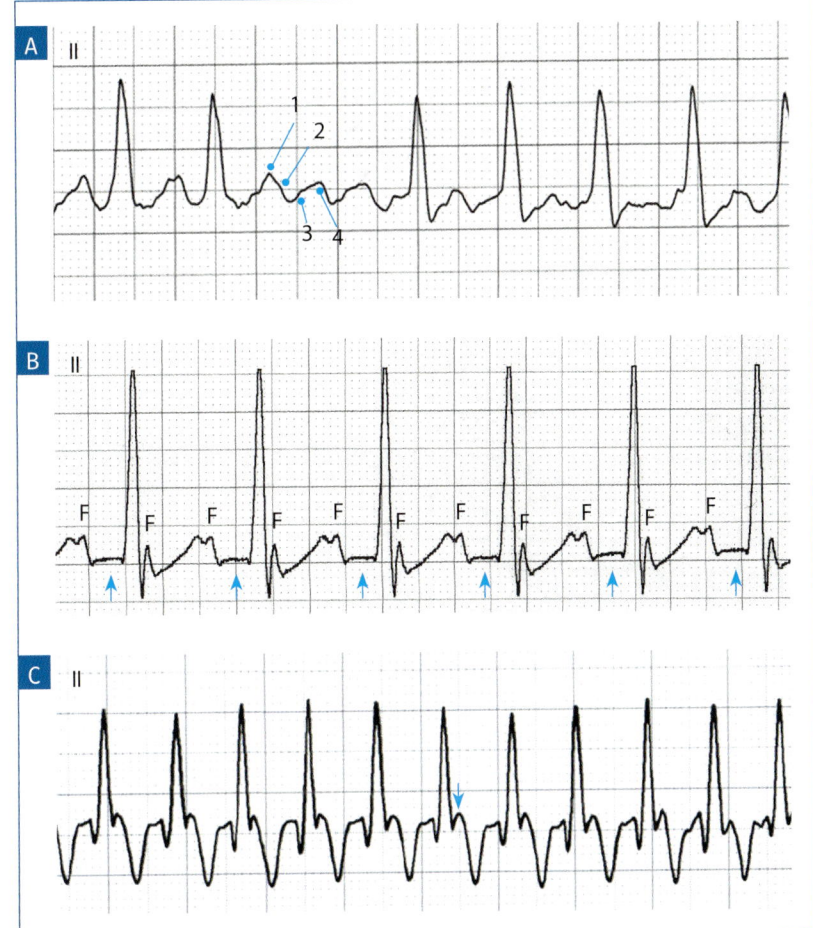

Figure 8.15. Morphology of F waves in typical (A), typical reverse (B) and atypical atrial flutter (C) in dogs.
A) Typical atrial flutter. (Dog, Boxer, male, 12 years. Lead II - speed 50 mm/s - calibration 10 mm/1 mV). In typical atrial flutter, F waves are formed by: 1) a slow descending segment; 2) a rapid negative deflection; 3) a rapid rise; 4) a small positive cusp. The QRS complexes are usually narrow with a duration of 60 ms.
B) Typical reverse atrial flutter. (Dog, English Setter, male, 8 years. Lead II - speed 50 mm/s - calibration 10 mm / 1 mV).
B) Typical reverse atrial flutter with an atrioventricular conduction ratio of 2:1. Note the morphology of F waves that have a positive polarity and rounded appearance in lead II. There are segments of the isoelectric line between two atrial deflections (arrows).
C) Atypical atrial flutter (right septal atrial flutter). (Dog, Bernese Mountain, male, 9 years. Lead II - speed 50 mm/s - calibration 10 mm/1 mV). Atypical atrial flutter with an atrioventricular conduction ratio of 1:1. Note the morphology of the F waves located in the ST segment of the previous QRS complex (arrow) that have a positive polarity and rounded appearance in lead II.

Chapter 8. Supraventricular tachycardias

> **BOX 8.11.**
> ### TYPICAL ATRIAL FLUTTER IN THE DOG
>
> **HEART RATE:** dependent on atrioventricular conduction ratio.
> **R-R INTERVAL:** irregular or rarely regular.
> **P WAVE:** absent; presence of F waves with a sawtooth pattern in the inferior leads; absence of isoelectric line between the atrial waves in all leads and rate faster than 300 bpm.
> **ATRIOVENTRICULAR CONDUCTION:** present with ratios from 1:1 to 6:1, more frequently with an even numerator, particularly 2:1.
> **FQ INTERVAL:** variable and difficult to measure.
> **QRS COMPLEX:** narrow (≤70 ms), unless concomitant functional or anatomical disorders of intraventricular conduction.
> **VENTRICULO-ATRIAL CONDUCTION:** absent.
> **BLOCKED BEATS:** present.
> **INITIATION AND TERMINATION MODALITY:** sudden.

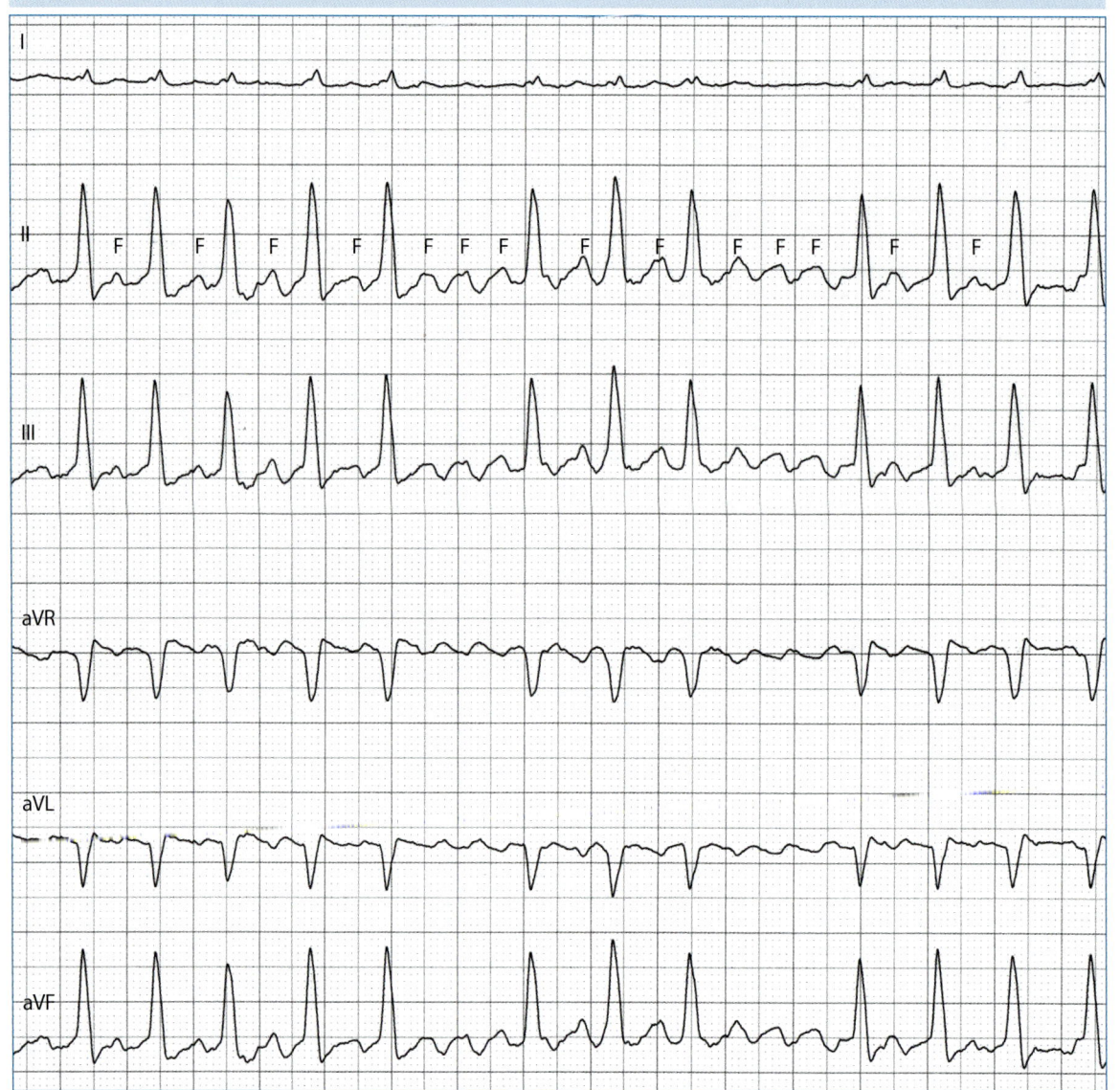

Dog, Boxer, male, 12 years.
Six limb leads (I, II, III, aVR, aVL, aVF) - speed 50 mm/s - calibration 10 mm/1 mV.

Notes: typical atrial flutter, ventricular rate of 240 bpm. F waves with a sawtooth appearance in the inferior leads; absent isoelectric line between atrial depolarizations in all leads; narrow QRS complexes (60 ms); atrioventricular conduction ratio from 1:1 to 6:1, in a progressive and regressive fashion.

Macro-reentrant atrial tachycardia (atrial flutter) | 171

> **BOX 8.12.**
> **REVERSE TYPICAL ATRIAL FLUTTER IN THE DOG**
>
> **HEART RATE:** dependent on atrioventricular conduction ratio.
> **R-R INTERVAL:** irregular or rarely regular.
> **P WAVE:** absent; presence of F waves with positive polarity in the inferior leads; segments of isoelectric line between the atrial waves and rate above 300 bpm.
> **ATRIOVENTRICULAR CONDUCTION:** present from 1:1 to 6:1, with greater ratios with even numerator more frequent, particularly the 2:1 ratio.
> **FQ INTERVAL:** variable and difficult to measure.
> **QRS COMPLEX:** narrow (≤70 ms), unless concomitant functional or anatomical disorders of intraventricular conduction.
> **VENTRICULO-ATRIAL CONDUCTION:** absent.
> **BLOCKED BEATS:** present.
> **INITIATION AND TERMINATION MODALITY:** sudden.

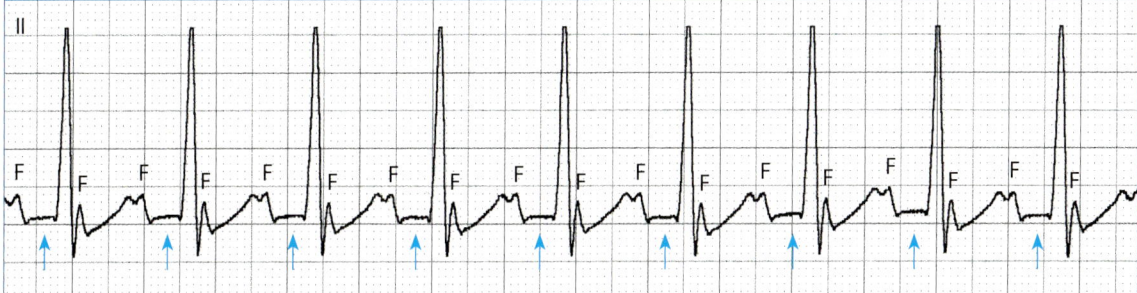

Dog, English Setter, Male, 8 years.
Lead II -speed 50 mm/s - calibration 10 mm/1 mV.

Notes: reverse typical atrial flutter, with a ventricular rate of 180 bpm. Note the presence of F waves with positive polarity in the inferior leads, the presence of an isoelectric line between the atrial waves (arrows); narrow QRS complexes (45 ms) and a fixed atrioventricular conduction ratio of 2:1.

The regularity of the atrial cycle length is explained by the fixed position and length of the reentrant circuit.

Although it has been suggested that it is the atrial activation preceding the last fully visible F wave in front of the QRS complex that is conducted to the ventricles, practically it is not possible to determine with certainty the beginning of the atrial cycle, and therefore it is not possible to identify the atrioventricular conduction interval (F-Q interval). The ventricular response rate depends on the atrial rate, and the refractory period and conduction times within the atrioventricular node. The F waves are conducted to the ventricles with various atrioventricular conduction ratios from 2:1 to 6:1. Atrial impulses blocked in the atrioventricular node can impact the conduction velocity of subsequent atrial impulses to the ventricles (*concealed conduction*) (see p. 16). The ventricular rate during atrial flutter can be regular or irregular, depending on the atrioventricular conduction ratio. A common atrial to ventricular conduction ratio during atrial flutter is 2:1 (Box 8.12); a less common ratio is 1:1. In the former case, every other atrial depolarization is conducted to the ventricles; in the latter case all atrial impulses are conducted through the atrioventricular node to the ventricles. The occurrence of atrial flutter with 1:1 atrioventricular conduction may result from: a low atrial rate, high sympathetic tone, a short refractory period of the atrioventricular node or the presence of an accessory pathway. Conduction ratios with an even numerator (2:1, 4:1, 6:1) are more common than those with an odd numerator (3:1, 5:1). During atrial flutter, changes in conduction ratios can occur: they are called *progressive conduction block* if the change is from a low to a high conduction relationship, and *regressive block* if the change is from a high to a low conduction ratio (Box 8.11).

The QRS complex has normal morphology and duration (≤70 ms in dogs) unless there is a pre-existing bundle branch block, tachycardia rate-dependent aberrant conduction or ventricular pre-excitation.

Intermittent or sustained intra-ventricular aberrancy is favored by a 1:1 conduction ratio with a fast atrial rate or by the presence of sequences of long and short R-R intervals (Ashman's phenomenon), for example when the atrioventricular conduction changes from 4:1 to 2:1.

Atypical or non-cavotricuspid isthmus-dependent atrial flutter

The term atypical atrial flutter is used to describe non-cavotricuspid isthmus-dependent macro-reentrant atrial tachycardias. The area of slow conduction is located in a different region of the atrium. Depending on the location of this isthmus two atypical atrial flutters have so far been described in dogs:

- right septal atrial flutter, and
- right atrial free wall flutter without prior atriotomy (non-scar-related atrial flutter).

The right posterior free wall and the middle portion of the inter-atrial septum are important arrhythmogenic substrates due to the presence of the *crista terminalis*, a line of transverse conduction block, and the bilaminate muscular structure of the inter-atrial septum which induces longitudinal and transverse conduction delays. Right septal atrial flutter is commonly observed in the Bernese Mountain dog in the absence of structural heart disease, while right atrial free wall flutter is found in large breed dogs with myocardial disease. Although right atrial free wall flutters frequently form around an atriotomy scar in people, this is not the case in dogs.

The electrocardiographic characteristics of *atypical atrial flutters* (Fig. 8.15C, Box 8.13) include regular and identical flutter waves (F waves) with an atrial rate that ranges around 280 bpm in dogs. The F waves are positive in the inferior leads (II, III, and aVF) and usually found in the previous ST segment.

F-F intervals are regular and the isoelectric line is visible between consecutive F waves due to the presence of electrically silent areas within the anatomical circuit.

The atrioventricular conduction ratio varies from 1:1 to 2:1, although progressive and regressive ratios of atrioventricular conduction can be detected rarely.

The QRS complex has normal morphology and duration (≤70 ms in dogs) unless there is a pre-existing bundle branch block, tachycardia rate-dependent aberrant conduction or ventricular pre-excitation.

Other types of atrial flutter

Other types of atrial flutter have been described. Controversy exists regarding the classifications of rhythms of atrial flutter that do not fit into the anatomically defined cavotricuspid isthmus-dependent or independent atrial flutters. The instability of these types of atrial flutter have made it difficult to study the anatomy and mechanism of the reentrant pathway. These rhythms may in fact be due to electrophysiologic effects without structural pathology. Often characterized by a very rapid atrial rate of greater than 450 bpm it can transition between atrial fibrillation, atrial flutter or sinus rhythm. The underlying mechanism is considered a functional reentry in a rhythm previously described by Wells as a *type II atrial flutter*; this type of atrial flutter usually occurs in the presence of high vagal tone. Moreover, the flutter can vacillate with atrial fibrillation.

The electrocardiographic features of functional (without anatomic pathology) flutter include: F waves with variable morphology, but usually positive in the inferior leads (II, III and aVF) with no isoelectric line between consecutive F waves; a very rapid atrial rate (greater than 450 bpm); variable F-F intervals. The arrhythmia is unstable and rapidly returns to atrial fibrillation, type I atrial flutter or sinus rhythm (Fig. 8.16).

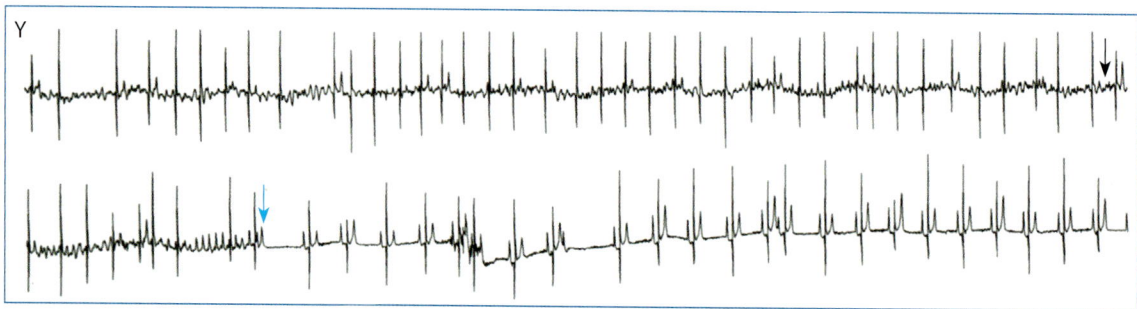

Figure 8.16. Type II Wells atrial flutter. (Dog, mongrel, female, 10 years - Holter lead Y - speed 7.5 mm/s - calibration 2 mm/1 mV). During the first part of the tracing the dominant rhythm is a paroxysmal atrial fibrillation that suddenly organizes into a type II atrial flutter (black arrow). Note the presence of rapid atrial depolarizations (482 bpm) with variable morphology, sudden onset and termination (blue arrow), followed by spontaneous cardioversion into sinus rhythm.

Macro-reentrant atrial tachycardia (atrial flutter)

BOX 8.13.
ATYPICAL ATRIAL FLUTTER IN THE DOG

HEART RATE: dependent on atrioventricular conduction ratio.
R-R INTERVAL: irregular or rarely regular.
P WAVE: absent; presence of F waves with positive polarity in the inferior leads, areas of isoelectric line between the atrial waves and rate usually around 280 bpm.
ATRIOVENTRICULAR CONDUCTION: present from 1:1 to 6:1, with greater conduction ratios with even numerator more frequent, particularly the 2:1 ratio.

FQ INTERVAL: variable and difficult to measure.
QRS COMPLEX: narrow (≤ 70 ms), unless concomitant functional or anatomical disorders of intraventricular conduction.
VENTRICULO-ATRIAL CONDUCTION: absent.
BLOCKED BEATS: present.
INITIATION AND TERMINATION MODALITY: sudden.

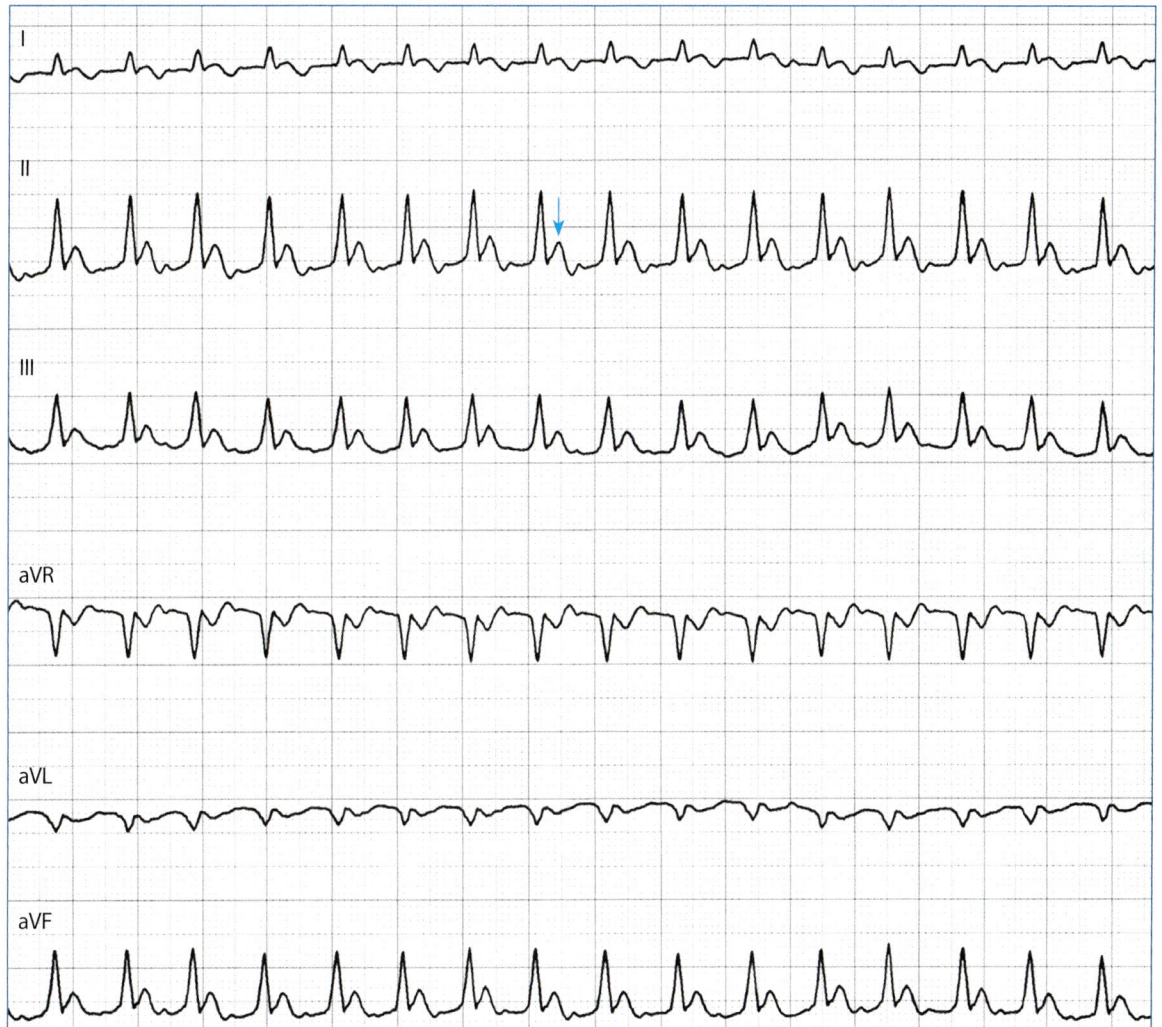

Dog, Bernese Mountain, male, 7 years.
Six limb leads (I, II, III, aVR, aVL, aVF) - speed 50 mm/s - calibration 10 mm/1 mV.

Notes: atypical atrial flutter, with a ventricular rate of 280 bpm. Note the presence of F waves in the ST segment of preceding QRS complexes (arrow) with positive polarity in the inferior leads; the presence of an isoelectric line between atrial waves; narrow QRS complexes (50 ms) and a fixed atrioventricular conduction ratio of 1:1. The presence of a positive atrial depolarisation wave in the preceding ST segment with a rate around 280 bpm and 1.1 atrioventricular conduction enables the differentiation between typical and atypical atrial flutters.

Atrial fibrillation

Atrial fibrillation is characterized by extremely rapid and uncoordinated atrial activity with loss of atrial contraction.

Atrial fibrillation can be classified according to its duration as:
- paroxysmal, when self-limiting,
- persistent, when it is not self-limiting but it can be terminated via electrical or pharmacological cardioversión, and
- permanent, when it persists long-term in animals who are not candidates for electrical cardioversion, or if cardioversion was performed but failed to terminate the arrhythmia.

The electrophysiological mechanisms proposed to explain the induction and maintenance of atrial fibrillation include rapidly discharging ectopic foci and reentry. The reentrant circuits can be single or multiple. When ectopic foci are involved they are frequently located in the myocardial sleeve that extends in the walls of the pulmonary veins. Triggered activity is the most common mechanism responsible for these ectopies, which can not only initiate but also perpetuate atrial fibrillation. Factors that promote reentry include a dispersion of refractoriness, short atrial refractory period, fibrosis and atrial enlargement. A short refractory period allows smaller circuits to remain stable in the long-term, fibrosis can serve as their anchoring points, and a large atrial surface can support a higher number of reentry waves. At least in people, it is believed that the natural history of atrial fibrillation is a progression from paroxysmal to persistent and then to permanent atrial fibrillation due to the anatomical and electrical remodeling of the atrial myocardium that result from the arrhythmia itself. In dogs, paroxysmal atrial fibrillation has been reported secondary to excessive vagal stimulation, for example secondary to the administration of opioids for sedation (Fig. 8.17). Indeed, vagal stimulation causes a reduction in the duration of the action potential of cardiac myocytes which is heterogeneously distributed throughout the atria and, therefore, creates an environment favorable to reentrant arrhythmias.

Atrial fibrillation is more common in medium-sized and large breed dogs, likely because a large atrial surface is necessary for the perpetuation of the arrhythmia. Atrial fibrillation is also commonly associated with heart diseases that cause atrial dilatation, such as chronic valvular disease, dilated cardiomyopathy, myocarditis, patent ductus arteriosus, ventricular septal defects, mitral and tricuspid dysplasia and end-stage aortic and pulmonic stenosis. In giant breeds (Great Dane, Saint Bernard, Newfoundland, Dogue de Bordeaux, Irish Wolfhound), a form of atrial fibrillation called *lone atrial fibrillation* (or primary atrial fibrillation) occurs without obvious structural cardiac disease. It is likely triggered by focal atrial tachycardia arising within the tributary veins of the atria, and anatomical or functional atrial flutter. Although rare in cats, atrial fibrillation can occur in the presence of marked atrial dilatation secondary to cardiomyopathies (hypertrophic, restrictive or dilated).

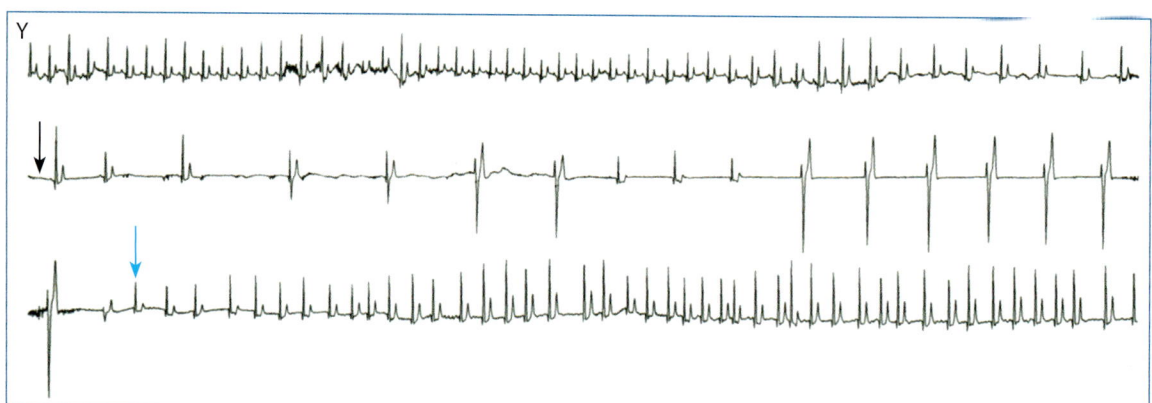

Figure 8.17. Vagal atrial fibrillation. (Dog, Boxer, male, 9 years - Holter lead Y- speed 7.5 mm/s - calibration 2 mm/mV. The first part of the tracing reveals a sinus rhythm with an average ventricular rate of 153 bpm, followed by a progressive sinus bradycardia, then a sinus arrest lasting 16 s (black arrow) and an escape ventricular rhythm (average ventricular rate of 55 bpm). After the period of sinus arrest there is paroxysmal atrial fibrillation with an average ventricular heart rate of 166 bpm occurs (blue arrow).

The electrocardiographic characteristics of atrial fibrillation include a narrow QRS complex tachycardia (≤70 ms in dogs and ≤40 ms in cats) unless aberrant conduction or a preexisting anatomical intraventricular conduction block is present. During atrial fibrillation, the R-R intervals are always irregular, P waves are absent and replaced by fibrillation waves (f waves). The number of f waves that can travel through the atrioventricular node and activate the ventricles defines the *ventricular response rate*. The ventricular response is determined by the influence of the autonomic nervous system on the conduction properties of the atrioventricular node. The ventricular response rate is lower in dogs with lone atrial fibrillation, and usually rapid in the presence of advanced structural cardiac disease and heart failure. The average ventricular response typically varies between 130 and 260 bpm in dogs and 200 and 280 bpm in cats (Boxes 8.14 and 8.15).

The f waves reflect the chaotic and continuously variable atrial activation. These f waves have variable morphology and voltage, a rate of 400 to 600 bpm and are continuous, which eliminates the isoelectric line between them. The f waves are usually visualized better in leads II and V_1. The finding of f waves with a large amplitude suggests atrial enlargement or a recent onset arrhythmia. It is important to note that the f waves are not always visible on the surface electrocardiogram, because of their small amplitude or the impact of the filters selected during the recording to remove high frequency, small amplitude signals secondary to skeletal muscle noise. For this reason, the diagnosis of atrial fibrillation is not usually based on the presence of f waves, but rather an irregular ventricular rhythm and absent P waves.

The presence of irregular R-R intervals is the key criterion used to diagnose atrial fibrillation. The irregular ventricular response rate is due to the variability of the number of impulses that can cross the atrioventricular node because of the refractory period of the junctional region and the intensity of the atrial impulses. The atrioventricular node has the property of *decremental conduction*, which causes the electrical impulses to progressively lose their ability to excite contiguous tissue as they propagate deeper in the node. As a result, the less intense atrial impulses, although they reach the atrioventricular node in an excitable state, dissipate inside the atrioventricular node (*concealed conduction*) and cause a prolongation of the refractory period of the node. This prolongation of the refractory period delays or blocks the next fibrillation wave. Due to the effects of decremental and concealed conduction in the atrioventricular node, atrial fibrillation is characterized by irregular R-R intervals (Fig. 8.18).

Atrial fibrillation only has regular R-R intervals if it is associated with third-degree atrioventricular block (Box 8.16). In this case the ventricular rhythm is an escape rhythm with a rate and a morphology of the QRS complexes that depends on the origin of the escape rhythm (junctional or ventricular).

During atrial fibrillation the QRS complexes appear normal in duration (<70 ms in dogs and <40 ms in cats), unless they are slightly prolonged by the presence of left ventricular enlargement or significantly prolonged by anatomical or functional intraventricular conduction delays.

Very commonly during atrial fibrillation the QRS complex amplitude varies slightly. This could be attributed to Brody's effect, which states that QRS complex amplitude is influenced by variations in intracardiac blood volume and the associated positional changes of the heart within the chest (Box 8.14).

Whenever one or more QRS complexes display a different morphology and a significantly increased duration (greater than 70 ms in dogs and greater than 40 ms in cats) during atrial fibrillation, three possibilities should be considered:
- aberrant intraventricular conduction of supraventricular impulses,
- ventricular ectopic beats, and
- ventricular pre-excitation.

During atrial fibrillation it is common to see intraventricular conduction aberrancy, which is tachycardia-dependent (or phase 3) aberrancy (see p. 286). This is explained by the different refractory periods of the left and right bundle branches. Under normal conditions, the right bundle branch has a longer refractory period than the left; in the presence of heart disease, the opposite is usually the case. The likelihood of aberrant intraventricular conduction is directly proportional to the difference in refractory period between the two branches.

Chapter 8. Supraventricular tachycardias

BOX 8.14.
ATRIAL FIBRILLATION IN THE DOG

HEART RATE: 130-260 bpm according to ventricular response.
R-R INTERVAL: irregular.
P WAVE: absent; presence of f waves of variable morphology and amplitude and rate from 400 to 600 bpm with the absence of an isoelectric line between them.
ATRIOVENTRICULAR CONDUCTION: present with variable conduction.
fQ INTERVAL: not evaluable.

QRS COMPLEX: narrow (≤70 ms), unless concomitant functional or anatomical disorders of intraventricular conduction.
VENTRICULO-ATRIAL CONDUCTION: absent.
BLOCKED BEATS: present; concealed conduction in the atrioventricular node.
INITIATION AND TERMINATION MODALITY: sudden in paroxysmal forms otherwise incessant behavior.

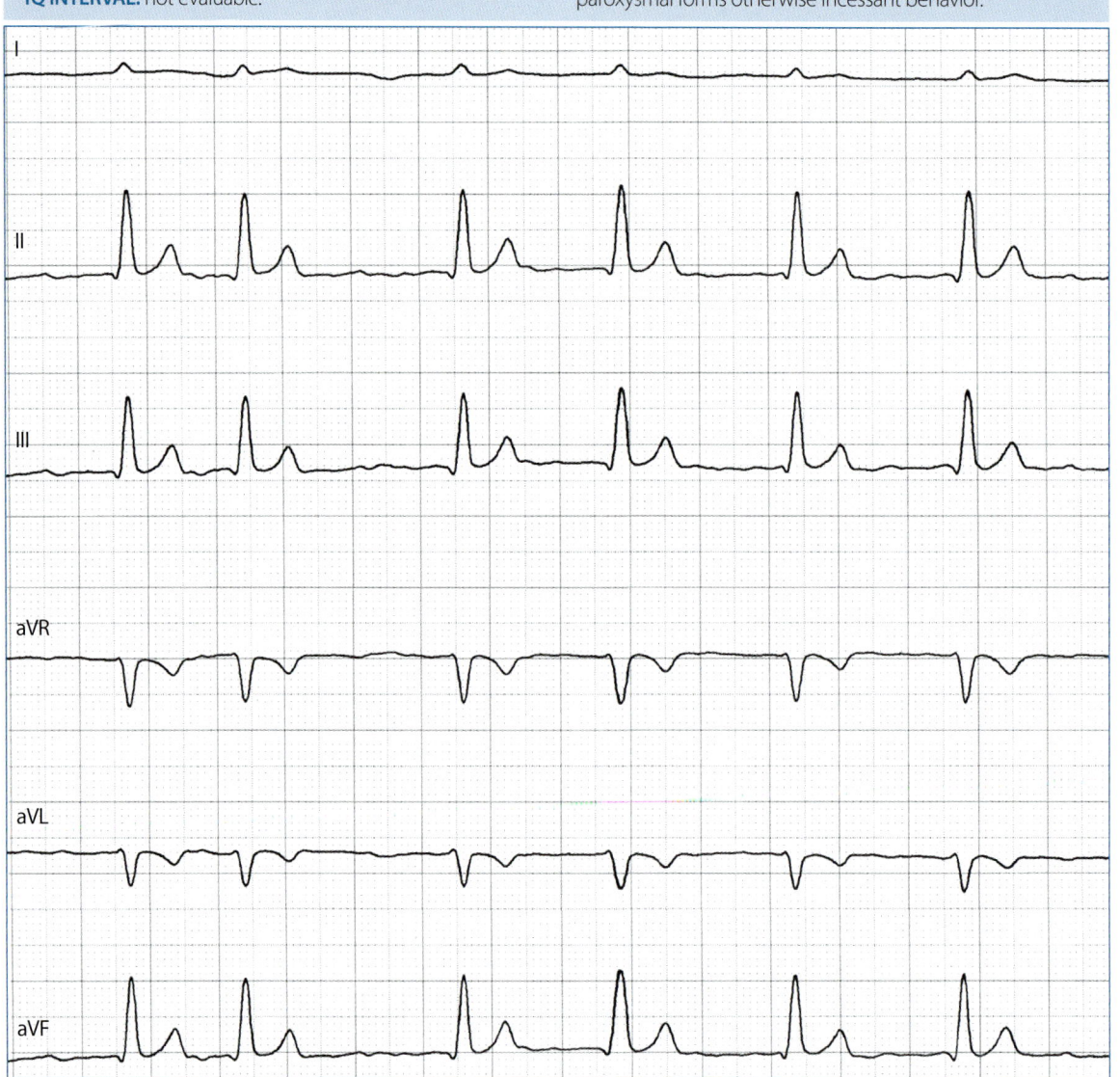

Dog, Bull Mastiff, male, 5 years.
Lead II - speed 50 mm/s - calibration 10 mm/1 mV.

Note: atrial fibrillation with ventricular rate of 180 bpm. f waves are present with variable amplitude and morphology; no isoelectric line can be detected between consecutive f waves; QRS complexes of normal duration (60 ms), but with the characteristic slurring on the descending limb of the R wave typical of intraventricular conduction delay secondary to structural cardiac diseases. The R-R intervals are irregular.

Atrial fibrillation

BOX 8.15.
ATRIAL FIBRILLATION IN THE CAT.

HEART RATE: 200-280 bpm according to ventricular response.
R-R INTERVAL: irregular.
P WAVE: absent; presence of f waves of variable morphology and amplitude and rate from 400 to 600 bpm with the absence of an isoelectric line between them.
ATRIOVENTRICULAR CONDUCTION: present, with variable conduction.
fQ INTERVAL: not evaluable.

QRS COMPLEX: narrow (<40 ms), unless concomitant functional or anatomical disorders of intraventricular conduction.
VENTRICULO-ATRIAL CONDUCTION: absent.
BLOCKED BEATS: present.
INITIATION AND TERMINATION MODALITY: sudden if paroxysmal (likely the most common form of atrial fibrillation in cats).

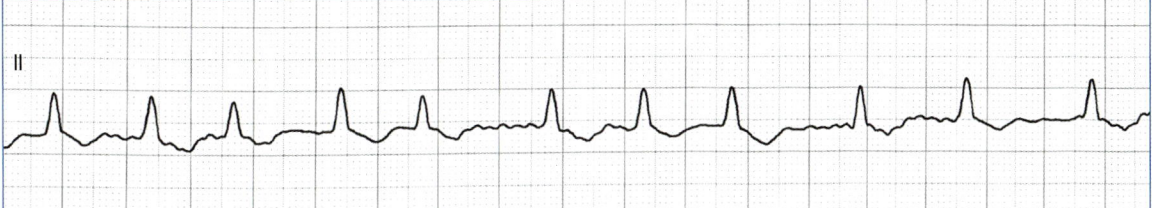

Cat, Domestic Short Hair, male, 5 years.
Lead II - speed 50 mm/s - calibration 10 mm/1 mV.

Notes: atrial fibrillation with a ventricular rate of 200 bpm. f waves are present with variable amplitude and morphology and without an isoelectric line between consecutive f waves, QRS complexes of normal duration (40 ms) and irregular R-R intervals.

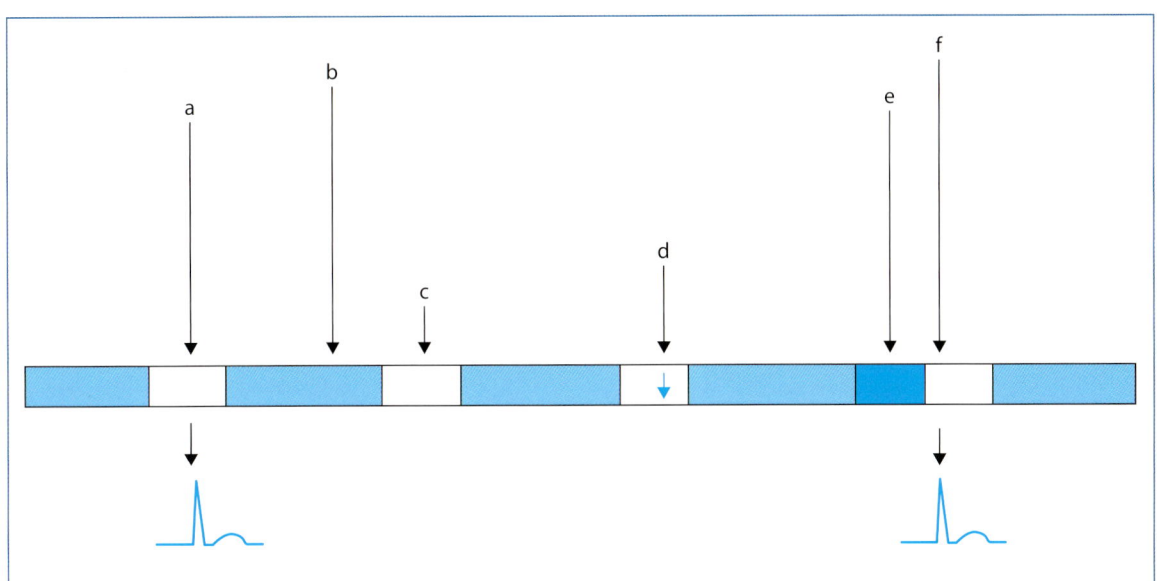

Figure 8.18. Mechanism of the variable ventricular response rate during atrial fibrillation. Impulse *a* falls in the excitable period of atrioventricular nodal tissue and has sufficient intensity to travel through the structure completely (first QRS complex). Conversely, impulse *b* meets the atrioventricular nodal tissues in a refractory state and, therefore, fails to generate ventricular depolarization. Impulse *c*, despite falling in the excitable period, does not have sufficient intensity to penetrate the atrioventricular node. Impulse *d*, however, has sufficient intensity and penetrates the atrioventricular node, but fails to emerge in the atrioventricular distal bundle (concealed conduction). The concealed conduction along the nodal structure of impulse *d* prolongs the refractory period so that the next impulse *e*, although of sufficient intensity, is blocked. Impulse *f*, falling at the end of the refractory period induced by concealed conduction of impulse *d*, is normally conducted and initiates ventricular depolarization (second QRS complex). *White bar*: period of excitability; *Blue bar*: refractory period.

Chapter 8. Supraventricular tachycardias

BOX 8.16.
ATRIAL FIBRILLATION WITH THIRD-DEGREE ATRIOVENTRICULAR BLOCK IN THE DOG

HEART RATE: variable and dependent on the firing rate of the subsidiary pacemaker.
R-R INTERVAL: regular.
P WAVE: absent; presence of f waves of variable morphology and amplitude and a rate from 400 to 600 bpm with absence of an isoelectric line between them.

ATRIOVENTRICULAR CONDUCTION: absent.
fQ INTERVAL: not evaluable.
QRS COMPLEX: narrow (≤70 ms) or wide depending on the location of the subsidiary pacemaker.
VENTRICULO-ATRIAL CONDUCTION: not evaluable.
BLOCKED BEATS: present.

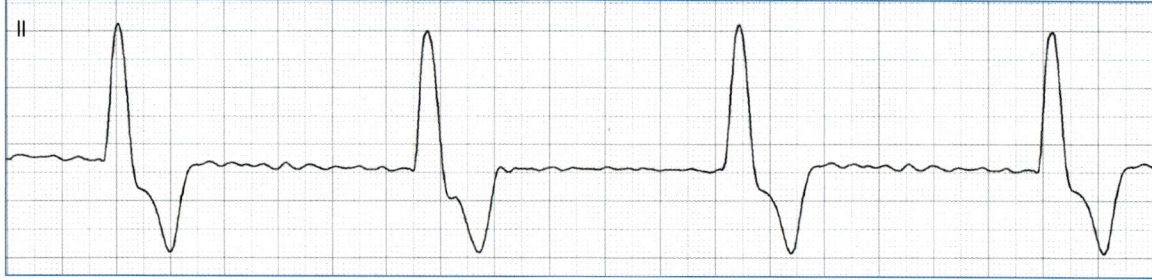

Dog, Labrador Retriever, male, 8 years.
Lead II - speed 50 mm/s - calibration 10 mm/1 mV.

Notes: atrial fibrillation with third-degree atrioventricular block and ventricular escape rhythm with a firing rate of 52 bpm. There are undulations of the isoelectric line compatible with f waves, wide QRS complexes (100 ms) and regular R-R intervals. Atrial potentials and atrial response to electrical stimuli are necessary to differentiate this rhythm from sinus standstill or atrial standstill.

During atrial fibrillation, the irregularity of the cycle length results in the alternation of long R-R and shorter R-R intervals. A relatively long R-R interval induces a prolongation of the refractory period of the conduction system. If a long R-R interval is followed by a short R-R interval, the resulting heartbeat may have an aberrant morphology, as the electrical impulse may be blocked along one bundle branch and only be conducted along the contralateral branch. QRS aberrancy caused by a long-short R-R interval sequence is called *Ashman's phenomenon* (Fig. 8.19). Aberrant intraventricular conduction can also persist over time (*linking phenomenon*) (see p. 288).

The differentiation between aberrant intraventricular conduction and ventricular ectopic beats is done by examining:
- the coupling interval of the wide QRS complex with the previous beat,
- the presence or absence of a pause after the wide QRS complex,
- the morphology of the wide QRS complex, and
- the tendency of the wide QRS complex beats to form groups.

Wide QRS complexes corresponding to ventricular ectopic beats typically have a fixed coupling interval, do not occur as a result of a long R-R/short R-R sequence (which is typical of Ashman's phenomenon), and are characterized by a post-extrasystolic pause caused by concealed retrograde conduction within the atrioventricular node. Moreover, the morphology of the wide beat on the 12-lead electrocardiogram is typical of ectopic ventricular beats, and they tend to cluster in couplets, triplets, or follow a bigeminal pattern (Fig. 8.20).

Wide QRS complexes resulting from aberrant intraventricular conduction have variable coupling intervals, occur during a characteristic long R-R/short R-R sequence and are not followed by a post-extrasystolic pause. Furthermore, their morphology on the 12-lead electrocardiogram has the characteristics of a bundle branch block and they do not organize in couplets, triplets or bigeminy.

Sequences of aberrant intraventricular conduction (linking) during atrial fibrillation can be differentiated from ventricular tachycardia using two basic criteria: the regularity of the R-R intervals and the presence of a pause after the last wide QRS complex. During

Atrial fibrillation

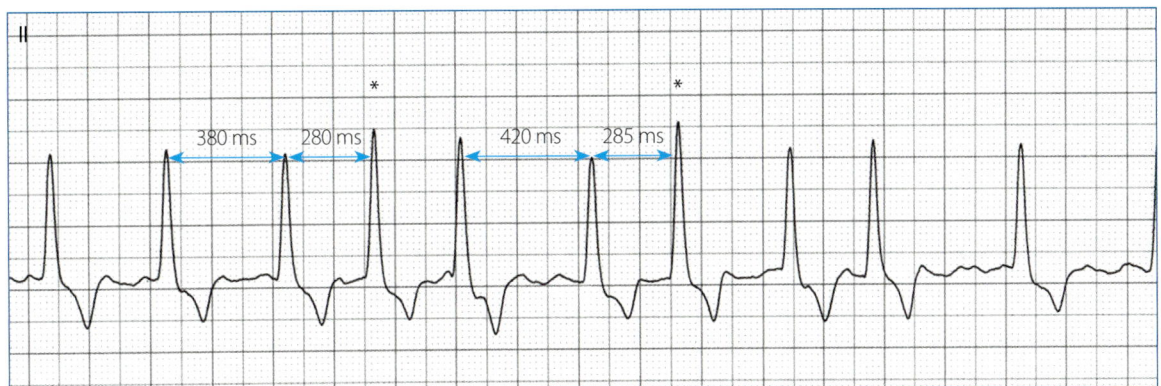

Figure 8.19. Atrial fibrillation with intraventricular aberrant conduction. This corresponds to tachycardia-dependent or phase 3 (Ashman's phenomenon) aberrancy (Dog, German Shepherd, female, 13 years. Lead II - speed 50 mm/s - calibration 10 mm/1 mV). The basic rhythm is an atrial fibrillation with a ventricular rate of 180 bpm. The third and sixth QRS complexes have increased amplitude and duration (80 ms) (*). Note the classical pattern of a long R-R interval followed by a short R-R interval preceding the aberrant beats.

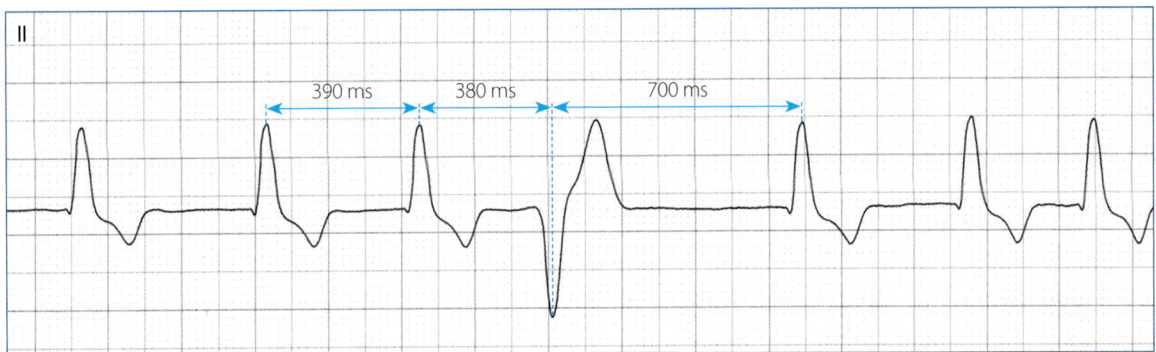

Figure 8.20. Atrial fibrillation with premature ventricular ectopic beat (Dog, mongrel, male, 11 years. Lead II - speed 50 mm/s - calibration 5 mm/1 mV). The basic rhythm is represented by an atrial fibrillation with a ventricular rate of 140 bpm. The fourth beat has an abnormal morphology with a right bundle branch block pattern. Note the absence of the typical sequence of a long R-R interval followed by a short R-R interval before the wide QRS complex. Also note the presence of a post-extrasystolic pause.

ventricular tachycardia, the R-R intervals are usually regular and the pause after the last wide QRS complex is typically long because of concealed retrograde conduction in the atrioventricular node (Fig. 8.21). Conversely, during atrial fibrillation with sustained aberrant intraventricular conduction, the R-R intervals are irregular and the pause after the last wide QRS complex is short (Fig. 8.22).

Fibrillatory conduction

Atrial fibrillatory conduction during irregular atrial tachycardias occurs when a portion of the atrial myocardium is unable to respond in a 1:1 fashion to rapid impulses originating from another part of the atrium. As a result, organized and chaotic electrical activity coexist in the atria. On the surface electrocardiogram, fibrillatory conduction is very difficult to differentiate from atrial fibrillation. Fibrillatory conduction is an unstable rhythm that usually follows periods of organized rhythm that suddenly returns to fibrillatory conduction (Fig. 8.23).

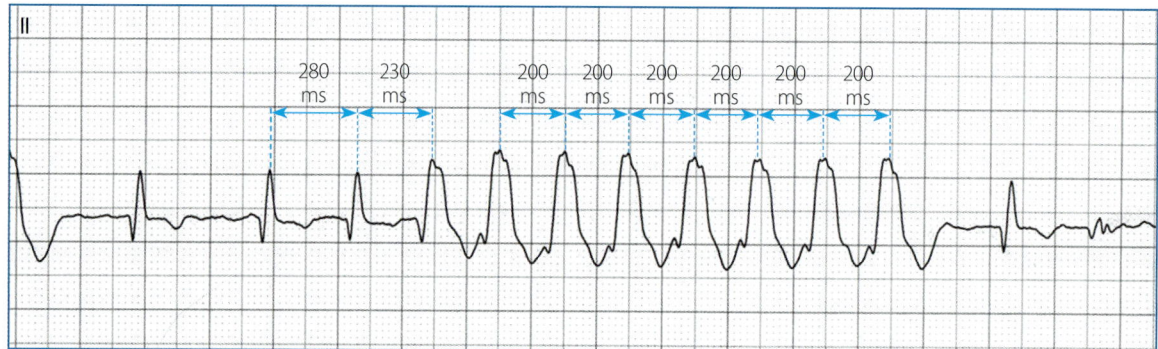

Figure 8.21. Atrial fibrillation with a run of non-sustained monomorphic ventricular tachycardia (Dog, Giant Schnauzer, male, 10 years. Lead II - speed 50 mm/s - calibration 5 mm/1 mV).
The first part of the tracing is represented by atrial fibrillation with a ventricular rate of 200 bpm. It is followed by a tachycardia with a left bundle branch block pattern and a rate of 310 bpm. The presence of a wide QRS tachycardia and regular R-R intervals and the absence of the long R-R/short R-R cycles before the onset of the tachycardia is suggestive of a non-sustained monomorphic ventricular tachycardia.

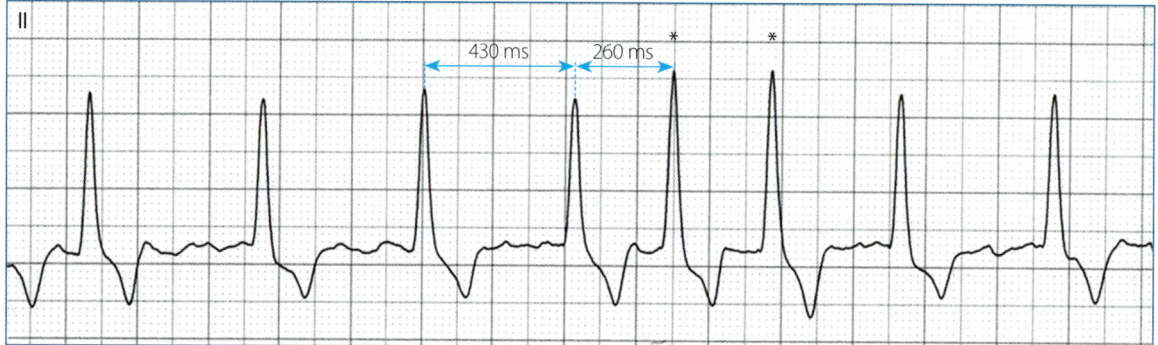

Figure 8.22. Atrial fibrillation with sustained intraventricular aberrancy or phase 3 *linking*. (Dog, German Shepherd, female, 13 years. Lead II - speed 50 mm/s - calibration 10 mm/mV).
The first part of the tracing is represented by atrial fibrillation with a ventricular rate of 135 bpm. Then two QRS complexes (*) with increased duration (80 ms) and amplitude are visible. The morphology of the QRS complexes and the presence of the classical long R-R/short R-R interval sequence is consistent with sustained intraventricular aberrancy (phase 3 *linking*).

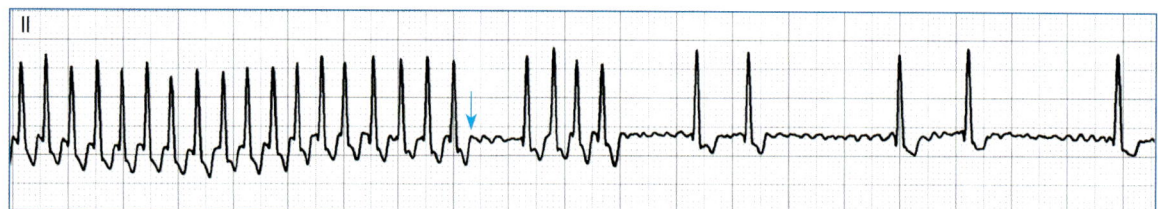

Figure 8.23. Fibrillatory conduction. (Dog, American Staffordshire, female, 10 years. Lead II - speed 25 mm/s - calibration 5 mm/mV). Note a narrow QRS complex tachycardia with regular R-R intervals and a rate of 330 bpm in the first part of the tracing. This tachycardia stops suddenly (arrow) and an irregular tachycardia begins with disorganized atrial activity characterized by the presence of f waves with variable morphology and amplitude and an average rate of 590 bpm compatible with fibrillatory conduction. After the pause, the tachycardia reorganizes for four beats and then degenerates again into fibrillatory conduction.

Differential diagnosis of narrow QRS complex tachycardias in the dog

Several electrocardiographic parameters can be used to differentiate the most common supraventricular tachycardias in dogs, including sinus tachycardia, atrial fibrillation, orthodromic atrioventricular reciprocating tachycardia, permanent junctional reciprocating tachycardia, focal junctional tachycardia, focal atrial tachycardia, and typical and atypical atrial flutter. They include:
- the atrial rate,
- the presence or absence of electrical alternans of the QRS complexes during tachycardia,
- the regularity or irregularity of the tachycardia cycle length,
- the presence or absence of P' waves during tachycardia,
- the relationship between P' waves and QRS complexes (RP'/P'R),
- the P' wave axis in the frontal plane,
- the atrioventricular conduction ratio,
- the ST segment and the T wave, and
- the presence or absence of ventricular pre-excitation.

Atrial rate

Sinus tachycardia has an atrial rate ranging from 180 to 280 bpm, focal atrial tachycardia from 210 to 330 bpm, typical atrial flutter from 350 to 450 bpm, atypical atrial flutter ranging from 280 to 350 bpm, atrial fibrillation from 400 to 600 bpm, orthodromic atrioventricular reciprocating tachycardia from 190 to 300 bpm, permanent junctional reciprocating tachycardia from 230 to 250 bpm and focal junctional tachycardia from 100 and 160 bpm.

QRS complex electric alternans

The presence of a beat-to-beat R wave amplitude variation greater than 0.1 mV in at least one lead during tachycardia supports the diagnosis of orthodromic atrioventricular reciprocating tachycardia or permanent junctional reciprocating tachycardia. Indeed, it occurs in two-thirds of cases of orthodromic atrioventricular reciprocating tachycardia. It is less common with focal atrial tachycardia (occurring in fewer than one-third of the cases). Alternans is more pronounced in leads II, III, aVF, V_3 and V_6 (Fig. 8.24).

Cycle length irregularity

A ≥20 ms variation of the length of the tachycardia cycle is characteristic of focal atrial tachycardia and atrial flutter. This electrocardiographic feature is caused by the irregularity of the discharge of the ectopic focus, by the presence of an atrioventricular block or by different atrioventricular conduction time related to impulse conduction through the fast or slow pathway (Fig. 8.25). During orthodromic reciprocating atrioventricular tachycardia, cycle length irregularity is less common and, if present, displays a pattern of beat-to-beat cycle length alternans, because of the presence of multiple accessory pathways or alternating conduction along the fast and slow atrioventricular nodal pathways.

Identification of the P' waves during tachycardia

In order to identify P' waves during tachycardia, it is helpful to compare the QRS-T complex morphology during sinus rhythm and during tachycardia in lead II. Depending on the type of tachycardia, P' waves can be present

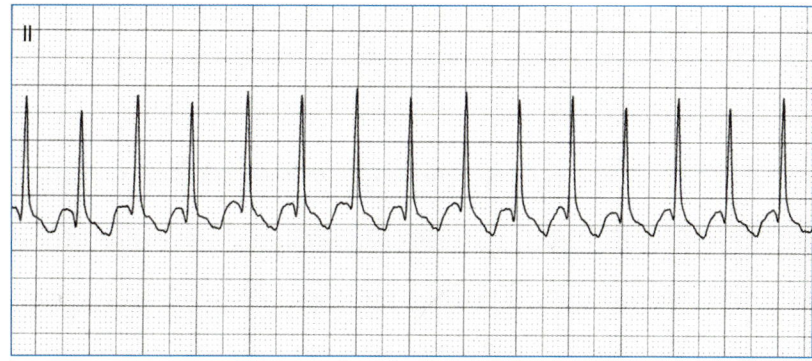

Figure 8.24. Electrical alternans during orthodromic atrioventricular reciprocating tachycardia. (Dog, Labrador Retriever, male, 2 years. Lead II - speed 50 mm/s - calibration 10 mm/1 mV).
The dominant rhythm is represented by an orthodromic atrioventricular reciprocating tachycardia with rate of 300 bpm. Note the electrical alternans characterized by a beat-to-beat variation of R wave amplitude greater than 0.1 mV (1 mm).

before or in the descending branch of the QRS complex, in the initial or final portion of the ST segment, in the ascending or descending branch of the T wave, or they might be found after the T wave (Fig. 8.26). Focal junctional tachycardia with 1:1 ventriculo-atrial conduction usually displays a negative P' wave in the initial portion of the previous ST segment forming a pseudo-S wave (Fig. 8.26A). During isorhythmic atrioventricular dissociation positive P waves can be found before or after the QRS complex (Fig. 8.26H). Orthodromic atrioventricular reciprocating tachycardia has visible P' waves, identifiable as a negative deflection in the initial part of the ST segment (Figs. 8.26B and 8.27A). Focal atrial tachycardia rarely displays a positive P' wave in the preceding ST

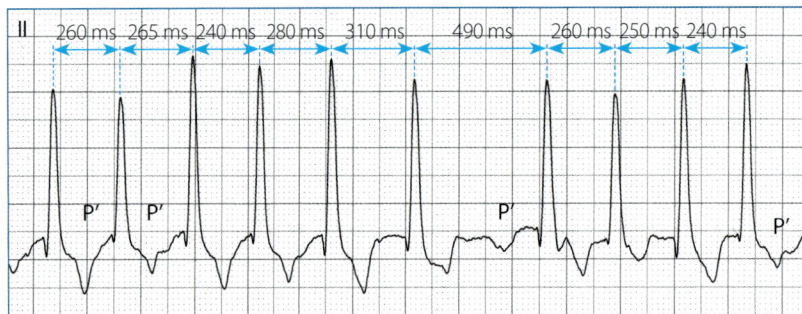

Figure 8.25. Cycle length irregularity during atrial tachycardia. (Dog, English Setter, male, 8 years. Lead II - speed 50 mm/s - calibration 10 mm/mV).

The dominant rhythm is an atrial tachycardia with a ventricular rate of 220 bpm. Note the variation of R-R interval durations, and P' waves that are occasionally visible.

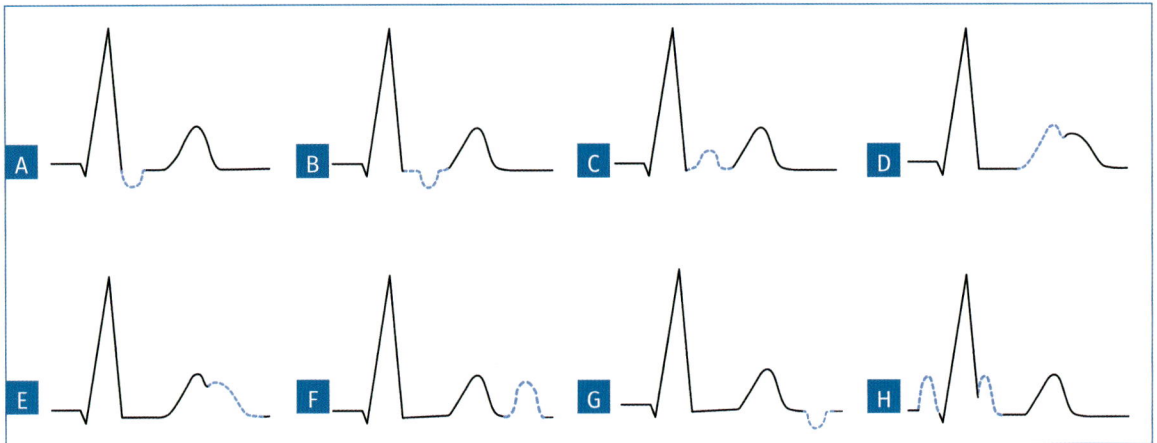

Figure 8.26. Electrocardiographic signs for identifying atrial depolarization (dashed blue line) during supraventricular tachycardia in lead II.
A) The atrial depolarization occurs at the onset of the ST segment, forming a pseudo S wave. It is a characteristic feature of focal junctional tachycardia with 1:1 ventriculo-atrial conduction.
B) The atrial depolarization occurs in the first portion of the ST segment. When the atrial depolarization is negative, orthodromic atrioventricular reciprocating tachycardia is the first differential diagnosis.
C) The atrial depolarization occurs in the first portion of the ST segment. When it is positive, either atrial flutter or atrial tachycardia should be considered.
D) The atrial depolarization is within the ascending branch of the T wave. This is a classical feature of focal atrial tachycardia.
E) The atrial depolarization is within the descending part of the T wave, giving a typical appearance of a bifid T wave (camel sign). This is a characteristic feature of focal atrial tachycardia.
F) The atrial depolarization falls after the T wave. If it is positive, sinus tachycardia is the first differential diagnosis.
G) The atrial depolarization falls after the T wave. If it is negative, permanent junctional reciprocating tachycardia should be considered.
H) The atrial depolarization falls just before or just after the QRS complex. The differential diagnoses include focal junctional tachycardia with isorhythmic atrioventricular dissociation and type I or II synchronization, or atrial flutter.

segment (Fig. 8.26C), which is more frequently found in the ascending or descending portion of the T wave, forming the so-called "camel sign" (Figs. 8.26D-E and 8.27B). Sinus tachycardia has positive P waves after the preceding T wave (Fig. 8.26F), while permanent junctional reciprocating tachycardia reveals negative P' waves following the preceding T wave (Fig. 8.26G).

During atrial flutter, P' waves are replaced by F waves, with or without interposition of the isoelectric line. The morphology of the F waves depends on the type of flutter and the direction of activation along the inter-atrial septum (see p. 169). F waves are usually visible either before or after the QRS complex depending on the atrioventricular conduction times and ratios (Fig. 8.26C-H).

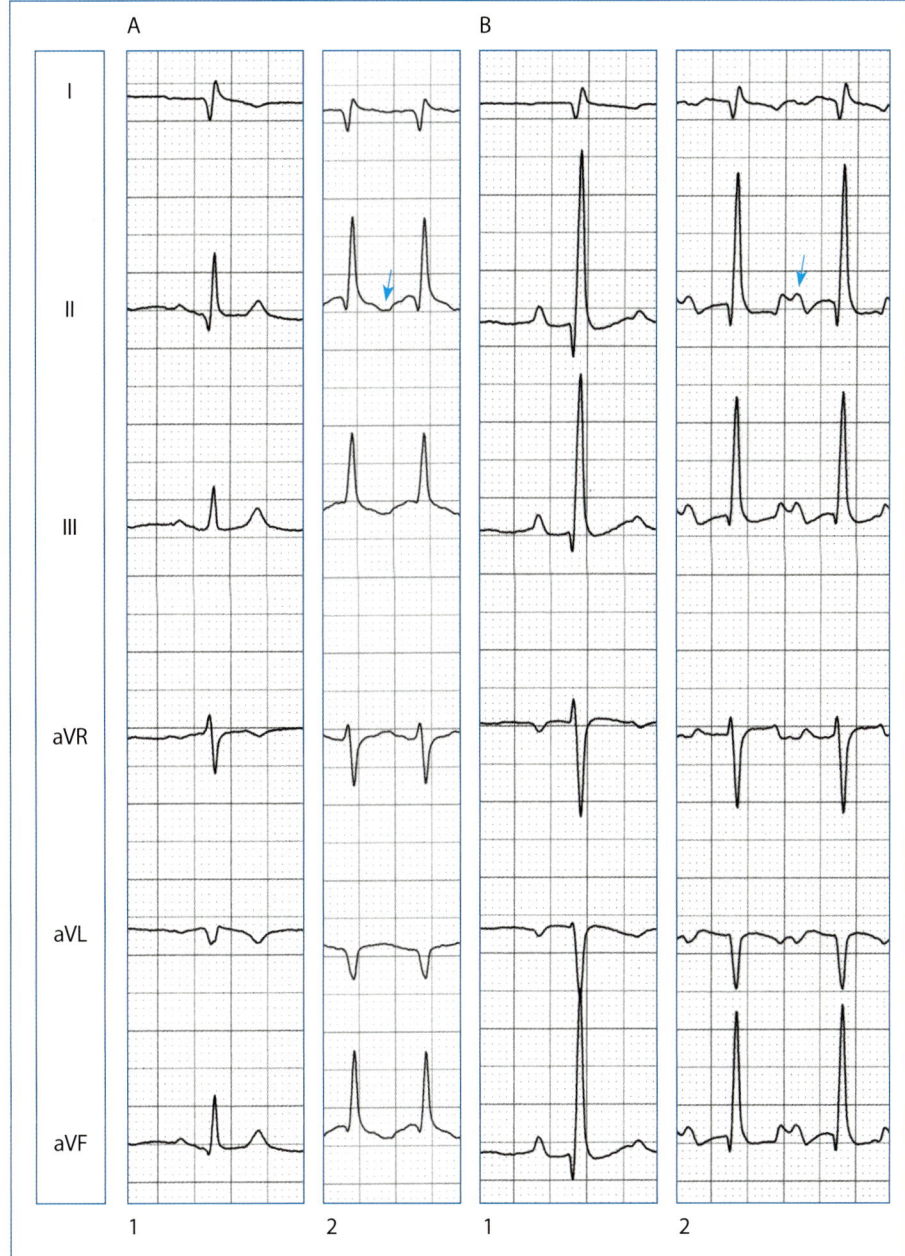

Figure 8.27. A) Identification of P' waves during orthodromic atrioventricular reciprocating tachycardia. (Dog, Labrador Retriever, male, 2 years. Six limb leads - speed 50 mm/s - calibration 5 mm/mV).
1. Sinus rhythm.
2. Orthodromic atrioventricular reciprocating tachycardia: note the presence of P' waves within the ST segment, altering its shape (arrow).

B) Identification of P' wave during focal atrial tachycardia. (Dog, Rottweiler, female, 9 months. Six limb leads - speed 50 mm/s - calibration 10 mm/mV).
1. Sinus rhythm.
2. Focal atrial tachycardia: note the presence of P' waves within the apex of the T wave (camel sign) (arrow).

The presence of an atrial depolarization, exactly equidistant between the preceding and subsequent QRS complexes, suggests that another atrial depolarization is hidden within the QRS complexes and is commonly found during atrial flutter with a 2:1 conduction ratio ("Bix rule") (Fig. 8.28).

During atrial fibrillation, there are no P waves, P' waves or F waves. The isoelectric line is replaced by f waves that represent the rapid and disorganized activation of portions of the atrial myocardium. f waves have variable morphology and voltage, are continuous and have a rate of 400 to 600 bpm.

Ratio of P waves to QRS complexes

The atrioventricular (P'R) and ventriculo-atrial (RP') conduction times and the RP'/P'R ratio are used to differentiate supraventricular tachycardias. For focal atrial tachycardias, although there is no retrograde conduction of the impulse from the ventricles to the atria, the length of the RP' interval and the ratio of the RP' interval to the P'R interval are used to differentiate them from other forms of supraventricular tachycardias. Tachycardias can be classified as short RP' or long RP' depending on the length of the segment. A short RP' segment corresponds to a ventriculo-atrial conduction time less than 50 % of the R-R interval that includes it. Otherwise it is classified as a long RP' tachycardia. Orthodromic atrioventricular reciprocating tachycardias, which usually have retrograde conduction through a fast accessory pathway, are characterized by a short RP' interval and a RP'/P'R ratio of less than 0.7. Focal atrial tachycardias and permanent junctional reciprocating tachycardia generally have a long RP' interval with a RP'/P'R ratio greater than 0.7 (Fig. 8.29).

P' wave axis in the frontal plane

Once the P' wave has been identified, its axis in the frontal plane during tachycardia needs to be evaluated. This measure is used to differentiate reciprocating tachycardias from focal atrial tachycardias and sinus tachycardia. In the case of reciprocating tachycardias, the axis is directed toward the upper right quadrant with ST elevation in aVR (in all cases) (Fig. 8.27A); in the case of focal atrial tachycardias, the axis is typically superior-inferior (two-thirds of the dogs) (Fig. 8.27B) while sinus tachycardia has an axis between –18 ° and +90 ° in the dog and between +0 ° and +90 ° in the cat. Focal junctional tachycardia displays sinus P waves during isorhythmic atrioventricular dissociation and negative P waves with a concentric inferior-to-superior axis (from –80 ° to –100 °) during 1:1 ventriculo-atrial conduction.

Atrioventricular conduction ratio

For diagnostic purposes, the presence of Wenckebach-type (Mobitz I) second-degree atrioventricular block is an important point to differentiate non-atrioventricular nodal-dependent tachycardia (sinus tachycardia, focal atrial tachycardia, and atrial flutter) from atrioventricular nodal-dependent tachycardia (orthodromic atrioventricular

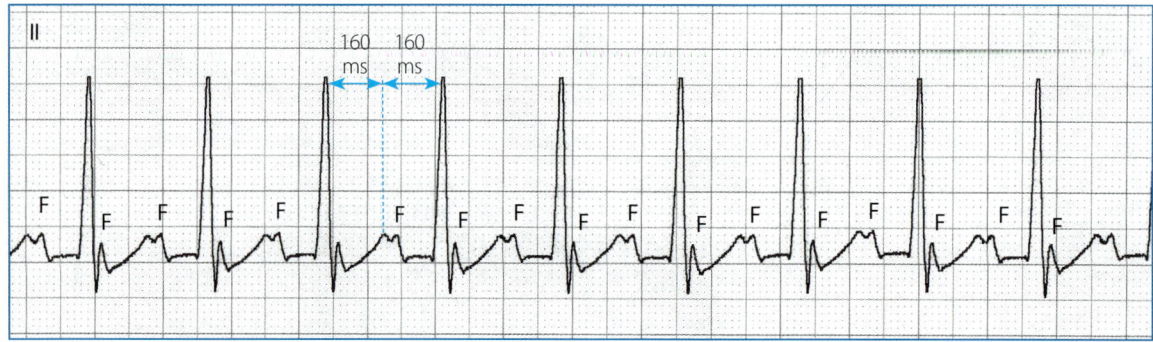

Figure 8.28. Typical reverse atrial flutter with a 2:1 atrioventricular conduction ratio. (Dog, English Setter, male, 10 years. Lead II - speed 50 mm/s - calibration 10 mm/1 mV).
The dominant rhythm is represented by a reverse typical atrial flutter with a 2:1 atrioventricular conduction ratio. Note that the F wave peak falls exactly at an equidistant point between the previous and the next R wave (Bix rule). This electrocardiographic finding is strongly suspicious of atrial flutter with an atrioventricular conduction ratio of 2:1.

reciprocating tachycardia and permanent junctional reciprocating tachycardia). Indeed, atrioventricular block can be present in the former group of arrhythmias, while it is never present during reciprocating tachycardias, because conduction through the atrioventricular node is required for the arrhythmia to persist over time. However, the presence of different atrioventricular conduction ratios is much more frequent during focal atrial tachycardia and atrial flutter, especially when the atrial rate is elevated.

The presence of atrioventricular conduction blocks is, therefore, diagnostic of focal atrial tachycardia (present in approximately 20 % to 25 % of cases) (Fig. 8.12) or atrial flutter (Boxes 8.11 and 8.12, Fig. 8.15A-B). The occurrence of atrioventricular block may be an isolated event, or may present with conduction ratios from 2:1 to a higher ratio, as often happens with atrial flutter. Focal junctional tachycardia is the only supraventricular tachycardia that can have atrioventricular dissociation with different degrees of synchronization (Fig. 8.2 B-C).

ST segment and the T wave

Approximately 60 % of cases of orthodromic atrioventricular reciprocating tachycardia display marked alterations of the ST segment and T wave, largely attributable to the presence of retro-conducted P' waves, and possibly to an electrical gradient persisting during the ST segment (mechanical systole) because of differences in action potential duration in various regions of the heart.

Ventricular pre-excitation

Ventricular pre-excitation, which confirms the presence of an accessory atrioventricular conduction pathway, is present in approximately 30 % of dogs with orthodromic atrioventricular reciprocating tachycardia. 70 % of dogs with orthodromic atrioventricular reciprocating tachycardia and all dogs with permanent junctional reciprocating tachycardia have accessory pathways with unidirectional retrograde conduction (concealed pathways) and therefore do not have ventricular pre-excitation during sinus rhythm. During focal junctional tachycardia with isorhythmic atrioventricular dissociation and type II synchronization (Fig. 8.2C) the short PQ interval can mimic ventricular pre-excitation. The variation of the PQ interval over time, the absence of a δ wave, the narrow QRS complexes, normal ST segment and T wave are used to rule out ventricular pre-excitation.

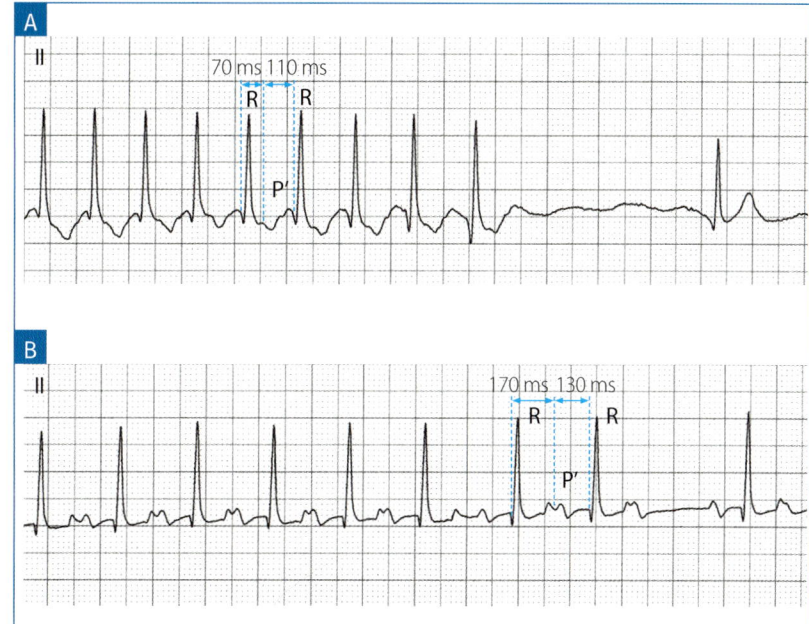

Figure 8.29. RP' interval and RP'/P'R ratio during orthodromic atrioventricular reciprocating tachycardia and focal atrial tachycardia.
A) (Dog, Labrador Retriever, male, 2 years. Lead II - speed 50 mm/s - calibration 10 mm/1 mV). Orthodromic atrioventricular reciprocating tachycardia characterized by a short RP' interval (less than half of the R-R interval duration) with a RP'/P'R ratio of 0.63 (RP' interval: 70 ms - P'R interval: 110 ms - R-R interval: 180 ms).
B) (Dog, Rottweiler, female, 8 months. Lead II - speed 50 mm/s - calibration 10 mm/1 mV). Focal atrial tachycardia characterized by a long RP' interval (more than half of the R-R interval length) with a RP'/P'R ratio of 1.3 (RP' interval: 170 ms - P'R interval: 130 ms - R-R interval: 300 ms).

Suggested readings

1. Allessie MA, Lammers WJEP, Bonke FIM, et al. Intra-atrial reentry as a mechanism for atrial flutter induced by acetylcholine and rapid pacing in the dog. *Circulation* 1984; 70:123-135.
2. Amoore JN. The Brody effect and change of volume of the heart. *J Electrocardiol* 1985; 18:71-75.
3. Atkins CE, Kanter R, Wright K, et al. Orthodromic reciprocating tachycardia and heart failure in a dog with a concealed posteroseptal accessory pathway. *J Vet Intern Med* 1995; 9:43-49.
4. De Bakker JMT, Ho SY, Hocini M. Basic and clinical electrophysiology of pulmonary veins ectopy. *Cardiovasc Res* 2002; 54;287-294.
5. Bun SS, Latcu DG, Marchlinski F, et al. Atrial flutter: more than just one of a kind. *Eur Heart J* 2015; 36:2356-2363.
6. Blomstrom-Lundqvist C, Scheinman MM, Aliot EM, et al. ACC/AHA/ESC Guidelines for the management of patients with supraventricular arrhythmias-executive summary. A report of the American College of Cardiology/American Heart Association Task Force on Practice Guidelines and the European Society of Cardiology Committee for Practice Guidelines (writing committee to develop guidelines for the management of patients with supraventricular arrhythmias) developed in collaboration with NASPE-Heart Rhythm Society. *J Am Coll Cardiol* 2003; 42:1493-1531.
7. Boineau JP, Schuessler RB, Mooney CR, et al. Natural and evoked atrial flutter due to circus movement in dogs. Role of abnormal atrial pathways, slow conduction, nonuniform refractory period distribution and premature beats. *Am J Cardiol* 1980; 45:1167-1181.
8. Boyden PA. Activation sequence during atrial flutter in dogs with surgically induced right atrial enlargement: I. Observations during sustained rhythms. *Circ Res* 1988; 62:596-608.
9. Cosío FG. Atrial flutter update. *Card Electrophysiol Rev* 2002; 6:356-364.
10. Côté E, Harpster NK, Laste NJ, et al. Atrial fibrillation in cats: 50 cases (1979-2002). *J Am Vet Med Assoc* 2004; 225:256-260.
11. Damato AN, Lau SH. His bundle rhythms. *Circulation* 1969; 40:527-534.
12. De Madron E, Kadish A, Spear JF, et al. Incessant atrial tachycardias in a dog with tricuspid dysplasia. Clinical management and electrophysiology. *J Vet Intern Med* 1987; 1:163-169.
13. Foster SF, Hunt GB, Thomas SP et al. Tachycardia-induced cardiomyopathy in a young Boxer dog with supraventricular tachycardia due to an accessory pathway. *Aust Vet J* 2006;84; 326-331.
14. Gandhi SK, Bromberg BI, Rodefeld MD, et al. Spontaneous atrial flutter in a chronic canine model of the modified Fontan operation. *J Am Coll Cardiol* 1997; 30:1095-1103.
15. Guglielmini C, Chetboul V, Pietra M, et al. Influence of left atrial enlargement and body weight on the development of atrial fibrillation: retrospective study on 205 dogs. *Vet J* 2000; 160:235-241.
16. Haissaguerre M, Jais P, Shah DC, et al. Spontaneous initiation of atrial fibrillation by ectopic beats originating in the pulmonary veins. *N Engl J Med* 1998; 339:659–666.
17. Hill BL, Tilley LP. Ventricular pre-excitation in seven dogs and nine cats. *J Am Vet Med Assoc* 1985; 187:1026-1031.
18. Khan R. Identifying and understanding the role of pulmonary vein activity in atrial fibrillation. *Cardiovasc Res* 2004; 64:387-394.
19. Kirchhof P, Benussi S, Kotecha D et al. 2016 ESC Guidelines for the management of atrial fibrillation developed in collaboration with EACTS. *Eur Heart J* 2016; 37: 2893-2962.
20. Kornreich BG, Moise NS. Right atrioventricular valve malformation in dogs and cats: an electrocardiographic survey with emphasis on splintered QRS complexes. *J Vet Intern Med* 1997; 11:226-230.
21. Iwasaki YK, Nishida K, Kato T, et al. Atrial fibrillation pathophysiology. Implications for management. *Circulation* 2011; 124:2264-2274.
22. Levy MN, Edflstein J. The mechanism of synchronization in isorhythmic AV dissociation: II. Clinical studies. *Circulation* 1970; 42:689-699.
23. Lin FY, Lo HM, Cheng JJ. Experimentally created atrioventricular node reentrant tachycardia in the dog: evidence of a brake system for nodal reeentry in the anterior inter-atrial septum. *J Am Coll Cardiol* 1993; 22:1541-1547.
24. Lo HM, Lin FY, Cheng JJ, et al. Anatomic substrate of the experimentally-created atrioventricular node re-entrant tachycardia in the dog. *Int J Cardiol* 1995; 51:273-282.
25. Meijler FL, Van der Tweel I. Comparative study of atrial fibrillation and AV conduction in mammals. *Heart Vessels Suppl* 1987; 2:24-31.
26. Moore EN. Observations on concealed conduction in atrial fibrillation. *Circ Res* 1967; 21:201-208.
27. Page RL, Joglar JA, Caldwell MA, et al. 2015 ACC/AHA/HRS guideline for the management of adult patients with supraventricular tachycardia: Executive summary: A Report of the American College of Cardiology/American Heart Association Task Force on Clinical Practice Guidelines and the Heart Rhythm Society. *Heart Rhythm* 2016; 13:92-135.
28. Pariaut R, Moïse NS, Koetje BD, et al. Evaluation of atrial fibrillation induced during anesthesia with fentanyl and pentobarbital in German Shepherd Dogs with inherited arrhythmias. *Am J Vet Res* 2008; 69:1434-1445.

29. Perego M, Ramera L, Santilli RA. Isorhythmic atrioventricular dissociation in Labrador Retrievers. *J Vet Intern Med* 2012; 26:320-325.
30. Perry JC. Junctional ectopic tachycardia: epidemiology, pathophysiology, primary prevention, immediate evaluation and management, long- term management and experimental and theoretical developments. *Cardiac Electrophysiol Rev* 1997; 1/2:76-78.
31. Porteiro Vazquez DM, Perego M, Santos Luis, et al. Paroxysmal atrial fibrillation in seven dogs with presumed neurally-mediated syncope. *J Vet Cardiol* 2016,18:1-9.
32. Santilli RA, Bussadori C. Orthodromic incessant atrioventricular reciprocating tachycardia in a dog. *J Vet Cardiol* 2000; 2:23-27.
33. Santilli RA, Spadacini G, Moretti P, et al. Radiofrequency catheter ablation of concealed accessory pathways in two dogs with symptomatic atrioventricular reciprocating tachycardia. *J Vet Cardiol* 2006; 8:157-165.
34. Santilli RA, Spadacini G, Moretti P, et al. Anatomic distribution and electrophysiologic properties of accessory atrioventricular pathways in dogs. *J Am Vet Med Assoc* 2007; 231:393-398.
35. Santilli RA, Spadacini G, Crosara S, et al. Utility of 12-lead electrocardiogram in differentiating paroxysmal supraventricular tachycardias in the dog. *J Vet Inter Med* 2008; 22:915-923.
36. Santilli RA, Perego M, Perini A, et al. Radiofrequency catheter ablation of cavo-tricuspid isthmus as treatment of atrial flutter in two dogs. *J Vet Cardiol* 2010; 12:59-66.
37. Santilli RA, Perego M, Perini A, et al. Electrophysiologic characteristics and topographic distribution of focal atrial tachycardias in dogs. *J Vet Intern Med* 2010; 24:539-545.
38. Santilli RA, Critelli M, Baron Toaldo M. ECG of the month. Pre-excited atrial fibrillation in a dog with an atrioventricular accessory pathway. *J Am Vet Med Assoc* 2010;237: 1142-1144. 2010;24:1-9. Note double reference.
39. Santilli RA, Diana A, Baron Toaldo M. Orthodromic atrioventricular reciprocating tachycardia conducted with intraventricular conduction disturbance mimicking ventricular tachycardia in an English Bulldog. *J Vet Cardiol* 2012; 14:363-370.
40. Santilli RA. Atrial depolarization waves localization on surface electrocardiogram in dogs with supraventricular arrhythmias. ACVIM Forum, Seattle, WA 2013; 1:174.
41. Santilli RA, Santos LFN, Perego M. Permanent junctional reciprocating tachycardia in a dog. *J Vet Cardiol* 2013; 15:225-230.
42. Santilli RA, Ramera L, Perego M, et al. Radiofrequency catheter ablation of atypical atrial flutter in five dogs. *J Vet Cardiol* 2014; 16:9-17.
43. Saoudi N, Cosio F, Waldo A, et al. A classification of atrial flutter and regular atrial tachycardia according to electrophysiological mechanisms and anatomical bases. *Eur Heart J* 2001; 22:1162-1182.
44. Schoels W, Gough WB, Restivo M, et al. Circus movement atrial flutter in the canine sterile pericarditis model. Activation patterns during initiation, termination, and sustained reentry in vivo. *Circ Res* 1990; 67:35-50.
45. Shi XM, Yuan HT, Guo HY, et al. Electrophysiologic characteristics of paroxysmal atrial fibrillation originating from superior vena cava: a clinical analysis of 30 cases. *Int J Clin Exp Med* 2015; 8:240-248.
46. Tan AY, Zhou S, Ogawa M, et al. Neural mechanisms of paroxysmal atrial fibrillation and paroxysmal atrial tachycardia in ambulatory canines. *Circulation* 2008; 118:916-925.
47. Tyszko C, Bright JM, Swist SL. Recurrent supraventricular arrhythmias in a dog with atrial myocarditis and gastritis. *J Small Anim Pract* 2007; 48:335-338.
48. Urthaler F, Neely BH, Hageman GR. Atrioventricular junctional tachycardia during heart block. *J Am Coll Cardiol* 1986; 8:657-660.
49. Vit P, Richig JW. Ventricular preexcitation in a dog. *J Am Vet Med Assoc* 1985; 187:584-585.
50. Waldo AL. Mechanisms of atrial fibrillation, atrial flutter, and ectopic atrial tachycardia-A brief review. *Circulation* 1987; 75:37-40.
51. Waldo AL, Vitikainen KJ, Harris PD, et al. The mechanism of synchronization in isorhythmic AV dissociation: some observations on the morphology and polarity of the P wave during retrograde capture atria. *Circulation* 1968; 38:880-898.
52. Wells JL, MacLean WAH, James TN, et al. Characterization of atrial flutter. Studies in man after open heart surgery using fixed atrial electrodes. *Circulation* 1979; 60:665-673.
53. Wright KN, Atkins CE, Kanter R. Supraventricular tachycardia in four young dogs. *J Am Vet Med Assoc* 1996; 208:75-80.
54. Wright KN, Mehdirad AA, Giacobbe P, et al. Radiofrequency catheter ablation of atrioventricular accessory pathways in 3 dogs with subse- quent resolution of tachycardia-induced cardiomyopathy. *J Vet Intern Med* 1999; 13:361-371.
55. Zipes DP, Rothbaum DA, DeJoseph RL. Pre-excitation syndrome. *Cardiovasc Clin* 1974; 6:209-243.

Ventricular ectopic beats and rhythms

Ventricular ectopic beats and rhythms are the most common arrhythmias in dogs and cats. They originate from the ventricular specialized conduction tissue (bundle of His, bundle branches and Purkinje network) or from the ventricular working myocardium. Ventricular ectopic beats and rhythms occur in structurally normal hearts, but more commonly in the presence of cardiac or systemic diseases. Their electrophysiological mechanisms include enhanced automaticity, triggered activity and anatomical or functional reentrant circuits.

Ventricular ectopic beats

Ventricular ectopic beats are spontaneous ventricular depolarizations. They are also called *premature ventricular beats*, *premature ventricular complexes*, *ventricular premature complexes* or extrasystoles when they occur earlier than expected based on the preceding sequence of R-R intervals. They are called *escape beats* if they occur after a long pause. Escape beats reflect the activity of subsidiary pacemakers whenever the dominant pacemaker fails to generate impulses or depolarizes at a slower rate than the pacemaker cells within the ventricles. When more than three ventricular escape beats occur successively, they form an *idioventricular rhythm* (or *escape rhythm*). The escape rate varies with the location of the Purkinje fibers that are firing. Studies in the dog have documented that Purkinje fibers in the left ventricle fire at a faster rate than those in the right ventricle. Most commonly the escape rhythm rate from the ventricles in the dog is between 20 and 40 bpm, although rates approaching 60 bpm can occur depending upon the location of the Purkinje fibers, the age of the dog and even, to some degree, sympathetic influences.

Common structural cardiac diseases that can present with ventricular arrhythmias include cardiomyopathies, myocardial trauma, myocarditis, pericarditis, myocardial ischemia, congenital heart diseases (subaortic stenosis, pulmonic stenosis) and cardiac neoplasia. A non-exhaustive list of systemic diseases that frequently trigger ventricular premature beats includes: gastric dilatation-volvulus, splenic tumors or torsion, pleural effusion, pyometra, prostatitis, pancreatitis, hyper or hypothyroidism, anemia, uremia, endotoxemia, diabetes mellitus, stress and anxiety. Administration of dobutamine, dopamine, isoproterenol, atropine, high doses of digoxin and certain anesthetics and sedatives may trigger ventricular premature beats and rhythms. Ventricular escape beats occur with pauses secondary to sinus node dysfunction, atrioventricular block, a high level of vagal tone secondary to systemic diseases or drugs.

Ventricular ectopic beats do not propagate through the normal conduction system, but instead electrical impulses travel from working myocytes to working myocytes to depolarize both ventricles. The resulting prolonged depolarization of the ventricular myocardium is responsible for the increased duration (greater than 70 ms in dogs and greater than 40 ms in cats) of the QRS complexes and their abnormal configuration that markedly differs from beats that use the ventricular conduction system. The term "wide and bizarre" has been used to describe complexes that originate from the ventricle; however, simply saying that the QRS complex has a "different" morphology from a supraventricular complex likely represents a better electrophysiological understanding. Moreover, ventricular complexes in the cat may have only subtle differences from those of supraventricular complexes making the term "bizarre" to describe the ventricular complexes misleading. Additionally, complexes from the ventricle can have a varied appearance depending upon where in the ventricle they originate (right versus left ventricle, intra-atrial septum versus free wall, base versus apex) (see p. 191). Ventricular ectopic beats that originate in the Hisian region can depolarize the ventricles through the His-Purkinje system, which results in a QRS complex of normal duration. The QRS complex of ventricular ectopic beats originating in the right ventricle has a left bundle branch block morphology, i.e. a large positive deflection in the inferior leads (II, III and aVF) and in the left precordial leads (V_2-V_6); the depolarization wavefront travels in a right-to-left, anterior-to-posterior and superior-to-inferior direction (Fig. 9.1A). The QRS complex of ventricular ectopic beats originating in the left ventricle displays a right bundle branch block morphology, i.e. a larger negative deflection in the inferior leads (II, III, and aVF) and in the left precordial leads (V_2-V_6); the depolarization wavefront travels in a left-to-right, posterior-to-anterior and inferior-to-superior direction (Fig. 9.1B). It should be noted that the morphology of ventricular premature complexes can vary from the classical right and left bundle branch block patterns. The repolarization phase of ventricular ectopic beats is also altered and results in a T wave of increased duration and amplitude, which typically has the opposite polarity to that of the QRS complex (Fig. 9.1A-B).

The morphology of ventricular ectopic beats can be constant or vary on the surface electrocardiogram. When all the beats have the same morphology, they are described as *monomorphic*; otherwise, they are called *polymorphic* or *multiform*. Monomorphic ventricular ectopic beats usually indicate that the ventricular impulses arise from the same location with similar conduction pathways, whereas polymorphic beats arise from various locations or have variable conduction pathways. On occasion, the wavefront of ventricular ectopic depolarization collides with the impulse originating in the sinus node, forming a QRS complex with intermediate morphology (*fusion beat*).

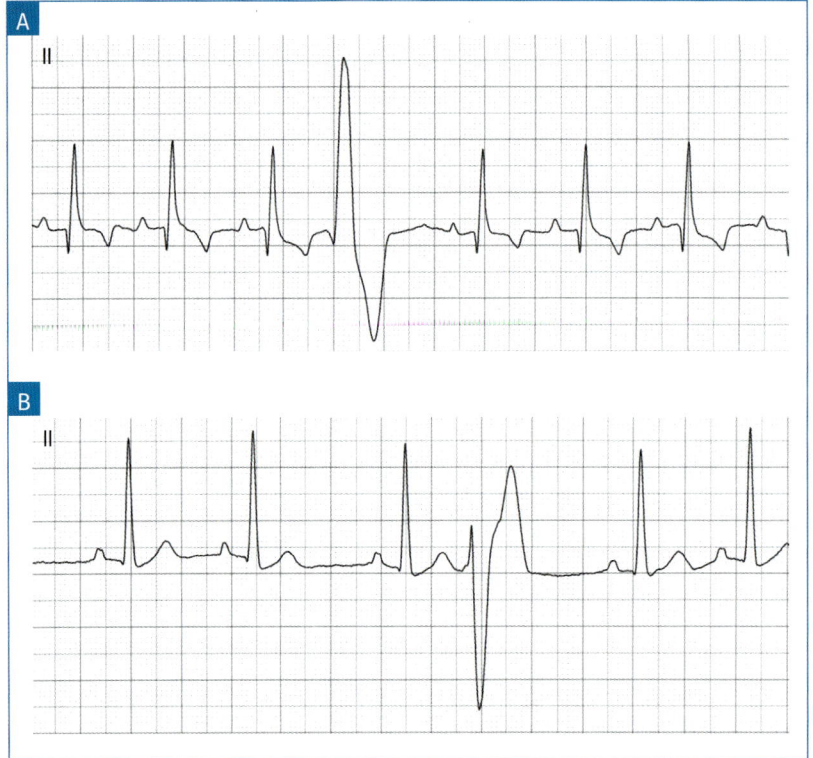

Figure 9.1. Morphology of ventricular ectopic beats.

A) Right ventricular ectopic beat. (Dog, Boxer, male, 7 years. Lead II - speed 50 mm/s - calibration 10 mm/1 mV).
The underlying rhythm is sinus tachycardia with a rate of 150 bpm. The fourth QRS complex is wide with a duration of 120 ms and an abnormal configuration. In lead II, the large amplitude deflection is positive and is followed by a large amplitude T wave with the opposite polarity.

B) Left ventricular ectopic beat. (Dog, German Shepherd, male, 8 years. Lead II - speed 50 mm/s - calibration 10 mm/1 mV).
The underlying rhythm is sinus arrhythmia with a rate of 110 bpm. The fourth QRS complex is wide with a duration of 100 ms and an abnormal configuration. In lead II, the large amplitude deflection is negative and is followed by a large amplitude T wave with the opposite polarity.

Ventricular ectopic depolarizations occur independently of normal sinus node activity. Consequently, there is atrioventricular dissociation: sinus P waves, if visible, do not have any relationship with the ventricular ectopic beats. In some cases, impulses from ventricular ectopic beats or rhythms travel in a retrograde manner through the atrioventricular node and depolarize the atria. This is called *ventriculo-atrial* retro-conduction. The ability of consecutive ventricular ectopic beats to conduct retrogradely varies, and results in different beat-to-beat conduction ratios, for example 1:1 (when every beat conducts retrogradely) or 2:1 (when every other ventricular beat conducts retrogradely). The retrograde P' waves can be detected within the initial portion of the ST segment. The P' waves have a negative polarity in the inferior leads (II, III and aVF) and a mean electrical axis in the frontal plane between −80 ° and −100 °. In this case, the retrograde conduction is defined as concentric (see p. 17) (Fig. 9.2).

Sites of origin of ventricular ectopic beats

Ventricular ectopic beats and rhythms originate within the ventricular working myocardium or the specialized ventricular conduction tissue. The arrhythmogenic mechanisms of these rhythm disorders include foci with enhanced automaticity, anatomical or functional reentrant circuits and triggered activity.

In dogs, electrophysiological studies have found various morphologies for the ventricular ectopic beats and rhythms based on their site of origin:

- the Hisian region,
- left ventricular region:
  - apical,
  - septal,
  - left ventricular outflow tract, and
  - left ventricular inflow;
- right ventricular region:
  - apical,
  - septal, and
  - right ventricular outflow tract.

Hisian ventricular beats and rhythms

Ectopic beats and rhythms originating from the Hisian region are characterized by a QRS complex of short duration (≤70 ms in dogs and ≤40 ms in cats), an electrical axis in the frontal plane between +60 ° and +80 ° and an abnormal configuration that differs from that of the normally conducted beats (Fig. 9.3).

Left ventricular beats and rhythms

Ectopic beats and rhythms originating from the left ventricle are the most common types in dogs and cats, and are generally secondary to systemic diseases or cardiac diseases that involve the left ventricle.

All the left ventricular ectopic beats and rhythms are characterized by a broad QRS complex (greater than 70 ms) with a right bundle branch block morphology and a larger negative deflection in the inferior leads (II, III and aVF). The mean electrical axis in the frontal plane is directed inferior-to-superior and to the right when these

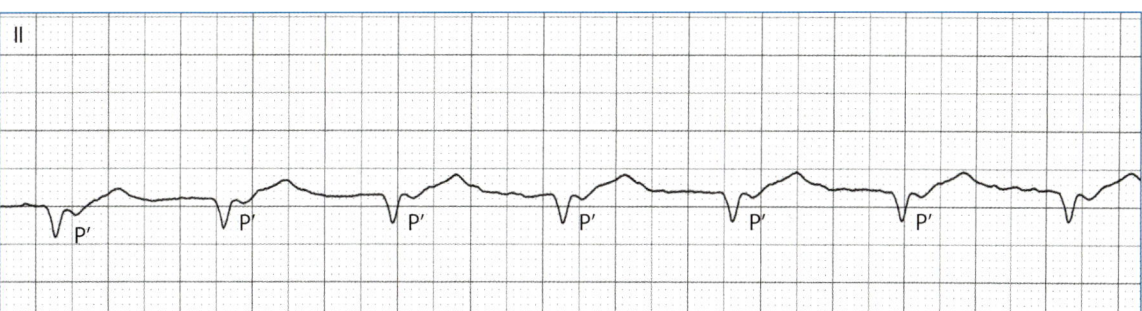

Figure 9.2. Idioventricular rhythm with ventriculo-atrial conduction in a 1:1 ratio (Cat, Domestic Shorthair, male, 1 year. Lead II - speed 50 mm/s - calibration 10 mm/1 mV).
Idioventricular rhythm with a rate of 130 bpm. The QRS complexes have an increased duration (45 ms) with an abnormal configuration, showing a wide negative deflection in lead II followed by a T wave with the opposite polarity. Note the presence of P' waves with negative polarity in the initial portion of the ST segment.

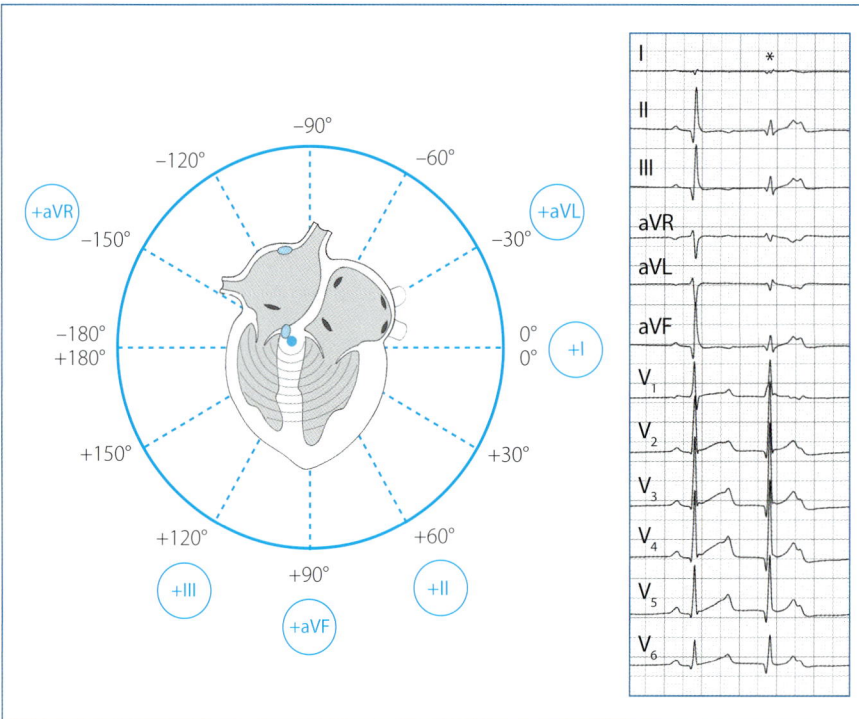

Figure 9.3. Ventricular ectopic beats originating from the Hisian region (*). The ventricular beats have an abnormal configuration compared to the sinus beat but a normal duration. The axis of the QRS complexes is shown in the frontal plane- speed 50 mm/s - calibration 10 mm/1 mV. See text for explanations.

beats originate from the apex, the septum or the inflow of the left ventricle. The mean electrical axis is however variable when the beats originate from the left ventricular outflow tract. Evaluation of the precordial leads enables recognition of beats originating in the left ventricular apex from their wider negative deflection compared to beats initiated in other parts of the ventricle (Fig. 9.4).

Right ventricular beats and rhythms

The morphology of right ventricular ectopic beats and rhythms can be used to differentiate beats originating from the apex, the septum and the right ventricular outflow tract. The detection of right-sided ectopic beats suggests the presence of arrhythmogenic right ventricular cardiomyopathy in some breeds (Boxer, English Bulldog) (see p. 227). Right ventricular ectopic beats and rhythms display a left bundle branch block morphology and, depending on the site of origin in the right ventricle, have additional characteristics:

- Beats originating in the right ventricular apex have a prolonged QRS complex (greater than 70 ms), with a wider positive deflection in the inferior leads (II, III and aVF) and a variable mean electrical axis in the frontal plane. The QRS complex is positive in lead I, negative in the precordial leads V_1 and V_2, and positive in the left precordial leads from V_3 to V_6 (Fig. 9.5).
- Beats originating in the right ventricular septum have a prolonged QRS complex (greater than 70 ms) with a wider positive deflection in the inferior leads (II, III and aVF) and a mean electrical axis in the frontal plane that is directed superior-to-inferior; lead I is usually positive; the right precordial lead (V_1) has a variable morphology, and the left precordial leads (V_2-V_6) are all positive (Fig. 9.6).
- Beats originating from the right ventricular outflow tract have a prolonged QRS complex (>70 ms), with a larger positive deflection in the inferior leads (II, III and aVF) and a mean electrical axis in the frontal plane directed superior-to-inferior. The QRS complex is negative in lead I when the beats originate in the anterior part of the outflow tract; it is negative, diphasic or isodiphasic when they have a more posterior origin. The QRS complex is negative in lead aVL if the site of origin is just below the pulmonary valve, and is positive

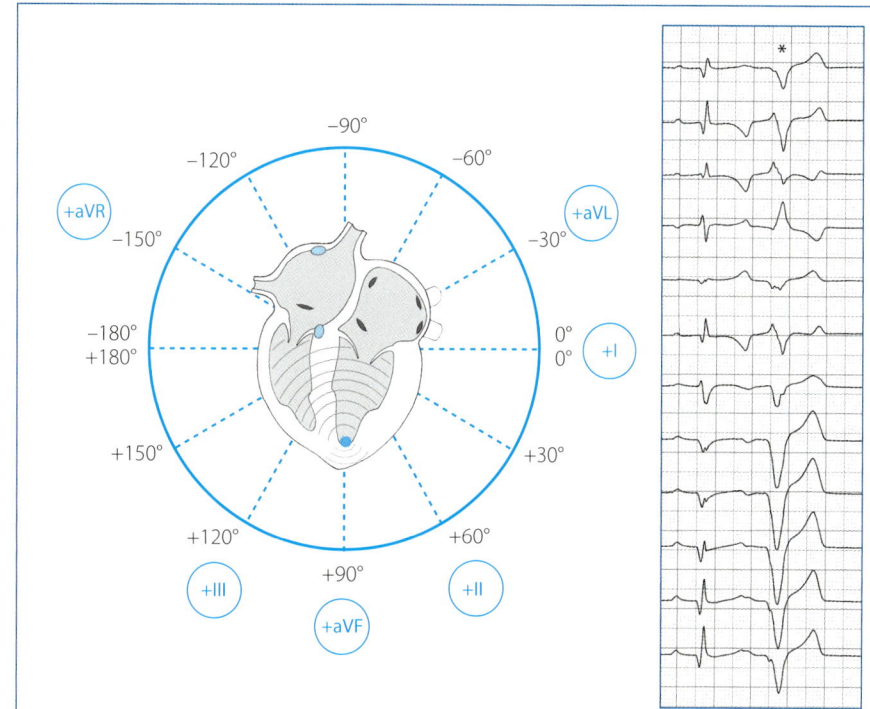

Figure 9.4. Ventricular ectopic beats originating from the apex of the left ventricle (*). Axis of the QRS complex in the frontal plane and morphology of ventricular ectopic beat in the 12-lead electrocardiogram - speed 50 mm/s - calibration 5 mm/1 mV. See text for explanations.

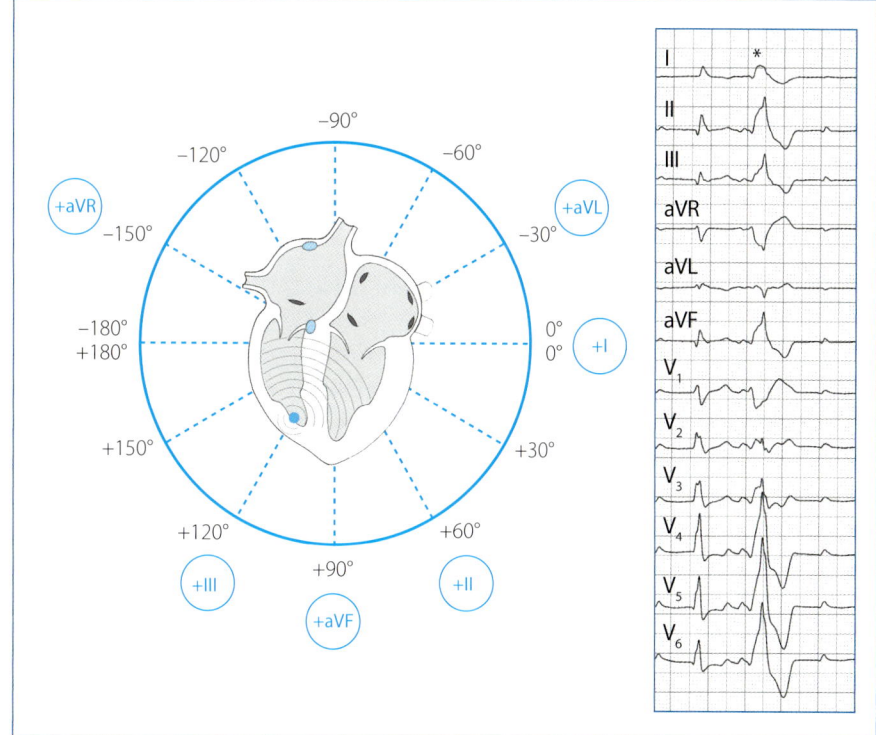

Figure 9.5. Ventricular ectopic beats originating from the apex of the right ventricle (*). Axis of the QRS complex in the frontal plane and morphology of ventricular ectopic beats in the 12-lead electrocardiogram - speed 50 mm/s - calibration 5 mm/1 mV. See text for explanations.

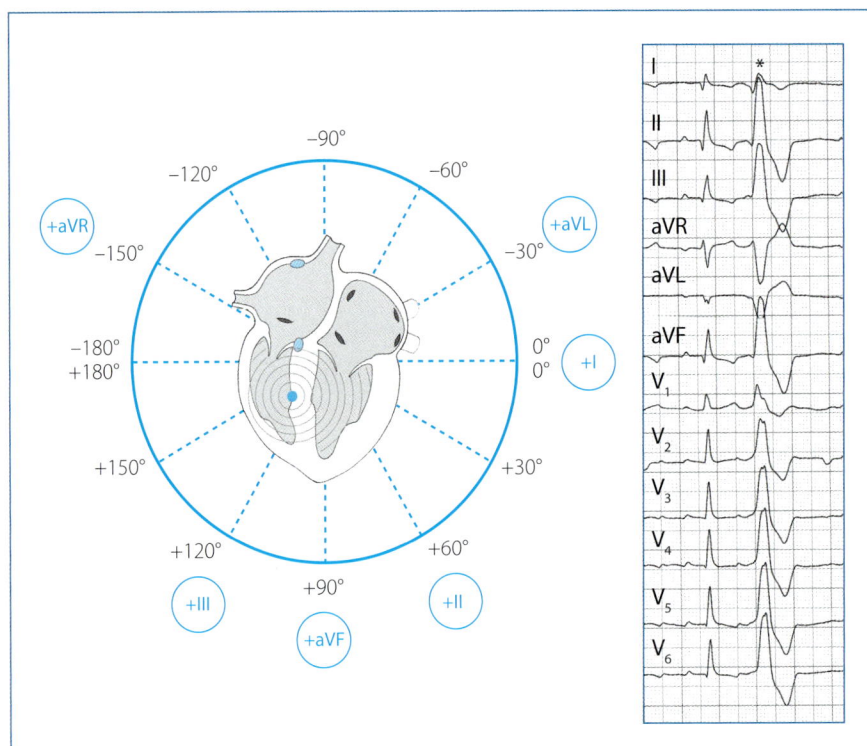

Figure 9.6. Ventricular ectopic beats originating from the right ventricular septum (*). Axis of the QRS complex in the frontal plane and morphology of ventricular ectopic beats in the 12-lead electrocardiogram - speed 50 mm/s - calibration 5 mm/1 mV. See text for explanations.

if the origin is further away from the valve. The presence of notches in the inferior leads (II, III and aVF) indicates a site of origin in the spiral aorticopulmonary septum between the pulmonary trunk and the aortic arch. The polarity of the QRS complex in the right precordial lead (V_1) is variable, while the polarity in the left precordial leads (V_2-V_6) is positive (Fig. 9.7).

Prematurity and organization of ventricular ectopic beats

The *coupling interval*, which is the interval between the R wave of the beat preceding the ectopic beat and the largest deflection of the ectopic QRS complex, defines the prematurity of the ventricular ectopic beat. It is called *premature* (Fig. 9.8) when the coupling interval is shorter than the interval between beats forming the underlying rhythm. Conversely, if the coupling interval between the ectopic beat and the preceding beat corresponds to the inherent rate of the ventricular pacemaker cells because of a failure of the underlying rhythm to activate the ventricles, it is defined as a ventricular *escape* beat (Fig. 9.9).

Ventricular premature beats have a fixed or relatively fixed coupling interval when the arrhythmogenic mechanism is a reentry, and more rarely when it is triggered activity or enhanced automaticity. The coupling interval is variable with ventricular parasystole (see p. 200).

Very short coupling intervals result in the onset of the premature ectopic beat to occur close to the peak of the T wave of the previous beat (*R-on-T phenomenon*) (Fig. 9.10). This portion of the T wave is known as the "vulnerable" period of ventricular repolarization and, theoretically, a premature beat occurring during this window of time could initiate ventricular fibrillation in the presence of an underlying structural or electrical cardiac disease. However, the probability that a ventricular arrhythmia degenerates into ventricular fibrillation is not determined solely by the timing of ventricular premature beats.

Ventricular ectopic beats can serve as triggers for tachyarrhythmias, including orthodromic atrioventricular reciprocating tachycardia, and reentrant ventricular tachycardias.

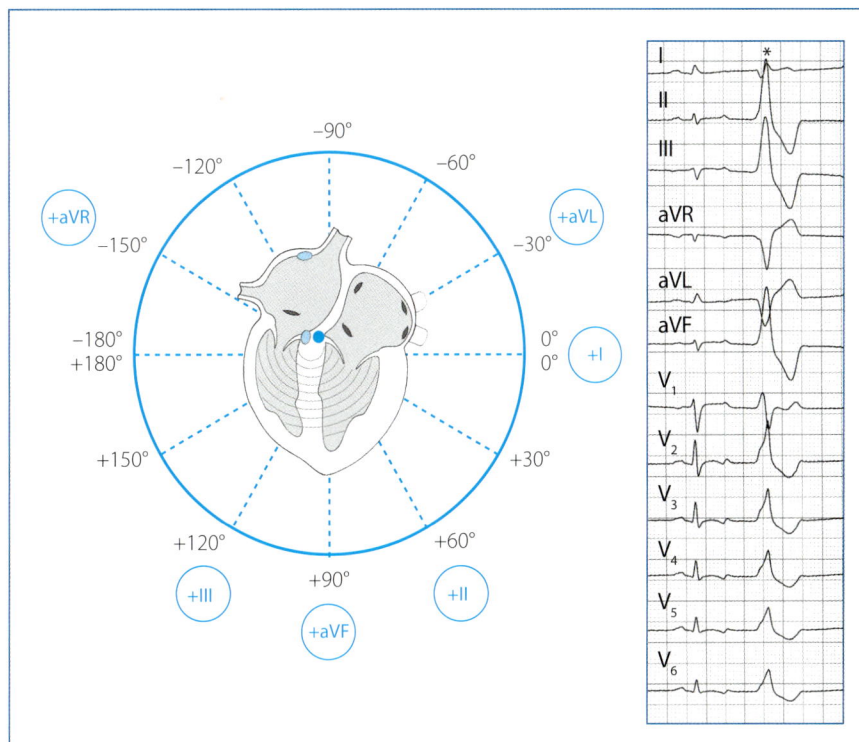

Figure 9.7. Ventricular ectopic beats originating from the right ventricular outflow tract (*). Axis and morphology of ventricular ectopic beats in the 12-lead electrocardiogram - speed 50 mm/s - calibration 5 mm/mV. See text for explanations.

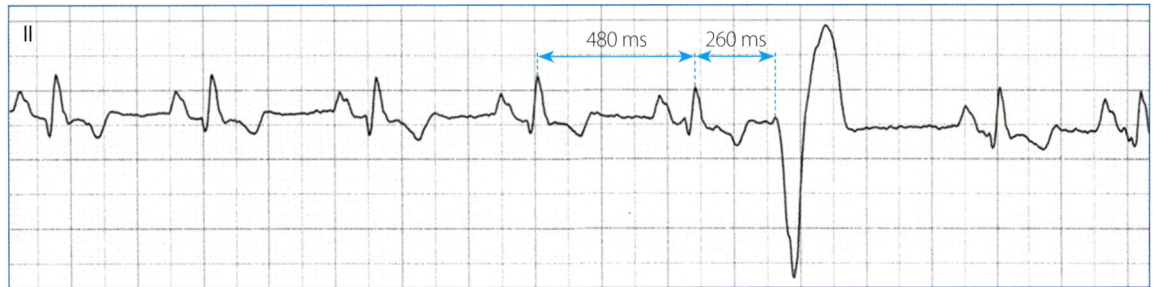

Figure 9.8. Ventricular premature beat (Dog, Doberman, male, 9 years. Lead II - speed 50 mm/s - calibration 10 mm/1 mV). The underlying rhythm is a sinus rhythm with signs of left atrial and ventricular enlargement and a rate of 125 bpm. The fifth QRS complex has an increased duration (100 ms) and an abnormal configuration. The ventricular ectopic beat is premature because its coupling interval with the previous sinus beat is shorter (260 ms) than the basal R-R interval (480 ms).

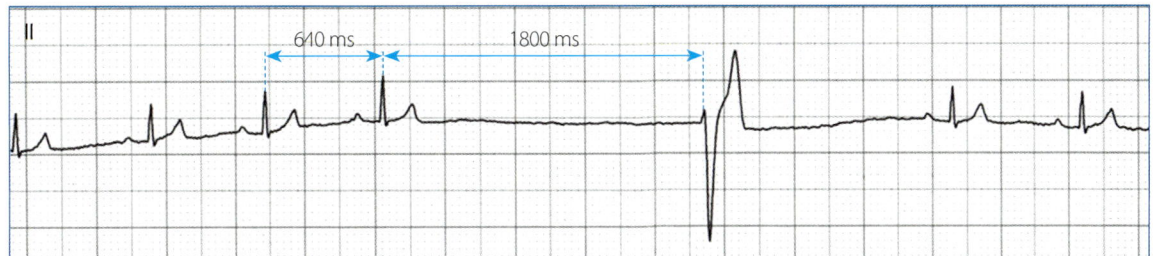

Figure 9.9. Ventricular escape beat (Dog, Boxer, male, 5 years. Lead II - speed 25 mm/s - calibration 10 mm/1 mV). The underlying rhythm is sinus with a rate of 90 bpm. The fourth QRS complex has an increased duration (90 ms) and an abnormal configuration. The ventricular ectopic beat is classified as an escape beat because its coupling interval is markedly longer (1800 ms) than the basal R-R interval (640 ms), and corresponds to the firing rate of the subsidiary ventricular pacemaker cells.

Premature ventricular beats are usually followed by a pause (*post-extrasystolic pause*). The post-extrasystolic pause is described as *compensatory* or *non-compensatory*, but this can only be determined if the underlying rhythm (usually sinus rhythm) is regular. Unfortunately, respiratory sinus arrhythmia is the typical rhythm in dogs, which results in a constant variation of the R-R intervals. The *pause* is described as *compensatory* if the interval that includes the premature beat is exactly twice the interval between two sinus beats of the underlying rhythm. A compensatory pause occurs when the ventricular premature beat does not conduct retrogradely through the atrioventricular node, and does not interfere with the activity of the sinus node. In this situation, the sinus beat following the ventricular premature beat reaches the atrioventricular node or the ventricles during its refractory period and does not, therefore, depolarize the ventricles. This P wave is not visible, because it is embedded within the QRS complex of the premature beat (Fig. 9.11).

The pause that follows a premature ventricular beat is called *non-compensatory* if the interval that includes the ectopic beat is less than twice the R-R interval between two beats of the underlying rhythm. A non-compensatory pause indicates that the ventricular ectopic beat

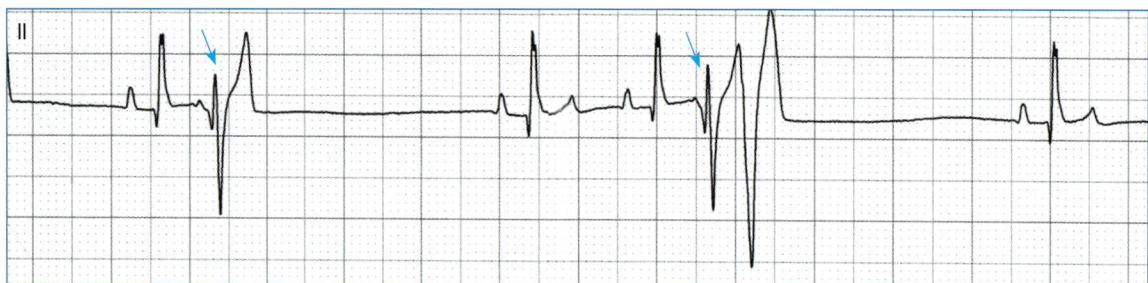

Figure 9.10. Ventricular premature beats with "R-on-T phenomenon" (Dog, German Shepherd, male, 9 months. Lead II - speed 25 mm/s - calibration 10 mm/1 mV).
The underlying rhythm is a respiratory sinus arrhythmia with a rate varying from 40 to 100 bpm. The second, fifth and sixth beats have an increased duration (80 ms) and abnormal configuration. The QRS complexes of the second and fifth beats (arrows) occur during the peak of the T wave of the preceding beat ("R-on-T phenomenon"). The fifth and sixth ventricular ectopic beats form a ventricular couplet.

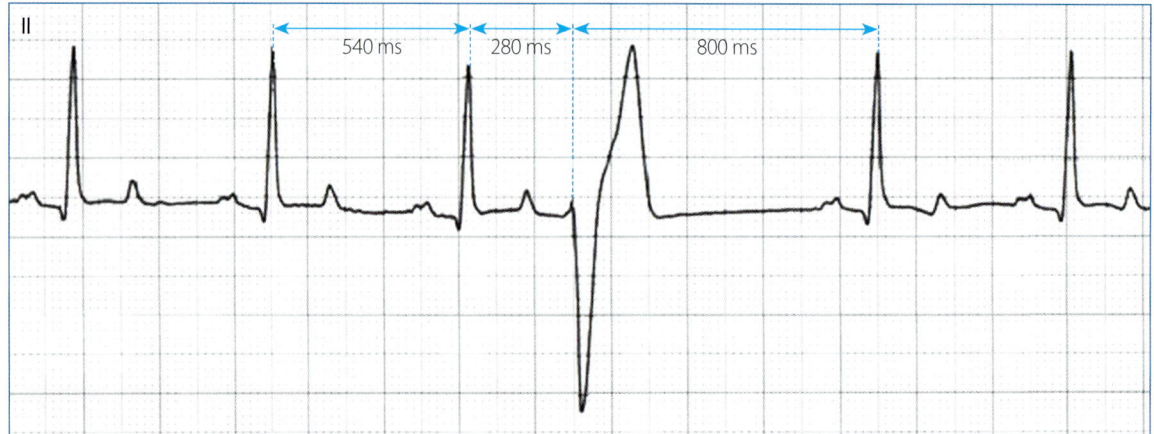

Figure 9.11. Ventricular premature beat with compensatory post-extrasystolic pause (Dog, Boxer, male, 10 years. Lead II - speed 50 mm/s - calibration 10 mm/1 mV).
The underlying rhythm is sinus in origin with signs of left atrial enlargement and a rate of 110 bpm. The fourth beat has an increased duration (80 ms) and abnormal configuration. The ventricular premature beat is followed by a post-extrasystolic pause of 800 ms. This pause is defined as compensatory since the interval that includes the ventricular premature beat (800 + 280 = 1080 ms) is twice the duration of the basal cycle (540 × 2 = 1080 ms). In dogs it is very often difficult to assess the characteristics of the post-extrasystolic pause due to the presence of sinus arrhythmia.

is conducted retrogradely through the atrioventricular node, reaching the atria and sinus node. The sinus node pacemaker is reset by this depolarization, which disrupts the regularity of the sinus rhythm (Fig. 9.12).

Ventricular premature beats are described as interpolated when they do not interfere with the underlying sinus rhythm. An interpolated ventricular beat indicates that the ventricular myocardium has been able to fully repolarize before the subsequent sinus beat, because the underlying sinus rhythm is slow or because the ectopic beat is very premature (short coupling interval) (Fig. 9.13). Frequently, interpolated ventricular beats conduct retrogradely until they are blocked inside the junctional area (*occult ventriculo-atrial conduction*). As a result, the sinus beat following the interpolated ventricular ectopic beat has a prolonged PQ interval, which reflects the delay in anterograde atrioventricular conduction caused by the occult retrograde conduction of the interpolated beat.

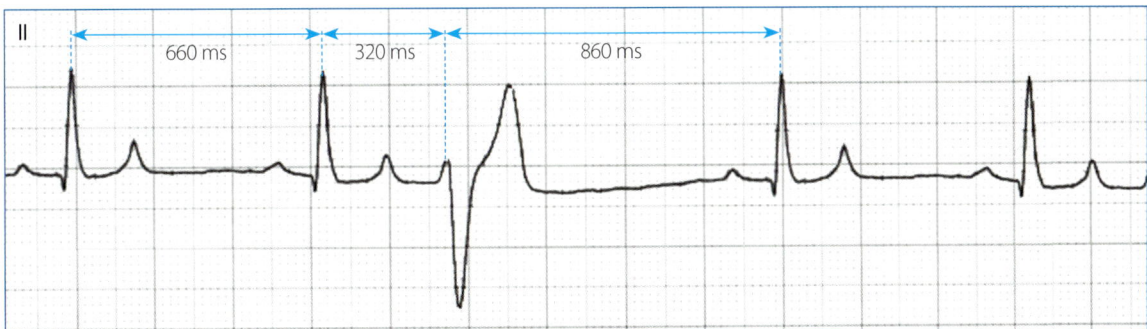

Figure 9.12. Ventricular premature beat with a non-compensatory post-extrasystolic pause (Dog, Doberman, male, 11 years. Lead II - speed 50 mm/s - calibration 5 mm/1 mV).
The underlying rhythm is a sinus rhythm with a rate of 90 bpm. The third beat has an increased duration (80 ms) and abnormal morphology. The premature ventricular beat is followed by a post-extrasystolic pause of 860 ms. This pause is defined as non-compensatory since the interval that includes the ventricular premature beat (320 + 860 ms = 1180 ms) is less than twice the duration of the basal cycle (660 × 2 = 1320 ms). In dogs it is very often difficult to assess the characteristics of the post-extrasystolic pause due to the presence of sinus arrhythmia.

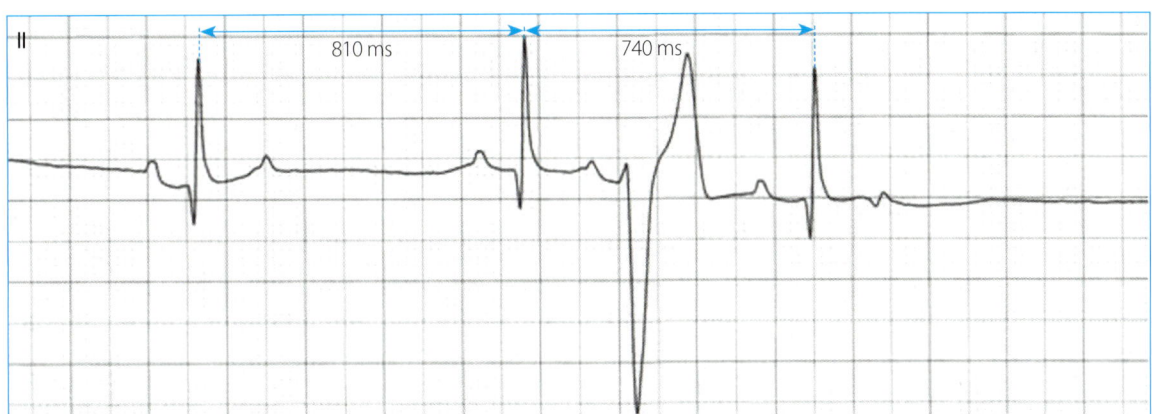

Figure 9.13. Interpolated ventricular premature beat (Dog, Labrador Retriever, male, 2 years. Lead II - speed 50 mm/s - calibration 10 mm/1 mV).
The underlying rhythm is a respiratory sinus arrhythmia with a rate of 75 bpm. The third beat has an increased duration (80 ms) and abnormal configuration. The ventricular premature beat is defined as interpolated because it occurs between two QRS complexes without interfering with the underlying rhythm. The interval that includes the ventricular premature beat is 740 ms, which is shorter than the preceding interval between two sinus beats (810 ms) as a result of sinus arrhythmia. Note the variable T wave morphology of the sinus beats suggesting repolarization abnormalities. In dogs it is very often difficult to assess the characteristics of the post-extrasystolic pause due to the presence of sinus arrhythmia.

Finally, when the interval that includes the premature beat exceeds twice the interval between two sinus beats, the pause following the premature beat is described as *supracompensatory*). This phenomenon is attributed to the depression of sinus node automaticity by the ventricular premature beat.

Ventricular premature beats may be isolated or occur with a variety of patterns, including bigeminy, trigeminy, quadrigeminy (*allorhythmias*), couplets, triplets and runs of ventricular tachycardia. *Ventricular bigeminy* corresponds to sinus beats alternating with ventricular premature beats in a 1:1 ratio (Fig. 9.14). Ventricular trigeminy corresponds to two sinus beats alternating with one ventricular premature beat. Quadrigeminy describes three sinus beats alternating with one ventricular premature beat. Two consecutive ventricular premature beats are called a couplet (Fig. 9.10), and three consecutive ventricular premature beats are called a triplet (Fig. 9.15). More than three consecutive ventricular ectopic beats are called idioventricular rhythm, accelerated idioventricular rhythm or ventricular tachycardia depending on their rate.

Four or more consecutive ventricular escape beats are described as ventricular escape rhythm or *idioventricular rhythm*. Ventricular escape rhythms occur when the ventricles are not depolarized by supraventricular impulses for at least several seconds. The cause can be sinus node dysfunction, or an atrioventricular block in the sub-Hisian segment of the atrioventricular conduction axis. Idioventricular rhythms originate from an unprotected automatic ventricular focus (subsidiary pacemaker), which means that the focus is usually inhibited by the presence of a more rapid supraventricular rhythm (*overdrive suppression*).

In some cases, idiopathic ventricular rhythms can be associated with concentric ventriculo-atrial retrograde conduction (see p. 17). Ventricular escape rhythms are usually regular, although some rate variation can be noted at the initiation of the rhythm because of the "warm-up" that characterizes automatic foci (Box 9.1).

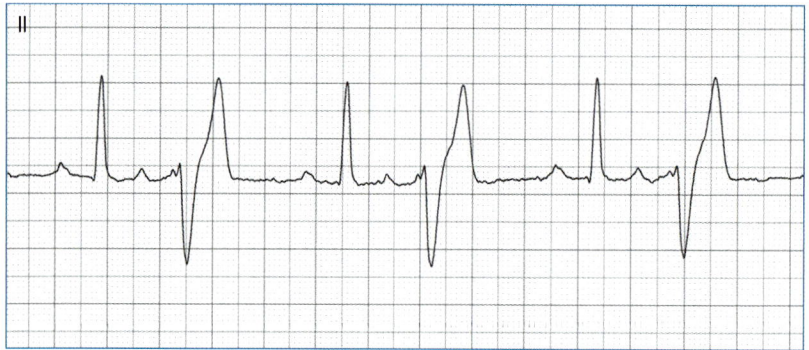

Figure 9.14. Ventricular bigeminy (Dog, Rottweiler, male, 1 year. Lead II - speed 50 mm/s - calibration 10 mm/1 mV).
The underlying rhythm is ventricular bigeminy, with sinus beats alternating with ventricular premature beats in a 1:1 ratio.

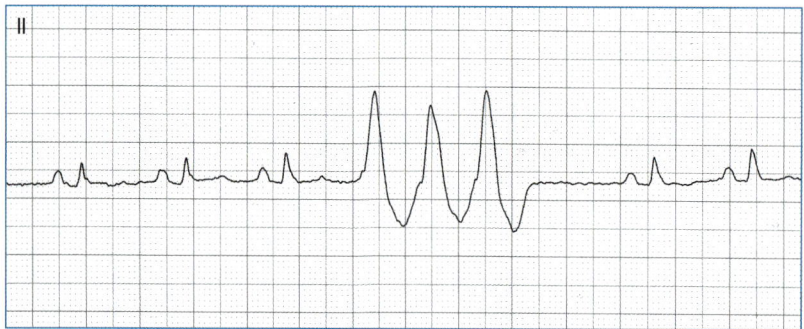

Figure 9.15. Ventricular triplet (Dog, English Bulldog, male, 9 years. Lead II - speed 50 mm/s - calibration 10 mm/1 mV).
The underlying rhythm is a sinus tachycardia with a rate of 160 bpm. The fourth, fifth and sixth beats have an increased duration (90 ms) and abnormal configuration. They form a sequence of three ventricular premature beats (a triplet) with a rate of 300 bpm.

Relationship between atrial and ventricular activation

Ventricular ectopic beats generate a depolarization wavefront that usually collides with impulses of supraventricular origin at the level of the atrioventricular junction. As a result, the supraventricular impulses fail to propagate to the ventricles and the ventricular ectopies do not conduct retrogradely to the atria. This event appears as atrioventricular dissociation on the electrocardiogram. If the timing between a ventricular ectopy and a sinus beat is such that the onset of the ventricular impulse occurs later after the P wave, it becomes more likely that the two depolarization wavefronts collide at the ventricular level rather than the atrioventricular junction. On the electrocardiogram, this is recognized as a *fusion beat*. A fusion beat is the result of partial depolarization of the ventricles by the sinus impulse travelling along the conduction system and by the ventricular beat travelling through the working myocardial cells. The QRS complex of the fusion beat has an intermediate morphology between that of the sinus beat and that of the ventricular ectopy; its duration is shorter than the ventricular ectopic beats (Fig. 9.16). The presence of fusion beats confirms the presence of atrioventricular dissociation.

When a premature ventricular ectopic beat is able to conduct retrogradely through the atrioventricular junction and is followed by a non-compensatory post-extrasystolic pause (indicating that it did not reset the sinus node pacemaker), evidence of concentric retrograde conduction may be seen as a P' wave within the ST segment of the ectopic ventricular beat with an electrical axis of −80 ° to −100 °, i.e. a negative P' in the inferior leads (II, III and aVF), and equally positive in aVR and aVL (Fig. 9.2).

BOX 9.1.
IDIOVENTRICULAR OR ESCAPE RHYTHM DURING THIRD-DEGREE ATRIOVENTRICULAR BLOCK

HEART RATE: ≤60 bpm.
R-R INTERVAL: regular.
P WAVE: presence of normal sinus P waves dissociated from the QRS complex.
ATRIOVENTRICULAR CONDUCTION: absent (atrioventricular dissociation).

PQ INTERVAL: variable.
QRS COMPLEX: wide (>70 ms) and different morphology from expected morphology of supraventricular origin.
VENTRICULO-ATRIAL CONDUCTION: absent or present with occasional conduction ratio from 1:1 to 2:1.
BLOCKED BEATS: all P waves.

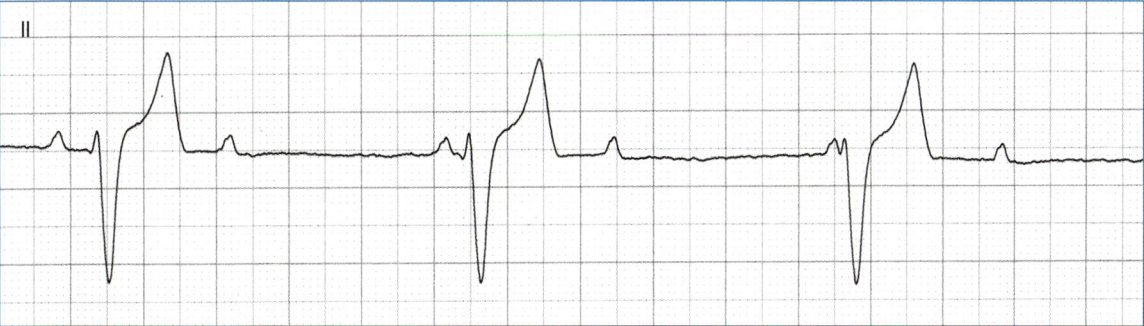

Dog, German Shepherd, female, 6 years.
Lead II - speed 50 mm/s - calibration 10 mm/1 mV.

Notes: idioventricular/escape rhythm during third-degree atrioventricular block. Broad QRS complexes are present with increased duration (80 ms) and abnormal configuration, with regular R-R intervals (escape rhythms are not always regular) and a discharge rate of 59 bpm. The P waves with sinus axis are dissociated from the QRS complex and have a discharge rate varying between 108 and 131 bpm. The irregularity of the P-P interval is caused by a mechanism known as ventriculo-phasic sinus arrhythmia. Given that sinus arrhythmia may still be the underlying rhythm in the dog, careful examination is required to determine whether a ventriculo-phasic sinus arrhythmia exists.

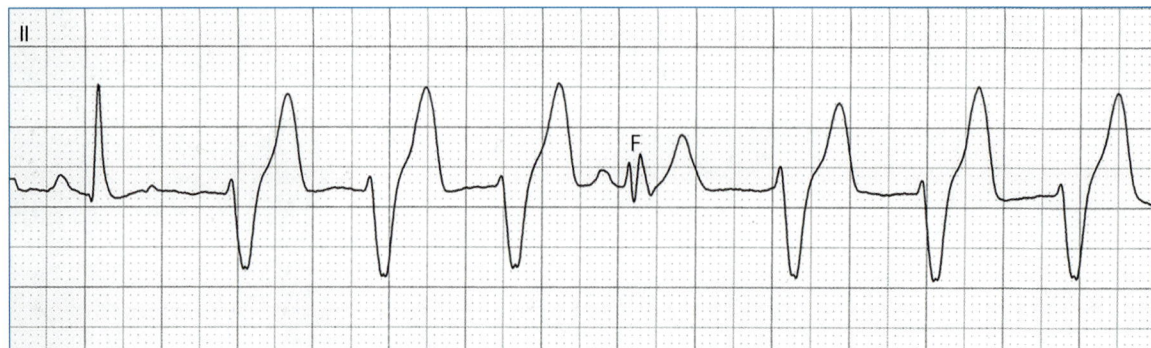

Figure 9.16. Fusion beat (Dog, Labrador Retriever, female, 12 years. Lead II - speed 50 mm/s - calibration 10 mm/1 mV). The underlying rhythm is ventricular in origin with a rate of 172 bpm. The first sinus beat is followed by three QRS complexes (93 ms) with a right bundle branch block morphology. After the fourth complex, a sinus P wave is followed by a QRS (F) complex of increased duration (80 ms) and intermediate morphology between the sinus beat and the ectopic beats (fusion beat).

Ventricular parasystole

Ventricular *parasystole* is a particular form of ventricular ectopic rhythm classically characterized by the presence of an automatic ventricular focus that is "protected" (not insulated) from the influence of the dominant rhythm (*entrance block*). Since its original description it has been learned that impulse formation may be due to automaticity or triggered activity. Additionally, it is unlikely that the protection is absolute because the rhythm is influenced by electrotonic potentials. Electrotonic potentials are typically generated by intervening sinus beats and can modulate the rate of the parasystolic focus. However, the entrance block is effective in protecting the fixed ventricular parasystolic rhythm from overdrive suppression by the leading pacemaker (usually sinus rhythm). Therefore, during classical ventricular parasystole, parasystolic impulses occur at regular intervals irrespective of the underlying rhythm, and their ability to generate a QRS complex depends on the excitability of the myocardium at the time the impulse is generated.

A varying coupling interval, fusion beats and mathematically related intervals between complexes are the three classic components that describe the parasystolic rhythm. To make the diagnosis of parasystole the ventricular beat interval is measured and is indicated by X-X which is the non-modulated ectopic cycle length. This X-X does not have an intervening sinus beat.

Unfortunately it is uncommon to identify such an interval easily. More commonly the basic parasystolic interval is calculated by measuring multiple intervals and the non-modulated parasystolic fixed interval is calculated as the basic integer. Because modulation of the parasystolic rhythm occurs commonly there will be some differences in the exact multiple relationship. Modulation occurs when sinus beats interrupt the X-X interval and is designated as X-R-X. Modulation is dictated by the X-R interval. When a sinus beat occurs early (before 50 % of the cycle interval) in the X-X interval the next parasystolic beat will be delayed, whereas when a sinus beat occurs late (after more than 50 % of the cycle interval) in the X-X interval the next parasystolic beat will occur early. A graph (known as a phase response curve) of the normalized values (intervals represented as a percentage of the ectopic cycle length), with X-R % on the x-axis and the X-R-X % on the y-axis, shows this biphasic phenomenon. A triphasic phase response curve can be seen during supernormal conduction. It should be pointed out that the behavior of the inter-ectopic interval is more difficult to predict when there is more than one intervening sinus beat. These effects have been studied experimentally in the dog. Another, important factor concerning modulation is the location of the parasystolic site.

Additional characteristics of parasystolic rhythm include parasystolic entrainment and intermittent parasystole. In an entrained parasystolic rhythm the non-parasystolic beats (usually sinus beats) can change the parasystolic rate so that it is equal, faster or slower than the non-parasystolic rates. An intermittent parasystolic rhythm is one whereby the sinus beats reset the parasystolic cycle length and where the parasystolic site is variably active or not. However the latter may also be a function of modulation.

Figure 9.17 shows the two components necessary to make the diagnosis of a parasystolic rhythm with varying coupling intervals and a constant interval between ventricular beats; however, there are intervening sinus beats so that the true interectopic interval is unknown. A key to the diagnosis of ventricular parasystole is to examine very long recordings in an attempt to identify all components and to look for modulation, which is common.

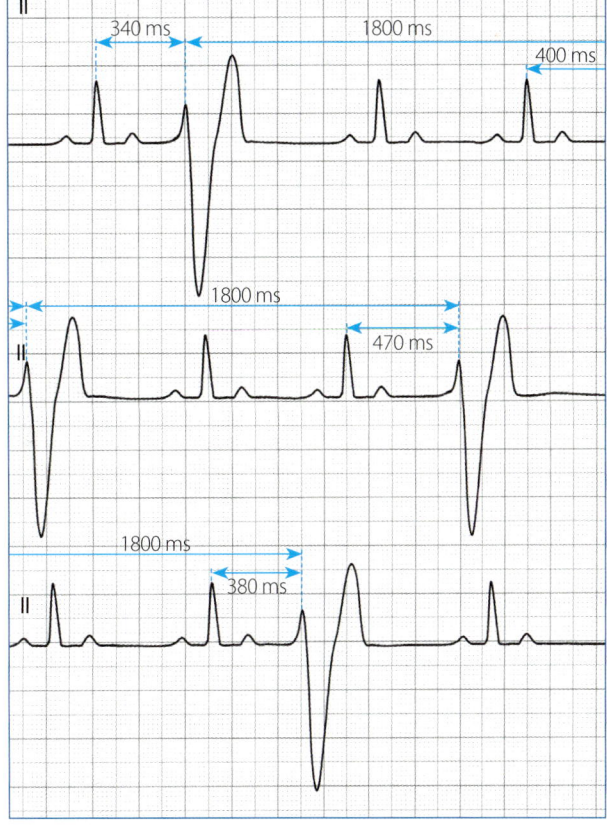

Figure 9.17. Ventricular parasystole (Dog, mongrel, male, 12 years. Lead II - speed 50 mm/s - calibration 10 mm/1 mV). The underlying rhythm is sinus in origin with a rate of 95 bpm. The second, fifth, eighth and eleventh QRS complexes have abnormal morphology (90 ms); the coupling interval between the sinus beats and the ectopic beats is variable (from 340 to 370 ms); the interectopic interval is constant (1800 ms).

Suggested readings

1. Boyden PA, Dun W, Robinson RB. Cardiac Purkinje fibers and arrhythmias; the GK Moe award lecture 2015. *Heart Rhythm* 2016; 13:1172-1181.
2. Castellanow A, Saoudi N, Moleiro F, Myerburg RJ. Parasystole. Cardiac Electrophysiology From Cell to Bedside 3rd edition. DP Zipes and J Jalife. WB Saunders Company 2000; 690-694.
3. Foster PR, Elharrar V, Zipes DP. Accelerated ventricular escapes induced in the intact dog by barium, strontium and calcium. *J Pharmacol Exp Ther* 1977; 200:373-383.
4. Han J. The concepts of reentrant activity responsible for ectopic rhythms. *Am J Cardiol* 1971; 28:253-262.
5. Issa ZF, Rosenberger J, Groh WJ, et al. Ischemic ventricular arrhythmias during heart failure: a canine model to replicate clinical events. *Heart Rhythm* 2005; 2:979-983.
6. James TN, Isobe JH, Urthaler F. Correlative electrophysiological and anatomical studies concerning the site of origin of escape rhythm during complete atrioventricular block in the dog. *Circ Res* 1979; 45:108-119.
7. Joshi S, Wilber DJ. Ablation of idiopathic right ventricular outflow tract tachycardia: current perspectives. *J Cardiovasc Electrophysiol* 2005; 16:S52-S58.
8. Kabell G, Scherlag BJ, Brachmann J, et al. Ventricular arrhythmias following one-stage and two-stage coronary reperfusion: evidence for both reentry and enhanced automaticity. *J Electrocardiol* 1985; 18:87-96.
9. Kraus MS, Moïse NS, Rishniw M, et al. Morphology of ventricular arrhythmias in the Boxer as measured by 12-lead electrocardiography with pace-mapping comparison. *J Vet Intern Med* 2002; 16:153-158.
10. Lown B, Wolf M. Approaches to sudden death from coronary heart disease. *Circulation* 1971; 44:130-142.
11. Marino DJ, Matthiesen DT, Fox PR, et al. Ventricular arrhythmias in dogs undergoing splenectomy: a prospective study. *Vet Surg* 1994; 23:101-106.
12. Meurs KM, Spier AW, Miller MW, et al. Familiar ventricular arrhythmias in boxers. *J Vet Intern Med* 1999; 13:437-439.
13. Meurs KM, Spier AW, Wright NA, et al. Comparison of in-hospital versus 24-hour ambulatory electrocardiography for detection of ventricular premature complexes in mature Boxers. *J Am Vet Med Assoc* 2001; 218:222-224.
14. Moore EN, Spear JF. Experimental studies on the facilitation of AV conduction by ectopic beats in dogs and rabbits. *Circ Res* 1971; 29:29-39.
15. Peiss CN, Spurgeon HA. Origin of initial escape beat during graded vagal stimulation. *J Electrocardiol* 1975; 8:25-29.
16. Plotnikov AN, Sosunov EA, Qu J, et al. Biological pacemaker implanted in canine left bundle branch provides ventricular escape rhythms that have physiologically acceptable rates. *Circulation* 2004; 109:506-512.
17. Santilli RA, Bontempi LV, Perego M, et al. Outflow tract segmental arrhythmogenic right ventricular cardiomyopathy in an English Bulldog. *J Vet Cardiol* 2009; 11:47-51.
18. Santilli RA, Bontempi LV, Perego M. Ventricular tachycardia in English Bulldog with localized right ventricular outflow tract enlargement. *J Small Anim Pract* 2011; 52:574-580.
19. Savard P, Roberge FA, Perry JB, et al. Representation of cardiac electrical activity by a moving dipole for normal and ectopic beats in the intact dog. *Circ Res* 1980; 46:415-425.
20. Sideris DA, Toumanidis ST, Stringli TN, et al. Anatomical origin of pressure-related ventricular ectopic rhythms. *Int J Cardiol* 1992; 37:365-372.
21. Sosunov EA, Anyukhovsky E. Differential effects of ivabradine and ryanodine on pacemaker activity in canine sinus node and Purkinje fibers. *J Cardiovasc Electrophysiol* 2012; 23:650-655.
22. Spach MS, Barr RC. Analysis of ventricular activation and repolarization from intramural and epicardial potential distributions for ectopic beats in the intact dog. *Circ Res* 1975; 37:830-843.
23. Taccardi B, Arisi G, Macchi E, et al. A new intracavitary probe for detecting the site of origin of ectopic ventricular beats during one cardiac cycle. *Circulation* 1987; 75:272-281.
24. Vasalle M, Cummins M, Castro C, et al. The relationship between overdrive suppression and overdrive excitation in venticular pacemaker in dogs. *Circ Res* 1976; 38:367-374.
25. Vos MA, Gorgels AP, de Wit B, et al. Premature escape beats. A model for triggered activity in the intact heart? *Circulation* 1990; 82:213-224.
26. Zhou J, Scherlag BJ, Yamanashi W, et al. Experimental model simulating right ventricular outflow tract tachycardia: a novel technique to initiate RVOT-VT. *J Cardiovasc Electrophysiol* 2006; 17:771-775.

CHAPTER 10

Ventricular arrhythmias

Ventricular arrhythmias originate from cardiac structures distal to the non-penetrating portion of the distal atrioventricular bundle. These structures include the region of the His bundle, the ventricular myocardium, the right bundle branch, the left bundle branch and its anterior and posterior subdivisions, the Purkinje fibers, the left and right ventricular outflow tracts, the sinus of Valsalva of the aortic valve, and possibly the pulmonary artery. Ventricular tachycardia can be arbitrarily defined as more than three consecutive ventricular ectopic beats at a rate that exceeds the inherent escape rhythm rate of subsidiary pacemaker cells of the ventricular tissue. However, clinicians often use the term "ventricular tachycardia" to describe ventricular rhythms with rapid heart rates capable of causing hemodynamic compromise and requiring treatment. Nevertheless, the definition of a rhythm disturbance is based on electrocardiographic and electrophysiologic characterizations and not treatment criteria. Although it can sometimes be challenging to differentiate between ventricular and supraventricular tachycardias, the typical morphology of ventricular ectopic beats is that of a broad QRS complex (greater than 70 ms in the dog and 40 ms in the cat) with a T wave that has an opposite direction to the main deflection of the QRS complex. The latter is also described as discordance between the QRS complex and the T wave.

Defining tachycardia

In the strictest terms, a ventricular tachycardia is any rhythm from ventricular tissues that exceeds the subsidiary pacemaker rate. In the dog, the rate of firing of ventricular subsidiary pacemaker cells is approximately 30 to 40 bpm, whereas it is 100 to 140 bpm in the cat. However, for clarity in clinical communications, specific terms are used to described ventricular rates and include *idioventricular rhythms*, *accelerated idioventricular rhythms* and *ventricular tachycardia*. In the literature concerning tachyarrhythmias in people, the definition of an *accelerated idioventricular rhythm* is one whose rate is within 10 % of the underlying sinus rhythm. A ventricular rhythm below this heart rate range is termed an *idioventricular rhythm*, while a ventricular rhythm above this heart rate is termed *ventricular tachycardia*. A fundamental question concerning the clinical value of this definition is: what is considered the underlying sinus rhythm? Is the underlying sinus rhythm that which should be present or that which is present? The definition is problematic because the answer to this question is unclear. For example, many dogs with arrhythmias do not have heart failure and have a normal underlying sinus rate. Conversely, some dogs have ventricular tachycardia triggered by excitement, which is associated with fast sinus rates. That is, it is possible that a dog with a sinus rate of 200 bpm during excitement and a ventricular rate of 210 bpm would have the latter rhythm diagnosed as an accelerated idioventricular rhythm, when it is actually ventricular tachycardia?

Although defining an accelerated idioventricular rhythm can be arbitrary, some guidance in establishing the approximate rate range can come from an understanding of the inherent sinus node heart rate distribution in the dog (data from cats are more limited). The normal heart rate range in humans depends on their age and physical condition but ranges from 60 to 100 bpm. In humans, an accelerated idioventricular rhythm is diagnosed when the heart rate is less than 100 bpm (within 10 %

of the underlying sinus rate). Based on the data derived from 178 Holter recordings of dogs of various breeds with normal sinus function, the average heart rate of the dog is 83 ± 11.8 bpm (upper 95 % confidence interval 86 bpm, median 81 bpm). The average heart rate range in the home environment for the dog based on these data is, therefore, 60 to 100 bpm. The range of heart rates from 10 % below to two-standard deviations above this mean is ~54 to 117 bpm. Rounding these numbers would, therefore, mean that a idioventricular/ventricular escape rhythm rate would be less than 60 bpm (less than 40 bpm in most dogs), accelerated idioventricular rhythm 60 to 120 bpm and ventricular tachycardia greater than 120 bpm. However, some cardiologists prefer to use the term accelerated idioventricular rhythm with rates up to 140 to 160 bpm and ventricular tachycardia for rates faster than 160 bpm. Others prefer to characterize ventricular tachycardia as slow or rapid. The range of ventricular tachycardia is usually 160 to 350 bpm in the dog. Examples in the progression of defining ventricular rhythms illustrate the difficulty in making absolute rate definitions (Fig. 10.1). When viewing these arrhythmias, the underlying sinus rhythm rate should also be noted. In some cases, particularly in polymorphic ventricular tachycardias in young dogs, rates as high as 450 bpm have been documented.

Describing tachycardia

There are different types of ventricular tachyarrhythmia, including monomorphic ventricular tachycardia, pleomorphic tachycardia, polymorphic ventricular tachycardia, bidirectional ventricular tachycardia and ventricular fibrillation. The attributes monomorphic, pleomorphic, polymorphic and bidirectional refer to the stable or variable morphology of the ventricular beats on the electrocardiogram during an episode of tachycardia. *Monomorphic* tachycardias are characterized by a single QRS complex morphology; *pleomorphic* tachycardias display different QRS complex morphologies (usually two), but the QRS complexes do not change on a beat-to-beat basis (each QRS morphology is represented by at least five or six consecutive beats); *polymorphic* tachycardias display beat-to-beat variation of the QRS complex morphology, which reflects a continuous change in the sequence of ventricular activation; *bidirectional* tachycardias show a beat-to-beat polarity switch of the QRS complex in the frontal plane.

Ventricular tachycardias can also be described by their "behavior" as non-sustained, sustained, repetitive, permanent (or incessant), or paroxysmal. Non-sustained tachycardias last less than 30 s, whereas sustained tachycardias exceed 30 s. Permanent or incessant ventricular tachycardias are sustained for most of the day. Repetitive ventricular tachycardias are characterized by frequent ventricular ectopic beats and non-sustained runs interspersed between sinus beats. A ventricular storm is said to be present when a hemodynamically unstable ventricular tachycardia that requires intravenous treatment occurs repeatedly during a 24-hour period. Ventricular tachycardia is called paroxysmal when it has an abrupt onset and termination.

Finally, ventricular rhythms that lead to significant hemodynamic compromise and the loss of a palpable arterial pulse are described as pulseless ventricular tachycardias.

This chapter includes a detailed description of the following arrhythmias:
- Monomorphic ventricular tachycardias:
    - accelerated idioventricular rhythm,
    - non-sustained monomorphic ventricular tachycardia,
    - repetitive monomorphic ventricular tachycardia,
    - sustained monomorphic ventricular tachycardia, and
    - ventricular flutter.
- Polymorphic ventricular tachycardias:
    - non-sustained polymorphic ventricular tachycardia,
    - repetitive polymorphic ventricular tachycardia, and
    - Torsade de pointes.
- Bidirectional ventricular tachycardia.
- Ventricular fibrillation.

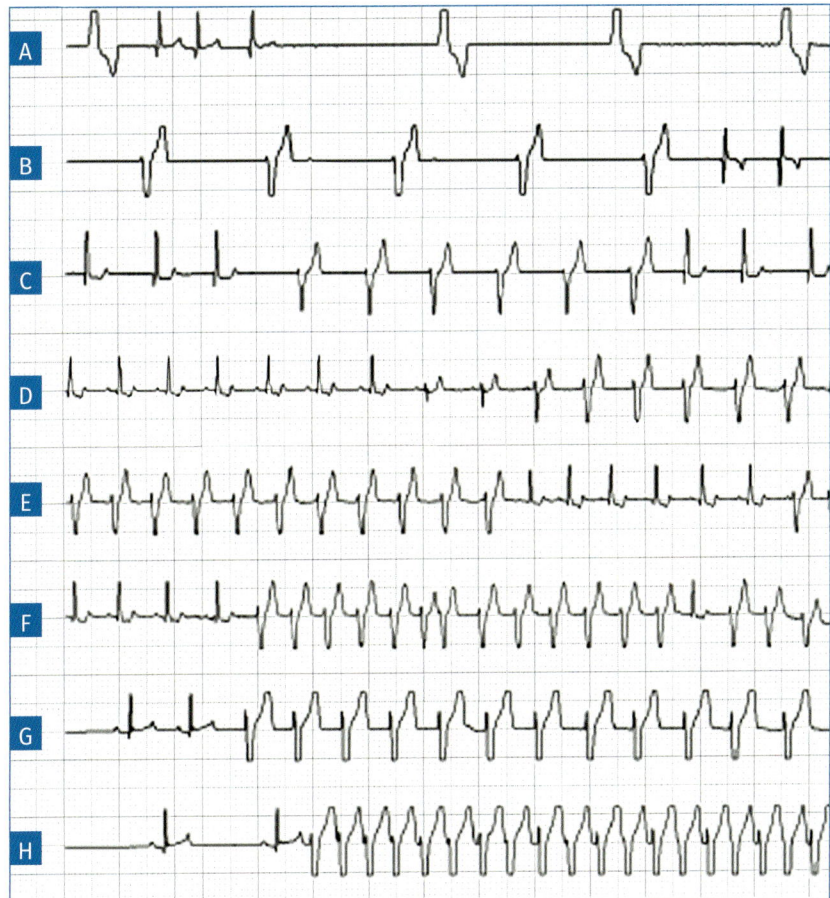

Figure 10.1. Electrocardiographic examples of ventricular rhythms at varying rates (Dog. Lead Y from a 24-hour electrocardiographic recording full disclosure image). When a ventricular rhythm is that of a high-rate escape rhythm or ventricular tachycardia the diagnosis is not as difficult as it is when the rate is between 120 and 160 bpm. In this latter range, accelerated idioventricular rhythm must be differentiated from a slow ventricular tachycardia. Most authors agree that the gray zone for distinguishing between accelerated idioventricular rhythm and ventricular tachycardia is somewhere between 120 and 160 bpm.

A) Recording from a dog with high degree atrioventricular block during atrial fibrillation. The ventricular rate is, on average, 37 bpm, which approximates the inherent rate of ventricular Purkinje cells. Idioventricular rhythm or escape rhythm.

B) Recording from a dog with a ventricular rate of 53 bpm, which exceeds the "usual" inherent ventricular rate. Ventricular escape rhythm or idioventricular rhythm rates can vary with the age of a dog and underlying disease, but are usually between 20 and 40 bpm.

C) Recording from a dog with a ventricular rate of 100 bpm, which is within 10 % of the rate of the underlying sinus rhythm (97 to 115 bpm on the tracing). Accelerated idioventricular rhythm.

D) Recording from a dog with an average ventricular rate of 128 bpm, which approximates that of the sinus rhythm resulting in numerous fusion beats. The ventricular rate is within 10 % of the sinus rate at that time and that of the average rate for a dog. Accelerated idioventricular rhythm.

E) Recording from a dog with an average ventricular rate of 160 bpm, which approximates the elevated sinus rate here but which is well above the resting sinus rate of the dog. Because of these characteristics some would call this rhythm an accelerated idioventricular rhythm whereas others would call it ventricular tachycardia.

F) Recording made 10 minutes after that shown in E with an average ventricular rate of 203 bpm. It is interesting that this dog had a ventricular rhythm with the same morphology but a slower rate as that shown in E. It is important not to misdiagnose a slow ventricular tachycardia as an accelerated idioventricular rhythm, because the clinical importance of the former may be revealed with further examination. Ventricular tachycardia.

G) Recording from a dog with an average ventricular rate of 137 bpm. Accelerated idioventricular rhythm or slow ventricular tachycardia?

H) Recording from a dog with a ventricular rate of 245 bpm. This is a recording from the same dog as in (G), taken a few minutes later. Ventricular tachycardia.

Monomorphic ventricular tachycardias

Monomorphic ventricular tachycardias are defined as a sequence of four or more ventricular ectopic beats. The QRS complexes are commonly described as "wide and bizarre"; however, the term "bizarre" is ambiguous, with a connotation that the morphology is extremely irregular. Moreover, how irregular in appearance a QRS complex must be to be classified as bizarre is open to interpretation. It is usually true that ventricular ectopic beats have a prolonged QRS (greater than 70 ms in dogs and greater than 40 ms in cats), but the altered QRS morphology is better described as simply being different from that of normally conducted beats. Their mean electrical axis in the frontal plane is variable depending on their site of origin. All the ventricular beats of a monomorphic ventricular tachycardia share the same morphology.

Monomorphic ventricular tachycardias are classified according to their duration as sustained or non-sustained, and based on their behavior as incessant, repetitive, paroxysmal or non-paroxysmal.

Reentry is the most common electrophysiological mechanism responsible for monomorphic ventricular tachycardias, although triggered activity and abnormal automaticity cannot be ruled out. It is usually not possible to determine with absolute certainty the electrophysiological mechanism of an arrhythmia from an electrocardiographic recording.

The mechanism of reentry which is likely responsible for many of the monomorphic ventricular tachycardias is usually based on an anatomical substrate defined by areas of fibrosis and slow conduction (see p. 99). In addition to a substrate, triggers and modulating factors are considered to be necessary for the initiation and maintenance of arrhythmia. This concept was developed by Philippe Coumel, a French electrophysiologist, and for this reason, the three factors involved in the genesis of arrhythmias are usually identified as the "Coumel's triangle" (Fig. 10.2). The arrhythmia trigger is usually a ventricular ectopy. Common modulating factors include autonomic system imbalance, electrolyte abnormalities and excessive wall stress from volume and pressure overload. Among these various factors, elevations in sympathetic tone have a major role in the initiation and maintenance of arrhythmias. Adrenergic system activation increases cell automaticity and triggered activity, and can promote dispersion of refractoriness in the ventricular myocardium. The action of the sympathetic nervous system is mediated by the release of norepinephrine from the sympathetic fibers, and by circulating epinephrine released by the adrenal cortex. Neurogenic stimulation is active for a short period and its action is non-uniform because of the heterogeneous distribution of the sympathetic efferents to the ventricles. In contrast, the action of circulating catecholamines is more gradual, lasts longer and affects the different cardiac chambers equally. During exercise and sleep, large variations in autonomic tone can trigger arrhythmias, especially in animals with heart failure.

Monomorphic ventricular tachycardias are common with structural cardiac diseases, including dilated cardiomyopathy, arrhythmogenic right ventricular cardiomyopathy, ischemic cardiomyopathy, hypertrophic cardiomyopathy, restrictive cardiomyopathy, myocarditis, congenital and acquired valvular disease with congestive heart failure and cardiac neoplasia. They also accompany systemic diseases, including gastric dilation and volvulus, splenic tumors and torsion, neurologic disorders, pyometra, prostatitis, pancreatitis, anemia, uremia, endotoxemia, autoimmune diseases, electrolyte and

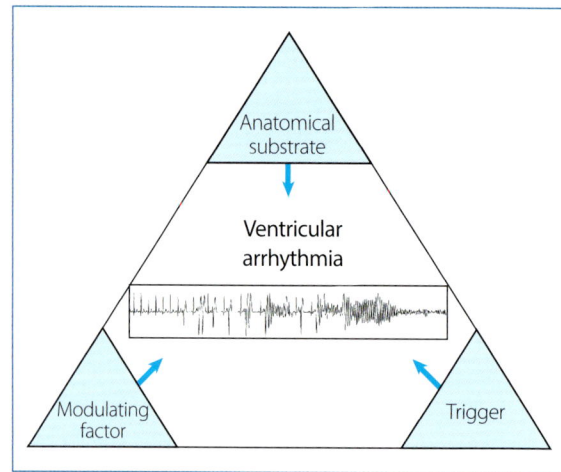

Figure 10.2. Coumel's triangle of arrhythmogenesis. Each vertex of the triangle corresponds to an etiopathogenic factor that contributes to the formation of arrhythmias: an anatomical substrate, triggers, and modulating factors. See text for explanations.

acid-base imbalances, and endocrinopathies. Monomorphic ventricular tachycardia can also result from trauma. Finally, antiarrhythmic drugs, chemotherapeutic agents, anesthetics and sedatives can trigger monomorphic ventricular tachycardias. It is worth noting that monomorphic ventricular tachycardia is rare in the absence of structural or systemic cardiac disease.

The electrocardiographic characteristics of monomorphic ventricular tachycardias include:
- wide QRS complexes (greater than 70 ms in dogs and greater than 40 ms in cats) with a single morphology in all leads,
- ventricular rate (usual rate 120 to 350 bpm); a cut-off of greater than 160 bpm can be used to distinguish them from accelerated idioventricular rhythm,
- usually regular R-R intervals (although the R-R interval may be more irregular at the beginning of a run),
- atrioventricular dissociation, and
- possible ventriculo-atrial retrograde conduction with a 1:1 to 2:1 ratio.

Monomorphic ventricular tachycardias have wide QRS complexes (greater than 70 ms in dogs and greater than 40 ms in cats) (Fig. 10.3) that differ markedly from normally conducted beats because electrical impulses form in the ventricles and have to travel within the working myocardium instead of the specialized intraventricular conduction system. Narrow (normal duration) QRS complex ventricular tachycardia is possible if the origin of the arrhythmia is in the Hisian region or the interventricular septum, and the impulse travels along the specialized conduction tissue for most of its path in the ventricles. However, even in this case, the morphology of the QRS complex typically differs from that of a normally conducted sinus beat. The main characteristic of monomorphic ventricular tachycardias is that all the QRS complexes are identical (*uniform*) when examined within each of the leads. In some cases, variations in morphology can be observed from one episode of stable tachycardia to the next, or during a single episode. These changes are described as *pleomorphism* (Fig. 10.4). Typically, there are sequences of at least five or six consecutive identical QRS complexes before a change in morphology becomes apparent. This phenomenon is thought to reflect a change in the path of activation of the ventricular myocardium in response to a change in the exit site of an anatomical reentrant circuit.

Depending on the site of origin of the arrhythmia, QRS complexes can have a left bundle branch block morphology with a wide, positive dominant deflection in the inferior leads (II, III and aVF) and in the left precordial leads (V_2-V_6) (Fig. 10.5), or a right bundle branch block morphology with a wide, negative dominant deflection in the inferior leads (II, III and aVF) and in the left precordial leads (V_2-V_6) (Fig. 10.6). Tachycardias with left bundle branch block morphology typically originate from the right ventricle, whereas those with a right bundle branch block morphology originate from the left ventricle. Although the terms left and right bundle branch block morphology are used to describe these arrhythmias, a detailed evaluation of the electrocardiogram reveals that the morphology of the QRS complexes during tachycardia does not completely match the characteristics of the QRS complexes during a typical bundle branch block,

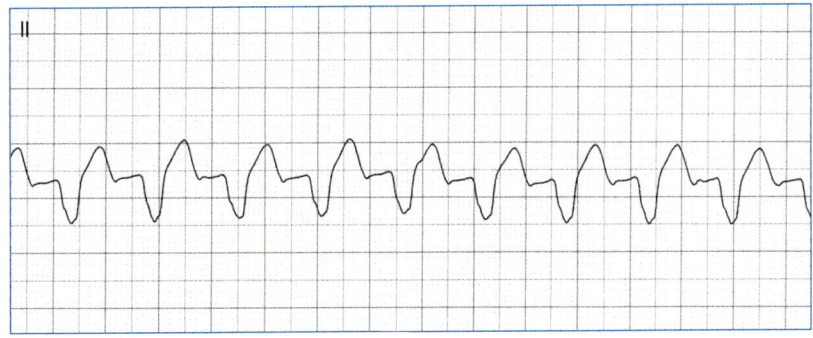

Figure 10.3. Monomorphic ventricular tachycardia (Dog, Labrador Retriever, male, 10 years. Lead II - speed 50 mm/s - calibration 5 mm/1 mV). The basal rhythm is a monomorphic ventricular tachycardia with a discharge rate of 190 bpm. Note the presence of wide QRS complexes (90 ms) with bizarre morphology. The QRS complexes have a single, uniform morphology. The R-R intervals are regular (320 ms).

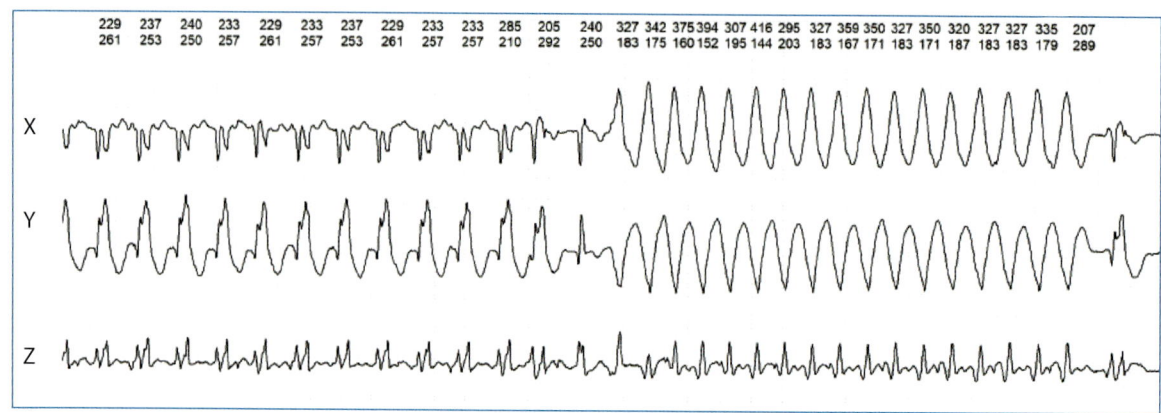

Figure 10.4. Monomorphic ventricular tachycardia with pleomorphism (Dog. Leads X, Y and Z from a 24-hour Holter recording - 8-second strip - calibration 5 mm/1 mV). The top set of numbers is the heart rate and the bottom set is the R-R interval. This electrocardiogram shows two different morphologies of ventricular tachycardia; however, the morphology is not continuously changing, which differentiates this rhythm, described as pleomorphic, from one that is polymorphic (ventricular tachycardia that changes on a beat-by-beat basis). Note the sinus beat separating the two rhythms.

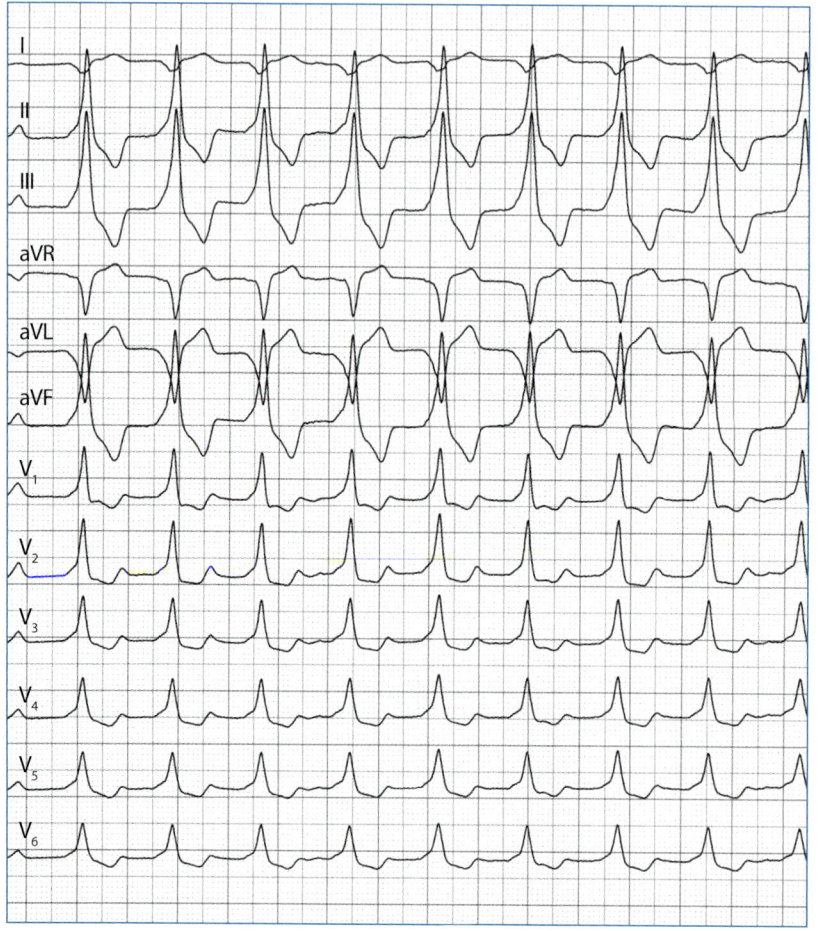

Figure 10.5. Monomorphic ventricular tachycardia with left bundle branch block type morphology (Dog, Siberian Husky, female, 2 years. Twelve leads (I, II, III, aVR, aVL, aVF, V_1, V_2, V_3, V_4, V_5, V_6) - speed 50 mm/s - calibration 5 mm/1 mV).

The basal rhythm is a monomorphic ventricular tachycardia with a ventricular rate of 185 bpm. The QRS complexes have an increased duration (100 ms) and left bundle branch block morphology with a larger positive deflection in the inferior leads (II, III and aVF) and left precordial leads (from V_2 to V_6). Note the presence of precordial positive concordance (V_1 = V_2-V_6). The R-R intervals are regular with a duration of 325 ms.

especially in lead V_1. That is, during ventricular tachycardia the QRS complex typically has the same polarity as the other precordial leads. This is referred to as *precordial concordance*, where V_1 through V_6 have a dominant deflection with the same polarity. English Bulldogs with arrhythmogenic right ventricular cardiomyopathy often have ventricular tachycardia arising from the right ventricular outflow tract with a left bundle branch morphology and precordial discordance (see p. 228). In such cases, since the QRS morphology in the 12-lead electrocardiogram is very similar to that of a supraventricular tachycardia conducted with bundle branch block, the identification of atrioventricular dissociation on the electrocardiogram becomes critical to establish a diagnosis of ventricular tachycardia.

Although most monomorphic ventricular tachycardias are regular, small variations in R-R cycle length can be present. These may be due, for example, to changes in the discharge rate of an automatic focus, or the electrophysiologic characteristics of a reentrant circuit.

Atrioventricular dissociation is a distinctive feature of ventricular tachycardias. On the electrocardiogram, atrioventricular dissociation is revealed by an analysis of the relationship between P waves and QRS complexes, or by the presence of fusion and capture beats.

The term atrioventricular dissociation refers to the concomitant but independent activation of the atria and ventricles. During atrioventricular dissociation, electrical impulses responsible for atrial activation do not reach the ventricles because they are in a refractory state.

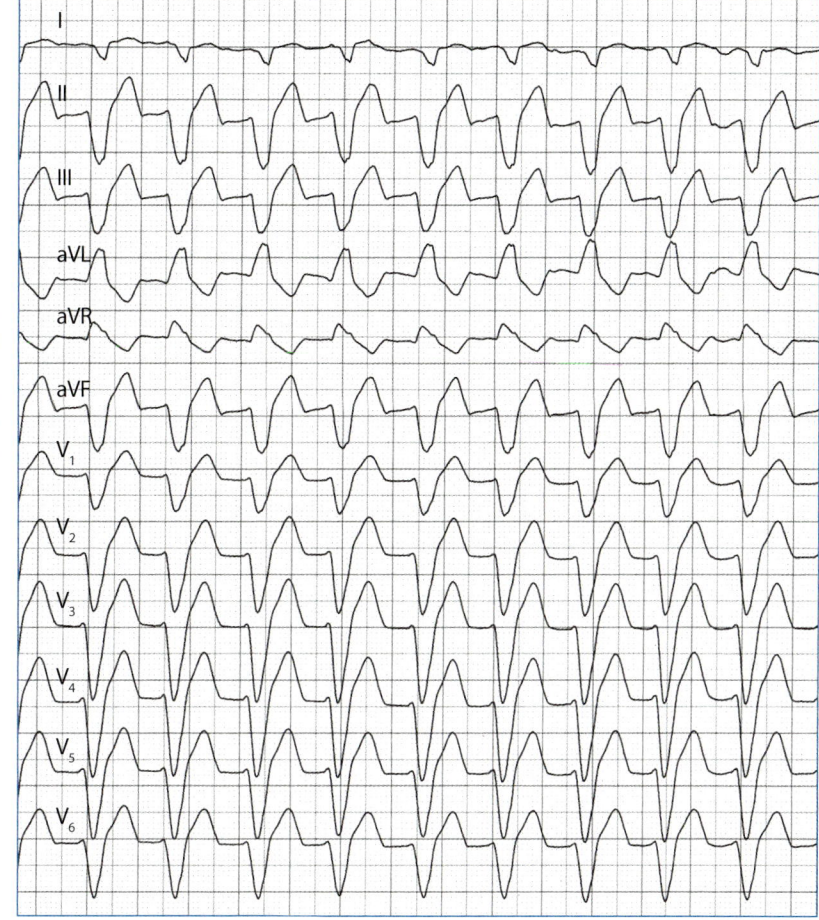

Figure 10.6. Monomorphic ventricular tachycardia with right bundle branch block type morphology (Dog, Labrador Retriever, male, 10 years. Twelve leads (I, II, III, aVR, aVL, aVF, V_1, V_2, V_3, V_4, V_5, V_6) - speed 50 mm/s - calibration 5 mm/1 mV).
The basal rhythm is a monomorphic ventricular tachycardia with a ventricular rate of 190 bpm. The QRS complexes have an increased duration (95 ms) and right bundle branch block morphology with the widest negative deflection occurring in the inferior leads (II, III and aVF) and in the left precordial leads (from V_2 to V_6). Note the presence of precordial negative concordance. The R-R intervals are regular with a duration of 320 ms.

As a result, sinus P waves can sometimes be seen before, after or within QRS complexes, without any fixed relationship between the atrial and ventricular waveforms. It is common that sinus P waves distort the ST segment, the T wave or the descending branch of the R wave (Fig. 10.7). However, variations in the ST segment and T wave morphology can also reflect alterations in repolarization during ventricular tachycardia, and notches in the descending segment of the R wave can occur secondary to changes in the direction of ventricular depolarization. This alteration of R wave morphology should not be confused with the J wave, which is visible at the end of the QRS complex (see p. 46).

In many electrocardiographic recordings during ventricular tachycardia, the presence of atrial activity is masked by the QRS-T complexes, which makes it more difficult to confirm the presence of atrioventricular dissociation. Other signs that support the presence of atrioventricular dissociation are fusion beats and intermittent capture beats. A *fusion beat* reflects the simultaneous activation of the ventricles by a supraventricular impulse (usually sinus in origin) and a ventricular ectopic beat. On the electrocardiogram, the QRS complex is preceded by a P wave and has an intermediate morphology between a normal QRS complex and the ectopic QRS complex (Fig. 10.8). The fusion beat does not interfere with the regularity of the tachycardia. A *capture beat* corresponds to a supraventricular impulse (usually sinus beat) that activates (or "captures") the ventricles before the subsequent ventricular ectopic beat. A capture beat has a P wave and a normal or slightly aberrant QRS complex morphology. It interferes with the regularity of the tachycardia, as it occurs at a faster rate than the tachycardia cycle length (Fig. 10.8).

On occasion, ventriculo-atrial retrograde conduction occurs in a 1:1 to 2:1 pattern. It appears on the electrocardiogram as a concentric retrograde ventriculo-atrial conduction, with P' waves inscribed within the ST segment of the ectopic ventricular beat. These P' waves that activate the atria from the atrioventricular junction have negative polarity in the inferior leads (II, III and aVF) and equally positive polarity in aVL and aVR, which corresponds to a mean electrical axis between –80 ° and –100 ° (Fig. 10.9).

The next section details the characteristics of the different types of monomorphic ventricular tachycardias including:
- accelerated idioventricular rhythm,
- non-sustained monomorphic ventricular tachycardia,
- repetitive monomorphic ventricular tachycardia,
- sustained monomorphic ventricular tachycardia, and
- ventricular flutter.

Accelerated idioventricular rhythm

An accelerated idioventricular rhythm is a ventricular ectopic rhythm formed by four or more ventricular beats with a rate that exceeds the depolarization rate of Purkinje fibers and is within 10 % of the underlying sinus rhythm it is competing with. In the dog, the rate is frequently approximately 60 to 120 bpm, but can reach up to 160 bpm. As described above, this suggested rate range for an accelerated idioventricular rhythm in the dog is based on a 10 % variation of two standard deviations of the mean heart rate (mean rate 83 bpm; median rate 81 bpm) in dogs with normal sinus node function.

Based on experimental studies the mechanism responsible for accelerated idioventricular rhythms is likely abnormal automaticity from a single focus within the Purkinje network, but reentry or triggered activity from delayed after-depolarization is also possible. In humans, triggered activity is more likely when accelerated idioventricular rhythms occur during post-ischemia reperfusion. In humans it is considered a benign arrhythmia, which is hemodynamically well-tolerated unless severe myocardial ischemia is present. It can also occur in association with digitalis toxicity.

On the electrocardiogram, an accelerated idioventricular rhythm is recognized by a sequence of four or more broad QRS complexes (greater than 70 ms in dogs and greater than 40 ms in cats) which frequently have a right bundle branch block morphology. In most cases, the morphology of the QRS complexes remains constant in any single lead, although pleomorphism can be present. Because the rate of this arrhythmia is very close to the rate of the underlying sinus beats, the two rhythms may be seen to "compete" on the electrocardiogram. When the sinus rate exceeds the rate of the ventricular ectopies, the arrhythmia dissipates. Conversely,

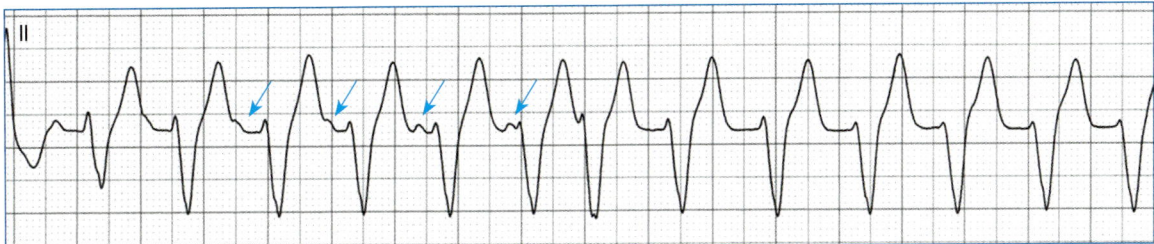

Figure 10.7. Monomorphic ventricular tachycardia with atrioventricular dissociation (Dog, Maremmano Shepherd, male, 6 years old. Lead II - speed 50 mm/s - calibration 5 mm/1 mV).
The basal rhythm is a monomorphic ventricular tachycardia with a discharge rate between 230 and 300 bpm. The QRS complexes have an increased duration (80 mms) and a morphology of right bundle branch block type. Note the presence of sinus P waves (arrows) dissociated from the ectopic QRS complexes with variable PQ intervals. The R-R intervals are irregular with a duration of 200 to 260 ms.

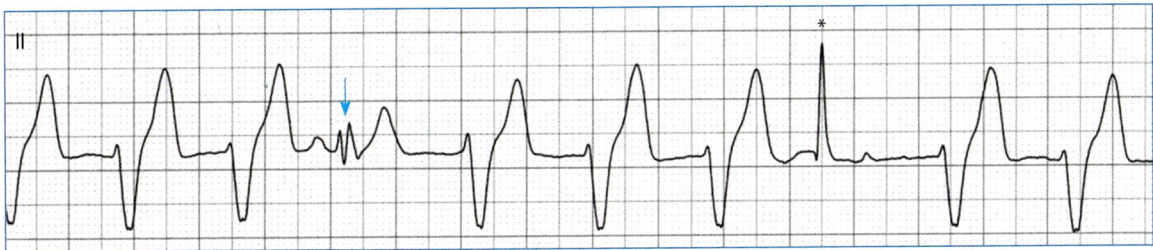

Figure 10.8. Monomorphic ventricular tachycardia with fusion beats and intermittent capture beats (Dog, Labrador Retriever, female, 9 years. Lead II - speed 50 mm/s - calibration 10 mm/1 mV).
The first, second, fourth, fifth, sixth and eighth QRS complexes have increased duration (80 ms) and a right bundle branch block-type morphology. The R-R intervals are irregular with a duration of between 320 and 370 ms. Note the presence of a fusion beat (arrow) with an intermediate morphology between the sinus QRS complex and the ectopic QRS complex and an intermittent capture beat (*) interrupting the tachycardia.

Figure 10.9. Accelerated idioventricular rhythm with 1:1 retro-conduction (Dog, Labrador Retriever, female, 11 years. Limb leads (I, II, III, aVR, aVL, aVF) - speed 50 mm/s - calibration 10 mm/1 mV).
The basal rhythm is an idioventricular accelerated rhythm with a ventricular rate of 158 bpm. The QRS complexes have increased duration (90 ms) and a right bundle branch block-type morphology. Note the presence of atrial retro-conduction characterized by concentric retrograde P' waves (arrows) inscribed in the ST segment. The P' waves show negative polarity in the inferior leads (II, III and aVF) and are equally positive in aVR and aVL with the electrical axis in the frontal plane being −90 °. The R-R intervals are regular with a duration of 380 ms.

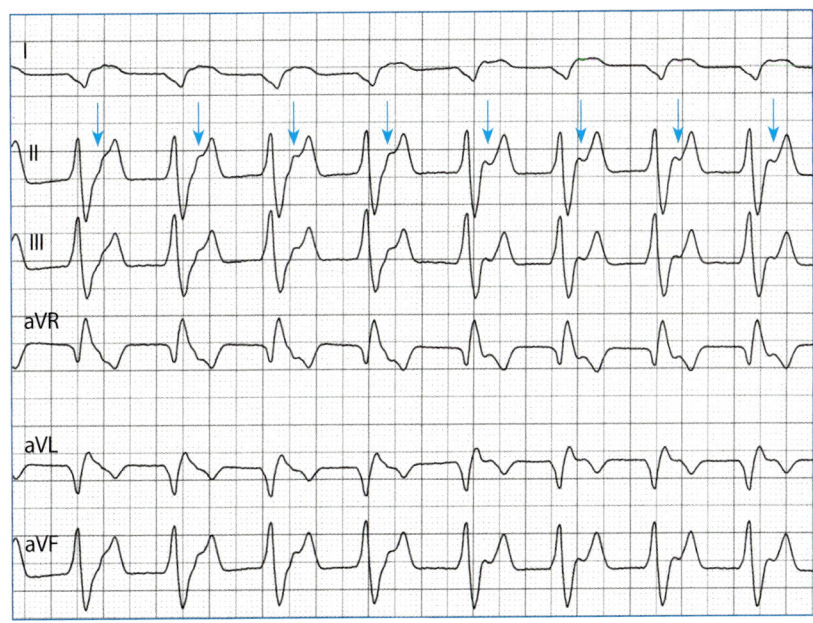

during periods of slower sinus rate, for example during sleep, the accelerated idioventricular rhythm becomes the dominant rhythm. Frequently the accelerated idioventricular rhythm begins and ends with a fusion beat, which demonstrates the competition between the two pacing sites to gain control of the ventricular rate. Another consequence of the presence of two rhythms with similar rates is periods of isorhythmic atrioventricular dissociation. These are characterized by the presence of P waves with a sinus axis that are dissociated from the ectopic QRS complexes but follow various patterns of synchronization (see p. 150). On occasion, ventriculo-atrial retrograde conduction occurs, particularly when the discharge rate of the ventricular ectopic rhythm exceeds the firing rate of the sinus node. Upon initiation, the rate of the ectopic rhythm usually increases gradually, which is common for automatic foci. Finally, accelerated idioventricular rhythms are non-sustained and repetitive, unless the sinus node rate is markedly depressed and the accelerated idioventricular rhythm becomes the dominant rhythm (Boxes 10.1 and 10.2).

Non-sustained monomorphic ventricular tachycardia

Non-sustained monomorphic ventricular tachycardia is characterized by the presence of runs of four or more premature ventricular ectopic beats with a single morphology in each lead, although pleomorphism can occasionally be present; its rate usually ranges between 160 to 350 bpm in both dogs and cats and it terminates spontaneously within 30 s. It should also be mentioned that the mechanism that initiates ventricular tachycardia may not be the same as the mechanism that continues the rhythm; thus, a monomorphic ventricular tachycardia may be initiated by a couple of beats of different morphology (Fig.10.10). Non-sustained monomorphic ventricular tachycardia is frequently paroxysmal, namely it starts and ends abruptly (Fig. 10.11).

Repetitive monomorphic ventricular tachycardia

Repetitive monomorphic ventricular tachycardia is characterized by repeated episodes of non-sustained or sustained monomorphic ventricular tachycardia. A few sinus beats or short periods of sinus rhythm are interspersed between episodes (Fig. 10.12). Isolated ventricular premature beats, couplets and triplets that share the morphology of the QRS complexes during tachycardia can be present. The arrhythmia usually begins with a progressive shortening of the R-R intervals ("warm-up") and there is progressive lengthening of the R-R intervals when it terminates ("cool-down"). However, paroxysmal forms of repetitive monomorphic ventricular tachycardia can occur.

The likely mechanism of this arrhythmia in people is triggered activity from delayed after-depolarizations. The arrhythmia is more frequent during periods of elevated sympathetic tone (for example during exercise), which promotes delayed after-depolarizations by shortening the action potential and increasing intracellular calcium concentration. The mechanism in dogs is unkown.

Sustained monomorphic ventricular tachycardia

Sustained monomorphic ventricular tachycardia is a sequence of ventricular premature beats that display a single morphology in each lead, have a rate above 160 bpm in dogs and cats, and last more than 30 s. If the tachycardia lasts for most of the day (for example more than 12 hours), it is called incessant (Box 10.3). Pleomorphism can be present.

The most common electrophysiological mechanism responsible for sustained monomorphic ventricular tachycardia is reentry.

Different degrees of hemodynamic compromise result from monomorphic ventricular tachycardia including syncope, weakness, cardiogenic shock and arrhythmia-induced cardiomyopathy.

Dog, Great Dane, male, 7 years.
Limb leads (I, II, III, aVR, aVL, aVF) - speed 50 mm/s - calibration 5 mm/1 mV.

Note: accelerated idioventricular rhythm with a rate of 160 bpm. Note the presence of wide QRS complex (80 ms) with a single and uniform left bundle branch block morphology. The R-R intervals are regular with a duration of 375 ms. P waves (arrows) with sinus axis, dissociated from the QRS complex with a rate similar to the ventricular rate.

Monomorphic ventricular tachycardias

BOX 10.1.
ACCELERATED IDIOVENTRICULAR RHYTHM IN THE DOG

HEART RATE: 60-160 bpm.
R-R INTERVAL: usually regular.
P WAVE: present with sinus axis if periods of sinus rhythm or isorhythmic atrioventricular dissociation or P' waves with concentric inferior-superior axis during ventriculo-atrial conduction
ATRIOVENTRICULAR CONDUCTION: absent.
PQ INTERVAL: variable.
QRS COMPLEX: wide (>70 ms) with right or left bundle branch block morphology; usually monomorphic, occasional pleomorphism. Presence of fusion beats or intermittent capture beats.
VENTRICULO-ATRIAL CONDUCTION: absent or rarely present with conduction ratio from 1:1 to 2:1.
BLOCKED BEATS: yes, sinus P waves occuring when the ventricles are refractory, unless a fusion beat occurs.
ONSET AND TERMINATION: gradual, often with fusion beats or capture beats. The onset is characterized by a long coupling interval.

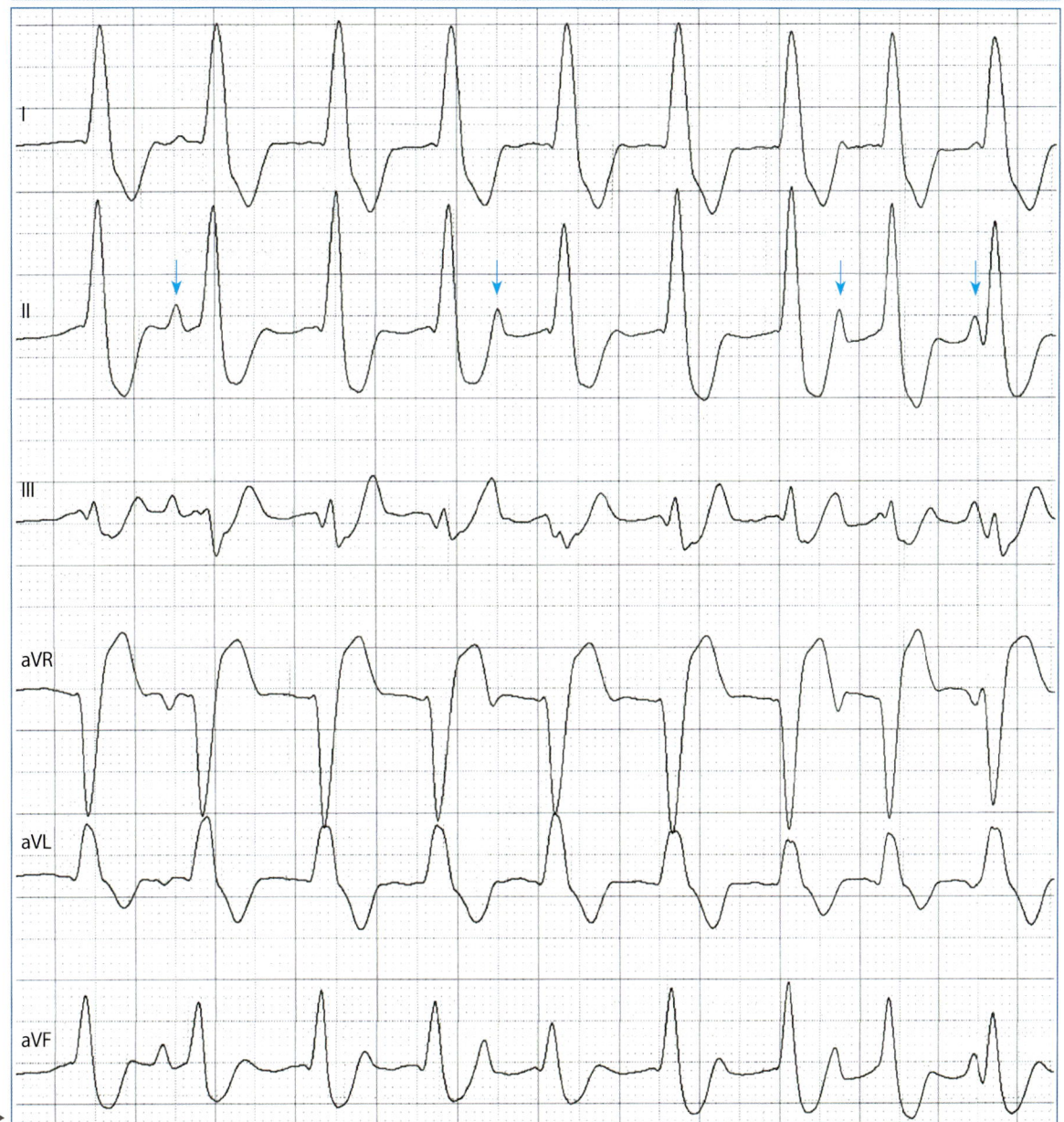

Chapter 10. Ventricular arrhythmias

> **BOX 10.2.**
> **ACCELERATED IDIOVENTRICULAR RHYTHM IN THE CAT**
>
> **HEART RATE:** 60-160 bpm. Usually within 10 % of the rate of the underlying sinus rhythm.
> **R-R INTERVAL:** usually regular.
> **P WAVE:** present with sinus axis during periods of sinus rhythm and isorhythmic atrioventricular dissociation or P' waves with concentric inferior-superior axis during ventriculo-atrial conduction.
> **ATRIOVENTRICULAR CONDUCTION:** absent.
> **PQ INTERVAL:** variable.
> **QRS COMPLEX:** wide (>40 ms) with right or left bundle branch block morphology; usually monomorphic, occasional pleomorphism.
> Presence of fusion beats or intermittent capture beats.
> **VENTRICULO-ATRIAL CONDUCTION:** rarely present with conduction ratio from 1:1 to 2:1.
> **BLOCKED BEATS:** yes, sinus P waves occurring when the ventricles are refractory, unless a fusion beat occurs.
> **ONSET AND TERMINATION:** gradual, often with fusion beats and capture beats. The onset is characterized by a long coupling interval.
>
>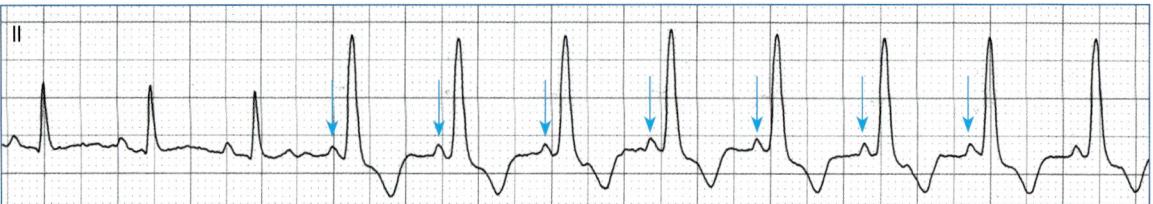
>
> Cat, Russian Blue, male, 8 months.
> Lead II - speed 50 mm/s - calibration 10 mm/1 mV.
>
> Notes: idioventricular accelerated rhythm with a rate of 176 bpm. The first 3 beats are sinus with a frequency of 180 bpm, followed by an accelerated idioventricular rhythm characterized by wide QRS complexes (60 ms) with a single, uniform left bundle branch block morphology. The R-R intervals are regular with a duration of 340 ms. P waves (arrows) with sinus axis are dissociated from the QRS complexes, with an atrial rate similar to the ventricular rate and with a constant PQ interval, corresponding to isorhythmic atrioventricular dissociation with type II synchronization.

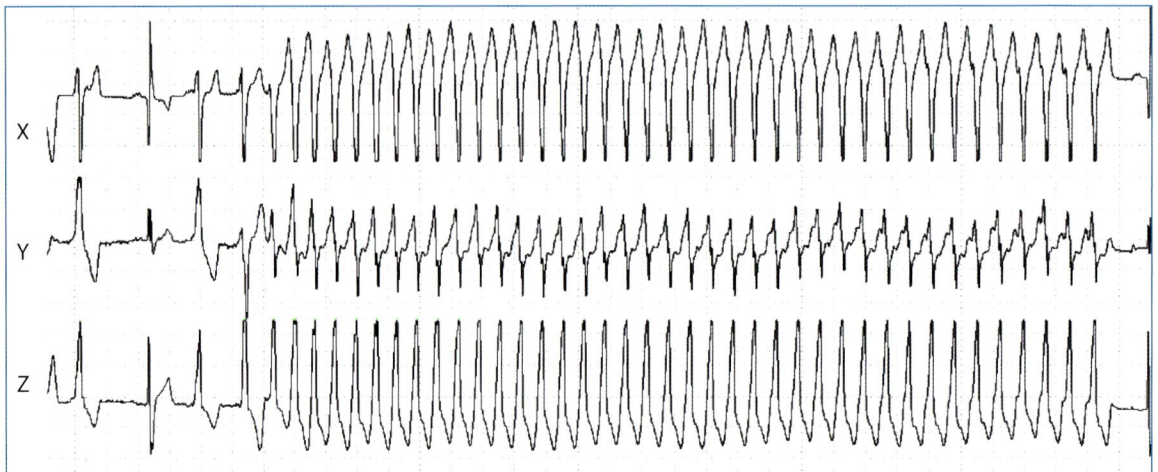

Figure 10.10. Non-sustained monomorphic ventricular tachycardia. (Dog. Leads X, Y and Z from a 24-hour electrocardiographic recording full disclosure image). This electrocardiogram illustrates a monomorphic ventricular tachycardia that is initiated by three ventricular complexes (beats 3, 4 and 5 from the left) following a sinus beat (capture beat) which have different morphology and R-R intervals. This type of pattern is relatively common when examining ventricular arrhythmias on 24-hour Holter recordings from dogs. The exact mechanism underlying this observation is unknown, because electrophysiological studies are not yet available. Possibilities include the stabilization of a reentrant loop or two different mechanisms responsible for the initial polymorphic beats and the subsequent monomorphic ventricular tachycardia. Often this type of pattern can be seen repeating throughout a 24-hour recording.

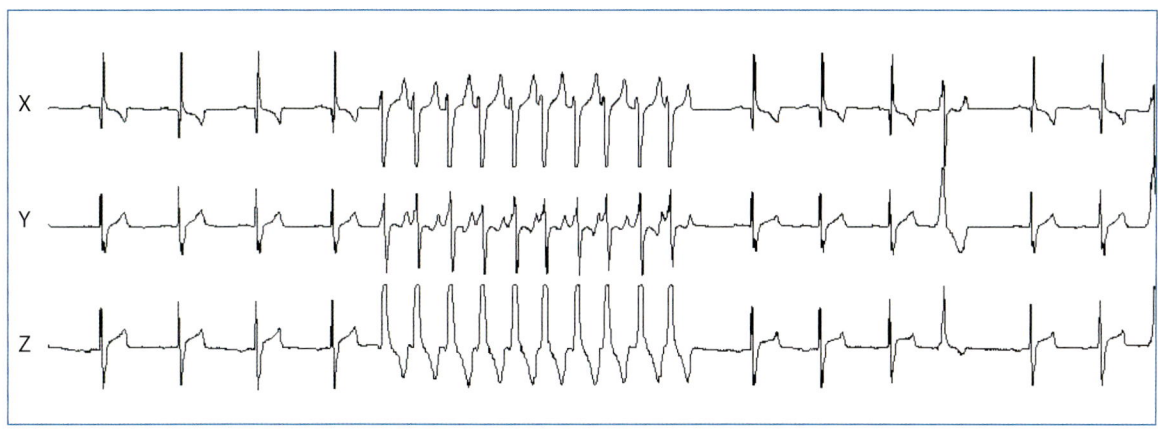

Figure 10.11. Paroxysmal non-sustained monomorphic ventricular tachycardia. (Dog. Leads X, Y and Z from a 24-hour electrocardiographic recording). A brief run of ventricular tachycardia begins and stops abruptly. Note the single ventricular premature beat (third beat from the right) that has a different morphology from those involved in the run of ventricular tachycardia.

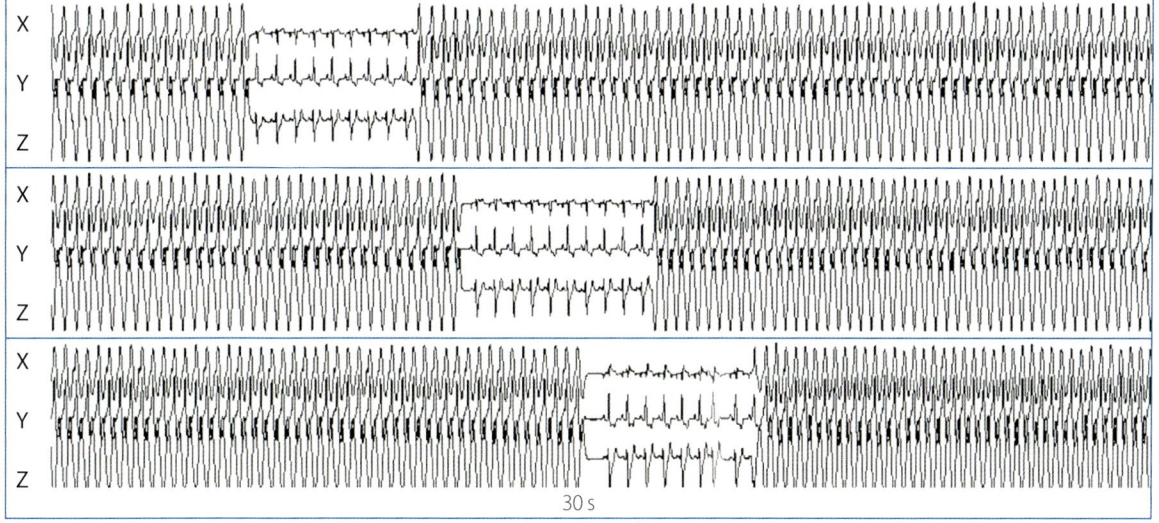

Figure 10.12. Repetitive monomorphic ventricular tachycardia. (Dog. Leads X, Y and Z from a 24-hour electrocardiographic recording). Runs of ventricular tachycardia are interrupted by sinus rhythm, but the ectopic rhythm repeats and repeats.

Ventricular flutter

Ventricular flutter is a rapid and regular monomorphic ventricular tachycardia characterized by a sinusoidal waveform, which, at least in some leads, does not allow the distinction between QRS complexes and T waves. Moreover, it is not possible to identify the isoelectric line between two QRST complexes. In veterinary medicine a specific cutoff rate has not been established to separate ventricular flutter from monomorphic ventricular tachycardia, although, in dogs and cats, rates above 350 bpm are needed to obtain the typical electrocardiographic appearance of this arrhythmia (Fig. 10.13). It is important to note that ventricular flutter is not a well-defined entity, other than being a very rapid ventricular tachycardia.

Ventricular flutter is associated with severe hemodynamic compromise, is non-sustained with a paroxysmal behavior, and frequently degenerates into ventricular fibrillation. Ventricular flutter is a pulseless ventricular tachycardia and its occurrence is always considered a cardiac emergency.

BOX 10.3.
SUSTAINED MONOMORPHIC VENTRICULAR TACHYCARDIA IN THE DOG

HEART RATE: 160-350 bpm.
R-R INTERVAL: usually regular.
P WAVE: present, sinus axis during atrioventricular dissociation, otherwise P' waves with inferior-superior concentric axis during ventriculo-atrial conduction.
ATRIOVENTRICULAR CONDUCTION: absent.
PQ INTERVAL: variable.
QRS COMPLEX: wide (>70 ms) with right bundle branch block or left bundle branch block morphology, uniform with occasional pleomorphism. Occasional presence of fusion beats or capture beats.
VENTRICULO-ATRIAL CONDUCTION: absent or occasionally present with conduction ratios from 1:1 to 2:1.
BLOCKED BEATS: yes, all the P sinus waves during the tachycardia, unless a fusion or intermittent capture beats occur.
ONSET AND TERMINATION: sudden.

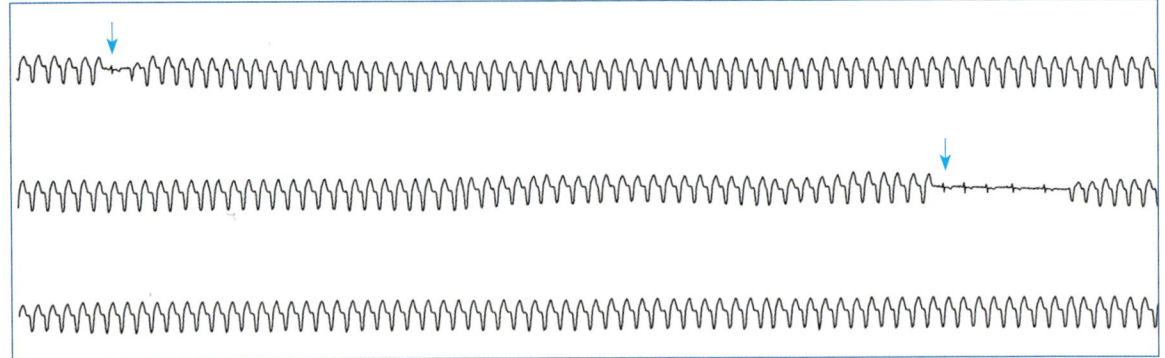

Dog, Doberman, Male, 6 years.
Holter monitoring, lead Y - speed 7.5 mm/s - calibration 2 mm/1 mV - Each line corresponds to 20 s of recording.

Notes: sustained monomorphic ventricular tachycardia with a frequency of 230 bpm. The episode of ventricular tachycardia is characterized by wide QRS complexes (90 ms) with a uniform right bundle branch block morphology. This tachycardia is sustained because it lasts more than 30 s. On two occasions, the ventricular tachycardia is interrupted by capture beats (arrows).

Polymorphic ventricular tachycardia

Polymorphic ventricular tachycardia is defined as a sequence of four or more ventricular premature beats with a rate above an arbitrary cutoff of 160 bpm in both dogs and cats and wide QRS complexes with variable morphology on a beat-to-beat basis. R-R intervals are usually slightly irregular.

Polymorphic ventricular tachycardias associated with QT (or QTU) segment prolongation are called *torsade de pointes* (French for "twisting of the points"). Polymorphic ventricular tachycardias in the absence of QT segment prolongation can be observed in animals with or without underlying structural cardiac disease. Catecholaminergic polymorphic ventricular tachycardia, and familial ventricular tachycardia in German Shepherd dogs are the most common examples of polymorphic ventricular tachycardia not associated with a long QT segment or structural cardiac disease. Polymorphic ventricular tachycardia with a normal QT segment can also occur with arrhythmogenic right ventricular cardiomyopathy, dilated cardiomyopathy and severe myocardial hypertrophy. Torsade de pointes-like polymorphic ventricular tachycardia has the electrocardiographic characteristics of torsade de pointes but the QT segment is normal during periods of sinus rhythm.

Polymorphic ventricular tachycardias are described by their duration as sustained or non-sustained, and by their behavior as incessant or repetitive.

Polymorphic ventricular tachycardia can result from reentry and triggered activity. Specifically, repetitive polymorphic ventricular tachycardia, which has been described in German Shepherd dogs is likely initiated by early after-depolarizations arising from the Purkinje fibers, and possibly maintained by a reentrant mechanism. Catecholaminergic polymorphic ventricular tachycardia

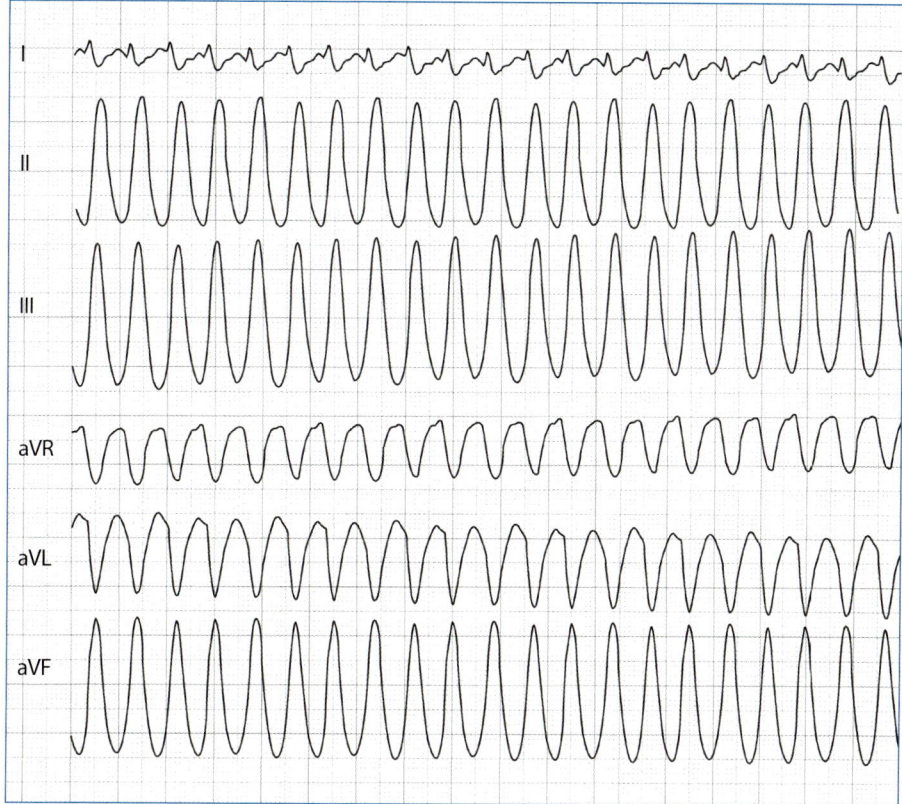

Figure 10.13. Ventricular flutter. (Dog. Six-lead electrocardiographic recording - speed 50 mm/s - calibration 5 mm/1 mV). The heart rate in this dog is approximately 365 bpm and it is difficult to delineate the QRS complex and T waves. It is also difficult to determine whether this is rapid monomorphic ventricular tachycardia or ventricular flutter.

is induced by triggered activity from delayed after-depolarizations. Torsade de pointes is initiated by early after-depolarizations secondary to delayed ventricular repolarization, which appears as a prolonged QT segment on the surface electrocardiogram. QT segment prolongation in people has been associated with mutations of genes coding for ion channel proteins, electrolyte disturbances (hypokalemia) and marked bradycardia.

The electrocardiographic findings during polymorphic ventricular tachycardia include:
- wide QRS complexes (greater than 70 ms in dogs and greater than 40 ms in cats) with beat-to-beat variation in morphology in all leads; it is important to realize that when a single lead is examined QRS complexes may look monomorphic, so they must be examined in all the leads,
- ventricular rate of 160 to 450 bpm (usually) in dogs and cats,
- irregular R-R intervals,
- atrioventricular dissociation, and
- possible 1:1 to 2:1 ventriculo-atrial conduction.

The next section describes the following different types of polymorphic ventricular tachycardia in detail:
- non-sustained polymorphic ventricular tachycardia,
- repetitive polymorphic ventricular tachycardia,
- sustained polymorphic ventricular tachycardia, and
- torsade de pointes.

Non-sustained polymorphic ventricular tachycardia

This tachycardia is formed by a sequence of four or more premature ventricular ectopic beats with a ventricular rate of 160 to 450 bpm in both dogs and cats and a beat-to-beat variation in QRS morphology in all leads. The tachycardia terminates spontaneously within 30 s and its behavior is usually paroxysmal (Fig. 10.14).

218 | Chapter 10. Ventricular arrhythmias

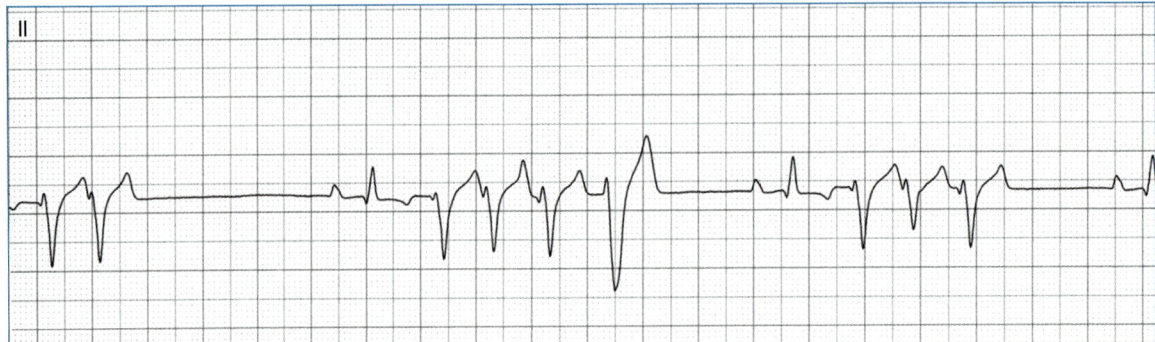

Figure 10.14. Non-sustained, repetitive, polymorphic ventricular tachycardia, (Dog, German Shepherd, female, 1 year. Lead II - speed 50 mm/s - calibration 5 mm/1 mV).
The first and sixth QRS complexes are sinus beats. These complexes are followed by premature ventricular ectopic beats organized, respectively, in a non-sustained run of ventricular tachycardia and in a triplet with a rate between 250 and 330 bpm. The QRS complexes have an increased duration (80 ms) with unstable morphology with beat-to-beat variations. R-R intervals are irregular and last between 180 and 240 ms. The polymorphic ventricular tachycardia is bradycardia-dependent and its onset is preceded by a long R-R interval.

Repetitive polymorphic ventricular tachycardia

Repetitive polymorphic ventricular tachycardia is characterized by repeated non-sustained or sustained episodes of polymorphic ventricular tachycardia. A few sinus beats or periods of normal sinus rhythm are interspersed between the episodes of tachycardia (Fig. 10.15). This type of tachycardia is characteristic of inherited ventricular arrhythmia in German Shepherd dogs. It is frequently accompanied by isolated premature ventricular ectopic beats, couplets and triplets. In this disease, the QRS complexes commonly have a right bundle branch block morphology, with a wider negative dominant deflection in the inferior leads (II, III and aVF) and in the left precordial leads (V_2-V_6).

Sustained polymorphic ventricular tachycardia

Sustained polymorphic ventricular tachycardia is characterized by a sequence of ventricular premature beats with a ventricular rate from 160 to 450 bpm, beat-to-beat variation in QRS morphology in all leads, and a duration that exceeds 30 s. The term sustained is also frequently used to describe polymorphic ventricular tachycardias that trigger syncope independently of their duration.

This form of ventricular tachycardia has not yet been described in dogs. In humans, it corresponds to catecholaminergic polymorphic ventricular tachycardia.

Torsade de pointes

Torsade de pointes is a polymorphic ventricular tachycardia associated with a prolonged QT segment during sinus rhythm. Torsade de pointes is a French term that can be translated as "twisting of the points", because the QRS complexes seem to rotate along an imaginary baseline on the electrocardiogram. The polarity of the QRS complexes therefore gradually varies between positive and negative values. The characteristic pattern of torsade de pointes may not be obvious in all leads. It is therefore critical to record a 6- or 12-lead electrocardiogram. On occasion, runs of monomorphic ventricular tachycardia may occur during torsade de pointes. A range of heart rates during torsade de pointes has not been established for dogs and cats, but it is likely that rates can exceed 500 bpm in dogs. Although, the heart rate is extremely rapid during this arrhythmia, a certain degree of organization of the electrical activity is still present in the ventricles.

The occurrence of torsade de pointes in human beings is associated with prolongation of the QT (or QTU) segment secondary to mutations of genes coding for ion channel proteins, electrolyte abnormalities (hypokalemia, hypomagnesemia, hypocalcemia), drugs (class Ia and III anti-arrhythmic agents, tricyclic antidepressants, phenothiazines, cisapride, erythromycin, haloperidol, and antihistamines) and extreme bradycardia (sinus bradycardia, sino-atrial block, sinus arrest, atrial silence or advanced atrioventricular block).

Polymorphic ventricular tachycardia

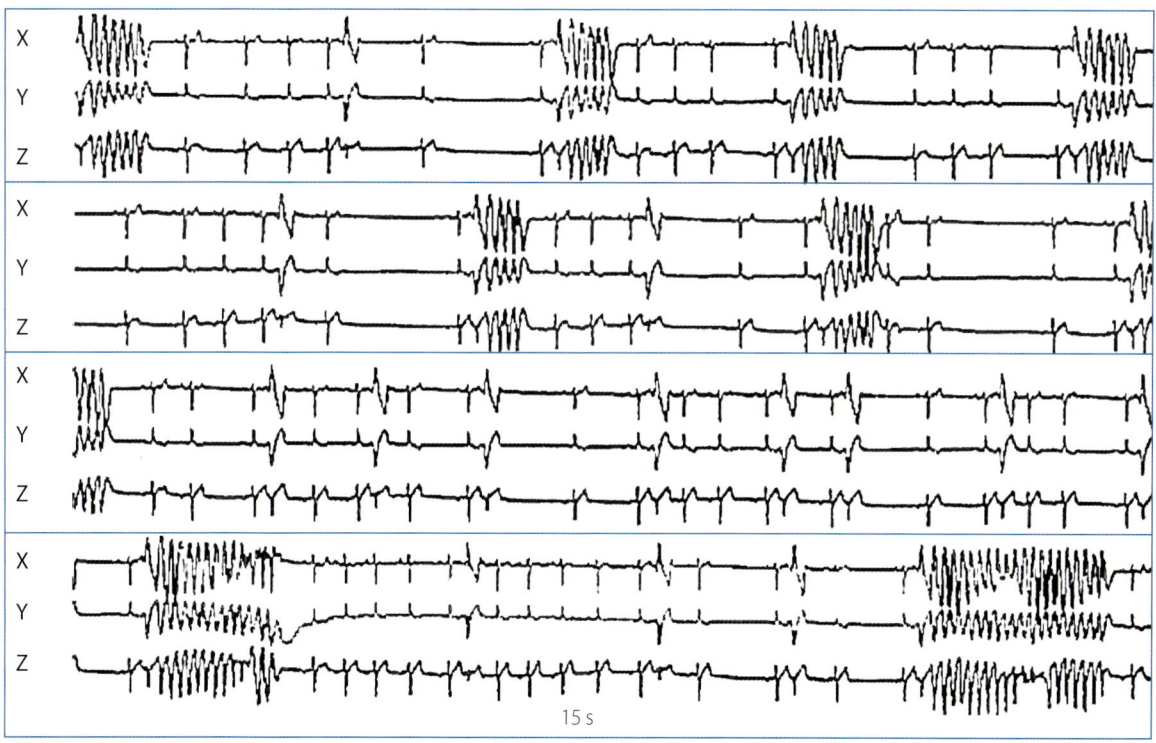

Figure 10.15. Repetitive polymorphic ventricular tachycardia. (Dog. Leads X, Y and Z from a 24-hour electrocardiographic recording full disclosure image).
Non-sustained runs of polymorphic ventricular tachycardia were recorded in a 7-month-old German Shepherd dog with inherited ventricular arrhythmias. Often the runs of ventricular tachycardia are preceded by longer sinus intervals. These runs of ventricular tachycardia were most prominent during sleep when the greatest number of long R-R intervals were present. The mechanism for these arrhythmias was determined to be early after-depolarizations.

Torsade de pointes is frequently triggered by a short-long-short sequence of beat intervals. The sequence starts with a ventricular premature beat that is followed by a post-ectopic pause before the next sinus beat. The long diastolic interval preceding the sinus beat results in prolongation of its QT segment (corresponding to prolongation of the ventricular myocyte action potential duration) triggering early after-depolarizations and initiating the tachycardia. Because not all regions of the ventricular myocardium are equally affected by the prolongation of action potential duration, the ventricles become electrically heterogeneous, which creates a substrate for maintaining the arrhythmia (see p. 97).

The electrocardiographic characteristics of torsade de pointes include a sequence of four or more ventricular ectopic beats with QRS complexes of continuously changing morphology, amplitude and polarity which seem to rotate around the axis formed by the baseline of the tracing. The mean ventricular rate during torsade de pointes in dogs could be greater than 500 bpm and R-R intervals are mostly regular. As for any other ventricular tachycardia atrioventricular dissociation is present but very difficult to identify because the baseline is not visible between QRS complexes. Although beat-to-beat variation of the morphology of the QRS complexes is a distinctive electrocardiographic feature of torsade de pointes, other electrocardiographic features that are useful to reach the diagnosis include a prolonged QT or QTU segment during sinus rhythm, a low baseline heart rate, a short-long-short sequence of beat cycle lengths just prior to the tachycardia, and T wave or U wave abnormalities and alternans. Rhythms that precede torsade de pointes include sinus bradycardia, sino-atrial block, sinus arrest, atrial standstill and third-degree atrioventricular block. Torsade de pointes is also frequently preceded by a period of ventricular bigeminy, with macro T wave alternans, which initiates the typical short-long-short sequence of beat cycle length variation before the tachycardia (Fig. 10.16).

Torsade de pointes can occur as brief paroxysms of tachycardia that terminate spontaneously, although it can also degenerate into ventricular fibrillation (Box 10.4). In dogs, it is more common to see polymorphic ventricular tachycardia that has the characteristics of torsade de pointes at the exception of a prolonged QT segment during sinus rhythm.

Bidirectional ventricular tachycardia

Bidirectional ventricular tachycardia is a sequence of four or more ventricular premature beats, with wide QRS complexes (greater than 70 ms in dogs and greater than 40 ms in cats) and beat-to-beat alternation of the ventricular complex morphology in the frontal plane.

The term bidirectional ventricular tachycardia refers to a heterogeneous group of arrhythmias that have similar electrocardiographic appearance, but are caused by different electrophysiologic mechanisms. The most common form of bidirectional ventricular tachycardia reported in people is secondary to digitalis toxicity. In the absence of digoxin toxicity, it is likely a manifestation of catecholaminergic polymorphic ventricular tachycardia.

Bidirectional ventricular tachycardia associated with digitalis toxicity is caused by enhanced automaticity of two or more foci, or a single ectopic focus with aberrant conduction, which propagates alternatively along the anterior and posterior fascicles of the left bundle branch. Delayed after-depolarizations have also been suggested as the arrhythmogenic mechanism for bidirectional ventricular tachycardia during digitalis toxicity.

The electrocardiographic features of bidirectional ventricular tachycardia include a sequence of four or more wide QRS complexes (greater than 70 ms in dogs and greater than 40 ms in cats) and beat-to-beat alternation of QRS complex morphology between a left and a right bundle branch block pattern. The R-R intervals are usually regular. There is atrioventricular dissociation or, occasionally, ventriculo-atrial retrograde conduction with a 1:1 to 2:1 ratio. Bidirectional ventricular tachycardia has a gradual onset, is sustained or non-sustained, and repetitive or incessant (Fig. 10.17).

Ventricular fibrillation

Ventricular fibrillation is an extremely rapid and apparently disorganized electrical activity in the ventricles. During ventricular fibrillation, the ventricular myocardium is simultaneously activated by a large number of rapid and continuously changing electrical wavefronts, associated with a complete loss of organized cardiac contraction. The electrocardiogram of ventricular fibrillation is characterized by the absence of clearly defined QRS complexes, which are replaced by a succession of irregular and rapid undulations of the baseline. Ventricular fibrillation leads to rapid loss of consciousness and death within minutes unless rapid access to electrical defibrillation is available.

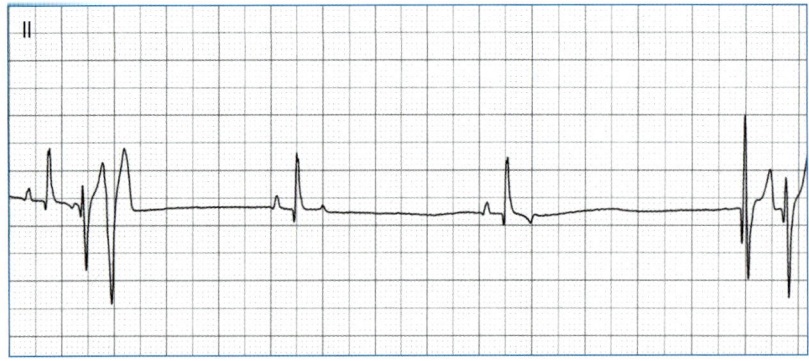

Figure 10.16. Macroscopic T-wave alternans with long QT interval (Dog, mixed breed, male, 4 years. Lead II - speed 25 mm/s - calibration 10 mm/1 mV).
The first, fourth and fifth QRS complexes are sinus. The first complex is followed by a couplet of ventricular ectopic beats with two different morphologies and a duration of 85 ms. Note the beat-to-beat variation of the T wave polarity and the presence of a prolonged QT interval (250 ms).

Historically, Wiggers described four temporal phases for ventricular fibrillation based on the direct observation of the surface of the dog's fibrillating heart: stage 1, or tachysystolic phase, lasted less than 1 s and corresponded to large amplitude ventricular contractions; stage 2, or the stage of convulsive incoordination, from 1 to 40 s after initiation; stage 3, or the stage of tremulous incoordination, from 40 s to 3 min; and finally, stage 4, or the stage of atonic incoordination. On the electrocardiogram, phase 1 is characterized by three to ten regular and repeatable large amplitude fluctuations of the baseline, which correspond to rapid ventricular

---

BOX 10.4.
POLYMORPHIC VENTRICULAR TACHYCARDIA MIMICKING TORSADE DES POINTES IN THE DOG

HEART RATE: >500 bpm.
R-R INTERVAL: usually regular.
P WAVE: present, sinus axis, dissociated from the QRS complex and usually not visible during the tachycardia.
ATRIOVENTRICULAR CONDUCTION: absent during the tachycardia.
PQ INTERVAL: not present.

QRS COMPLEX: wide (>70 ms) with variable morphology, and the appearance of rotating along an axis formed by the baseline of the tracing.
VENTRICULO-ATRIAL CONDUCTION: rarely detectable.
BLOCKED BEATS: yes, all the sinus P waves during tachycardia. However, usually not detectable.
ONSET AND TERMINATION: sudden onset preceded by the classic sequence short-long-short cycle length.

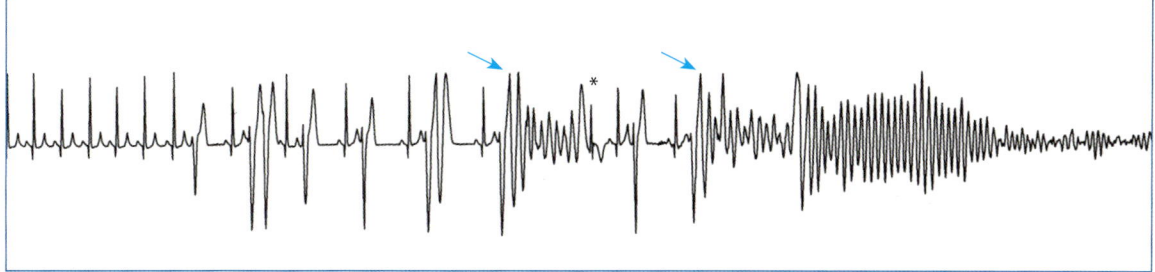

Dog, Labrador Retriever, male, 3 years
Holter monitoring, lead Y - speed 7.5 mm/s - calibration 2 mm/1 mV.

Notes: polymorphic ventricular tachycardia mimicking "torsade des pointes" with a rate of 750 bpm. Two episodes (arrows) of tachycardia are characterized by QRS complexes with continuously changing morphology, amplitude and polarity. The QRS complexes seem to rotate around an axis formed by the baseline. Both episodes are preceded by a ventricular premature beat with a short coupling interval that ends a short-long-short sequence. Also note before the first episode, the occurrence of premature ventricular ectopic beats arranged in couplets and bigeminy. This first episode is self-limiting and is interrupted by a capture beat (*), while the second episode degenerates into ventricular fibrillation.

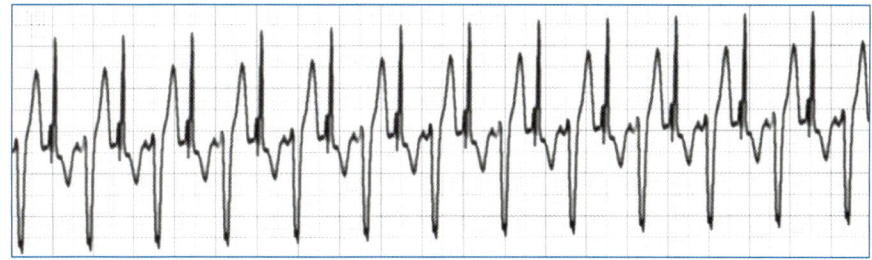

Figure 10.17. Bidirectional ventricular tachycardia (Dog, mixed-breed, male, 12 years. Lead II - speed 25 mm/s - calibration 10 mm/1 mV). Note the sequence of wide QRS complexes with a beat-to-beat alternation between a right bundle branch block morphology (80 ms) and left bundle branch block morphology (80 ms). The R-R intervals during tachycardia are regular with a cycle length of 340 ms.

tachycardia/flutter at the onset of fibrillation. The rhythm then becomes more irregular as the activation rate increases. The number of waveforms exceeds 600/min during phase 2 and is between 1100 and 1700/min during phase 3. Finally, phase 4 is associated with very small fluctuations of the baseline and rates below 400/min. Other descriptions of the stages of ventricular fibrillation based on rate and organization of the arrhythmia have been proposed, and support the initial observations made by Wiggers. Specifically, it appears that the reduction in fibrillation rate approximately two to three minutes after the onset of the arrhythmia, also indicates the time point beyond which intervention to terminate ventricular fibrillation is likely to fail. The effect of duration on the electrophysiological characteristics of ventricular fibrillation is largely attributed to ischemia and autonomic dysfunction secondary to the absence of myocardial perfusion during the arrhythmia.

Ventricular fibrillation is thought to be the most common cause of arrhythmia-related death in animals with structural cardiac disease and decreased contractility, including dilated cardiomyopathy, arrhythmogenic right ventricular cardiomyopathy, hypertrophic cardiomyopathy, myocarditis, ischemic cardiomyopathy, or acquired and congenital valvular diseases that lead to severe ventricular remodeling. Ventricular fibrillation can also result from electrolyte imbalances, alteration of autonomic tone, supraventricular arrhythmias conducting antegradely via an accessory pathway, electrical shock, cardiac trauma, inappropriate defibrillation or unsynchronized electrical cardioversion. A predisposition to sudden cardiac death from ventricular fibrillation has been identified in young German Shepherd dogs with familial ventricular arrhythmia.

The electrocardiographic features of ventricular fibrillation include rapid oscillations of the isoelectric line, and absent P waves, QRS complexes and T waves. The oscillations are of variable amplitude (*coarse versus fine ventricular fibrillation*) and their cycle length varies between 35 and 150 ms. Ventricular fibrillation is often preceded by arrhythmias that serve as triggers, including ventricular premature beats, monomorphic or polymorphic ventricular tachycardia and, less commonly, supraventricular tachycardias. Other electrocardiographic abnormalities that can be detected before the initiation of ventricular fibrillation include a prolongation of the QT segment and microvolt T wave alternans, which can only be identified by applying advanced analytic techniques to the electrocardiographic signal (Figs. 10.18, 10.19A and 10.19B).

Ventricular tachycardia without structural cardiac disease

It is estimated that approximately 10 % of human patients with ventricular tachycardia do not show evidence of structural cardiac disease. Ventricular arrhythmias and related syndromes that occur in the absence of structural cardiac disease include monomorphic ventricular premature beats originating from the right ventricle, ventricular tachycardia of the outflow tract of the right ventricle, ventricular tachycardia of the outflow tract of the left ventricle, idiopathic ventricular tachycardia of the left ventricle, idiopathic ventricular tachycardia sensitive to propranolol, catecholaminergic polymorphic ventricular tachycardia, Brugada syndrome, and congenital long QT syndrome.

Catecholaminergic polymorphic ventricular tachycardia, Brugada syndrome and long QT syndrome are inherited diseases caused in humans by mutations of genes coding for membrane ion channel proteins. Other idiopathic tachycardias that occur in the absence of structural cardiac disease do not seem to be inherited. These forms of tachycardia are classified according to the ventricle of origin, the response to pharmacologic tests or their association with the level of circulating catecholamines. Idiopathic ventricular tachycardias are monomorphic and can be sustained, non-sustained or repetitive.

So far in dogs, only three ventricular rhythm disorders have been recognized in the absence of structural cardiac disease: inherited ventricular arrhythmia in German Shepherd dogs, a form of congenital long QT syndrome in Springer Spaniels and a ventricular arrhythmia in Rhodesian Ridgebacks. Other breeds can be affected by the same arrhythmic disorders.

Figure 10.18. Ventricular fibrillation. (Dog. Leads X, Y and Z from a 24-hour electrocardiographic recording).
A run of rapid monomorphic ventricular tachycardia degenerating into ventricular fibrillation.

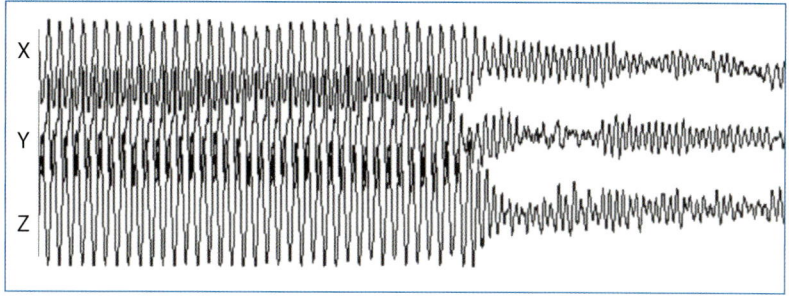

Figure 10.19. Ventricular fibrillation. (Dog. Leads X, Y and Z from a 24-hour electrocardiographic recording).
A) A monomorphic accelerated idioventricular rhythm (rate 80 bpm) is interrupted by a closely coupled premature ventricular complex, which initiates a short run of polymorphic ventricular tachycardia that degenerates into ventricular fibrillation. Note the coarseness of the ventricular fibrillation. The amplitude of the deflections becomes progressively smaller.
B) Induction of ventricular fibrillation with a low energy electrical shock timed to the peak of the T wave (vulnerable period) of a sinus beat in a dog during implantable cardioverter defibrillator testing. The shock is followed by a brief episode of rapid ventricular tachycardia corresponding to stage 1 (tachysystolic stage) of ventricular fibrillation described by Wiggers. The rhythm then transitions to ventricular fibrillation (stage 2). Progression to stage 3 (not displayed in this figure) is associated with an increase in ventricular fibrillation waveform frequency.

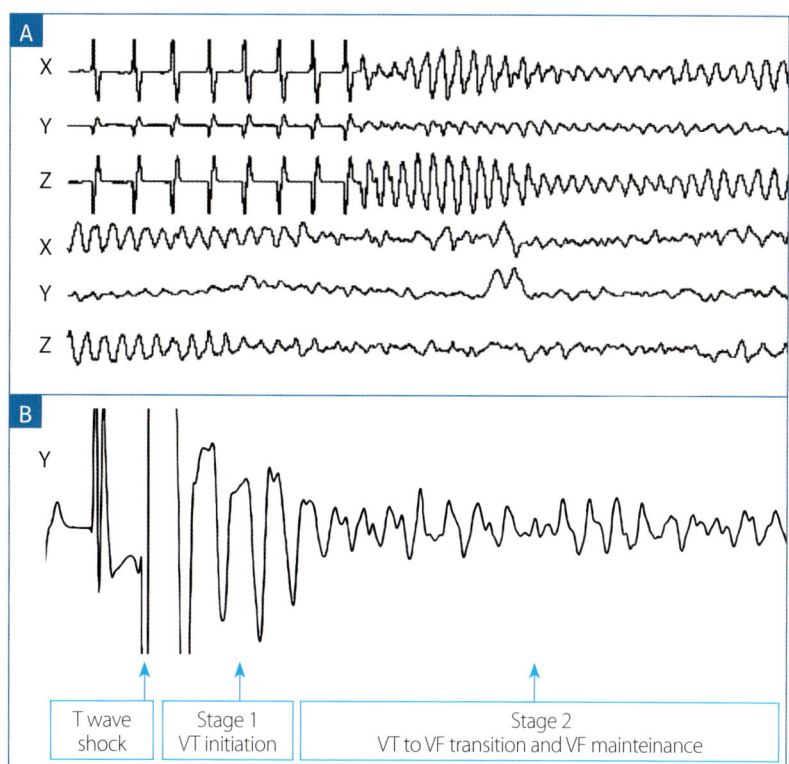

Inherited ventricular arrhythmia in German Shepherd dogs

Inherited ventricular arrhythmia in German Shepherd dogs is a repetitive, non-sustained polymorphic ventricular tachycardia. Its onset is usually around 12 weeks of age. The arrhythmia tends to worsen until approximately the age of 24 to 30 weeks and then the ventricular load and severity decline such that by the age of 18 months most affected dogs have had a substantial decrease in ventricular arrhythmias. By approximately 2 years of age most dogs will have few to no ectopies. Sudden cardiac death usually occurs within the first 4 to 18 months with a peak period of vulnerability between 4 and 12 months. It is more common that an affected dog will die during sleep, specifically in the early hours of the morning, or during recovery after a short period of exercise. Based on 24-hour electrocardiographic monitoring this disorder has a wide phenotypic range with some affected dogs having only a few premature ventricular complexes and others having tens of thousands. In addition to the variation in the total ventricular load the types of arrhythmia differ and include the following:

- Single ventricular premature complexes.
- Extended periods of time in ventricular bigeminy.
- Singlets, couplets and triplets.
- Rare salvos of non-sustained polymorphic ventricular tachycardia.
- Frequent runs of non-sustained repetitive very rapid (rates faster than 300 bpm) polymorphic ventricular tachycardia.
    - Dangerous runs with low total ventricular load (less than 10 % ventricular ectopy).
    - Dangerous runs with high total ventricular load (more than 25 % ventricular ectopy).
- Occasional sustained runs of monomorphic ventricular tachycardia.
- Infrequent premature atrial beats or short runs of atrial tachycardia.

The age at onset of these arrhythmias is variable and several 24-hour electrocardiographic recordings, beginning at approximately 4 months of age and separated by approximately 4-6 weeks, may therefore be needed to identify dogs at risk. Furthermore, identification of an affected dog requires 24-hour Holter monitoring and not in-hospital electrocardiography alone because the arrhythmias, and particularly ventricular tachycardia, may not occur during a short recording. In-hospital or Holter monitoring reveals that the polymorphic ventricular tachycardia is primarily pause-dependent (Fig.10.15) and the frequency is greatest during sleep. Single premature ventricular complexes, although more common in sleep may occur with or without a preceding pause. It should be noted that pacing severely affected dogs to prevent pauses does decrease the number of ventricular ectopies, but sudden death can still occur. If a dog has no arrhythmias identified by 12 months of age, it is unaffected, although if the animal is from an affected litter, it is still possible to produce affected offspring. The exact mode of inheritance has not been determined, nor has a mutation been discovered. Dogs with more than 10 runs of polymorphic ventricular tachycardia identified on any 24-hour Holter recording have a 50 % chance of sudden death. In contrast, dogs that have been assessed adequately by Holter and are free of any polymorphic ventricular tachycardia have a very remote chance of dying. Consequently, usually only dogs with frequent ventricular tachycardia (more than 3 premature complexes in a row) require treatment until full adulthood. Because repeated recordings are needed to diagnose these arrhythmias, provocation of the arrhythmias in certain situations may be helpful. Sedation or anesthesia that slows the heart rate will often expose an affected dog. Administration of phenylephrine to sedated dogs will also effectively expose affected animals. Although drugs that slow heart rate provoke the arrhythmias, these are very responsive to intravenous lidocaine. Adult dogs that were affected at a young age are not at risk of arrhythmic death. This disease is not associated with clinical signs, echocardiographic evidence of structural or functional disease or hematological abnormalities. In addition, the gross anatomy and histology of the heart are normal. Electron microscopy has identified ultrastructural changes in the mitochondria although these changes were not different from those seen with tachycardiomyopathy. However, even in the most severely affected dogs clinical recognition of tachycardiomyopathy is rare. This may be related to the amount of time a dog has high numbers of ectopies.

Polymorphic ventricular arrhythmias in German Shepherd dogs have been associated with abnormal sympathetic innervation of the myocardium, especially alpha-1 adrenergic fibers in the anterior portion of the interventricular septum and some regions of the left ventricular free wall. This could result in heterogeneity of the refractory periods within the ventricles and create a substrate that promotes arrhythmias. In addition, early after-depolarizations originating in the Purkinje fibers have been shown to initiate the tachycardia, although its maintenance could be dependent on a reentrant mechanism. Early after-depolarizations are more likely when the baseline action potential is prolonged. Accordingly, their origin in the Purkinje fibers can be in part explained by these cells having longer action potentials than other myocytes at baseline. It is also in agreement with the onset of the arrhythmia during bradycardia or after pauses, as a slow heart rate prolongs the action potential of myocytes. Delayed after-depolarizations were identified in dogs with monomorphic sustained ventricular tachycardia that occurred with faster heart rates. Finally, alterations in repolarizing currents, more specifically I_{to}, have been identified in affected dogs, and abnormalities in Ca^{2+} cycling contribute to the prolongation of the plateau phase of the action potential.

There is strong evidence to support the notion that the onset of ventricular arrhythmias is influenced by fluctuations in autonomic tone. Indeed, it has been shown that the frequency and severity of the arrhythmia increase during rapid eye movement (REM) sleep, which is a phase characterized by an abrupt interruption of high parasympathetic tone by adrenergic discharges.

The electrocardiographic characteristics of the inherited ventricular arrhythmia in German Shepherd dogs include ventricular premature beats with a predominantly right bundle branch block morphology, that is QRS complexes with a large negative deflection in the inferior leads (II, III and aVF) and a positive deflection in aVR and aVL; the left precordial leads (V_2-V_6) also display QRS complexes with a large negative deflection. These ventricular premature beats are often organized in couplets, triplets and short runs of ventricular tachycardia. In approximately 85 % of the cases, the ventricular tachycardia is rapid (rate above 300 bpm), polymorphic, non-sustained and repetitive. In approximately 15 % of the cases, the ventricular tachycardia is sustained, monomorphic and slower (approximately 200 bpm). The polymorphic form of ventricular tachycardia is bradycardia-dependent, in other words it is triggered by a long R-R interval. Conversely, the monomorphic form of ventricular tachycardia occurs during periods of elevated sinus rate. During longer runs of polymorphic ventricular tachycardia (approximately 15 to 30 ventricular premature beats), the arrhythmia mimics torsade de pointes. However, this arrhythmia is not associated with QT segment prolongation, although abnormalities in the T wave have been documented reflecting an abnormality in repolarization (Figs. 10.14 and 10.15).

Congenital long QT syndrome in the dog

Sudden death associated with increased activity and attributed to an inherited form of long QT syndrome has been documented in a family of English Springer Spaniels. The abnormal repolarization was believed to be due to a mutation of the *KCNQ1* gene as all dogs were heterozygous for the mutation. The *KCNQ1* gene codes for the alpha subunit of the potassium channel responsible for the I_{Ks} current. In humans, this gene is responsible for the most common type of long QT syndrome, long QT 1 syndrome, also known as Romano-Ward syndrome. Prolongation of action potential duration promotes early after-depolarizations and dispersion of refractoriness within the ventricular myocardium, as repolarization is altered to various degrees in epicardial, mid-myocardial and endocardial myocytes. All dogs carrying the mutation had a QT/TQ ratio greater than 1 (normal value usually less than 1), and the QT interval typically exceeded 260 ms (Fig. 10.20). In addition, a large biphasic T wave was also present in at least some leads (usually lead II), reflecting heterogeneous ventricular repolarization.

Ventricular arrhythmia and sudden death in Rhodesian Ridgebacks

Sudden death has been reported in a small number of apparently healthy male and female Rhodesian Ridgebacks between the age of 7 and 12 months. Death occurred during sleep or following a period of increased activity. No cardiovascular abnormalities were detected on necropsy. Evaluation of related dogs revealed ventricular arrhythmias that were more frequent and more complex (single ventricular premature beats, couplets, ventricular

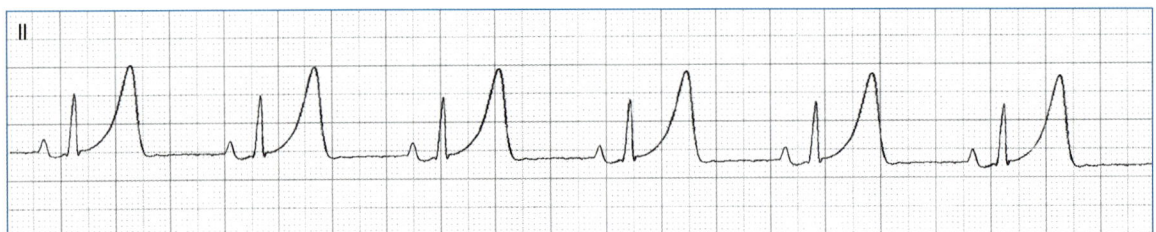

Figure 10.20. Congenital long QT syndrome (Dog, Springer Spaniel, female, 1 year. Lead II - speed 50 mm/s - calibration 10 mm/1 mV). The underlying rhythm is a sinus rhythm with a rate of 90 bpm. The P waves and QRS complexes have normal duration and axis in the frontal plane. The QT interval is severely prolonged at 300 ms. T waves have an abnormal morphology, including an increased amplitude and symmetrical branches.

tachycardia) in the littermates than in adult dogs. The exact cause of death was not identified. Based on the dogs' pedigree, the mode of inheritance was suspected to be autosomal recessive or autosomal dominant with incomplete penetrance.

Electrocardiographic findings characteristic of this familial arrhythmia include isolated polymorphic beats, couplets, allorhythmias and very commonly repetitive non-sustained episodes of polymorphic ventricular tachycardia. The arrhythmias commonly occur during rest or sleep and are abolished by a fast heart rate (Fig. 10.21). Many of the electrocardiographic characteristics found in Rhodesian Ridgeback puppies were very similar to those of the inherited arrhythmias identified in German Shepherd dogs. It should be noted that other breeds (e.g. Labrador Retrievers, Golden Retrievers) have also been found to have similar electrocardiographic phenotypes.

Ventricular tachycardia during familial dilated cardiomyopathy

Familial dilated cardiomyopathy is a myocardial disorder characterized by left ventricular or biventricular dilation and markedly decreased systolic function. Dilated cardiomyopathy is the second most prevalent heart disease in dogs after degenerative mitral valve disease. This myocardial disorder is known to be inherited in several breeds such as the Doberman, Great Dane, Newfoundland, Airedale Terrier, Labrador Retriever, St. Bernard, Pointer, Irish Wolfhound, Dalmatian, German Shepherd dog, American and English Cocker Spaniel, and finally the Portuguese Water Dog. Dogs with dilated cardiomyopathy have a propensity to ventricular arrhythmias and sudden cardiac death.

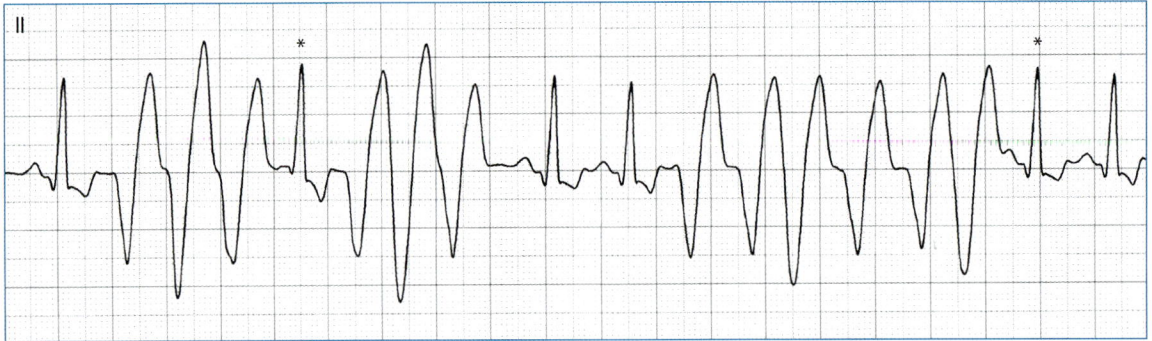

Figure 10.21. Familial ventricular arrhythmias in Rhodesian Ridgebacks (Dog, Rhodesian Ridgeback, male, 8 months. Lead II - speed 50 mm/s - calibration 10 mm/1 mV).
The underlying rhythm is a sinus rhythm. This is interrupted by triplets and runs of non-sustained polymorphic ventricular tachycardia with a QRS morphology that varies on a beat-to-beat basis and has a prolonged duration of 100 ms. The second and the fifth sinus beats (*) are capture beats.

Ventricular arrhythmias in the presence of dilated cardiomyopathy can result from enhanced automaticity, triggered activity and reentry. Alterations of ventricular geometry can form the substrate for anatomical reentry. Increased wall tension, reduction in the ventricular refractory period secondary to myocardial fiber stretching, high levels of circulating catecholamines and electrolyte disturbances also contribute to these arrhythmias.

Bundle branch reentrant ventricular tachycardia has been reported in humans with dilated cardiomyopathy and a left bundle branch block during sinus rhythm. This type of tachycardia might explain the characteristics of ventricular tachycardia in the Boxer, which is a macro-reentrant tachycardia characterized by anterograde conduction along the right bundle branch and retrograde conduction along the left bundle branch. It has the characteristics of a monomorphic ventricular tachycardia with left bundle branch block morphology. In humans it is associated with syncope and a risk of sudden death if it degenerates into ventricular fibrillation.

Ventricular arrhythmias are frequent in Dobermans with dilated cardiomyopathy. The rate of progression of the disease is variable, but typically it worsens rapidly and carries a poor prognosis if it occurs in younger dogs; its rate of progression is slower and it is associated with a better prognosis when the age of onset is 6 or 7 years. In Dobermans, clinical signs follow a long period called the subclinical or occult period during which one third of dogs die suddenly; the remaining cases are more likely to develop congestive heart failure. Electrocardiographic predictors of sudden cardiac death are the presence of ventricular tachycardia and the coupling interval of ventricular premature complexes (≤230 ms). Dobermans are frequently screened using 24-hour Holter monitoring to detect ventricular arrhythmias with the hope of identifying affected dogs before the onset of systolic dysfunction with the goal of excluding such dogs from breeding. Treatment of severe ventricular arrhythmias is problematic because of the poor systolic function in most affected dogs. Repeated evaluation is required not only to ascertain the effectiveness of treatment, but to identify pro-arrhythmic effects.

The electrocardiographic characteristics of ventricular arrhythmias during dilated cardiomyopathy include: premature ventricular ectopic beats usually with a right bundle branch block morphology, which can be organized in couplets, triplets, bigeminy, trigeminy, and non-sustained, repetitive, or sustained runs of monomorphic ventricular tachycardia. In some cases, monomorphic ventricular tachycardia is incessant. Other affected dogs can have non-sustained polymorphic ventricular tachycardia. The QRS complexes usually have a larger negative deflection in the inferior leads (II, III and aVF) and positive dominant deflection in aVR and aVL. The QRS complexes in the left precordial leads (V_2-V_6) have large negative deflections.

Ventricular tachycardias during arrhythmogenic cardiomyopathy

Arrhythmogenic (right ventricular) cardiomyopathy is a primary familial disease of the heart muscle, in which there are anatomical and functional alterations of the right and often also the left ventricle, resulting in progressive myocardial atrophy with fibro-adipose replacement. Familial arrhythmogenic cardiomyopathy has been described in Boxers and English Bulldogs, with sporadic forms documented in the German Dachshund, Bullmastiff, Siberian Husky, Labrador Retriever, and also in cats including Burmese, Birman and Domestic Shorthair.

In Boxers, arrhythmogenic right ventricular cardiomyopathy has an autosomal dominant mode of transmission. The disease is usually described to progress according to three stages. In the first stage, ventricular arrhythmias are present in the absence of clinical signs. In the second phase, dogs experience syncope and in some cases die suddenly, likely from ventricular fibrillation. This lethal arrhythmia is usually preceded by monomorphic ventricular tachycardia at a rate exceeding 200 to 300 bpm. Although affected dogs can die suddenly, many dogs live for years with the arrhythmia when efforts are made to control the occurrence of dangerous ventricular tachycardia. It is true that we do not know whether treatment extends life; however, the clinical signs of syncope are often documented to decrease in individual dogs as the arrhythmic load and severity decrease. Holter monitoring is required to manage the arrhythmias because in-hospital electrocardiography is usually inadequate. It is important to remember that the number and severity of the ventricular ectopy can vary by as much as 85 % on repeated day-to-day 24-hour recordings. Antiarrhythmic treatment must, therefore, produce a corresponding reduction in frequency to be able to be considered effective. Sotalol is often effective, but if not the addition of mexiletine may be helpful. Follow-up is required over months to years as the ventricular load and severity of the arrhythmia can increase and Boxers may develop concomitant supraventricular tachyarrhythmias. When the ventricular arrhythmias become multiform it is essential to examine the cardiac structure and function because these rhythms are often associated with disease extension to the left ventricle as dogs enter the third stage of the disease, which includes systolic dysfunction and congestive heart failure.

This disease has a broad phenotypic spectrum. Although a mutation in the striatin gene has been identified in affected Boxers, the fact that some dogs with a characteristic arrhythmic profile are negative for the mutation, indicates that other factors play a role. Nevertheless, it does appear that dogs homozygous for the gene mutation have more severe arrhythmias. In addition to the variation in the total ventricular load, the types of arrhythmia differ and include the following:
- single ventricular premature beats,
- couplets and triplets,
- nonsustained or sustained runs of monomorphic ventricular tachycardia that may or may not be repetitive, and
- occasional bradyarrhythmias and asystolic pauses that lead to syncope.

Most ventricular ectopic beats have a left bundle branch block morphology, that is QRS complexes with the widest positive deflection in the inferior leads (II, III and aVF) and in the left precordial leads (V_2-V_6). QRS complexes in leads I and V_1 have variable polarity depending on their site of origin in the right ventricle.

A particular variant of arrhythmogenic cardiomyopathy is a segmental form recognized in English Bulldogs. In these dogs, echocardiography reveals an aneurysmal dilation of the right ventricular outflow tract and a rapid and incessant monomorphic ventricular tachycardia.

This tachycardia usually has a left bundle branch block morphology with a superior-to-inferior axis, and a rate between 200 and 290 bpm. Accordingly, QRS complexes have their widest positive deflection in the inferior leads (II, III and aVF) and in the left precordial leads (V_2-V_6), and variable polarity in leads I, aVL and V_1 according to the site of origin within the right ventricular outflow tract (Figs. 10.22 and 10.23). Specifically, when ventricular tachycardia originates from the caudal free wall of the right ventricular outflow tract, lead I appears positive, leads II, III and aVF positive with notched R waves, lead aVL negative, lead V_1 negative and leads V_2-V_6 positive. A positive deflection in lead aVL suggests that the tachycardia arises within 2 cm of the pulmonary valve. When ventricular tachycardia originates from the cranial/septal portion of the right ventricular outflow tract lead I appears negative, leads II, III and aVF positive, lead aVL negative, lead V_1 isodiphasic and leads V_2-V_6 positive.

In cats with right ventricular arrhythmogenic cardiomyopathy, arrhythmias include ventricular premature beats with variable morphology, as well as monomorphic and polymorphic ventricular tachycardias.

Ventricular tachycardias during myocarditis

Ventricular arrhythmias are often a major recognized clinical feature of myocarditis. Although the specific diagnosis of myocarditis (which is different from endocarditis) is proven by endomyocardial biopsy or at postmortem examination, the use of troponin I has greatly facilitated the recognition of this disease in the presence of ventricular arrhythmias. Some affected dogs have markedly elevated concentrations of troponin I while others have more modest increases. This is the case in cats as well. In both dogs and in cats, myocarditis can result in progressive systolic dysfunction and various rhythm disturbances in addition to ventricular arrhythmias depending on the stage of the disease. Although the etiology cannot be determined in most cases, reported causes of myocarditis include viruses, protozoa, bacteria, fungi and non-infectious factors such as autoimmune reactions, toxins, and trauma. In particular *Bartonella* spp. has been isolated from the heart of the dog with inflammatory

Figure 10.22. Ventricular arrhythmias during arrhythmogenic right ventricular cardiomyopathy (Dog, English Bulldog, male, 9 years. Twelve leads (I, II, III, aVR, aVL, aVF, V_1, V_2, V_3, V_4, V_5, V_6) - speed 50 mm/s - calibration 5 mm/1 mV).

The dominant rhythm is a wide QRS tachycardia (QRS duration 100 ms) with a stable left bundle branch block type morphology and a ventricular rate of 250 bpm. Despite the concordance between the inferior limb leads and left precordial leads and the precordial discordance ($V_1 \neq V_2$-V_6), the diagnosis of sustained monomorphic ventricular tachycardia is based on the presence of atrioventricular dissociation (arrows). According to the morphology of the QRS complex the ventricular tachycardia probably originates from the caudal free wall of the right ventricular outflow tract since lead I appears positive, leads II, III and aVF positive with notched R waves, lead aVL negative, lead V_1 negative and leads V_2-V_6 positive.

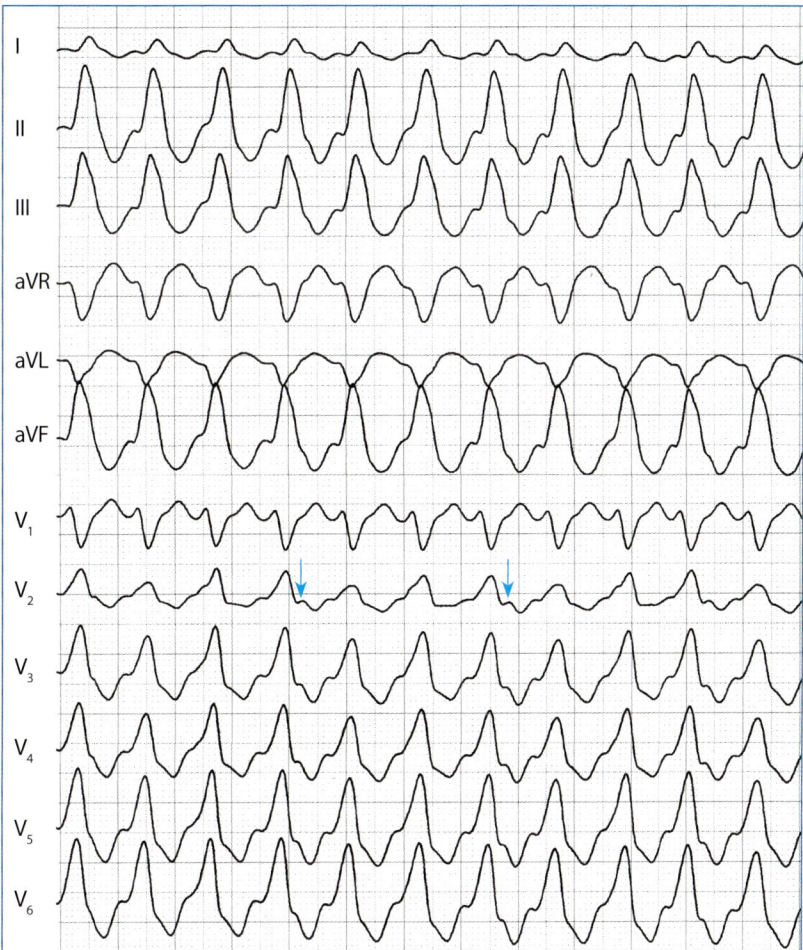

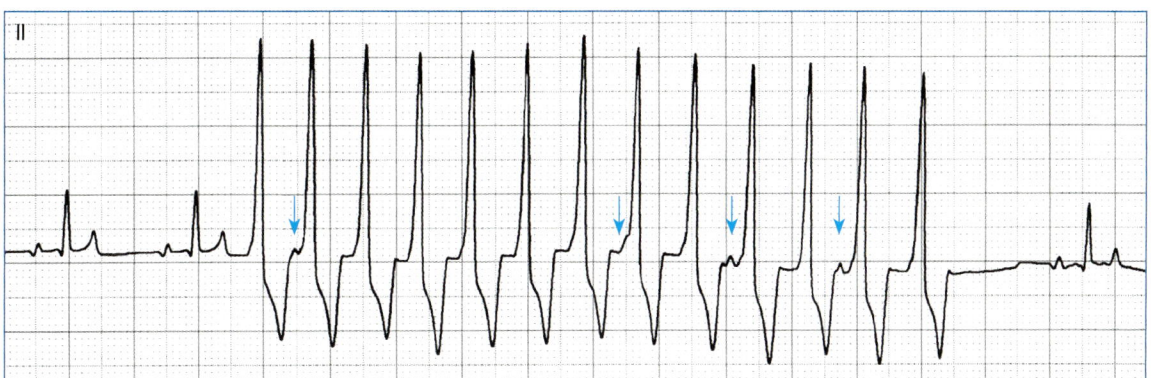

Figure 10.23. Ventricular arrhythmias during arrhythmogenic right ventricular cardiomyopathy (Dog, Boxer, male, 8 years. Lead II - speed 25 mm/s - calibration 10 mm/1 mV).
In the first part of the tracing normal sinus beats are present with a rate of 75 bpm. After the second beat there is a run of non-sustained monomorphic ventricular tachycardia with a ventricular rate of approximately 195 bpm and a left bundle branch block morphology. The duration of the QRS complex is 90 ms. Note the presence of sinus P waves (arrows) dissociated from the QRS complexes.

cardiomyopathy and in the cat with pyogranulomatous myocarditis and diaphragmatic myositis.

In the acute phase of myocarditis, acute necrosis and edema are induced by the replication of microorganisms and by cytotoxic molecules released by massive white blood cell infiltration. As a result, different degrees of atrioventricular and intraventricular block, supraventricular and ventricular arrhythmias can be present, including supraventricular and ventricular premature complexes, focal atrial tachycardia, accelerated idioventricular rhythm and various forms of ventricular tachycardia. Dogs with third-degree atrioventricular block requiring pacemaker implantation should likely be screened for myocarditis by determining troponin I levels. This is especially true if tachyarrhythmias are noted at the same time. In some dogs heart block resolves while arrhythmias persist. The chronic stage of myocarditis corresponds to replacement fibrosis and typically the development of a dilated cardiomyopathy phenotype. Arrhythmias continue to be detected but atrioventricular block is rare. Supraventricular and particularly ventricular arrhythmias can be documented. Supraventricular arrhythmias include atrial fibrillation, atrial flutter and focal atrial tachycardia. It should be noted that in some cases of myocarditis, it can be very difficult to control the ventricular arrhythmias with antiarrhythmic drugs. Dogs with therapeutically non-responsive ventricular tachycardia have been documented to develop ventricular fibrillation and die. Although controversial, some dogs respond to corticosteroids, as determined by the number of arrhythmias and troponin I levels.

Ventricular tachycardia during ischemic cardiomyopathy

Myocardial infarction in dogs is rare; however, in cats with hypertrophic cardiomyopathy, small vessel disease resulting in myocardial infarction of the left ventricular apex and left ventricular free wall has been repeatedly documented. The occurrence of *myocardial infarction* can trigger monomorphic sustained ventricular tachycardias that use the infarcted area as the anatomical substrate. The extent of myocardial necrosis and the degree of systolic dysfunction are the most important determinants of post-infarct arrhythmias.

Disease processes associated with myocardial infarction include severe hypertrophy, coronary arteriosclerosis and severe hypothyroidism. Ventricular tachycardias originate from myocytes localized within the extensive ischemic region where impulse conduction velocity is reduced and heterogeneous due to gap junction abnormalities.

Ventricular tachycardia during ventricular hypertrophy

Ventricular tachycardia may develop in dogs and cats with primary hypertrophic cardiomyopathy or with diseases that cause myocardial hypertrophy. Hypertrophic cardiomyopathy is a primary disorder of the myocardium characterized by concentric left ventricular hypertrophy in the absence of increased afterload. Hypertrophic cardiomyopathy is often the result of a genetic mutation and has been linked to the disease in some Maine Coon and Ragdoll cats. It is a familial disease in Persians, Norwegian cats, and also Dalmatians and Golden Retrievers.

In animals with hypertrophic cardiomyopathy, contributing factors to ventricular arrhythmias include the disorganized architecture of the left ventricular myocardium and the presence of ischemic areas. In this disease, the risk of myocardial ischemia is increased by the presence of coronary artery arteriosclerosis. In addition, ventricular tachycardia could be triggered by acute dynamic obstruction within the left ventricular outflow tract.

Arrhythmias are also reported with ventricular hypertrophy secondary to pressure overload, including subaortic stenosis, pulmonary valve stenosis, and systemic or pulmonary hypertension. Arrhythmias are triggered by a combination of ischemia and increased sympathetic tone. In addition, ventricular hypertrophy is associated with increased myocardial fibrosis, a decrease in the number and function of the gap junctions, and a mismatch between blood supply and volume of muscle. The three main electrophysiological mechanisms for arrhythmias can be present in subjects with ventricular hypertrophy. Arrhythmias caused by abnormal automaticity originate from ischemic cells, which have low resting membrane potential values and can be the source of ventricular ectopic beats or ventricular tachycardia. Reentrant arrhythmias are promoted by the presence of fibrosis, areas of slow conduction and the increase dispersion of the refractory periods within the ventricular myocardium.

Ventricular tachycardias occurring with hypertrophic cardiomyopathy may be non-sustained, repetitive and monomorphic. QRS complexes typically have a right bundle branch block morphology, with the widest negative deflection in the inferior leads (II, III and aVF) and positive deflections in aVR and aVL. The left precordial leads (V_2-V_6) display a QRS complex with a wide negative deflection.

Ventricular tachycardia during congestive heart failure

Ventricular tachyarrhythmias are frequent in large breed dogs with congestive heart failure and less common in small breed dogs. The underlying heart disease likely explains this difference. Large breed dogs are more likely to have primary myocardial disease that results in congestive heart failure while small breed dogs develop congestive heart failure primarily because of atrioventricular valve degeneration. Ventricular arrhythmia develops secondary to myocardial remodeling, including fibrosis, hypertrophy and local ischemia. It is modulated by electrolyte disorders, high concentrations of circulating catecholamines and increased wall tension. Specifically with heart failure, there is a prolongation of repolarization secondary to a reduction in the rectifying K⁺ currents I_{k1} and I_{to} leading to a dispersion of refractoriness, which promotes reentrant mechanisms. Excessive myocardial fiber stretching secondary to increased wall stress can induce arrhythmias via enhanced automaticity or delayed after-depolarizations.

In dogs with degenerative mitral valve disease, ventricular arrhythmias may occur but are usually benign. Some factors associated with valve disease that could trigger arrhythmias include the change in mechanical forces between the valve apparatus and the ventricles. For example, traction on the endocardium by the chordae tendineae causes prolongation of the refractory period in the cells of the papillary muscles. The ventricular premature beats that occur with degenerative valve disease usually have a right bundle branch block morphology.

Ventricular tachycardias during systemic diseases

Abdominal and systemic diseases can be associated with ventricular tachyarrhythmias. They usually correspond to an accelerated idioventricular rhythm (see p. 297).

Differential diagnosis of wide QRS complex tachycardia

The QRS complex reflects the depolarization wavefront within the working ventricular myocardium. The duration of the QRS complex is therefore the time necessary for the activation wavefront to excite the entire ventricular myocardium. Any factor that induces a delay in the activation of a small or larger portion of the ventricular mass is reflected by an increase in the duration of the QRS complex and an alteration of its morphology. These factors include electrical impulses originating within the ventricular myocardium, the conduction of a supraventricular impulse with an anatomical or functional intraventricular block (*aberrancy*) and the conduction of a supraventricular impulse along an atrioventricular accessory pathway (pre-excited tachycardia). The arrhythmias that appear as wide QRS complex tachycardias include:
- ventricular tachycardia,
- supraventricular tachycardia conducted with aberrancy or a preexisting anatomical bundle branch block, and
- supraventricular tachycardia conducted via an accessory pathway (pre-excited tachycardia).

One of the biggest challenges of electrocardiographic interpretation is the differentiation between the different types of wide QRS complex tachycardias. Several clinical and electrocardiographic criteria can be used to make an accurate diagnosis, although only intracardiac electrophysiological studies can provide a definitive diagnosis in some cases.

First, the medical history is important to identify the presence of structural cardiac disease that is associated with a higher probability that a wide QRS complex tachycardia is ventricular in origin. Similarly, if an animal has already been diagnosed with ventricular pre-excitation based on an electrocardiogram obtained during sinus rhythm, there is a higher probability that the wide QRS tachycardia episode is supraventricular in origin with aberrant conduction or pre-excitation.

It is extremely helpful when QRS complexes can be compared during sinus rhythm and during the tachycardia. This is unfortunately not possible when the arrhythmia is incessant. Features to take into account include (Table 10.1):
- the duration of the QRS complex,
- the ventricular rate,
- evidence of atrioventricular dissociation,
- regularity of the R-R intervals,
- the morphology and the axis of the QRS complex in the 12-lead electrocardiogram,
- the presence of concordance or discordance between the limb leads (I, II,III and aVF) and the left precordial leads (V_2-V_6), and
- the presence of precordial concordance (V_1 has the same polarity as V_2-V_6) or discordance (the polarity of V_1 is different from that of V_2-V_6).

A tachycardia is defined as a wide QRS complex tachycardia when the duration of the QRS complexes is greater than 70 ms in dogs and 40 ms in cats. A cutoff has not been established to differentiate supraventricular from ventricular tachycardias based on the duration of the QRS complex, although a duration greater than 100 ms suggests pre-excited supraventricular tachycardia.

The heart rate is another parameter that can be useful to differentiate supraventricular from ventricular tachyarrhythmias. Supraventricular tachyarrhythmias rarely exceed 300 to 350 bpm; a rate above 350 bpm is more likely with ventricular tachycardia.

The presence of atrioventricular dissociation confirms the presence of a ventricular rhythm that is independent from the supraventricular structures. There are three signs of atrioventricular dissociation: P waves with a sinus axis that are not related to wide QRS complexes, fusion beats and capture beats.

The presence of regular R-R intervals during a wide QRS tachycardia suggests the diagnosis of monomorphic ventricular tachycardia or supraventricular tachycardia conducted with aberrancy. Conversely, irregular R-R intervals suggest pre-excited atrial fibrillation or atrial fibrillation conducting with aberrancy. It is important to note however that the initiation of a run of ventricular tachycardia may have a few beats during which the R-R interval is irregular or even have a variable morphology before a monomorphic ventricular tachycardia stabilizes into a consistent form and rhythm.

The morphology and the axis of the QRS complex in the limb leads and the morphology of the QRS complex in the precordial leads play crucial roles in differentiating a tachycardia conducted with aberrancy or preexisting bundle branch block from a ventricular tachycardia and from a pre-excited supraventricular tachycardia.

QRS complexes of supraventricular tachycardias conducted with aberrancy or a preexisting bundle branch block should display the classic right bundle branch block or left bundle branch block pattern in the 12-lead electrocardiogram. In other words, the characteristic morphology of a bundle branch block should be present both in the limb leads and the precordial leads. Thus, the QRS complexes have a dominant deflection with the same polarity in the limb leads (I, II, III and AVF) and the left precordial leads. In addition, the polarity in V_1 is opposite to that of the other precordial leads (precordial discordance): with a right bundle branch block pattern, the main deflection of V_1 is positive and displays a typical Rr' or rR' morphology whereas the left chest leads are mostly negative; V_1 is negative and the left chest leads have a wide positive deflection with a left bundle branch block pattern (Fig 10.24A).

Conversely, discordance between the limb leads and the left precordial leads (V_2-V_6) is typically present with monomorphic ventricular tachycardia (Fig. 10.24B). Ventricular tachycardia is also the most likely diagnosis in the presence of precordial concordance (all precordial leads positive or negative) (Fig. 10.24C). It is important to keep in mind that precordial lead placement on the animal's chest can affect the polarity of these leads. Ideally, lead V_1 records the depolarization of the right ventricle and the other precordial leads record the depolarization of the left ventricle. However, depending on the animal's thoracic conformation and position of the heart, the V_1 lead placed in the standard position of the fifth right

TABLE 10.1. Differential diagnosis of wide QRS complex tachycardia in dogs.
Twelve leads (I, II, III, aVR, aVL, aVF, V_1, V_2, V_3, V_4, V_5, V_6) - speed 50 mm/s - calibration 5 mm/1 mV.

Electrocardiographic parameters	Ventricular tachycardia	Supraventricular tachycardia conducted with aberrancy or prior bundle branch block	Pre-excited supraventricular tachycardia
QRS duration	>70 ms	> 70 ms	> 100 ms
Ventricular rate	120-450 bpm	180-330 bpm	> 350 bpm
Atrioventricular dissociation	Present	Absent	Absent
R-R intervals	Regular or irregular	Regular or irregular	Irregular only in case of pre-excited atrial fibrillation
Morphology of the QRS complex in limb leads and precordial leads	Presence of limb lead (I, II, III, aVF) and left precordial lead (V_2-V_6) discordance and/or precordial concordance (same QRS polarity V_1 and V_2-V_6). Bulldog with right ventricular outflow tract tachycardia can be an exception to this rule (see text for explanation). In case of left bundle branch block morphology usually qR pattern from V_3 to V_6.	Presence of limb lead (I, II, III, aVF) and left precordial lead (V_2-V_6) concordance and/or precordial discordance (V_1 polarity different from V_2-V_6). In case of left bundle branch block R pattern from V_2 to V_6 in case of truncular block, and qR pattern in case of post-divisional block.	Presence of limb lead (I, II, III, aVF) and left precordial (V_2-V_6) lead concordance and/or precordial discordance (V_1 polarity different from V_2-V_6) and R complex from V_2 to V_6.

intercostal space does not always record the activation of the right ventricle, but rather the depolarization of the left ventricle. As a result, precordial concordance can be present in some supraventricular tachycardias with wide QRS complexes. Santilli proposed a more cranial placement of lead V_1 in the first right intercostal space at the level of costo-chondral junction in order to obtain a more reliable recording of right ventricular activation in all canine thoracic morphotypes. This modified lead system should improve the ability to differentiate wide QRS complex tachycardias in the dog (see p. 32).

Another way to differentiate supraventricular from ventricular tachycardias is to consider the mean electrical axis of the QRS complexes. A mean electrical axis of the QRS complex in the frontal plane oriented between –80 ° and –110 ° is suggestive of a ventricular tachycardia. Left axis deviation of a QRS complex that is less pronounced during tachycardia than during sinus rhythm is also suggestive of ventricular tachycardia.

Finally, the morphology of the QRS complexes can help with the diagnosis of a wide complex tachycardia. Obvious changes in QRS complex morphology are more likely consistent with monomorphic ventricular tachycardia with pleomorphism, polymorphic ventricular or bidirectional tachycardia. The presence of QRS complexes with a wide positive deflection and a qR morphology in the left precordial leads (V_2-V_6) excludes pre-excited supraventricular tachycardias. Indeed, with pre-excited supraventricular tachycardia the presence of the accessory pathway results in ventricular activation from the base to the cardiac apex, and therefore QRS complexes have their widest positive deflection in the left precordial leads (V_2 to V_6). However, pre-excited supraventricular tachycardias do not result in a qR morphology, because the septal activation wavefront is not present. Moreover, identification of the characteristic δ (*delta*) wave in the initial portion of the QRS complex is another sign of pre-excited supraventricular tachycardia. Lastly, a wide supraventricular tachycardia in the presence of a post-divisional left bundle branch block can be recognized by the presence of QRS complexes with a qR morphology in the left precordial leads (V_2-V_6).

Determining the danger of ventricular tachycardias

The characteristics of various ventricular tachycardias have been presented; however, what are the features of such rhythms that make them dangerous? The following points are critical and can alter the assessment and conclusions of a particular electrocardiographic recording:

- *Underlying myocardial function*. An abnormal rhythm is better tolerated when structure and function are preserved.
- *Circumstances during the electrocardiographic recording*. As the autonomic nervous system is a critical player in the development of arrhythmias, environmental circumstances that evoke the clinical arrhythmia should ideally be reproduced in order to capture an arrhythmia that may be causing clinical signs. For example, a dog with a few ventricular premature complexes during an electrocardiographic recording may not show a rapid ventricular tachycardia which would be apparent if the dog were to exercise.
- *Adequate duration of electrocardiographic recording*. Electronic electrocardiography is now the norm and this permits more prolonged recordings in the hospital. Arrhythmias are often intermittent and the longer the observation period, the more likely it is to identify a ventricular tachycardia. Of course, some arrhythmic events are uncommon and require longer-term monitoring beginning with 24-hour Holter monitoring, event recorders, or implantable loop recorders.
- *Changes with time*. When an arrhythmia in an animal is identified and disease processes are ongoing appropriate follow-up is mandatory to understand risks. For example, an idioventricular rhythm may accelerate and change to a hemodynamically unstable rapid ventricular tachycardia. Alternatively, an animal that is recovering from an arrhythmia-producing process may need treatment only temporarily, or the severity of the ventricular tachycardia in a young German Shepherd dog may not have peaked unless arrhythmic identification occurs in a subsequent 24-hour Holter monitoring.

- *Pro-arrhythmic effects.* Although seemingly uncommon in the dog, pro-arrhythmic effects have been identified in individual patients. Some of these may be predicted as possible, for example, when treating a German Shepherd puppy with sotalol, while others are surprising. It is always important to ascertain whether or not an increase in ventricular arrhythmias is the result of treatment or progression of a disease.

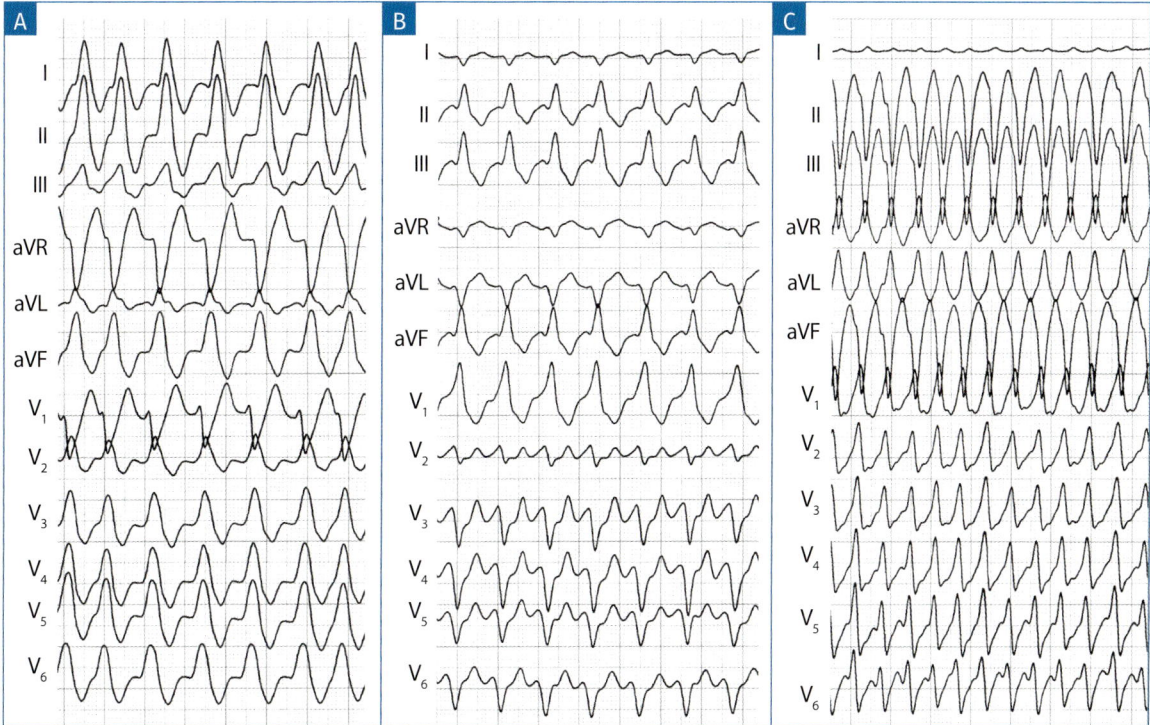

Figure 10.24. A) Persistent atrial fibrillation conducted with truncular left bundle branch block (Dog, American Staffordshire, male, 8 years. Twelve leads (I, II, III, aVR, aVL, aVF) - speed 50 mm/s - calibration 5 mm/1 mV).
Note the presence of wide QRS complexes (85 ms) with a rapid (280 bpm) and irregular ventricular rate. There is left bundle branch block morphology with QRS complexes positive in the limb (I, II, III and aVF) and left precordial (V_2-V_6) leads (concordance between limb and left precordial leads) and V_1 is negative (precordial discordance, $V_1 \neq V_2$-V_6). The electrocardiographic pattern is suggestive of a supraventricular tachycardia conducted with bundle branch block.
B) Monomorphic ventricular tachycardia (Dog, Boxer, female, 9 years. Twelve leads (I, II, III, aVR, aVL, aVF, V_1, V_2, V_3, V_4, V_5, V_6) - speed 50 mm/s - calibration 5 mm/1 mV).
Note the presence of wide QRS complexes (80 ms) with a rapid (285 bpm) and regular ventricular rate. There is left bundle branch block morphology with QRS complexes positive in the inferior leads (II, III and aVF) but negative in lead I and in the left precordial leads (V_2-V_6) (discordance between limb and left precordial leads). V_1 is positive (precordial concordance, $V_1 = V_2$-V_6). The electrocardiographic pattern is suggestive of a ventricular tachycardia with left bundle branch block morphology because of the discordance between the limb leads and precordial leads and precordial concordance.
C) Monomorphic ventricular tachycardia (Dog, German Shepherd, female, 2 years. Twelve leads (I, II, III, aVR, aVL, aVF, V_1, V_2, V_3, V_4, V_5, V_6) - speed 50 mm/s - calibration 5 mm/1 mV).
Note the presence of wide QRS complexes (80 ms) with a rapid (480 bpm) and regular ventricular rate. There is right bundle branch block morphology with negative QRS complexes in the inferior (II, III and aVF) leads but positive in I, V_1, V_2, V_3, V_4, V_5 and V_6 (discordance between limb and precordial leads and precordial concordance, $V_1 = V_2$-V_6). The electrocardiographic pattern is suggestive of a ventricular tachycardia with right bundle branch block morphology because of the discordance of QRS morphology between limb leads and precordial leads and the presence of precordial concordance.

The following are features which may suggest that a ventricular arrhythmia is dangerous and warrants consideration of treatment. There are two possible causes of death in animals with ventricular tachycardia. One is that the ventricular tachycardia degenerates into the fatal rhythm of ventricular fibrillation, the other is that asystole (e.g. strong Bezold-Jarisch reflex) occurs rather than ventricular fibrillation. Of course, there is always great variability, but these can serve as guidelines.

- *Rate and duration of ventricular tachycardia.* Rate is likely one of the most important factors in determining whether an arrhythmia is dangerous. The faster the rate, the less hemodynamically stable the cardiovascular system with an adequate generation of blood pressure, cardiac output, perfusion and myocardial oxygenation. The exact rate above which a ventricular tachycardia is considered dangerous varies because it depends on the hemodynamic status (e.g. the blood pressure) as this determines perfusion of the brain, heart and kidneys. Rate is also connected to the duration of the ventricular tachycardia. A very short non-sustained run of ventricular tachycardia at a rate of 450 bpm is unlikely to cause hemodynamic compromise, but the underlying mechanism may trigger ventricular fibrillation from this extremely rapid rate. The longer a run of ventricular tachycardia persists at a high rate, the more likely it is to have detrimental consequences either in the short term or the long term. However, 24-hour Holter recordings have revealed that dogs with sufficient myocardial functional reserve can survive hours or days with a fairly rapid ventricular tachycardia. It is known that tachycardiomyopathy can result from rapid rhythms. The faster the ventricular tachycardia, the quicker the tachycardiomyopathy develops.
- *Ventricular load.* The risk of death from a ventricular arrhythmia is, of course, the obvious immediate concern in animals with a rapid and sustained ventricular tachycardia; however, a more protracted consequence of loss of myocardial function is the development of large numbers of premature ventricular complexes or multiples (couplets, triplets, runs of three to five beats of ventricular tachycardia) which can lead to congestive heart failure and death. The assessment of ventricular load is ideally done by a 24-hour ambulatory electrocardiogram (Holter monitoring). In human beings the likelihood of development of tachycardiomyopathy increases when the ventricular load, defined by the percent of any form of ventricular premature complex, exceeds approximately 25 % of all QRS complexes in a 24-hour period. The percentage in the dog is unknown; however, this approximate number provides at least some guideline. Nevertheless, it should be kept in mind that 25 % is a large number of abnormal beats. For a dog with an average heart rate over a 24-hour period of 80 bpm this is approximately 28,000 ventricular ectopic beats. It should be emphasized that the decision to treat based on the number of ventricular ectopic beats is made on a case-by-case basis because of the multiple factors that must be considered. In general, more than 25 % ventricular ectopic complexes warrants therapy and in general, treatment is likely not necessary if there are fewer than 10 % ventricular ectopic beats and they are primarily singlets with only a few multiples. The gray zone for individual care lies between these two cutoffs.
- *Multiform ventricular complexes.* It is possible that ventricular complexes arising from different regions of the heart are more likely to induce tachycardiomyopathy than a singular focus. However, we do not have data to support this hypothesis in the dog.
- *Coupling intervals.* Some ventricular arrhythmias may not be characterized by even non-sustained runs of ventricular tachycardia but instead singlets, couplets, and triplets that have very short coupling intervals (and thus, a rapid rate). Such short coupling intervals could fall into the category of the described danger of R-on-T. It is true that there is a vulnerable period during repolarization in which an electrical impulse of a premature complex could suddenly induce ventricular fibrillation. Although the coupling interval is evaluated during the assessment of a ventricular arrhythmia and its related level of danger, identification and definition of R-on-T is difficult and imprecise in dogs and cats.

Suggested readings

1. Aliot M, Stevenson WG, Almendral-Garrote JM, et al. EHRA/HRS expert consensus on catheter ablation of ventricular arrhythmias. *Europace* 2009; 11:771-817.
2. Basso C, Fox PR, Meurs KM, et al. Arrhythmogenic right ventricular cardiomyopathy causing sudden cardiac death in Boxer dogs: a new animal model of human disease. *Circulation* 2004; 109:1180-1185.
3. Baty CJ, Sweet DC, Keene BW. Torsades de pointes-like polymorphic ventricular tachycardia in a dog. *J Vet Intern Med* 1994; 8:439-442.
4. Baumwart RD, Meurs KM, Atkins CE, et al. Clinical, echocardiographic, and electrocardiographic abnormalities in Boxers with cardiomyopathy and left ventricular systolic dysfunction: 48 cases (1985-2003). *J Am Vet Med Assoc* 2005; 226:1102-1104.
5. Bonometti C, Hwang C, Hough D, et al. Interaction between strong electrical stimulation and reentrant wavefronts in canine ventricular fibrillation. *Circ Res* 1995; 77:407-416.
6. Breitschwerdt EB, Atkins CE, Brown TT, et al. *Bartonella vinsonii* subsp. *berkhoffii* and related members of the alpha subdivision of the Proteobacteria in dogs with cardiac arrhythmias, endocarditis and myocarditis. *J Clin Microbiol* 1999; 37:3618-3626.
7. Bright JM, McEntee M. Isolated right ventricular cardiomyopathy in a dog. *J Am Vet Med Assoc* 1995; 207:64-66.
8. Brugada P, Brugada J, Mont L, et al. A new approach to the differential diagnosis of a regular tachycardia with a wide QRS complex. *Circulation* 1991; 83:1649-1659.
9. Côté E, Jaeger R. Ventricular tachyarrhythmias in 106 cats: associated structural cardiac disorders. *J Vet Intern Med* 2008; 22:1444-1446.
10. Cruickshank J, Quaas RL, Junya Li, et al. Genetic analysis of ventricular arrhythmia afflicting young German Shepherd dogs. *J Vet Int Med* 2009; 23:264-270.
11. Dae M, Ursell P, Lee R, et al. Heterogeneous sympathetic innervation in German Shepherd dogs with inherited ventricular arrhythmias and sudden death. *Circulation* 1997; 96:1337-1342.
12. Driehuys S, Van Winkle TJ, Sammarco CD, et al. Myocardial infarction in dogs and cats: 37 cases (1985-1994). *J Am Vet Med Assoc* 1998; 213:1444-1448.
13. Falk T, Jonsson L, Olsen LH, et al. Arteriosclerotic changes in the myocardium, lung and kidney in dogs with chronic congestive heart failure and myxomatous mitral valve disease. *Cardiovasc Pathol* 2006; 15:185-193.
14. Falk T, Jonsson L, Olsen LH, et al. Association between cardiac pathology and clinical, echocardiographic and electrocardiographic findings in dogs with chronic congestive heart failure. *Vet J* 2010; 185:68-74.
15. Fernandez del Palacio MJ, Bernal LJ, Bayon A, et al. Arrhythmogenic right ventricular dysplasia/cardiomyopathy in a Siberian Husky. *J Small Anim Pract* 2001; 42:137-142.
16. Fox PR, Maron BJ, Basso C, et al. Spontaneously occurring of arrhythmogenic right ventricular cardiomyopathy in the domestic cat: a new animal model of human disease. *Circulation* 2000; 102:1863–1870.
17. Freeman LC, Pacioretti LM, Moïse NS, et al. Decreased density of I_{to} in left ventricular myocytes from German Shepherd dogs with inherited arrhythmias. *J Cardiovasc Electrophysiol* 1997; 8:872-883.
18. Gelzer AMR, Kraus MS, Rishniw M, et al. Combination therapy with mexiletine and sotalol suppresses inherited ventricular arrhythmias in German Shepherd dogs better than mexiletine or sotalol monotherapy: a randomized crossover study. *J Vet Cardiol* 2010; 12:93-106.
19. Gilmour RF Jr, Moïse NS. Triggered activity as a mechanism for inherited ventricular arrhythmias in German Shepherd dogs. *J Am Coll Cardiol* 1996; 27:1526-1533.
20. Guglielmini C, Diana A, Civitella C, et al. Accelerated idioventricular rhythm in 9 dogs. *Vet Res Communications* 2006; 30:305-307.
21. Hadid C, Almendral J, Ortiz M, et al. Incidence, determinants and prognostic implications of true pleomorphism of ventricular tachycardia in ICD patients: a substudy of the DATAS trial. *Circ Arrhythm Electrophysiol* 2010; 4:33-42
22. Hanna MS, Coromilas J, Josephson ME, et al. Mechanisms of resetting reentrant circuits in canine ventricular tachycardia. *Circulation* 2001; 103:1148-1156.
23. Harvey AM, Battersby IA, Faena M, et al. Arrhythmogenic right ventricular cardiomyopathy in two cats. *J Small Anim Prac* 2005; 46,151-156.
24. Huand J, Rogers JM, Killingsworth CR, et al. Evolution of activation patterns during long-duration ventricular fibrillation in dogs. *Am J Physiol Heart Circ Physiol* 2004; 287:H1193-H1200.
25. Hunt GB, Malik R, Church DB. Ventricular tachycardia in the dog: a review of 28 consecutive cases. *Australian Veterinary Practitioner* 1990; 20:122-127.
26. Kagawa Y, Hirayama K, Uchida E, et al. Systemic atherosclerosis in dogs: Histopathological and immunohistochemical studies of atherosclerotic lesions. *J Comp Pathol* 1998; 118:195-206.
27. Kluser L, Holler PJ, Simak J, et al. Predictors of sudden cardiac death in Doberman Pinschers with dilated cardiomyopathy. *J Vet Intern Med* 2016; 30:722-732.
28. Kraus MS, Moïse NS, Rishniw M, et al. Morphology of ventricular arrhythmias in the Boxer described by 12-lead electrocardiography with pace mapping comparison. *J Vet Int Med* 2002; 16:153-158.
29. Janus I, Noszczyk-Nowak A, Nowak M, et al. Myocarditis in dogs: etiology, clinical and histopathological features (11 cases: 2007-2013). *Ir Vet J* 2014; 67:1-35
30. May PE. Ventricular fibrillation during anesthesia. *Vet Med Small Anim Clin* 1981; 76:309-313.
31. Marino DJ, Matthesian DT, Fox PR, et al. Ventricular arrhythmias in dogs undergoing splenectomy: a prospective study. *Vet Surg* 1994; 23:101-106.
32. Meurs KM. Boxer dog cardiomyopathy: an update. *Vet Clin North Am Small Anim Pract* 2004; 34:1235-1244.
33. Meurs KM, Spier AW, Miller MW, et al. Familial ventricular arrhythmias in boxers. *J Vet Intern Med* 1999; 13:437-439.

34. Meurs KM, Weidman JA, Rosenthal SL, et al. Ventricular arrhythmias in Rhodesian Ridgebacks with a family history of sudden death and results of a pedigree analysis for potential inheritance patterns. *J Am Vet Med Assoc* 2016; 248:1135-1138.
35. Moïse NS, Meyers-Wallen V, Flahive WJ, et al. Inherited ventricular arrhythmias and sudden death in German Shepherd dogs. *J Am Coll Cardiol* 1994; 24:233-243.
36. Moïse NS, Dugger DA, Brittain D, et al. Relationship of ventricular tachycardia to sleep/wakefulness in a model of sudden cardiac death. *Ped Res* 1996; 40:344-350.
37. Moïse NS, Moon PF, Flahive WJ, et al. Phenylephrine induced ventricular arrhythmias in dogs with inherited sudden death. *J Cardiovasc Electrophysiol* 1996; 7:217-230.
38. Moïse NS, Gilmour RF Jr, Riccio ML. An animal model of sudden arrhythmic death. *J Cardiovasc Electrophysiol* 1997; 8:98-103.
39. Moïse NS, Gilmour RF Jr, Riccio ML, et al. Diagnosis of inherited ventricular tachycardia in German Shepherd dogs. *J Am Vet Med Assoc* 1997; 210:403-410.
40. Moïse NS, Riccio ML, Kornreich B, et al. Age dependence of the development of ventricular arrhythmias in a canine model of sudden cardiac death. *Cardiovasc Res* 1997; 34:483-492.
41. Naito M, Michelson EL, Kaplinsky E, et al. Role of early cycle ventricular extrasystoles in initiation of ventricular tachycardia and fibrillation: evaluation of R on T phenomenon during acute ischemia in a canine model. *Am J Cardiol* 1982; 49:317-322.
42. Obreztchikova MN, Sosunov EA, Anyukhovsky EP, et al. Heterogeneous ventricular repolarization provides a substrate for arrhythmias in German shepherd model of spontaneous arrhythmic death. *Circulation* 2003; 108:1389-1394.
43. Ohad DG. Morphology of ventricular arrhythmias in the Boxer as measured by 12-lead electrocardiography with pace-mapping comparison. *J Vet Intern Med* 2002; 16:391.
44. Porteiro Vázquez DM, Perego M, Lombardo S, et al. Analysis of precordial lead system in dogs with different thoracic conformations. *J Vet Intern Med* 2017; 31:208.
45. Rosenbaum DS, Wilber DJ, Smith JM, et al. Local activation variability during monomorphic ventricular tachycardia in the dog. *Cardiovasc Res* 1992; 26:237-243.
46. Santilli RA, Bontempi LV, Perego M, et al. Outflow tract segmental arrhythmogenic right ventricular cardiomyopathy in an English Bulldog. *J Vet Cardiol* 2009; 11:47-51.
47. Santilli RA, Bontempi LV, Perego M. Ventricular tachycardia in English bulldog with localized right ventricular outflow tract enlargement. *J Small Anim Pract* 2011; 52:574-580.
48. Santilli RA, Perego M, Tursi M, et al. Role of right endomyocardial biopsy to characterize unexplained myocardial and rhythm disorders in the dog. *Proceeding 25th ECVIM-CA Congress* - Lisbon - P - 10-12 September 2015: 37.
49. Santilli RA, Battaia S, Perego M, et al. Bartonella-associated inflammatory cardiomyopathy in a dog. *J Vet Cardiol* 2017; 19:74-81.
50. Simpson KW, Bonagura JD, Eaton KA. Right ventricular cardiomyopathy in a dog. *J Vet Intern Med* 1994; 8:306-309.
51. Sosunov EA, Obreztchikova MN, Anyukhovsky EP, et al: Mechanisms of alpha-adrenergic potentiation of ventricular arrhythmias in German shepherd dogs with inherited arrhythmic sudden death. *Cardiovas Res* 2004; 61:715-723.
52. Spier AW, Meurs KM. Evaluation of spontaneous variability in the frequency of ventricular arrhythmias in Boxers with arrhythmogenic right ventricular cardiomyopathy. *J Am Vet Med Assoc* 2004; 224:538-541.
53. Spier AW, Meurs KM, Muir WW, et al. Correlation of QT dispersion with indices used to evaluate the severity of familial ventricular arrhyth- mias in Boxers. *Am J Vet Res* 2001; 62:1481-1485.
54. Srivathsan K, Lester SJ, Appleton CP. Ventricular tachycardia in the absence of structural heart disease. *Indian Pacing Electrophysiol J* 2005; 5:106-121.
55. Tsai J, Cao JM, Zhou S, et al. T wave alternans as a predictor of spontaneous ventricular tachycardia in a canine model of sudden cardiac death. *J Cardiovasc Electrophysiol* 2002; 13:51-55.
56. Varanat M, Broadhurst J, Linder KE, et al. Identification of *Bartonella henselae* in 2 cats with pyogranulomatous myocarditis and diaphragmatic myositis. *Vet Pathol* 2012; 49:608-611.
57. Vassalle M, Knob RE, Cummins M. An analysis of fast idioventricular rhythm in the dog. *Circ Res* 1977; 41:218-226.
58. Ware WA, Reina-Doreste Y, Stern JA, Meurs KM. Sudden death associated with QT interval prolongation and KCNQ1 gene mutation in a family of English Springer Spaniels. *J Vet Intern Med* 2015; 29:561-568.
59. Wiggers CJ The mechanism and nature of ventricular fibrillation. *Am Heart J* 1940; 20:399-412.

CHAPTER 11

Bradyarrhythmias

Bradyarrhythmia is the term used to describe rhythm disorders with a ventricular rate below the lower limit of the normal range for the animal considered. Bradyarrhythmias include:
- Sinus bradycardia:
  - Increased parasympathetic tone and reflex induced (physiological);
  - Sinus node dysfunction (pathological):
    - sinus bradycardia,
    - sinus arrest/exit block following tachycardia (tachycardia/bradycardia pattern), and
    - sinus arrest and sinus standstill.
  - Drug-induced (pharmacologic);
- Atrial standstill or atrioventricular muscular dystrophy.
- Sino-ventricular rhythm.
- Asystole or ventricular arrest.
- Pulseless electrical activity or electromechanical dissociation.

Other forms of bradyarrhythmias associated with other conduction blocks, including intra-atrial and atrioventricular blocks are described in chapter 12.

Sinus bradycardia

Sinus bradycardia has all the characteristics of sinus rhythm except for a heart rate in the awake animal below 60 bpm in dogs and 140 bpm in cats. Sinus bradycardia often results from a decrease in pacemaker cell automaticity within the sinus node. It can be classified as physiologic, pathologic or pharmacologic.

Physiologic sinus bradycardia: increased parasympathetic tone

Sinus bradycardia is the physiologic response that is due to an increase in parasympathetic (vagal) tone usually in conjunction with a withdrawal of sympathetic tone. Such situations include sleep or rest. In some animals, a sinus arrhythmia may become pronounced resulting in an average heart rate which is just below what is considered bradycardia. This may occur in brachycephalic breeds during deep breathing. In awake dogs the lower limit of 60 bpm is generally accepted; however, sleeping dogs often have lower heart rates. In general, most dogs will have a heart rate below 50 bpm for approximately 1 hour during a 24-hour Holter recording. This slow rate occurs during sleep and most commonly between midnight and 6 a.m. Comparative 24-hour heart rate and P-P/R-R interval patterning data between brachycephalic breeds and non-brachycephalic breeds has not been systematically investigated at this time. Clinicians often notice that brachycephalic breeds have a more pronounced sinus arrhythmia which is accentuated during periods of sleep. The reason hypothesized for this difference is the deeper breathing caused by obstructive upper airway problems. The appearance of a longer P-P/R-R interval when a dog takes a deep sigh is also of note. This can result in sinus pauses, usually lasting 2 to 4 s. Pauses longer than 4 s are uncommon.

Chronically increased parasympathetic tone (hypervagotonia) causing sinus bradycardia can occur because of pathologic conditions such as gastrointestinal diseases, urethral obstruction, chronic respiratory diseases, intracranial lesions, hypothermia, and hypoxia. It should be understood that this is a physiologic response of the heart to a pathologic condition. Animals presenting with sinus bradycardia, therefore, require careful examination to rule out primary causes that result in secondary slowing of the heart.

Physiologic sinus bradycardia: cardiovascular reflexes

Reflex sinus bradycardia (physiologic mechanism) most often goes unnoticed or can result in weakness, collapse, or syncope (transient loss of consciousness). Although based on a physiologic principle, dogs with exaggerated reflex responses that result in clinical signs would be considered abnormal. The most common of these reflexes are *situational vasovagal reflex*, *Bezold-Jarisch reflex* and *Cushing's reflex*.

Vasovagal reflex (situational)

A *vasovagal reflex* can be in response to a "situation" such as coughing, urination, vomiting, defecation, extreme emotion or other physiologic processes that heighten parasympathetic tone. It may be difficult to determine whether the clinical signs are the result of the severe bradycardia or hypotension, both of which occur with hypervagotonia. Clinicians note that suspected situational vasovagal reflex occurs more commonly in older dogs with chronic cardiac disease such as degenerative atrioventricular valve disease. In such clinical scenarios, the normal balance of sympathetic-parasympathetic interaction may be altered such that the consequences of acute autonomic change are not tolerated. When considering alterations in autonomic tone it is important to realize that background parasympathetic and sympathetic tone affect the neurocardiogenic response. It has been documented in anesthetized and awake dogs that elevations in sympathetic tone before a vagal stimulus will result in a more pronounced effect. This is known as *accentuated antagonism*. Specifically, if the background sympathetic tone is elevated, and, therefore, the heart rate is high, abrupt increases in vagal tone will have a more pronounced effect of slowing heart rate and decreasing blood pressure. Of course the sympathetic-parasympathetic interaction is temporally complex. Changes due to increased vagal tone can occur on a beat-to-beat basis while those of increased sympathetic tone are more sustained. However, "fade" of the vagal tone effect has been documented experimentally in dogs. With this background knowledge, it becomes more apparent why a careful historical account of what precedes the clinical signs of collapse or syncope may assist in making the correct diagnosis of reflex bradycardia. Often dogs suspected of having situational vasovagal reflex syncope have a period of excitement before the stimulus of the parasympathetic system. In such cases a sinus tachycardia is followed by a short period of gradual sinus slowing and then a long sinus pause with or without secondary pauses. Remember that although a sinus pause may be less than the expected duration for a loss of consciousness (longer than 8 s), multiple secondary pauses causing a protracted marked bradycardia also result in poor cerebral perfusion and syncope. Additionally, factors that cause the parasympathetic reflex for sinus slowing also can affect the dromotropic (conduction) properties of the atrioventricular node causing temporary atrioventricular block. Clinical situations that have been described include extreme excitement before urination or defecation, extreme anxiety followed by breath holding, and coughing after excited barking (Fig. 11.1) Depending on the individual dog and the situation, temporary atrioventricular block may occur in addition to sinus bradycardia (Fig. 11.2).

Bezold-Jarisch reflex

Another type of vasovagal response that is not dependent on a "behavior or situation" is the *Bezold-Jarisch reflex*. This reflex bradycardia develops as a response to an under-filled ventricle. Examples of circumstances that can result in low ventricular volumes include dehydration, severe pulmonic, aortic or subaortic stenosis and excessive tachycardia. Intracardiac C fibers are stimulated during vigorous ventricular contraction of the reduced volume chamber. This process increases parasympathetic output resulting in slowing of the heart rate that may be followed by extremely long sinus pauses with or without coexisting atrioventricular nodal block. Such bradycardia can result in near-syncope or syncope. An example in dogs whereby the Bezold-Jarisch reflex is the hypothesized mechanism for syncope is in Boxers with arrhythmogenic right ventricular cardiomyopathy that have very rapid ventricular tachycardia. The shortened period of diastole results in inadequate time

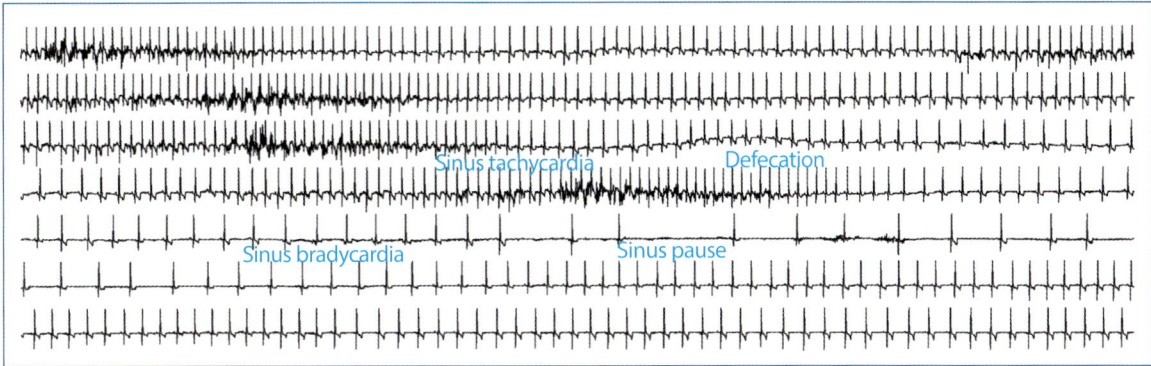

Figure 11.1. Electrocardiogram from a 24-hour Holter recording obtained in a small breed dog with a history of degenerative atrioventricular valve disease and experiencing weakness and "wobbly-behavior" after defecation. The excitement before the vagal stimulus of defecation is revealed by the sinus tachycardia that is then followed by a gradual slowing in heart rate followed by a sinus pause. Lead Y - speed 7.5 mm/s - calibration 2 mm/1 mV -. Each line corresponds to a 20 s recording.

for ventricular filling. Once the rapid contractions of the arrhythmia stop, there is sudden complete asystole because of the strong vagal stimulation and marked overdrive suppression of other subsidiary pacemakers. Episodes of ventricular tachycardia that follow such an event may not be similarly followed by long pauses, but instead by sinus tachycardia in response to the low blood pressure stimulating the baroreceptors to increase sympathetic tone. Several reasons may explain the varied sinus node responses following rapid ventricular tachycardia. The effects on the cardiovascular system due to autonomic nervous system input can change depending on the preceding balance in autonomic tone. For example, it is possible for the substrate of a Bezold-Jarisch reflex to exist, but the background sympathetic tone is such that the consequences of increased parasympathetic tone are not manifested after the ventricular tachycardia. Instead, a *post-vagal tachycardia* develops. Post-vagal tachycardia occurs following a strong parasympathetic stimulation which when stopped is followed by sinus tachycardia. The latter develops because the effects of increased parasympathetic output on sinus rate are rapid and occur on a beat-to-beat basis. However, if the consequences of high vagal tone have resulted in a reactive sympathetic stimulation (e.g. drop in systemic blood pressure stimulates the sympathetic efferents) then an "overshoot" of the rate occurs with a faster sinus tachycardia. This happens because of the more sustained effects of sympathetic tone. Although the above explanation is plausible, other reasons not associated with increased adrenergic stimulation have been forwarded and include an increase in sodium influx into sinus node cells caused by the hyperpolarization of these cells during and immediately following vagal stimulation. In dogs with suspected Bezold-Jarisch reflex syncope associated with ventricular tachycardia, elimination of clinical signs is successful with suppression of the arrhythmia. The mechanism is hypothesized to be the elimination of the long pauses following the ventricular tachycardia as the latter tachyarrhythmia is suppressed (Fig. 11.3).

Cushing's reflex

The *Cushing's reflex* (which has no association with hyperadrenocorticism) is identified in cases of neurologic lesions associated with increased intracranial pressure that exceeds the mean arterial pressure such that the cerebral arterioles are compressed and brain perfusion decreases. The central chemoreceptors in the medulla respond to the resulting decreased pH and increased PCO_2 with the activation of the sympathetic nervous system causing peripheral vasoconstriction and increase peripheral resistance. The systemic hypertension triggers the baroreceptors in the carotid arteries and aorta to stimulate the parasympathetic system. This then results in a slowing of the heart rate with extended periods of bradycardia because of continuous resetting of the reflex arc.

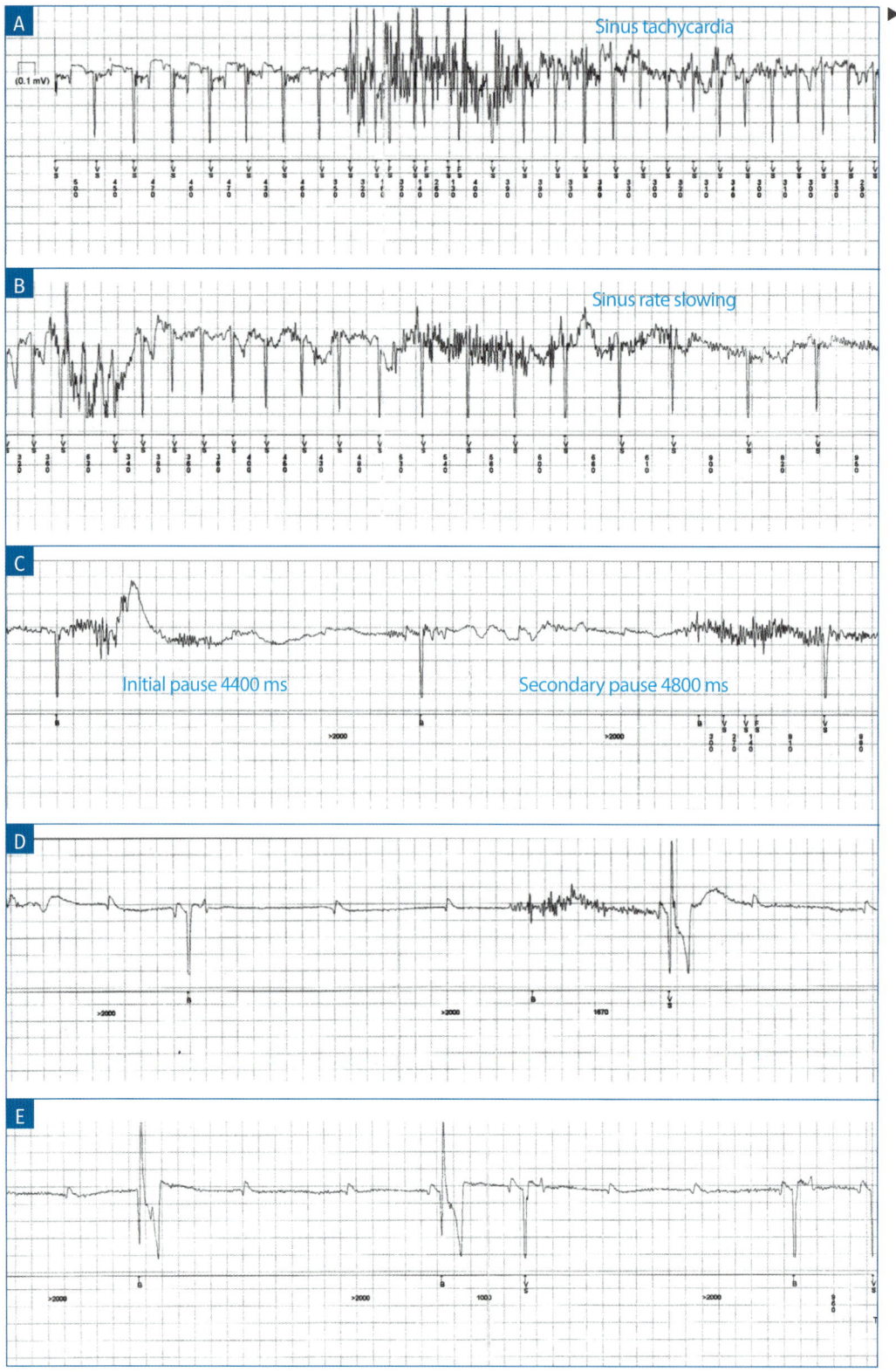

▶ **Figure 11.2.** Electrocardiographic recording downloaded from a subcutaneously implanted loop recorder (Medtronic REVEAL) in a nervous young dog with owner-separation anxiety. The owner had witnessed two syncopal events associated with excitement during the preceding year. The device was implanted after two 24-hour Holter recordings and other diagnostic tests had failed to explain the clinical signs. The recording demonstrates a tachycardia with motion artifact (A) followed by gradual slowing of heart rate (B) followed by an initial pause with a secondary pause separated by a single beat resulting in approximately 10 s (C) of inadequate cerebral perfusion. Although the owner only noted a single syncopal episode during the 5 months the REVEAL was implanted, 35 events had been stored with single and secondary pauses exceeding 8 s (several longer than 15 s). Recording strips D and E are from one of the other stored events with a tachycardia followed by a sinus bradycardia and then atrioventricular block (paper speed 25 mm/s).

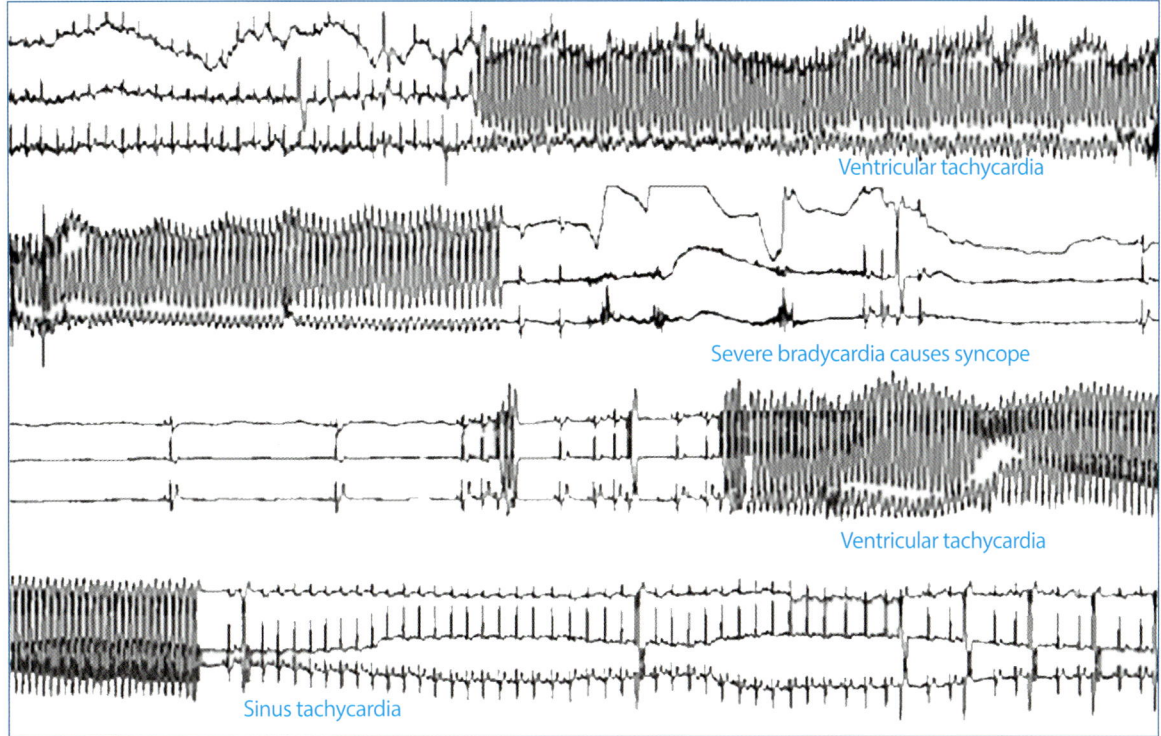

Figure 11.3. Electrocardiographic recording from a dog with repeated episodes of syncope. Rapid ventricular tachycardia with a rate faster than 300 bpm is followed by a severe bradycardia that causes a transient loss of consciousness. A second run of ventricular tachycardia is followed by a sinus tachycardia. The initial run of ventricular tachycardia is hypothesized to have evoked the Bezold-Jarisch reflex with a strong parasympathetic stimulation resulting in the severe bradycardia. However, the second run of ventricular tachycardia, which is not as protracted as the former is followed by a sinus tachycardia instead. Explanations for these differences may be related to the duration of the ventricular tachycardia influencing the degree of vagal stimulation due to stimulation of the C fibers or the background altered balance of autonomic tone that developed with the decreased blood pressure and perfusion that caused the syncope. Thus, the vagal stimulation during the second run of ventricular tachycardia was not manifest at the cessation of the arrhythmia, but instead a sinus tachycardia occurred at that time (post-vagal tachycardia). Lead Y - speed 7.5 mm/s - calibration 2 mm/1 mV. Each line corresponds to 20 s recording.

Sinus bradycardia: pathological

Pathological sinus bradycardia is caused by diseases of the sinus node and atrial myocardium. Theoretically any disease that may affect the heart could cause dysfunction of the sinus node or conduction to the atrial myocardium. In some dogs and cats dying of diseases such as cardiomyopathy, a sinus bradycardia is an ominous sign, although it may be indicative of the associated hypothermia of poor perfusion. Specific disease of the sinus node are discussed later in this chapter.

Sinus bradycardia: pharmacological

Finally, *pharmacological* sinus bradycardia is often caused by drug overdose, including digoxin, β-blockers and calcium channel blockers. It is also a common consequence of the use of alpha-2 agonists, sedation with opioids, and it can occur in response to the injection of intravenous contrast agents which causes a reflex bradycardia.

The electrocardiographic characteristics of sinus bradycardia are a ventricular rate below 60 bpm in dogs and 140 bpm in cats while awake, P waves with a sinus axis, normal of slightly prolonged PQ interval, with a duration of 60 to 130 ms in dogs and 50 to 90 ms in cats; QRS complexes have a normal morphology and duration (≤70 ms in dogs and ≤40 ms in cats) except in the presence of intraventricular conduction blocks. When the discharge rate of the sinus node is lower than the rate of the subsidiary pacemakers, junctional or ventricular escape ectopic beats or rhythms can become apparent on the electrocardiogram (Boxes 11.1 and 11.2), unless other mechanisms suppress these rescue beats or rhythms, as described above.

BOX 11.1.
SINUS BRADYCARDIA IN THE DOG

HEART RATE: <60 bpm.
R-R INTERVAL: regular unless sinus arrhythmia, sino-atrial block or sinus arrest present.
P WAVE: present, sinus axis.
ATRIOVENTRICULAR CONDUCTION: present.
PQ INTERVAL: normal.

QRS COMPLEX: normal (<70 ms), except if preexisting intraventricular conduction abnormalities, and if escape beats or rhythm present.
VENTRICULO-ATRIAL CONDUCTION: absent.
BLOCKED BEATS: absent unless second-degree atrioventricular block present.

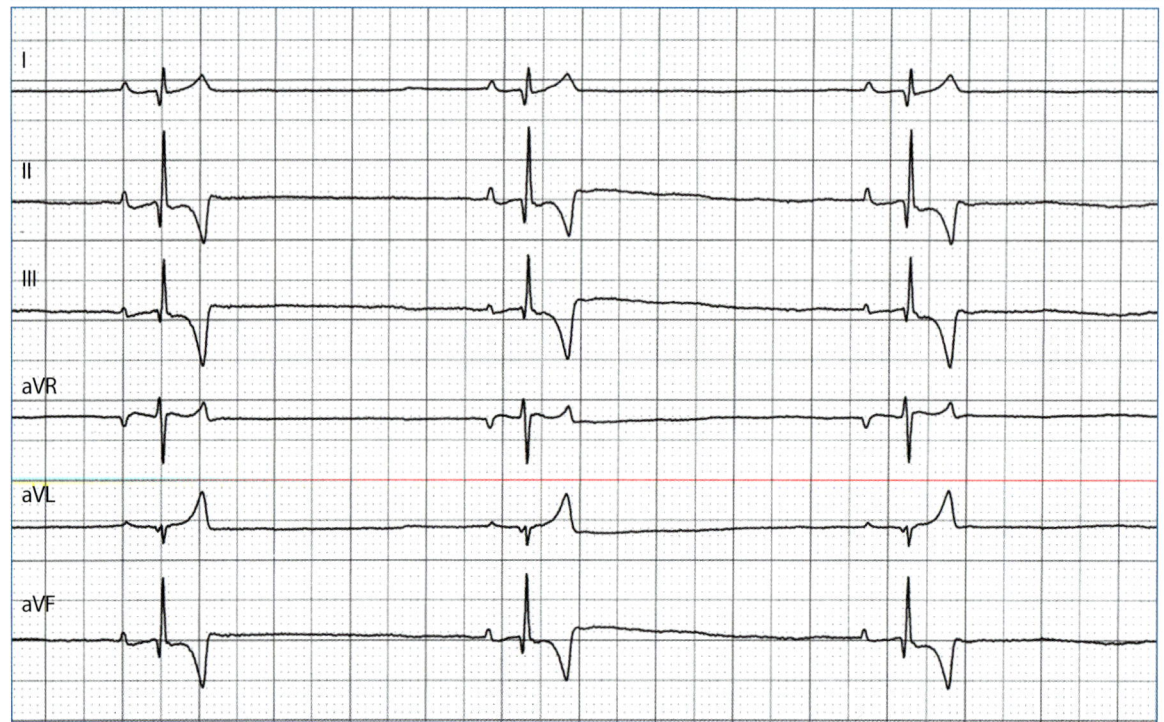

Dog, Rottweiler, female, 2 years.
Six limbs leads (I, II, III, aVR, aVL, aVF) - speed 25 mm/s - calibration 10 mm /1 mV.

Notes: sinus bradycardia with a rate of 60 bpm. P waves are visible with sinus axis, PQ interval are prolonged (220 ms), QRS complexes are normal.

Sinus arrest

Sinus arrest is a disorder of pacemaker cells automaticity characterized by unexpected interruption of sinus node activity for a variable period of time. On the electrocardiogram, it is recognized as an unexpected pause of the underlying sinus rhythm, often interrupted by an atrial, junctional or ventricular escape beat.

In dogs, sinus arrest may occur as a response to a physiologic or pathologic increase in vagal tone, neuro-mediated disorders or sinus node dysfunction. The pauses described with the autonomic reflexes discussed above are considered the result of sinus arrest.

In humans, the electrocardiogram during sinus arrest is characterized by a sinus rhythm interrupted by a pause, which is longer than twice the P-P interval between the preceding beats. In addition, the pause is not a multiple of the underlying P-P interval (Fig. 11.4). In dogs, the frequent occurrence of sinus arrhythmia, which results in a constant variation of the P-P interval, makes it difficult to apply this rule and to differentiate sinus arrest from sino-atrial block. The PQ interval is usually normal

---

BOX 11.2.
SINUS BRADYCARDIA IN THE CAT

HEART RATE: <140 bpm.
R-R INTERVAL: regular unless the presence of sinus arrhythmia, sino-atrial block or sinus arrest.
P WAVE: present, sinus axis.
ATRIOVENTRICULAR CONDUCTION: present.
PQ INTERVAL: normal or increased.

QRS COMPLEX: normal (<40 ms), except if preexisting intraventricular conduction abnormalities, and if escape beats or rhythm present.
VENTRICULO-ATRIAL CONDUCTION: absent.
BLOCKED BEATS: absent unless second-degree atrioventricular block present.

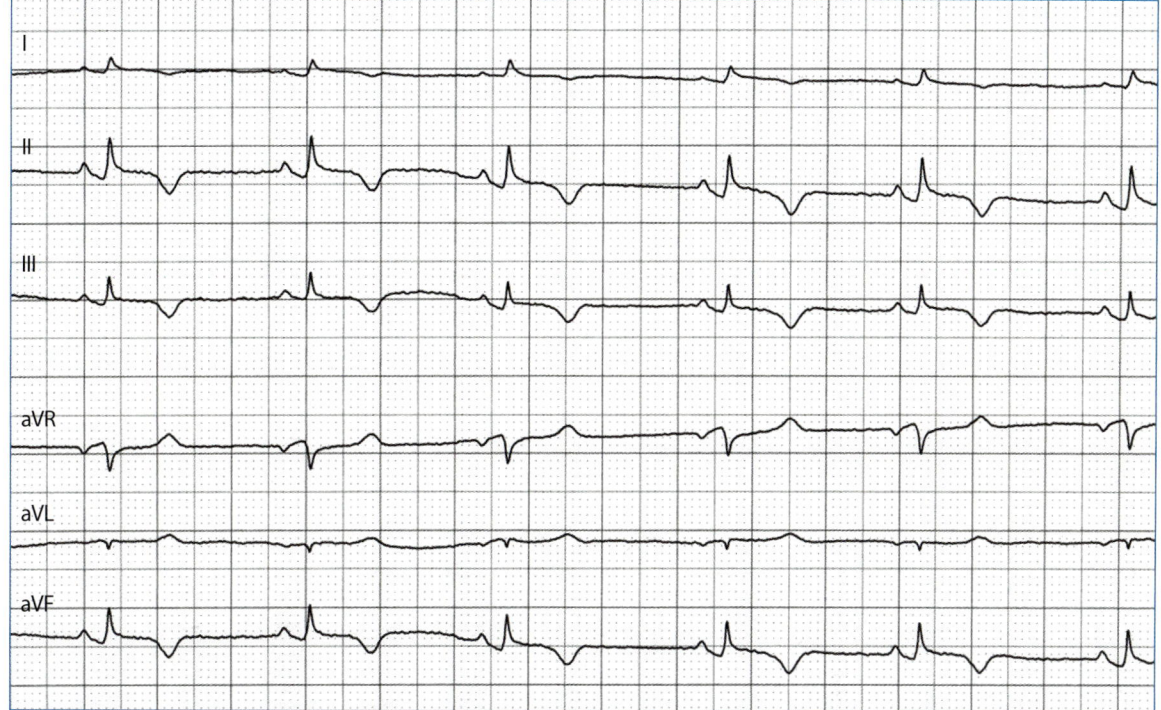

Cat, domestic shorthair, male, 8 years.
Six limbs leads (I, II, III, aVR, aVL, aVF) - speed 50 mm/s - calibration 10 mm/1 mV.

Notes: sinus bradycardia with a rate of 120 bpm. P waves are visible with sinus axis, normal PQ interval and QRS complexes, T wave large and negative and a long QT interval (>220 ms). T_a wave are also visible.

but can be slightly prolonged. The QRS complexes have a normal duration unless an intraventricular conduction block (fascicular or bundle branch block) is present. When ventricular escape beats are present, their morphology differs from the QRS complexes of the sinus beats. The ventricular rate depends on the rate of depolarization of the sinus node, the duration of the periods of sinus arrest and the site of origin of the escape rhythm (atrial versus junctional versus ventricular) (Box 11.3).

Sinus standstill

Sinus standstill describes a persistent or prolonged sinus arrest. During sinus standstill the heart rhythm is maintained by junctional escape rhythms, and less commonly atrial or ventricular escape rhythms.

Prolonged periods of sinus standstill with a junctional escape rhythm can be considered a feature of sick sinus syndrome (see below).

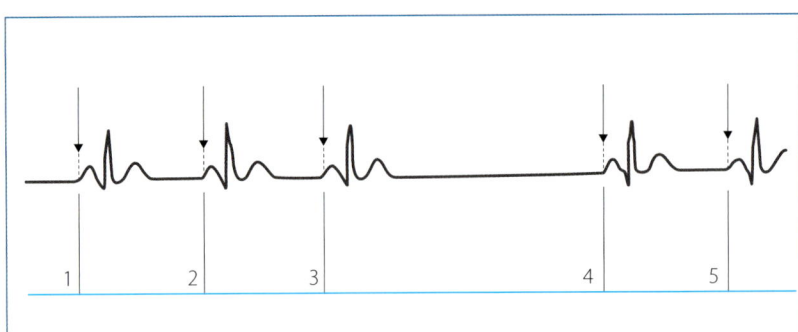

Figure 11.4. Schematic representation of sinus arrest. The arrows indicate the depolarization of the sinus node and coincide with the onset of the P wave. Every beat is normally conducted. After the third beat, the sinus node suddenly stops for a variable period of time and then resumes its normal activity. The interval between beats 3 and 4 is at least twice the basic cycle length but is not a multiple of the intervals between beats 1-2, 2-3 or 4-5.

BOX 11.3.
SINUS ARREST IN THE DOG

HEART RATE: variable.
R-R INTERVAL: irregular.
P WAVE: present, sinus axis, absent during the period of sinus arrest.
ATRIOVENTRICULAR CONDUCTION: present.
PQ INTERVAL: normal or increased.

QRS COMPLEX: normal (<70 ms), except if preexisting intraventricular conduction abnormalities, and if escape beats or rhythm present.
VENTRICULO-ATRIAL CONDUCTION: absent.
BLOCKED BEATS: absent.

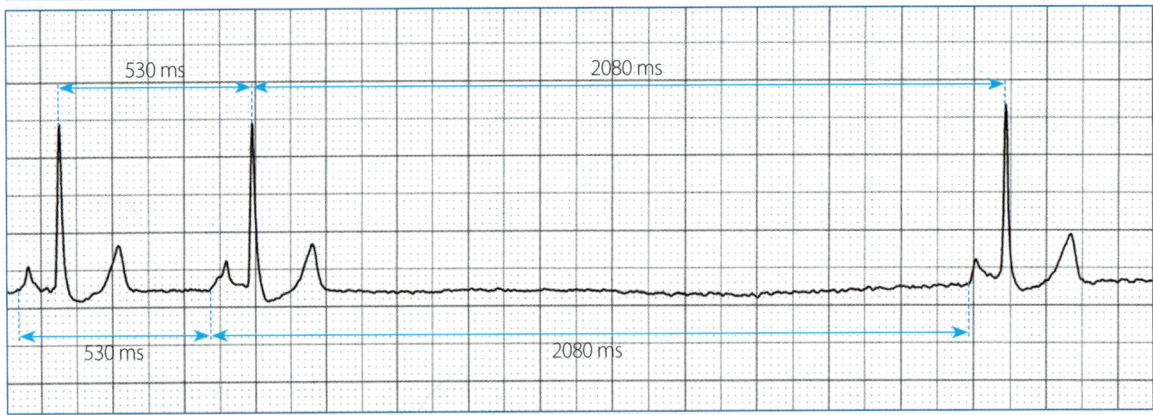

Dog, German Dachshund, female, 12 years.
Lead II- speed 50 mm/s - calibration 10 mm/1 mV.

Notes: sinus rhythm with a rate of 140 bpm and a period of sinus arrest lasting 2080 ms. The P-P interval, which includes the arrest, is equal to 3.8 times the average cycle length (530 ms).i

The electrocardiographic characteristics of sinus standstill include: absence of sinus P waves, QRS complexes of normal morphology and duration (≤70 ms in the dog and ≤40 ms in the cat) when the escape rhythm is junctional, or wide QRS complexes with a morphology that markedly differs from normally conducted beats when the escape rhythm originates in the ventricles, regular R-R intervals, and variable ventricular rate depending on the site of the escape rhythm. A feature of sinus standstill with a junctional escape rhythm is the presence of retrograde concentric atrial activation with ventriculo-atrial conduction ratio of 1:1. It appears as P' waves with an inferior-to-superior axis between −80° and −100° in the inferior leads (II, III, and aVF) within the first portion of the ST segment. They are usually described as pseudo-S waves (Box 11.4). Sinus standstill cannot be distinguished from third-degree sino-atrial block from the surface electrocardiogram (see p. 261).

Sinus node dysfunction or sick sinus syndrome

Sinus node dysfunction and *sick sinus syndrome* are commonly used to identify various rhythm abnormalities secondary to disorders of sinus node automaticity and sino-atrial conduction, and most likely dysfunction of the subsidiary cardiac pacemaker cells as well. This is a complex disorder that requires an understanding of its (1) definition (2) diagnostics, (3) clinical presentation, (4) possible etiologies and (5) specific electrocardiographic characteristics.

Definition

In veterinary medicine, a modification of the differentiating features of sinus node dysfunction and sick sinus syndrome can be adopted from that used in humans. In humans the term sinus node dysfunction is used to describe the electrocardiographic features of abnormal sinus node function in the absence of symptoms, and sick sinus syndrome is used when the person is experiencing symptoms associated with rhythm abnormalities. We can adopt these terms to separate dogs with and without clinical signs, realizing of course that because we are unaware of symptoms the differentiation is dependent on those observing the behavior. Importantly, older sedentary dogs without clinical signs but with a bradycardia, can have clear sinus node dysfunction that, if present in a human, would elicit the expression of symptoms. The term sinus node dysfunction will be used below because although obvious evidence of sinus node abnormality can be documented by electrocardiography, clinical signs may not be appreciated.

The criteria to diagnose sinus node dysfunction in the dog are developing as our understanding increases from more extensive evaluations. Of course, a diagnosis of sinus node dysfunction can be made from: (1) a routine electrocardiogram with the characteristics described below, but because of the complexity of the rhythms in this disorder it is helpful to have criteria from (2) 24-hour electrocardiographic recordings, (3) sinus node recovery times, and (4) pharmacological testing.

Diagnosis: electrocardiography

Electrocardiographic abnormalities that characterize sinus node dysfunction include sinus bradycardia with chronotropic incompetence, sinus arrest, sinus standstill and sino-atrial block. Most dogs can be correctly diagnosed from the electrocardiogram. At times the differentiation between a dog with high parasympathetic tone and a sinus bradycardia with sinus arrhythmia and a dog with sinus node dysfunction with sinus pauses that are excessive may be difficult. The entire clinical picture to obtain the correct diagnosis is important. Dogs with sinus node dysfunction may have sinus pauses usually between 2 and 8 s. These long pauses may be interrupted by either a very late sinus beat, junctional escape beat or ventricular escape beat. In advanced cases of sinus node dysfunction persistent sinus standstill is present with a rhythm of junctional or ventricular escapes. Some dogs will have supraventricular arrhythmias originating from the site near the sinus node or other locations throughout the atria based on P wave vector and morphology. Following brief or longer episodes of such tachycardia a pause occurs. Such pauses can be extremely long (>15 s) and result in syncope. Such a pattern in sinus node dysfunction is known as tachycardia-bradycardia syndrome (pattern). Therefore, electrocardiographic findings consistent with sinus node dysfunction include: sinus bradycardia (Box 11.1), sinus arrest that lasts from

BOX 11.4.
SINUS STANDSTILL IN THE DOG

HEART RATE: dependent on the firing rate of the escape rhythm.
R-R INTERVAL: regular.
P WAVE: absent.
ATRIOVENTRICULAR CONDUCTION: normal but only evident if atrial escape rhythm present.
PQ INTERVAL: absent. P'Q interval if atrial escape rhythm present.

QRS COMPLEX: normal (<70 ms), unless preexisting intraventricular conduction abnormalities, or escape beats or rhythm present.
VENTRICULO-ATRIAL CONDUCTION: present (ratio of 1:1) indicating the ability of the atrial myocardium to depolarize.
BLOCKED BEATS: absent.

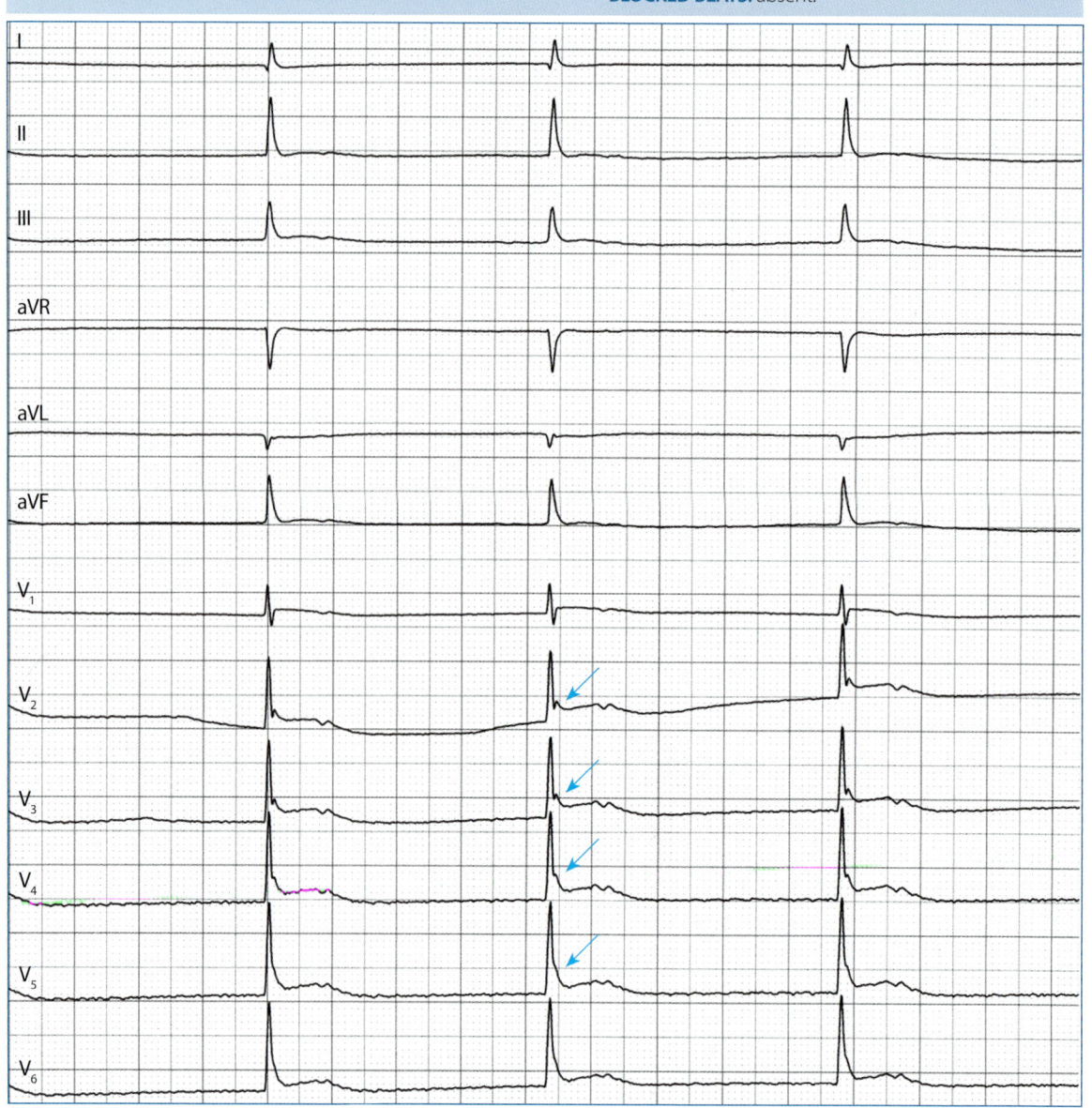

Dog, Labrador Retriever, female, 2 years.
Twelve leads (I, II, III, aVR, aVL, aVF, V_1, V_2, V_3, V_4, V_5, V_6) - speed 50 mm/s - calibration 5 mm/1 mV.

Notes: sinus standstill with junctional escape rhythm with a rate of 70 bpm. Note the absence of P waves and the presence of narrow QRS complexes (50 ms) originating at the atrioventricular junction. There is ventriculo-atrial conduction in a 1:1 ratio represented by the presence of P' waves in the initial portion of the ST segment, particularly evident from V_2 to V_5 (arrows).

2 to 8 s and ends with an escape beat (Box 11.3), sinus standstill with a junctional escape rhythm (Box 11.4), sino-atrial block of various degrees, periods of tachycardia followed by prolonged sinus pauses (Fig. 11.5) or periods of bradycardia followed by an idioventricular rhythm with a high firing rate. Sinus node dysfunction is often associated with various degrees of atrioventricular block and alteration of the subsidiary pacemaker automaticity, which explains the presence of pauses that extend beyond the normal pacing rate of ventricular escape beats.

Diagnosis: 24-hour Holter monitoring

A better understanding of the spectrum and type of bradycardias and tachycardias in sinus node dysfunction will come with more thorough evaluation of 24-hour ambulatory electrocardiography performed in the home environment, particularly with various perturbations to provoke exposure of abnormal rhythms. Holter monitoring is also a valuable diagnostic test when the diagnosis is questioned with regards to other reasons for sinus bradycardia, syncopal dogs are suspected of having sinus node dysfunction and to better understand if coexisting tachycardias are present.

From the evaluation of 24-hour electrocardiographic studies in normal and dogs with sinus node dysfunction the following are characteristics of affected dogs compared to normal dogs: sinus bradycardia of less than 50 bpm for longer than 4 hours, more than 3000 sinus pauses (consequence of sinus arrest, sino-atrial block or sinus standstill) exceeding 2 s in 24 hours, more than 3 pauses exceeding 4.5 s, or finally one pause exceeding 6 s (unless reflex response proven). Holter analysis reveals that the type and frequency of escape beats and rhythms are varied in these dogs. Some have very long intervals with a paucity of escape beats from either the junction or the ventricle, while others have many junctional escape beats activated at similar intervals to the delayed sinus P waves. Also, some dogs with sinus standstill can have only escape beats with no identifiable P waves. Other features of sinus node dysfunction include the presence of atrial arrhythmias. These tachyarrhythmias may have P waves similar in morphology and electrical axis to those of sinus P waves, varied morphology or negative polarity in lead II. The latter two rhythms are not problematic with regards to the diagnosis, but the former is a frequent diagnostic dilemma. Between the longer pauses the origin of the shorter P-P interval is difficult to know. Based on P wave morphology and the mildly tachycardic rates of 125-160 bpm the first assumption is a sinus origin; however, the behavior is abnormal with little variation in the cycle length. The clustering of the long P-P intervals and the short P-P intervals is not characteristic of the normal sinus arrhythmia seen in the dog. Thus, the question of whether such beats could originate as a sinus complex arrhythmia exists.

The beat-to-beat patterning described above presents a characteristic pattern in some dogs with sinus node dysfunction. These patterns are revealed by geometric heart rate variability tools such as the histogram, Poincaré plot and R-R interval tachogram (see p. 77). In addition to the obvious bradycardia the beat clustering is different when compared to normal dogs. Normal

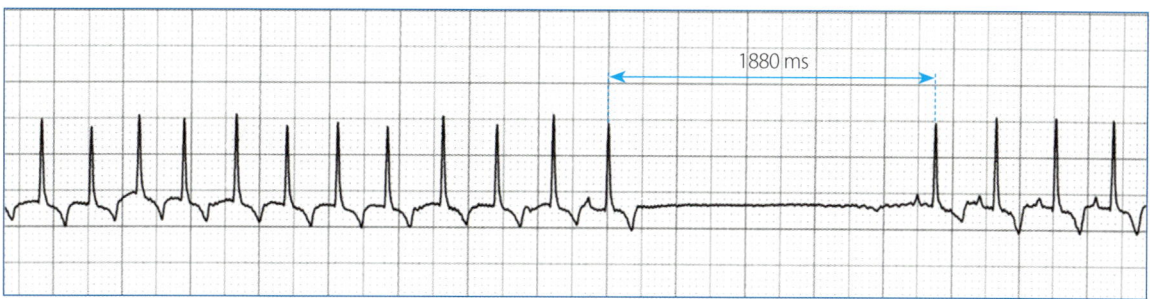

Figure 11.5. Sick sinus syndrome, tachycardia-bradycardia variant (Dog, Jack Russell Terrier, female, 10 years. Lead II - speed 25 mm/s - calibration 5 mm/1 mV).
In the first part of the tracing an atrial tachycardia with a firing rate of 215 bpm is present. The spontaneous termination of atrial tachycardia is not followed by the return of normal sinus node activity. Instead atrial tachycardia is followed by a prolonged asystolic pause lasting 1880 ms until sinus rhythm eventually resumes.

dogs with sinus arrhythmia tend to have a tachogram with double banding representing the R-R intervals (as a surrogate for the P-P intervals when there is atrial and ventricular association) with a very small number of R-R intervals between these two bands. Also, the slower heart rates of sinus arrhythmia are seen as double clusters (see p. 79). Dogs with sinus node dysfunction can have multiple clusters of beats that extend over a longer range of R-R intervals. This is appreciated in each of the geometric parameters. Other patterns of sinus node dysfunction are common but difficult to quantify as yet because of the difficulty in differentiating the sinus beats from ectopies with certainty (Fig. 11.6).

Diagnosis: sinus node recovery time

Sinus node recovery time and *corrected sinus node recovery time* have been used in humans in the electrophysiology laboratory to assist in the determination of normal sinus node function. The principle behind the determination of the sinus node recovery time is based on *overdrive suppression*. When the automaticity of pacemaker cells is inhibited by rapid pacing or rapid spontaneous heart rates, they are overdrive suppressed. This phenomenon occurs in both normal and abnormal cells but with a difference in the duration of the suppression. Importantly, the duration of suppression is dependent on the underlying heart rate or pacing rate. The latter influence is controlled with the corrected sinus node recovery time, which is the sinus node recovery time minus the basic pacing rate. Another means to correct for the basic cycle length is to divide the sinus node recovery time by the basic cycle length and multiply by 100 for a percentage which should not exceed 160 % in humans. To perform this test a catheter is positioned high in the right atrium and pacing is performed at a rate that is just slightly faster than the basic sinus rate. This pacing is continued for 30 s and then stopped, after which the interval between the last paced beat and the first sinus P wave is measured. With sinus node dysfunction the return of a sinus beat takes longer than in a normal dog. Studies of dogs with sinus node dysfunction compared to age-matched controls are lacking. Moreover, it is important to realize that although this test is commonly performed in humans, there is an overlap between normal and abnormal that can at times make interpretation of the results difficult. Consequently, further investigation is required in dogs, especially because variation in anesthetic protocols for performing this examination can influence the results. Certainly, however, electrocardiograms and 24-hour electrocardiographic monitoring of dogs with sinus node dysfunction can clearly have prolonged overdrive suppression of sinus node function following burst of supraventricular tachycardia.

Diagnosis: pharmacological tests

Sinus node automaticity and the integrity of the sinus node exit pathways can be studied with two pharmacological tests: the atropine response test and the determination of intrinsic sinus rhythm. It is important to realize that under certain circumstances these diagnostic tests may pose a risk. When a dog has a tachycardia/bradycardia pattern the administration of drugs that increase the propensity for tachycardia may lead to extreme overdrive suppression with excessive life-threatening sinus pauses or sinus arrest. Subcutaneous administration of atropine at a dose of 0.04 mg/kg in healthy dogs or bradycardic animals secondary to high vagal tone results in an increase of the sinus rate by at least 50 %, or above 140 bpm approximately 30 min after the injection. It should also be noted that some dogs will have a response within 15 min. Sinus node dysfunction is suspected when the heart rate does not increase within the expected time period, or if sinus node automaticity worsens after administration of atropine. However, many dogs with sinus node dysfunction have a normal response to the atropine test, which limits its use to distinguish healthy from affected dogs.

The intrinsic (or inherent) sinus rhythm is defined as the rate of depolarization of the P cells of the sinus node in the absence of autonomic influences. A pharmacological test can be used to block vagal and adrenergic tone simultaneously. This test is based on the administration of 0.01 mg/kg of propranolol intravenously over 1 min and 0.04 mg/kg of atropine intravenously over 2 min. The identification of a slow intrinsic sinus rhythm can be considered a sign of sinus node dysfunction. The intrinsic sinus rate of the dog is usually between 90 and 110 bpm. It must, however, be noted that the response to the test is influenced by the age of the dog. The use of this test is usually limited to the research laboratory, and

Sinus node dysfunction or sick sinus syndrome | 251

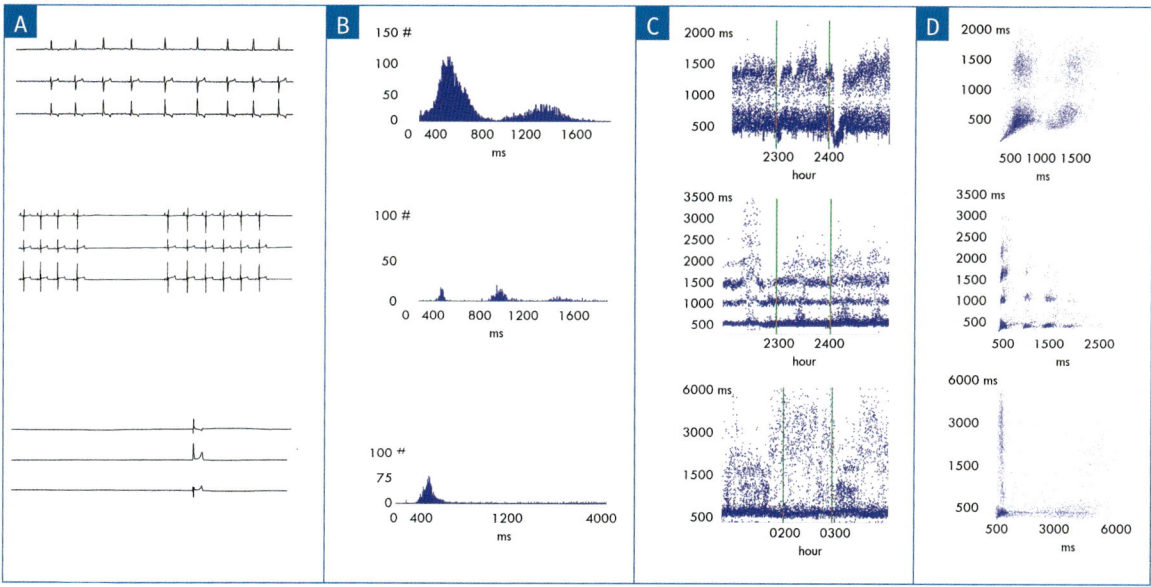

Figure 11.6. Comparison of Holter data in a normal dog and two dogs with sick sinus syndrome for 1 hour during the 24-hour recording. Shown for each dog is an electrocardiographic strip (A), histogram distribution of beats (B), tachogram of the R-R/P-P intervals (C) and the Poincaré plot (D). The blue bars on the tachogram indicate the hour examined with time of day on the X-axis.
In the top row a normal dog with sinus arrhythmia. The histogram shows the typical distribution of sinus beats. The tachogram shows clustering of beats in the 500 ms region, a paucity of beats between 750-1250 ms and then another cluster with longer intervals of greater than 1250 ms and mostly less than 1750 ms. The Poincaré plot which shows the beat to beat variability plotted as R-R interval versus the next beat (R-R interval + 1) demonstrates the normal beat clustering with the paucity of beats in the center.
In the middle row a dog with syncope caused by sick sinus syndrome. The electrocardiogram show more rapid rates with longer intervals between, illustrating the altered beat clustering. The histogram shows a multiple beat distribution. The tachogram shows several regions of beats with paucity of beats between. This type of pattern is suggestive of sinus node exit block. Moreover, the Poincaré plot shows clusters that approximate multiples of intervals, again supportive of exit block.
In the bottom row a dog with syncope caused by sick sinus syndrome. The electrocardiogram shows a long interval of sinus arrest with a single escape beat. The histogram shows a distribution with beats centered around 500 ms, but with many long intervals that are not clustering. The tachogram shows that long R-R intervals approach 6000 ms. The wide interval distribution is also seen in the Poincaré plot. It should be noted that in this recording the R waves were identified as "normal sinus complexes" because they were from the junction; thus, knowing for sure the beat clustering of sinus beats was not possible without extensive editing.

in clinical practice the diagnosis of sick sinus syndrome is based on the evaluation of a baseline electrocardiogram and 24-hour ambulatory Holter recording.

Clinical presentation

Dogs with sinus node dysfunction frequently have a common clinical presentation. The most common breeds afflicted with sinus node dysfunction include the Miniature Schnauzer, West Highland White Terrier, Cocker Spaniel, Cairn Terrier, Dachshund, and Pug. Some Boxers have also been documented with sinus node dysfunction but this disorder must be carefully differentiated from vasovagal situational bradycardia or Bezold-Jarisch reflex bradycardia in this breed given the frequency of ventricular tachycardia. Both sexes can be afflicted although female Miniature Schnauzers are more commonly diagnosed than males. It is rare in cats.

Middle-aged to elderly dogs are more commonly identified with sinus node dysfunction. Importantly, some loss of sinus node function is likely a factor of aging. Loss of sinus node chronotropic capacity is documented in older people such that "normal values" are age-adjusted. More advanced age changes commonly necessitate pacing in elderly people. No data exist, especially 24-hour recordings, to provide age-adjusted heart rates in the dog. A diagnosis can be made in many cases with routine electrocardiography, but more accurate appreciation of sinus node competency is obtained from 24-hour electrocardiography recordings via Holter monitoring when trying to assess elderly dogs.

In dogs, clinical signs include syncope, near-syncope, weakness and exercise intolerance. Frequently, dogs with sinus node dysfunction are only recognized when being evaluated for other problems or for pre-anesthesia screening for dental work or other procedures. Most frequently a sinus rate that is inconsistent with the dog's behavior is noted triggering further evaluation. For all cases differential diagnosis as described for sinus bradycardia applies.

Etiology

The etiology of sinus node dysfunction is likely not the same for each dog. Some may have advanced age or other disease-related dysfunction, while others may have as yet unproven inherited adult onset disease. Certainly given the specific breeds affected, the latter is a high probability. Structural abnormalities of the sinus node complex or micro-structural lesions of gap junctions and ion channels have been identified in humans with some studies in animals. Although in some affected dogs fibro-fatty replacement of nodal tissue has been documented, leaving only 30 % of the nodal cells and isolating the sinus node from the surrounding atrial myocardium, a clear link between sinus node dysfunction and fibrosis has not been established. Most old humans and dogs without sinus node dysfunction also have increased fibrosis. It is however known that in people the amount of fibrosis within the sinus node is inversely correlated with heart rate, and positively correlated with age. In addition, pathological upregulation of fibrosis within the sinus node may lead to tachycardia-bradycardia syndrome and sinus arrest on the electrocardiogram, possibly because it promotes sinus node reentry and exit blocks. Ageing is not only associated with increased fibrosis but also electrical remodelling. For example, an alteration of the expression of ion channels, including Na_v 1.5, and the Cx43 gap junctions in the periphery of the sinus node, which are critical elements for appropriate electrical coupling with the atrial myocardium, can result in sino-atrial exit block. Age-related changes of the L-type Ca^{2+} channel and the ryanodine receptor result in a reduction of the intrinsic heart rate in experimental animal models. In humans, familial sinus node dysfunction has been linked to point mutations or deletions within the HCN4 gene, resulting in bradycardia and paroxysmal atrial fibrillation. Mutations of the SCN5A gene resulting in sodium channel (Na_v 1.5) dysfunction have also been identified in humans.

As described above atrial arrhythmias are frequent in dogs with sinus node dysfunction and experimental animal models of atrial tachyarrhythmias showed that rapid atrial activity resulted in electrical remodeling within the sinus node based on an increase in sinus node recovery time and a reduction of the intrinsic sinus rate. In addition, the leading pacemaker cells shift caudally within the sinus node and become less sensitive to sympathetic stimulation. At the molecular level, there is a reduction in the expression of mRNA for HCN2 and HCN4 channel isoforms that are responsible for the I_f current in the sinus node.

Importantly, a component of autonomic imbalance could contribute or perhaps cause sinus node dysfunction.

Specific electrocardiographic characteristics

The amplitude and duration of P waves and QRS complexes are usually normal. Although some dogs may have a prolonged PQ interval, most are normal. The presence of a heart rate <60 bpm or sinus pauses with a duration greater than 2 s are not characteristic of sinus arrhythmia during recordings in clinical situation. Periods of sinus arrest with escape beats are identified. Supraventricular tachycardia followed by sinus pauses longer than 2 s are frequently noted. Although many normal dogs have pauses longer than 2 s with sinus arrhythmia, it is the pattern of the P-P intervals and the association with the pause that suggest the diagnosis of sinus node dysfunction.

Atrial standstill or atrioventricular muscular dystrophy

Atrial standstill also called *atrioventricular muscular dystrophy* is an electrical disorder characterized by fibrous replacement of the atrial myocardium with concomitant involvement of the sinus node and the internodal, inter-atrial and atrionodal conduction pathways. Atrial standstill was initially described in Springer Spaniels. The structural changes that characterize atrial standstill can be limited to one or both atria and occasionally extend to the left ventricle. Skeletal muscles are usually unaffected although atrial standstill can sometimes be a manifestation of fascio-scapulohumeral muscular dystrophy. On the basis of histopathological findings, atrioventricular muscular dystrophy can be divided into two forms: one associated with volume overload secondary to a structural cardiac disease, and the other secondary to neuromuscular myopathies, at least in dogs.

Histopathological evaluation reveals lymphocytic inflammation, fibrosis, fibro-elastosis and steatosis variably distributed to the atria, inter-atrial septum, sinus node, internodal pathways, atrioventricular node, His bundle and left ventricle. The progressive atrial fibrosis results in the inability of the atrial myocardium to depolarize and conduct impulses. As a result, the heart rhythm is maintained by subsidiary junctional or ventricular pacemakers.

Electrocardiographic characteristics of atrial standstill include an absence of P waves with a flat isoelectric line, or on occasion the presence of low amplitude P waves if the disease is confined to the left atrium, QRS complexes that have a normal morphology if they result from a junctional escape rhythm; they are wide and have an abnormal configuration compared to normally conducted beats if they originate in the ventricles. The heart rate is usually less than 60 bpm in dogs and 140 bpm in cats. R-R intervals are regular. The administration of atropine does not result in an increase in heart rate (Boxes 11.5 and 11.6).

Sino-ventricular rhythm

Severe hyperkalemia (8.5 and 10 mmol/L) brings resting membrane potential of atrial myocytes towards less negative values, to the point that it rises above the threshold potential. Atrial myocytes therefore remain in a constant depolarized state, are unexcitable and unable to conduct impulses. The electrical activity of the pacemaker cells of the sinus node, the *crista terminalis*, the Bachmann's bundle, the internodal and functional atrio-nodal pathways, the bundle of His and the ventricular myocardium are less affected by the elevated extracellular potassium concentration. The resulting rhythm is called *sino-ventricular conduction*. Sino-ventricular conduction is therefore initiated by the sinus node activity. The impulse then

BOX 11.5.
ATRIAL STANDSTILL OR ATRIOVENTRICULAR DYSTROPHY IN THE DOG

HEART RATE: <60 bpm.
R-R INTERVAL: regular.
P WAVE: absent.
ATRIOVENTRICULAR CONDUCTION: absent.
PQ INTERVAL: absent.

QRS COMPLEX: normal (<70 ms), except if preexisting intraventricular conduction abnormalities, and if escape beats or rhythm present.
VENTRICULO-ATRIAL CONDUCTION: absent.
BLOCKED BEATS: no.

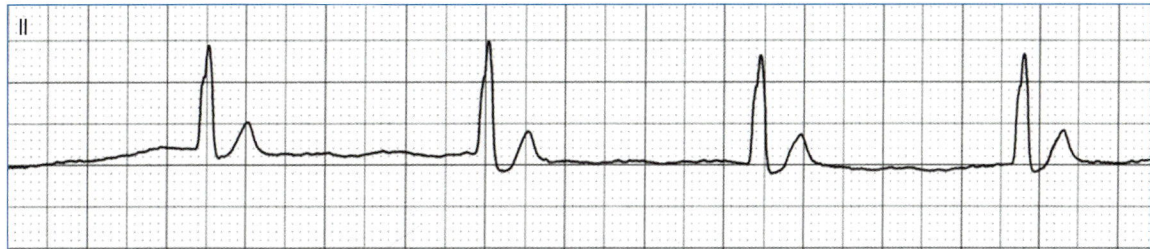

Dog, Labrador Retriever, male, 5 years.
Lead II - speed 25 mm/s - calibration 5 mm/1 mV.

Notes: atrial standstill with ventricular escape rhythm with a rate of 40 bpm. Note the absence of P waves, the presence of wide QRS complexes (100 ms) with regular R-R intervals (1410 ms).

BOX 11.6.
ATRIAL STANDSTILL IN THE CAT

HEART RATE: <140 bpm.
R-R INTERVAL: regular.
P WAVE: absent.
ATRIOVENTRICULAR CONDUCTION: absent.
PQ INTERVAL: absent.

QRS COMPLEX: normal (<40 ms), except if preexisting intraventricular conduction abnormalities, and if escape beats or rhythm present.
VENTRICULO-ATRIAL CONDUCTION: absent.
BLOCKED BEATS: no.

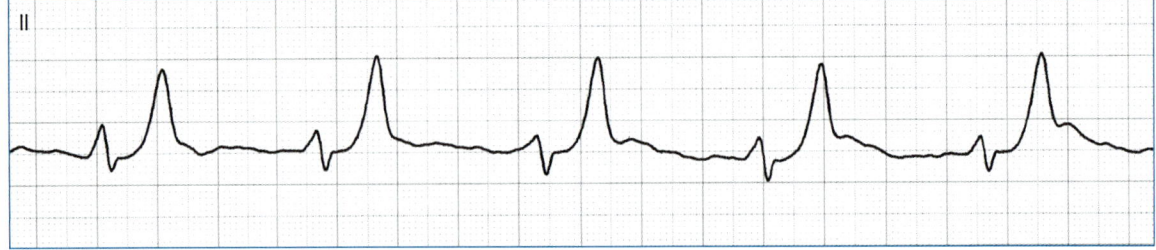

Cat, Maine Coon, female, 2 years.
Lead II- speed 50 mm/s - calibration 10 mm/1 mV.

Notes: atrial standstill with ventricular escape rhythm with a rate of 80 bpm. Note the absence of P waves, the presence of wide QRS complexes (60 ms) with regular R-R intervals (740 ms). As differential diagnosis, sino-ventricular conduction secondary to hyperkalemia should be considered..

propagates to the atrioventricular junction without triggering a depolarization of the atrial myocytes, and then reaches the ventricles.

In cases of extreme hyperkalemia (>11 mmol/L), sinus node automaticity can also be depressed and in this situation, the heart rhythm is usually dependent on junctional or ventricular escape rhythms. Sino-ventricular rhythm is completely reversible with resolution of the hyperkalemia (Box 11.7).

Sino-ventricular rhythms occur secondary to disorders associated with elevated serum potassium concentration, including hypoadrenocorticism (Addison's disease), obstruction or rupture of the urinary tract, oliguric and anuric renal failure, reperfusion following aortic thromboembolism, tumor lysis syndrome, and the administration of potassium penicillin G or potassium salts (potassium bromide).

The electrocardiographic characteristics of sino-ventricular rhythms include absence of P waves and QRS complexes with normal morphology but usually increased duration. The heart rate varies depending on the sinus automaticity, and R-R intervals can, therefore, be irregular. Finally, the T wave becomes symmetrical and peaked ("tented" T wave) (see p. 295).

Asystole or ventricular arrest

Asystole or ventricular arrest is the absence, for a variable period of time, of ventricular depolarizations and, consequently, of ventricular contractions. Asystole can result from the inability of the specialized cardiac conduction system to generate a ventricular depolarization. Usually, it is preceded by bradycardia, including sinus arrest, sinus standstill, sino-atrial block, complete atrioventricular block or atrial standstill with a junctional or ventricular escape rhythm. Asystole can follow a period of ventricular fibrillation. Extracardiac factors that affect the conduction system by causing myocardial hypoxia and cellular acidosis can also result in asystole. Examples include suffocation, massive pulmonary thromboembolism, end-stage hyperkalemia, hypothermia, overdose of sedatives, hypnotics or narcotics, and failure of an artificial pacemaker.

The electrocardiographic characteristics of asystole differ, depending on the underlying condition. There may be a temporary ventricular pause secondary to sino-atrial block, sinus arrest, sinus standstill or atrial standstill and atrioventricular block. In these cases, the pause is terminated by an escape beat (Fig. 11.7).

Asystole or ventricular arrest

BOX 11.7.
SINO-VENTRICULAR RHYTHM IN THE DOG

HEART RATE: depends on the rate of the sinus node.
R-R INTERVAL: depends on the regularity of the discharge rate of the sinus node.
P WAVE: absent.
ATRIOVENTRICULAR CONDUCTION: present without depolarization of the atrial working myocytes.
PQ INTERVAL: absent.
QRS COMPLEX: normal (<70 ms) or increased duration.
VENTRICULO-ATRIAL CONDUCTION: absent.
BLOCKED BEATS: absent.

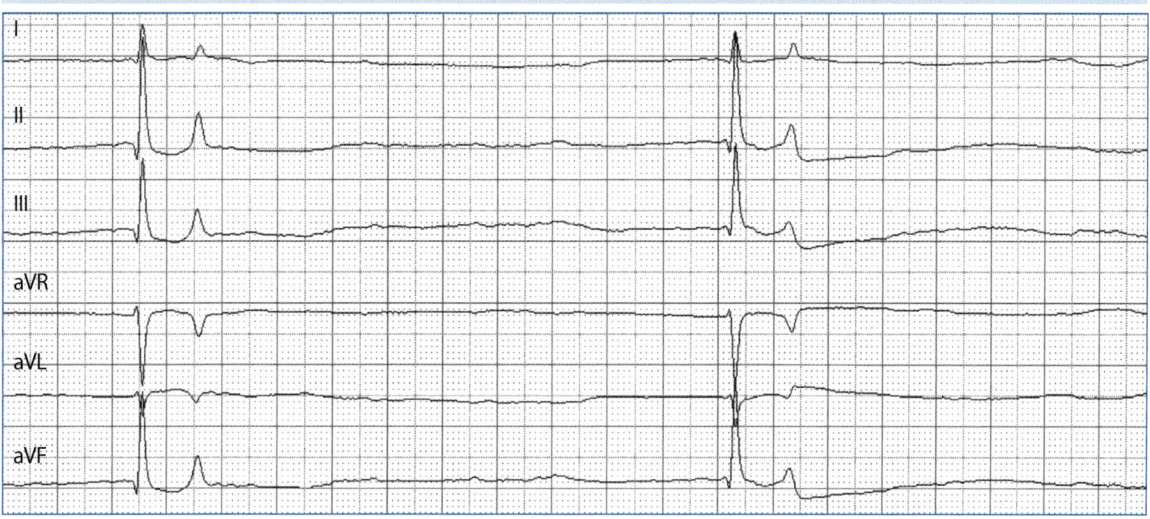

Dog, mixed breed, female, 6 years.
Lead- speed 50 mm / s - calibration 10 mm/1 mV.

Notes: sino-ventricular rhythm with a rate of 54 bpm. Note the absence of P waves and the presence of narrow QRS complexes (60 ms) with regular R-R intervals. Potassium level during the recording was >7.5 mEq/L.

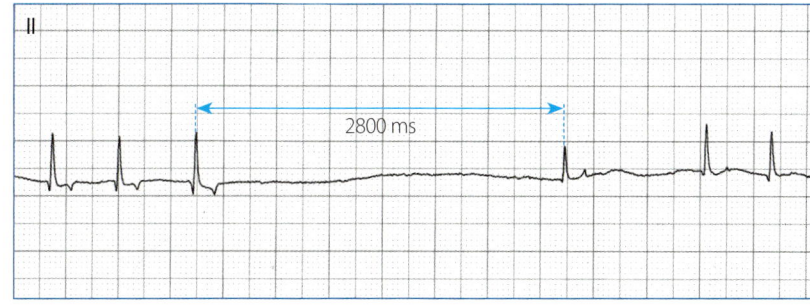

Figure 11.7. Temporary ventricular arrest during atrial standstill (Dog, mongrel, female, 6 years. Lead II - speed 25 mm/s - calibration 10 mm/1 mV).
The underlying rhythm is atrial standstill characterized by the absence of P waves and by narrow QRS complexes (60 ms). After the first three QRS complexes, there is a period of asystole lasting 2800 ms.

If the cause of the asystolic pause is atrioventricular block, P waves are still visible during the pause (Fig. 11.8). Alternatively, there may be a terminal rhythm following ventricular fibrillation or in association with hyperkalemia. In these cases, the isoelectric line is not interrupted by signs of electrical activity.

Pulseless electrical activity or electromechanical dissociation

Pulseless electrical activity is caused by the inability of the heart muscle to generate a contraction in response to ventricular depolarization; this phenomenon is therefore characterized by electrical activity detectable on the surface electrocardiogram in the absence of a femoral arterial pulse.

Pulseless electrical activity is confirmed when the electrical activity apparent on the electrocardiogram is not accompanied by ventricular systole. *Pseudo-pulseless electrical activity* however corresponds to the presence of electrocardiographic waves associated with pressure waveforms in the proximal aorta but the absence of a femoral pulse. This condition occurs when myocardial contractions are too weak to generate an adequate pulse, or severe peripheral vasodilatation is present.

Pulseless electrical activity is usually secondary to severe hypoxia induced by respiratory failure, massive pulmonary embolism, hypothermia, hyperkalemia, or by hypoxia present in the post-ventricular fibrillation period, or following ventricular defibrillation. The initial hypoxic insult causes a reduction of the inotropic capacity of the heart, which in turn promotes further loss of contractility due to cellular acidosis, hypoxia and increased vagal tone.

Pseudo-pulseless electrical activity occurs more frequently with severe hypovolemia, cardiac tamponade, tension pneumothorax, hypoglycemia and overdose of tricyclic antidepressant drugs.

The electrocardiographic characteristics of the true pulseless electrical activity are a slow and irregular rhythm with wide QRS complexes and absent P waves (Fig. 11.9).

Conversely, during pseudo-pulseless electrical activity, the rhythm is usually sinus with narrow QRS complexes, and the heart rate is elevated.

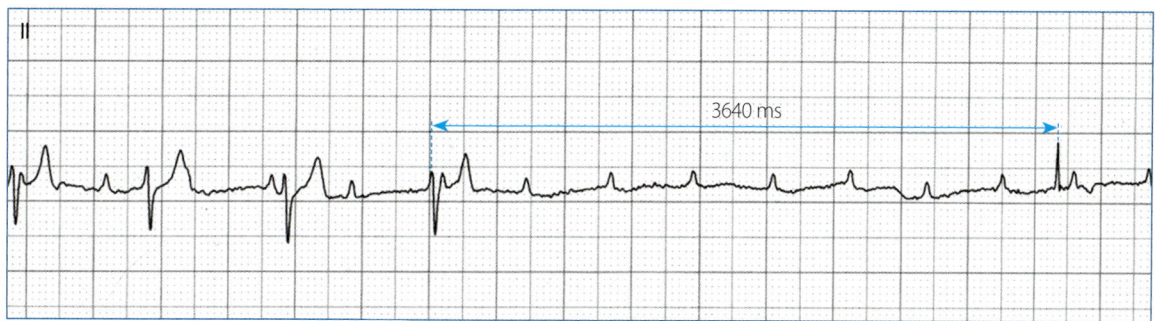

Figure 11.8. Temporary ventricular arrest during third-degree atrioventricular block (Dog, mongrel, female, 8 years. Lead II - speed 50 mm/s - calibration 5 mm/1 mV).

The underlying rhythm is a third-degree atrioventricular block with accelerated idioventricular rhythm and a rate of 75 bpm. After the third ventricular QRS complex, a period of ventricular arrest of 3640 ms occurs characterized by sinus P waves not associated with QRS complexes. The pause is interrupted by a QRS complex of different morphology, reflecting the presence of subsidiary pacemakers of variable origin.

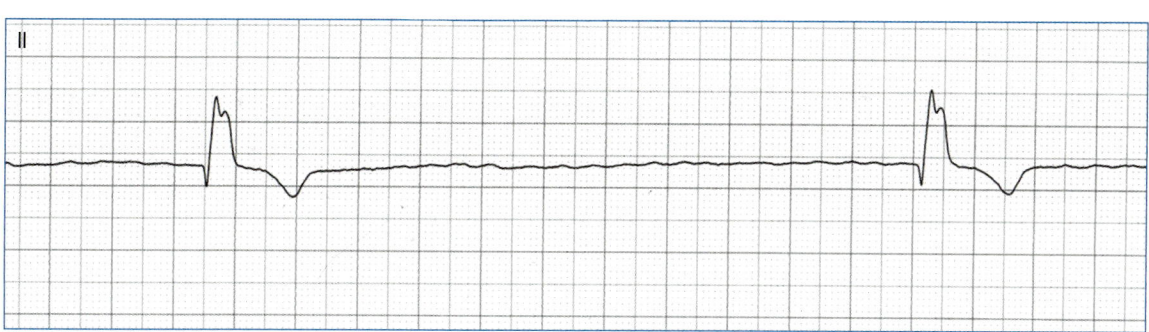

Figure 11.9. Pulseless electrical activity or electromechanical dissociation (Dog, mongrel, female, 14 years. Lead II - speed 25 mm/s - calibration 5 mm/1 mV).

The underlying rhythm is a ventricular escape rhythm with a firing rate of 13 bpm during terminal ventricular arrest. The electrocardiogram shows an isoelectric line without P waves, and QRS complexes with markedly prolonged duration (125 ms). The QRS complexes are not correlated with pressure waveforms.

Suggested readings

1. Auferdheide TP, Thakur RK, Stueven HA, et al. Electrocardiographic characteristics in EMD. *Resuscitation* 1989; 17:183-193.
2. Calvert CA, Jacobs GJ, Pickus CW. Bradycardia-associated episodic weakness, syncope, and aborted sudden death in cardiomyopathic Doberman Pinschers. *J Vet Intern Med* 1996; 1088-1093.
3. Cepse TA, Kalyanasundaram A, Hansen BJ, et al. Fibrosis: a structural modulator of sino-atrial node physiology and dysfunction. *Frontier in Physiology* 2015; 6:1-8.
4. Cervenec RM, Stauthammer CD, Fine H, Kellihan HB, Scansen BA. Survival time with pacemaker implantation for dogs diagnosed with persistent atrial standstill. *J Vet Cardiol* 2017; 19:240-246.
5. Childers HE. Atrial standstill in a dog. *J Am Vet Med Assoc* 1986; 188:140-141.
6. Choudhury M, Boyett MR, Morris GM. Biology of the sinus node and its disease. *Arrhythmia & Electrophysiol Rev* 2015; 4:28-34.
7. Collet M. Sinocarotid compression, and its use in cardiology of the dog. *Animal de Compagnie* 1978; 13:139-160.
8. Dobrzynski H, Boyett MR, Anderson RH. New insight into pacemaker activity promoting understanding of sick sinus syndrome. *Circulation* 2007; 115:1921-1932.
9. Elvan A, Wylie K, Zupes DP. Pacing-induced chronic atrial fibrillation impairs sinus node function in dogs: electrophysiological remodelling. *Circulation* 1996; 94:2953-2960.
10. Gavaghan BJ, Kittleson MD, McAloose D. Persistent atrial standstill in a cat. *Aust Vet J* 1999; 77:574-579.
11. Greco DS. Hypoadrenocorticism in small animals. *Clin Tech Small Anim Pract* 2007; 22:32-35.
12. Hamlin RL, Smetzer DL, Breznock EM. Sino-atrial syncope in Miniature Schnauzers. *J Am Vet Assoc* 1972; 161:1022-1028.
13. Ishikawa S, Sawada K, Tanahashi Y, et al. Experimental studies on sick sinus syndrome: relationship of extent of right atrial lesions to subsidiary pacemaker shift and its function. *Am Heart J* 1983; 105:593-602.
14. Jeraj K, Ogburn PN, Edwards WD, et al. Atrial standstill, myocarditis and destruction of cardiac conduction system: clinicopathologic correlation in a dog. *Am Heart J* 1980; 99:185-192.
15. Jochman-Edwards CM, Tilley LP, Lichtenberger M, et al. Electrocardiographic findings in Miniature Schnauzers with syncope. *J Vet Emerg Crit Care* 2002; 12:253-259.
16. Kavanagh K. Sick sinus syndrome in a Bull Terrier. *Can Vet J* 2002; 43:46-48.
17. Kelly PJ. Vagal bradycardia in a dog. *J S Afr Vet Assoc* 1985; 56:151.
18. Kittleson MD, Schukei TW. Sino-atrial block in a dog. *J Am Vet Med Assoc* 1980; 15;177:332-334.
19. Knowlton AI, Baer L. Cardiac failure in Addison's disease. *Am J Med* 1984; 74:829-836.
20. Larabee TM, Paradis NA, Bartsch J, et al. A swine model of pseudo-pulseless electrical activity induced by partial asphyxiation. *Resuscitation* 2008; 78:196-199.
21. Little C, Marshall C, Downs J. Addison's disease in the dog. *Vet Rec* 1989; 124:469-470.
22. Milanesi R, Bucchi A, Baruscotti M. The genetic basis for inherited forms of sino-atrial dysfunction and atrioventricular node dysfunction. *J Interv card Electrophysiol* 2015; 43:121-134.
23. Moneva-Jordan A, Corcoran BM, French A, et al. Sick sinus syndrome in nine West Highland White Terriers. *Vet Rec* 2001; 148:142-147.
24. Nakao S, Hirakawa A, Fukushima R, et al. The anatomical basis of bradycardia-tachycardia syndrome in elderly dogs with chronic degenerative valvular disease. *J Comp Path* 2012; 146:175-182.
25. Peterson ME, Kintzer PP, Kass HH. Pretreatment clinical and laboratory findings in dogs with hypoadrenocorticism: 225 cases (1979-1993). *J Am Vet Med Assoc* 1996; 208:85-91.
26. Robinson WF, Thompson RR, Clark WT. Sino-atrial arrest associated with primary atrial myocarditis in a dog. *J Small Anim Pract* 1981; 22:99-107.
27. Schmitt KE, Lefbom BK. Long-term management of atrial myopathy in two dogs with single chamber permanent transvenous pacemakers. *J Vet Cardiol* 2016; 18:187-193.
28. Shen WK, Wharton JM, Strauss HC. Mechanisms of bradyarrhythmias and blocks. *Hosp Pract* (Off Ed) 1988; 23:93-103,107-110.
29. Stramba-Badiale M, Vanoli E, De Ferrari GM, et al. Sympathetic-parasympathetic interaction and accentuated antagonism in conscious dogs. *Am J Physiol* 1991; 260:335-340.
30. Stueven HA, Aufderheide T, Thakur RK, et al. Defining electromechanical dissociation: morphologic presentation. *Resuscitation* 1989; 17:195-203.
31. Thomanson JD, Kraus MS, Fallaw TL, et al. Survival in 4 dogs with persistent atrial standstill treated by pacemaker implantation. *Can Vet J* 2016; 57:297-298.
32. Vincent JL, Thijs L, Weil MH, et al. Clinical and experimental studies on electromechanical dissociation. *Circulation* 1981; 64:18-27.
33. Waldo AL, Vitikainen KJ, Kaiser GA, et al. Atrial standstill secondary to atrial inexcitability (atrial quiescence) recognition and treatment following open-heart surgery. *Circulation* 1972; 46:690-697.
34. Ward JL, DeFrancesco TC, Tou SP, et al. Outcome and survival in canine sick sinus syndrome and sinus node dysfunction: 93 cases (2002-2014). *J Vet Cardiol* 2016; 18:199-212.
35. Wessalowski S, Abbott J, Borgarelli M, Tursi M. Presumptive partial atrial standstill secondary to atrial cardiomyopathy in a Greyhound. *J Vet Cardiol* 2017; 19:276-282.
36. Wright Kz, Hines DA, Bright JM. Cardiac electrophysiologic measurements in dogs before and after intravenous administration of atropine and propranolol. *Am J Vet Res* 1996; 57:1695-1701.

CHAPTER 12

Conduction disorders

The term *conduction* describes the propagation of an electrical impulse through heart muscle tissue. Delayed conduction and intermittent or permanent interruption of electrical impulse propagation is called *block*. Blocks can occur at the sino-atrial junction (first, second and third-degree sino-atrial block), within the atrial myocardium (intra-atrial block), at the level of the Bachmann's bundle (inter-atrial block), and finally within the atrioventricular node and intraventricular His-Purkinje system (first, second and third-degree atrioventricular blocks and bundle branch blocks). First-degree blocks correspond to the prolongation of the propagation of an impulse within a specific cardiac structure; second-degree blocks are an intermittent interruption of conduction; third-degree blocks are a permanent interruption of impulse conduction.

Disorders of atrial conduction

Disorders of atrial conduction include:
- sino-atrial blocks,
- intra-atrial delays and blocks, and
- inter-atrial blocks.

Most of these conduction abnormalities are features of sinus node dysfunction (or *sick sinus syndrome*) (see p. 247).

Sino-atrial block

A *sino-atrial block* results in a delay or an interruption of the transmission of electrical impulses between the sinus node and the atrial myocardium during normal sinus pacemaker activity. Theoretically, there are three forms of block (first, second and third-degree), but the typical presence of sinus arrhythmia in dogs makes it impossible to identify first-degree sino-atrial block, which is a slower than normal impulse propagation between the sinus node and the atrial myocardium. Second-degree sino-atrial block is a temporary interruption of sinus impulse conduction to the atrial myocardium. The pauses that characterize sino-atrial block are usually terminated by atrial or junctional escape beats, and uncommonly ventricular escape beats. Finally, third-degree sino-atrial block corresponds to the absence of conduction between the sinus node and atrium.

Sino-atrial block results from inflammation, degeneration of the sinus node or abnormalities in ion channel function (sick sinus syndrome), hypervagotonia, use of certain medications (digitalis, β-blockers, amiodarone, potassium, opioids) and increased intracranial pressure.

Second-degree sino-atrial block is characterized by an unexpected pause of the underlying sinus rhythm. The pause is frequently terminated by a sinus beat, and the duration of the pause is a multiple of the preceding P-P intervals. This rule does not apply if the pause is terminated by an escape beat, if the underlying rhythm is sinus arrhythmia or if variations of the PQ interval are also present. In the presence of a regular sinus rhythm, second-degree sino-atrial block can be differentiated from sinus arrest, because during sinus arrest the pause is longer than twice the underlying sinus rate and is not a multiple of the previous P-P intervals. However, it is not possible to differentiate sino-atrial block from sinus arrest when the underlying rhythm is irregular. During sino-atrial block the QRS complexes have normal morphology and duration, unless there is a pre-existing intraventricular block, or if an occasional ventricular escape beat occurs at the end of a pause (Fig. 12.1 and Box 12.1).

Figure 12.1. Sino-atrial block. The arrows indicate the sinus node depolarization and coincide with the beginning of a P wave. Beats 1, 2, 3, 5, 6 represent the sinus node depolarizations normally conducted to the atrioventricular node and to the ventricles. The sinus node depolarization corresponding to number 4, however, is not conducted. The P-P intervals that include the pause are twice the P-P intervals of the underlying sinus rhythm. These observations are valid only if the firing rate of the sinus node is regular, that is, if intervals 1-2, 2-3 and 5-6 are equal.

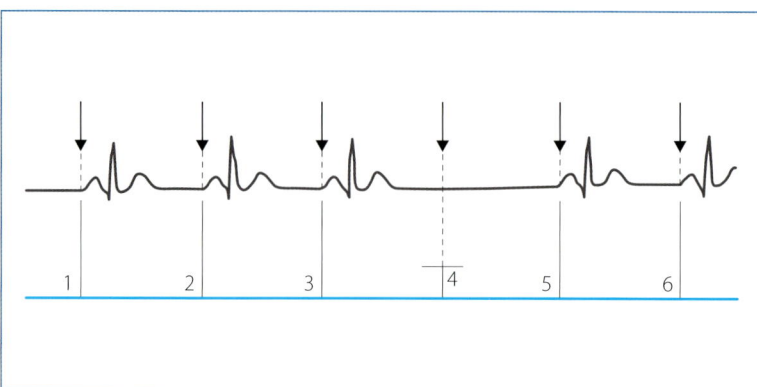

BOX 12.1.
SECOND-DEGREE SINO-ATRIAL BLOCK IN THE DOG

HEART RATE: variable.
R-R INTERVALS: regularly irregular.
P WAVE: present, sinus axis, absent during the period of sino-atrial block.
ATRIOVENTRICULAR CONDUCTION: present.
PQ INTERVAL: usually normal.

QRS COMPLEX: normal (<70 ms, unless presence of ventricular escape beats or previous functional conduction disorders).
VENTRICULO-ATRIAL CONDUCTION: absent.
BLOCKED BEATS: some, originating from the sinus node.

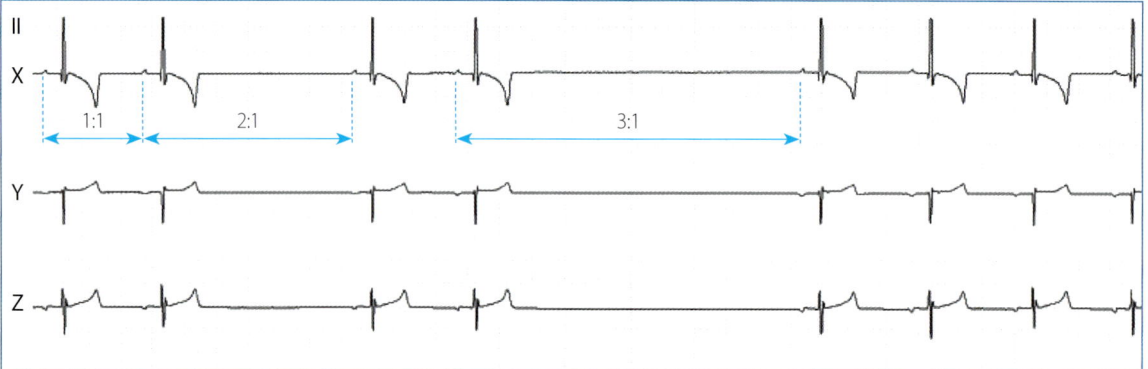

Dog, Miniature Schnauzer, male, 16 years.
Orthogonal leads X, Y, and Z from Holter recording (8 s strip).

Notes: second-degree sino-atrial block in a dog with sinus node dysfunction. The shortest identifiable P-P interval ranges from 621 ms to 683 ms (note that with a consistent PQ interval the R-R intervals serve as a surrogate for the P-P intervals). This ECG supports 2:1 and 3:1 sino-atrial block. Note that the variation in the multiples is approximately 10 %. This variation is realistic for what is identified in the dog given the modulation by the autonomic nervous system. It is rare to have exact multiples in canine sino-atrial block.

The electrocardiographic features of *third-degree sino-atrial block* include the absence of P waves and a junctional or ventricular escape rhythm as the underlying rhythm. Third-degree sino-atrial block with a junctional escape rhythm is indistinguishable from sinus standstill (see p. 246). Both rhythms are characterized by the absence of P waves and a junctional or ventricular escape rhythm with frequent 1:1 ventriculo-atrial retrograde conduction. Retrograde conduction appears as P' waves with an inferior-superior axis within the first portion of the ST segment, appearing as pseudo-S waves in the inferior leads (II, III, and aVF) (Box 12.2).

Disorders of atrial conduction

BOX 12.2.
THIRD-DEGREE SINO-ATRIAL BLOCK IN THE DOG

HEART RATE: dependent on the rate of the escape rhythm.
R-R INTERVALS: regular.
P WAVE: absent. Usually P' waves following the QRS complex, giving the appearance of pseudo-S waves in inferior leads.
ATRIOVENTRICULAR CONDUCTION: absent.
PQ INTERVAL: not evaluable.

QRS COMPLEX: normal (<70 ms), unless ventricular escape beats or rhythm present.
VENTRICULO-ATRIAL CONDUCTION: usually present (1:1) during junctional or ventricular escape rhythm.
BLOCKED BEATS: yes, all the impulses originating from the sinus node.

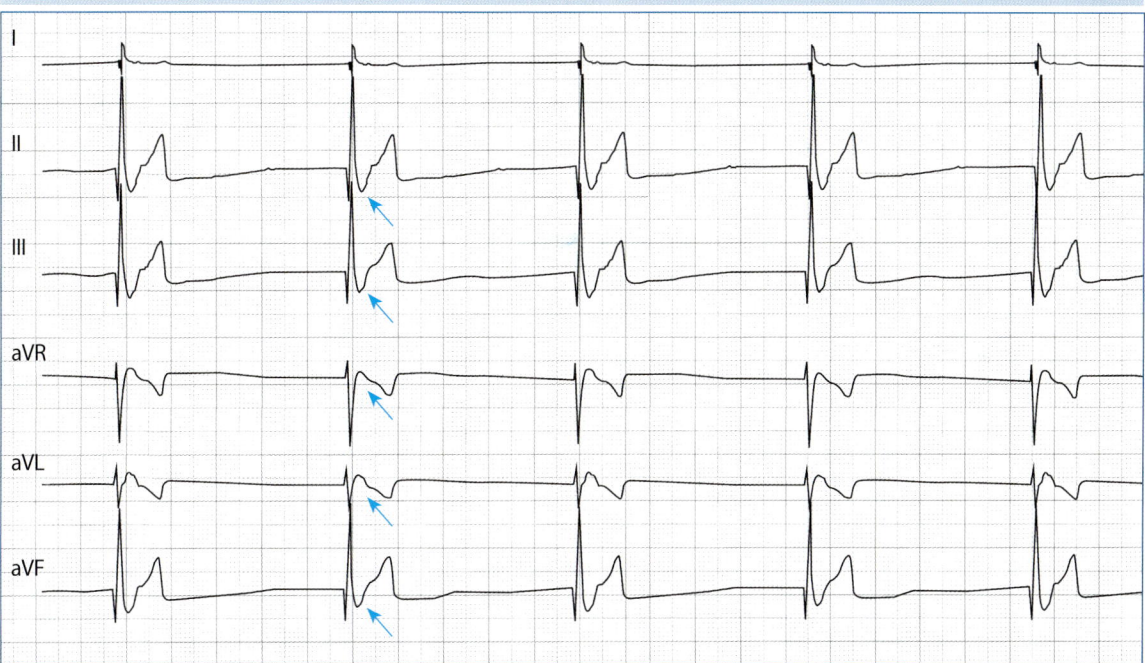

Dog, Dachshund, male, 10 years.
6-lead ECG - speed 50 mm/s - calibration 10 mm/1 mV.

Notes: third-degree sino-atrial block with junctional escape rhythm with a rate of 60 bpm. Note the absence of P waves and the presence of narrow QRS complexes (50 ms) with nodo-Hisian origin and 1:1 ventriculo-atrial conduction, characterized by the presence of P' waves inscribed in the initial portion of the ST segment (arrows). Note the polarity (vector) of the P wave in each of the leads, consistent with concentric retro-activation. The P wave of the last beat is more obscured by the QRS complex than the other 2 beats. On the surface electrocardiogram third-degree sino-atrial block is indistinguishable from sinus standstill.

Intra-atrial conduction delay or block

Intra-atrial conduction disorders encompass delays or blocks of intra-atrial conduction as a result of anatomical or functional obstacles to electrical impulse propagation. A contributor to these delays and blocks is anisotropic conduction, a variation of impulse propagation velocity depending on the direction of the impulse within the atrial myocardium. Anisotropic conduction promotes the formation of reentrant circuits.

Intra-atrial conduction block or delay can result from the administration of class I anti-arrhythmic drugs, hyperkalemia (usually when potassium concentration approaches 7.5 mmol/l), atrial fibrosis, or hypervagotonia. It is also frequently present in the period following electrical cardioversion of atrial fibrillation.

Intra-atrial conduction block or delay appears on the surface electrocardiogram as a wide and frequently bifid P wave lasting longer than 40 ms in dogs (≥50 ms in giant breed dogs) and ≥35 ms in cats, and/or PQ interval prolongation (>130 ms in dogs and >90 ms in cats) (Box 12.3). The QRS complex is normal in duration and morphology unless an intraventricular conduction block is present.

Inter-atrial conduction block

Inter-atrial conduction blocks result from slow conduction within the atrial myocardium or along specialized conduction pathways, such as the Bachmann's bundle and, rarely, the inferior fascicle.

Normal left atrial activation depends on Bachmann's bundle, the inferior fascicle and the atrial myocardium. In the presence of a *Bachmann's bundle block*, left atrial depolarization is delayed and a deviation of the direction of atrial activation occurs. As a result, the electrocardiographic features of a Bachmann's bundle block include the prolongation of P wave duration (>40 ms in dogs and >35 ms in cats), bifid P waves in leads I, II, aVR, aVF and diphasic P waves in aVL and III. It is not always possible to differentiate inter-atrial conduction block from intra-atrial conduction block from the surface electrocardiogram.

Atrioventricular blocks

Atrioventricular blocks range from a reduction in conduction velocity to the intermittent or complete interruption of impulse propagation across the atrioventricular junction.

Atrioventricular blocks are divided into:
- first-degree atrioventricular block,
- second-degree atrioventricular block, and
- third-degree atrioventricular block.

First-degree atrioventricular block

First-degree atrioventricular block is a delay of conduction as the electrical impulse travels through the atrioventricular junction. It appears on the electrocardiogram as

---

BOX 12.3.
INTRA-ATRIAL CONDUCTION DELAY OR BLOCK IN THE DOG

HEART RATE: dependent on the firing rate of the sinus node.
R-R INTERVALS: variable depending on the regularity of the sinus rhythm.
P WAVE: present, sinus axis and duration >40 ms; occasionally bifid morphology.

ATRIOVENTRICULAR CONDUCTION: present.
PQ INTERVAL: normal.
QRS COMPLEX: normal (<70 ms), unless preexisting intraventricular conduction disturbance.
VENTRICULO-ATRIAL CONDUCTION: absent.
BLOCKED BEATS: no.

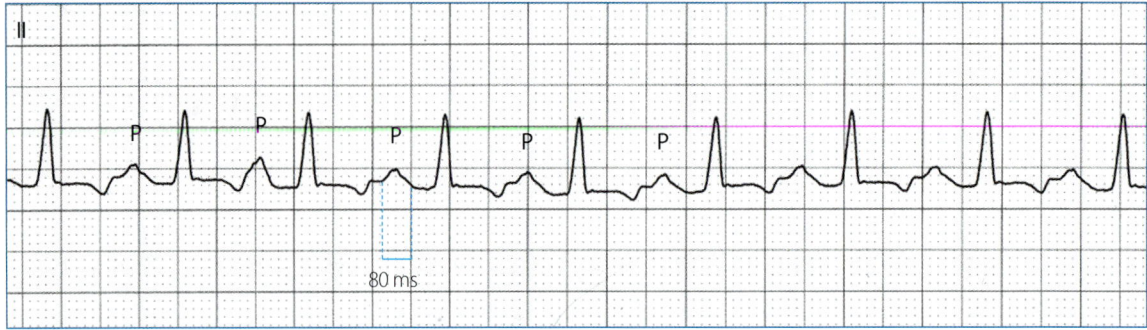

Dog, Newfoundland, female, 7 years.
Lead I - speed 50 mm/s - calibration 10 mm/1 mV.

Notes: sinus tachycardia with rate of 180 bpm, with intra-atrial conduction delay. The P waves have an increased duration (80 ms) and a bifid morphology.

a prolongation of the PQ interval. All the events between the formation of the impulse within the sinus node to the activation of the ventricles are included in the PQ interval: depolarization of the atrial myocardium, impulse propagation within the atrioventricular node, the His bundle and the proximal portion of the bundle branches. First-degree atrioventricular block can be described as intra-atrial, intra-nodal, intra-Hisian or infra-Hisian, but the site of the block cannot be determined from the surface electrocardiogram. A prolonged PQ interval may therefore reflect an alteration of conduction velocity within any of these structures.

First-degree atrioventricular block usually results from degenerative or inflammatory processes, neoplasia of the conduction system, drugs (digitalis, β-blockers, calcium channel blockers), electrolyte disturbances (hyperkaliemia) or hypervagotonia.

The electrocardiographic features of first-degree atrioventricular block are P waves with sinus axis and normal discharge rate, and prolonged PQ interval (>130 ms in dogs and >90 ms in cats). When the QRS complexes are normal in duration, an intra-atrial or intra-nodal conduction delay is more likely (Box 12.4). Conversely, if the QRS complexes are wide (>70 ms in dogs and >40 ms in cats) the conduction delay likely involves the His bundle, the proximal part of the right or left bundle, or a combination of several bundles.

Second-degree atrioventricular block

Second-degree atrioventricular block is an intermittent interruption of atrioventricular conduction, and is classified according to two electrocardiographic criteria: the mode of interruption of atrioventricular conduction and the ratio between successful atrioventricular conduction and atrioventricular block. This relationship is represented by a fraction with the number of conducted P waves in the numerator and the number of QRS complexes in the denominator (2:1, 3:1, 4:1, etc.). For example, a 3:1 block indicates that there are 3 P waves for every QRS complex, in other words 2 P waves are blocked and the third one is associated with a QRS complex.

BOX 12.4.
FIRST-DEGREE ATRIOVENTRICULAR BLOCK IN THE DOG

HEART RATE: dependent on the firing rate of the sinus node.
R-R INTERVALS: variable depending on the regularity of the sinus rhythm.
P WAVE: present, sinus axis.
ATRIOVENTRICULAR CONDUCTION: delayed.

PQ INTERVAL: prolonged (>130 ms).
QRS COMPLEX: normal (<70 ms) in the presence of intra-atrial and intranodal block; with a bundle branch block morphology if block involves the infra-Hisian region.
VENTRICULO-ATRIAL CONDUCTION: absent.
BLOCKED BEATS: no.

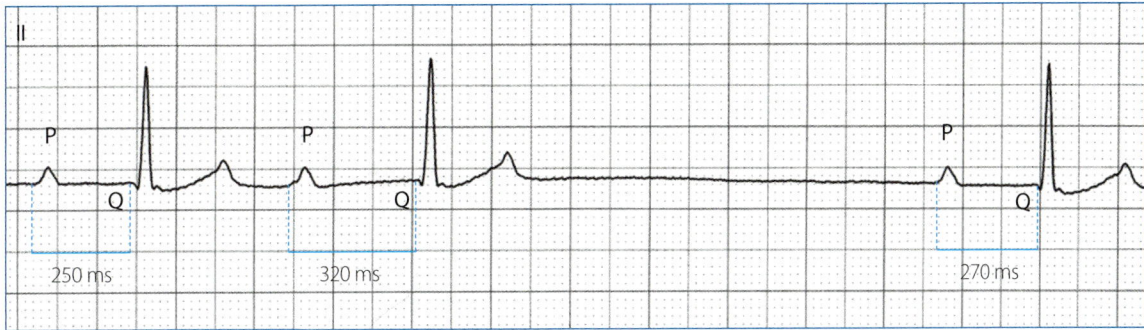

Dog, mongrel, male, 10 years.
Lead II- speed 50 mm/s - calibration 10 mm/1 mV.

Notes: respiratory sinus arrhythmia with a rate of 38-85 bpm with first-degree atrioventricular block. There are sinus P waves, prolonged PQ intervals with varying degrees of atrioventricular conduction prolongation (from 250 to 320 ms).

Second-degree atrioventricular blocks are divided into:
- Mobitz type I (or Wenckebach type),
- Mobitz type II,
- 2:1 block, and
- Advanced.

Second-degree atrioventricular block may be physiologic in young dogs between the age of 8 and 11 weeks or in situations of high vagal tone (e.g., secondary to chronic respiratory diseases). Physiologic blocks are always type I, although in normal puppies a sudden blocked P wave can occur. Pathologic blocks result from degenerative, inflammatory or neoplastic processes. In Pugs, a hereditary condition associated with a stenosis of the bundle of His has been described, but seems to be rare. Finally, digitalis overdose, opioids, β-blockers and calcium channel blockers can cause second-degree atrioventricular block.

It should be noted that when using the term second-degree atrioventricular block which is clinically often shortened to "second-degree heart block", the inference is that there is an underlying physiologic mechanism attributable to high vagal tone or to a disease process of this region of the conduction system. Consequently, the heart rate is often low. However, during supraventricular tachycardias that are independent of the atrioventricular nodal region, it is possible to have such a rhythm that is incompletely conducted to the ventricles. This atrioventricular nodal block is not due to high vagal tone nor to disease of this region. This is "functional block" (see below) and may be termed "tachycardia-dependent atrioventricular block". This type of conduction occurs simply because the rate is too high for the atrioventricular node to conduct for each atrial impulse. Therefore, when communicating about rhythms that are incompletely conducted to the ventricle the underlying rhythm should also be stated (e.g. sinus arrhythmia, sinus bradycardia, atrial tachycardia) for clarity of diagnosis.

Mobitz type I second-degree atrioventricular block (Wenckebach type)

In its typical form, Mobitz type I second-degree atrioventricular block is characterized by a progressive slowing of conduction velocity along the atrioventricular node leading to an increasing delay in sinus impulse propagation across the atrioventricular node until an impulse is blocked and does not initiate ventricular depolarization. The impulse following the blocked beat is usually conducted through the atrioventricular junction with a relatively normal conduction time. This pattern of conduction is also known as *Wenckebach phenomenon*.

The characteristic electrocardiographic findings of type I second-degree atrioventricular block include:
- a progressive prolongation of the PQ interval before the blocked P wave,
- the maximum change in PQ interval duration usually occurs with the second beat after the blocked P wave. The subsequent PQ intervals increase by a lower magnitude until the block,
- a reduction of R-R interval duration before the block (increase of the sinus rate),
- the PQ interval that follows the blocked P wave is shorter than the PQ of the beat that precedes the block, and
- the duration of the pause during the block is usually a multiple of the underlying P-P interval, unless sinus arrhythmia is present (which of course is the most common rhythm of the dog).

The mechanism for type I second-degree atrioventricular block is a progressive prolongation of the relative refractory period of the atrioventricular node that is proportional to the prematurity of the impulse traveling through it; the absolute refractory period of the tissue is normal (Fig. 12.2). The site of block is usually at the level of the atrioventricular node.

Type I second-degree atrioventricular block is further classified as *typical* or *atypical*. In its typical form, the progressive prolongation of the PQ before the blocked P wave is associated with a progressive shortening of the R-R intervals. The maximum variation in beat-to-beat PQ interval prolongation occurs between the first and the second conducted P waves of a series. The PQ interval that follows the blocked P wave is shorter than the PQ of the beat that precedes the block. The QRS complexes of the conducted beats usually have normal morphology and duration (Box 12.5).

The atypical form of block is frequent when the ratio of atrioventricular conduction is greater than 7:6. It is characterized by a PQ interval of variable duration, with the maximum prolongation of the PQ interval that does not affect the second beat after a blocked P wave and the absence of R-R interval shortening before a block. The PQ interval that follows the block remains shorter than the PQ that precedes it (Box 12.6).

Mobitz type II second-degree atrioventricular block

The essential characteristic of the Mobitz type II atrioventricular block is a fixed PQ interval for all the beats that precede and follow the blocked P waves (Fig. 12.2). This pattern on the electrocardiogram corresponds to a block in the Hisian or infra-Hisian region. As a result, at least in humans, the block at the level of the atrioventricular node is often associated with evidence of intraventricular conduction delays (bundle branch block).

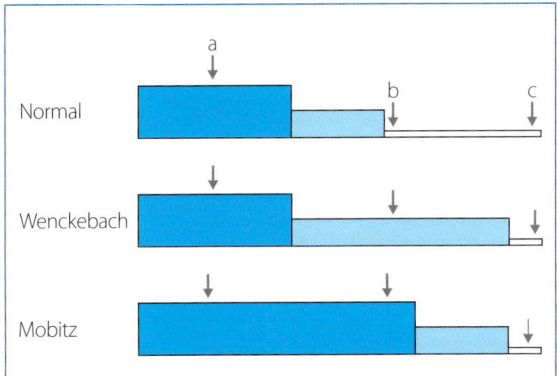

Figure 12.2. Electrophysiologic mechanisms of second-degree atrioventricular block, Mobitz type I (or Wenckebach type) and Mobitz type II. The diagram represents the refractory period of the atrioventricular node under normal conditions and during second-degree atrioventricular block type I (Wenckebach) and II. Mobitz type I or Wenckebach type second-degree atrioventricular block is characterized by a progressive prolongation of the relative refractory period (*light blue bar*), whereas Mobitz type II second-degree atrioventricular block is characterized by a marked prolongation of the absolute refractory period (*blue bar*). During Mobitz type I (Wenckebach type) atrioventricular block, the impulse occurs during the absolute refractory period (*blue bar*) and is then blocked; the impulse *b* occurs during the relative refractory period (*light blue bar*) and undergoes a conduction delay proportional to the prematurity of the impulse, while the impulse *c* occurs at the end of the refractory period and is then conducted without delay. During Mobitz type II second-degree atrioventricular block the impulses *a* and *b* fall in the absolute refractory period (*blue bar*) and are blocked, while the impulse *c* occurs at the end of the refractory period and is therefore conducted without delay.

The electrocardiographic characteristics of type II second-degree atrioventricular block include intermittent blocked P waves and a fixed PQ interval for the conducted impulses. The PQ interval can be normal or prolonged, as long as it remains the same before and after blocked P waves. The R-R intervals preceding the block are also regular, unless sinus arrhythmia is present. The QRS complex morphology can be consistent with a bundle branch block (Box 12.7).

2:1 second-degree atrioventricular block

This form of block is characterized by the alternation of a blocked P wave and a conducted P wave. In the absence of two consecutive conducted P waves, it is impossible to classify this block as Mobitz type I or type II. For this reason, it is considered a separate entity. The site of the block can be intranodal, Hisian or infra-Hisian. Normal duration QRS complexes (≤70 ms in dogs and ≤40 ms in cats) are more likely with a block at the level of the atrioventricular node. Whenever the QRS complex has the characteristics of a bundle branch block, the site of the block is more commonly in the His bundle and the infra-Hisian region. Atrioventricular block is frequently anatomical, in other words associated with a lesion of the conduction system, but it can also be functional when the atrial rate exceeds the time necessary for the atrioventricular node to recover from its refractory period. For example, functional 2:1 atrioventricular block is common with atrial flutter (see p. 171).

The electrocardiographic characteristics of 2:1 atrioventricular block include P waves with a sinus axis conducting across the atrioventricular node with a 2:1 ratio (one conducted P wave alternates with one blocked P wave). PQ intervals of conducted beats can be normal or prolonged; QRS complexes usually have normal morphology, but they can be wide in the presence of a distal area of block that affects the bundle branches. Ventriculo-phasic sinus arrhythmia is common with 2:1 second-degree atrioventricular block (Box 12.8) (see p. 81).

Advanced second-degree atrioventricular block

Advanced atrioventricular block is characterized by an atrium-to-ventricle conduction ratio greater than 2:1, i.e. two or more atrial depolarizations are blocked in sequence.

Chapter 12. Conduction disorders

BOX 12.5.
MOBITZ TYPE I SECOND-DEGREE ATRIOVENTRICULAR BLOCK (WENCKEBACH TYPE) IN THE DOG

HEART RATE: dependent on the firing rate of the sinus node and the atrioventricular conduction ratio.
R-R INTERVAL: regularly irregular.
P WAVE: present, sinus axis.
ATRIOVENTRICULAR CONDUCTION: variable (3:2, 4:3, 5:4, etc.).

PQ INTERVAL: variable, with the most pronounced change in PQ interval duration occurring with the second conducted P wave after the block.
QRS COMPLEX: normal (<70 ms).
VENTRICULO-ATRIAL CONDUCTION: absent.
BLOCKED BEATS: yes.

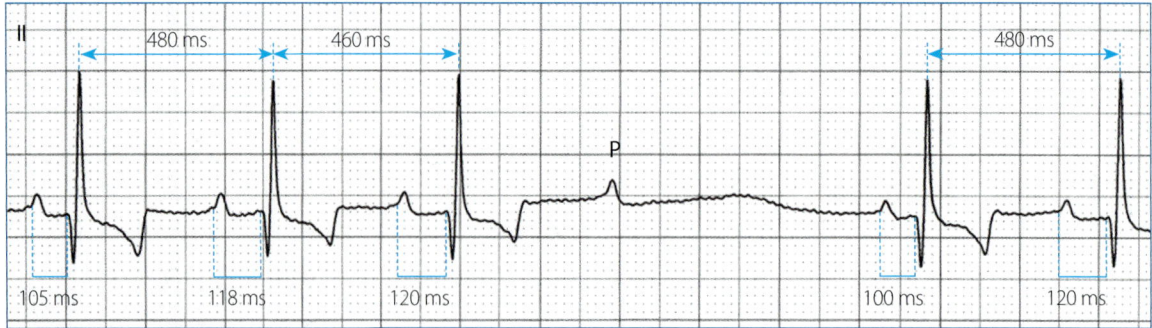

Dog, mongrel, male, 2 years
Lead II- speed 50 mm/s - calibration 10 mm/1 mV.

Notes: sinus rhythm with a rate of 120 bpm and type I second-degree atrioventricular block. Normal P waves with sinus axis are present, one of which is blocked. Before the block a gradual prolongation of the PQ interval is visible associated with a shortening of the R-R interval. The PQ interval that follows the block has a shorter duration (100 ms) than the PQ that precedes the block (120 ms).

Advanced second-degree atrioventricular blocks can be Hisian or infra-Hisian.

The electrocardiographic characteristics of advanced atrioventricular block include at least two consecutive P waves that fail to propagate across the atrioventricular junction, a normal or prolonged PQ interval, and a QRS complex morphology that is normal if the block is within the His bundle and has the characteristics of a bundle branch block if the block is infra-Hisian (Box 12.9). Ventriculo-phasic sinus arrhythmia is occasionally present (see p. 81).

A particular type of advanced atrioventricular block is associated with *alternating Wenckebach periods*. This phemomenon is characterized by a 2:1 second-degree atrioventricular block with a progressive prolongation of the PQ interval for the conducted P waves until the block worsens resulting in a more advanced block (e.g. 3:1, 4:1) (Fig. 12.3). Several mechanisms have been suggested to explain alternating Wenckebach periods, including two points of block: one more proximal at the atrioventricular node and one more distal at the bundle of His such that in this situation the manifestation of 2:1 block is proximal and the higher grade block more distal. A ventricular escape beat occasionally terminates these sequences of blocked P waves. Alternating Wenckebach periods are the manifestation of a functional block during supraventricular tachyarrhythmias, such as atrial flutter and atrial tachycardia.

The electrocardiographic characteristics of advanced second-degree atrioventricular blocks with alternating Wenckebach periods include blocked P waves with a sinus axis and an atrioventricular conduction ratio of 2:1 followed by periods of more advanced block such as periods of 3:1 or 4:1 ratio. The PQ interval of the beat that precedes the initiation of the 3:1 or 4:1 conduction ratio is longer than the PQ interval when atrioventricular conduction returns to 2:1. The QRS complexes have a normal morphology unless the site of the block is infra-Hisian, or if ventricular escape beats are present.

BOX 12.6.
ATYPICAL MOBITZ TYPE I SECOND-DEGREE ATRIOVENTRICULAR BLOCK IN THE DOG

HEART RATE: dependent on the firing rate of the sinus node and the atrioventricular conduction ratio.
R-R INTERVAL: regularly irregular.
P WAVE: present, sinus axis.
ATRIOVENTRICULAR CONDUCTION: variable (3:2, 4:3, 5:4, etc.).
PQ INTERVAL: variable, with the maximum change in PQ interval duration not occurring with the second beat after the block.
QRS COMPLEX: normal (<70 ms).
VENTRICULO-ATRIAL CONDUCTION: absent.
BLOCKED BEATS: yes.

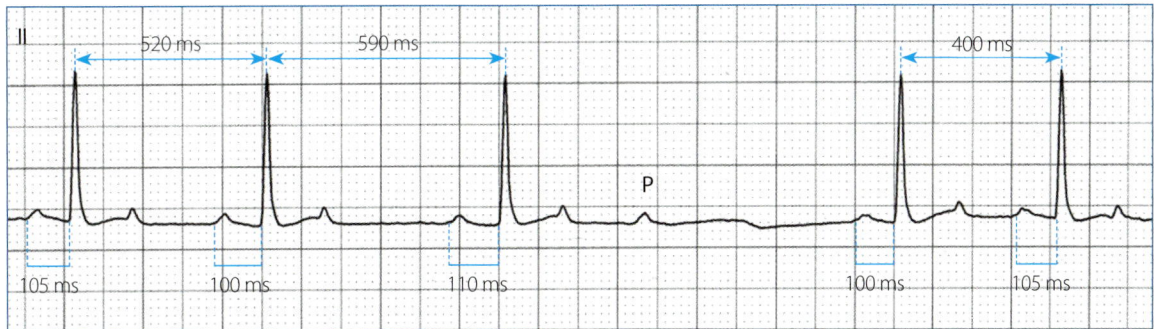

Dog, Cavalier King Charles Spaniel, female, 2 years.
Lead II - speed 50 mm/s - calibration 10 mm/1 mV.

Notes: sinus rhythm with a rate of 120 bpm and atypical type I (Wenckebach type) second-degree atrioventricular block. Normal P waves with sinus axis are present, one of which blocked (P). Note the absence of the progressive shortening of the R-R intervals preceding the non conducted P wave. The PQ interval that follows the block is less (100 ms) than the PQ interval that precedes it (110 ms).

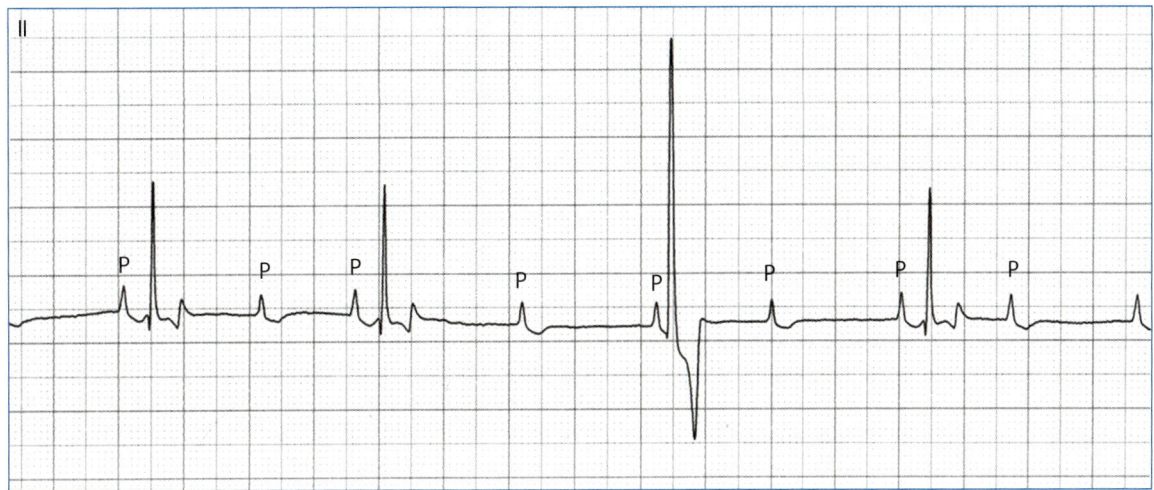

Figure 12.3. Alternating Wenckebach phenomenon during 2:1 second-degree atrioventricular block. (Dog, Afghan Greyhound, male, 13 years. Lead II - speed 25 mm/s - calibration 10 mm/1 mV.
The basic rhythm is a 2:1 second-degree atrioventricular block. Note that every other sinus P waves is blocked. After the second QRS complex, a period of advanced second-degree atrioventricular block occurs with an atrioventricular conduction ratio of 4:1. The third QRS complex is a ventricular escape beat. With greater conduction ratios (>3:1) the atrioventricular block is more likely to be more distal.

BOX 12.7.
MOBITZ TYPE II SECOND-DEGREE ATRIOVENTRICULAR BLOCK IN THE DOG

HEART RATE: dependent on the firing rate of the sinus node and the atrioventricular conduction ratio.
R-R INTERVAL: regularly irregular.
P WAVE: present, sinus axis.
ATRIOVENTRICULAR CONDUCTION: X:(X-1); for example 3:2, 4:3, 5:4, etc.
The ratio may be variable on rare occasions.
PQ INTERVAL: normal or prolonged but always constant.
QRS COMPLEX: normal (<70 ms) or often wide with a bundle branch block morphology.
VENTRICULO-ATRIAL CONDUCTION: absent.
BLOCKED BEATS: yes.

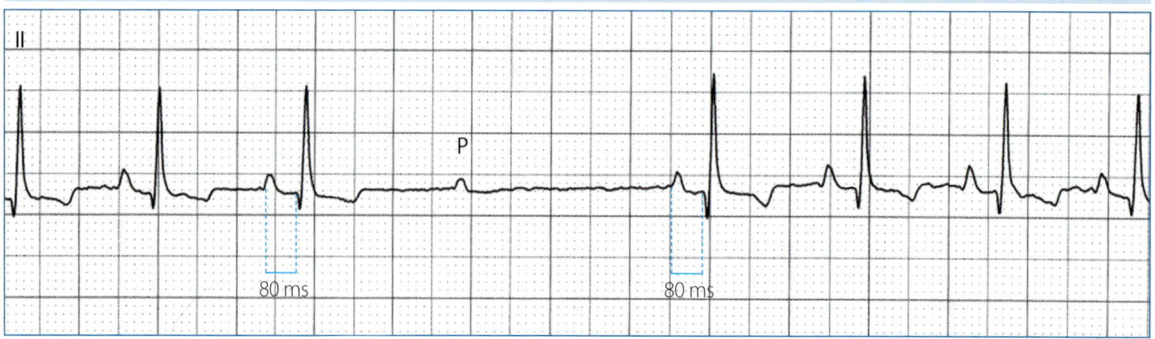

Dog, West Highland White Terrier, female, 14 years.
Lead II - speed 50 mm/s - calibration 10 mm/1 mV.

Notes: sinus tachycardia with a rate of 170 bpm with Mobitz type II second-degree atrioventricular block. Normal P waves with sinus axis are present, one of which is not followed by a QRS complex (P). The PQ interval preceding the block is equal to the PQ interval after the block (80 ms).

BOX 12.8.
2:1 SECOND-DEGREE ATRIOVENTRICULAR BLOCK IN THE DOG

HEART RATE: ventricular rate is half the sinus rate.
R-R INTERVAL: variable depending on the regularity of the sinus rhythm.
P WAVE: present, sinus axis.
ATRIOVENTRICULAR CONDUCTION: conduction with a 2:1 ratio.
PQ INTERVAL: normal or prolonged.
QRS COMPLEX: normal (<70 ms) or with bundle branch block type morphology.
VENTRICULO-ATRIAL CONDUCTION: absent.
BLOCKED BEATS: yes, every other P wave.

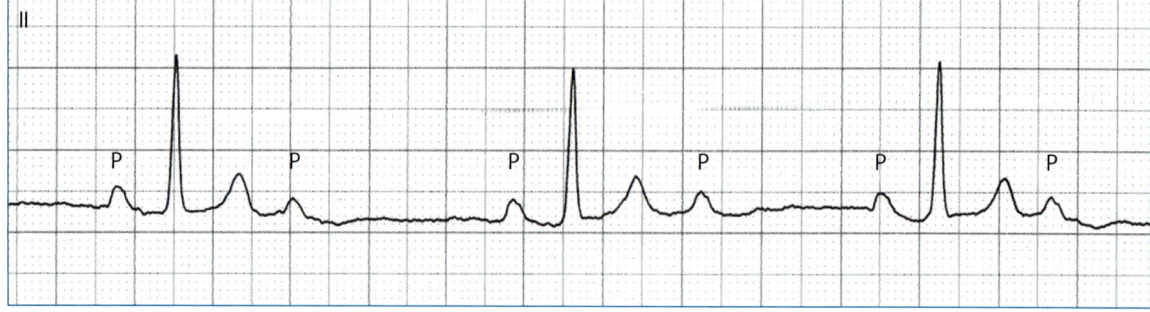

Dog, mongrel, male, 11 years.
Lead II - speed 50 mm/s - calibration 10 mm/1 mV.

Notes: 2:1 second-degree atrioventricular block. Normal P waves with sinus axis alternately blocked. The PQ interval and QRS complexes are normal. Ventriculo-phasic sinus arrhythmia is present.

> **BOX 12.9.**
> **ADVANCED SECOND-DEGREE ATRIOVENTRICULAR BLOCK IN THE DOG**
>
> **HEART RATE:** dependent on the firing rate of the sinus node and the atrioventricular conduction ratio.
> **R-R INTERVAL:** variable depending on the regularity of the sinus rhythm and the atrioventricular conduction ratio.
> **P WAVE:** present, sinus axis.
> **ATRIOVENTRICULAR CONDUCTION:** present, with a fixed or variable conduction ratio but always exceeding 2:1.
> **PQ INTERVAL:** normal or prolonged.
> **QRS COMPLEX:** normal (<70 ms) or with bundle branch block morphology.
> **VENTRICULO-ATRIAL CONDUCTION:** absent.
> **BLOCKED BEATS:** yes.

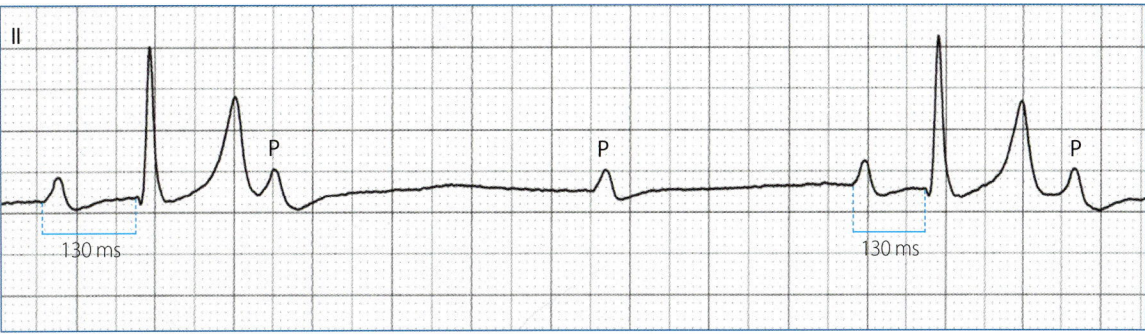

Dog, mongrel, male, 11 years.
Lead II- speed 50 mm/s - calibration 10 mm/1 mV.

Notes: advanced second-degree atrioventricular block. Normal blocked P waves with sinus axis are present, with an atrioventricular conduction ratio of 3:1. The PQ interval is normal. Ventriculo-phasic sinus arrhythmia is present.

Paroxysmal atrioventricular block

Paroxysmal atrioventricular block is characterized by a sudden/abrupt sustained atrioventricular block. The duration of this block varies, but often results in syncope or near-syncope. The definition of this type of conduction disturbance is variable in the literature. The period of atrioventricular block often begins with a premature atrial or ventricular complex and frequently ends with a ventricular escape complex. Paroxysmal atrioventricular block is believed to be due to infra-Hisian block, although the mechanism is unknown. Clinically, this type of block is more common in cats than dogs. Cats most often have syncope related to this type of block, rather than that of the more typical third-degree or complete atrioventricular block.

The electrocardiographic characteristics of paroxysmal atrioventricular block include conducted P waves with related QRS complexes and a consistent PQ interval which is abruptly interrupted by a series of P waves without associated QRS complex resulting in pauses of ventricular activity for extended periods (Fig. 12.4).

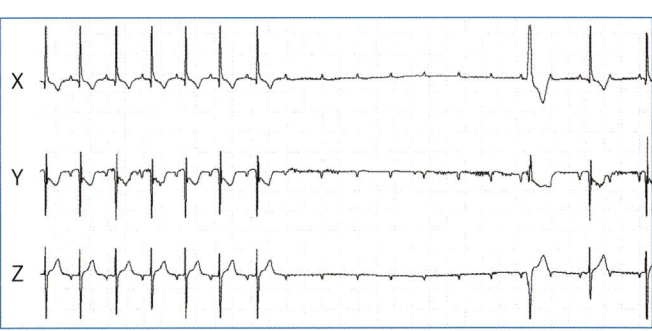

Figure 12.4. Electrocardiogram from a cat with syncope. Leads modified orthogonal X, Y and Z from 24-hour Holter recording 8 s strip. A presumed sinus rhythm with an average heart rate of 153 bpm and a consistent PQ interval precedes an abrupt atrioventricular block that resulted in a greater than 3 s pause. The pause is interrupted by a single ventricular escape beat. This electrocardiogram is an example of paroxysmal atrioventricular block. Top row of numbers indicates heart rate (bpm) and bottom row of numbers indicates R-R intervals (ms).

Third-degree atrioventricular block

During *third-degree* or *complete atrioventricular block*, no atrial impulse can reach the ventricles. Ventricular activation is dependent on a ventricular escape rhythm initiated by the subsidiary pacemaker cells. The duration and morphology of the QRS complexes that form the escape rhythm may give an indication of the site of block, since it is believed that the escape beats usually arise just distal to the site of block. Therefore, whenever the QRS complexes are narrow (≤70 ms in dogs, ≤40 ms in cats), the block is more likely situated in the intranodal or supra-Hisian region; conversely, a wide QRS complex (>70ms in dogs >40 ms in cats) suggests that the block is in the His region or infra-Hisian.

Third-degree atrioventricular block results in complete *atrioventricular dissociation*. Atrioventricular dissociation from the absence of antegrade conduction across the atrioventricular junction does not exclude the possibility of retrograde conduction of ventricular beats to the atrium. Atrioventricular dissociation is a feature of several arrhythmias and is not a clinical diagnosis.

It is usually difficult to determine the cause of third-degree atrioventricular block, although it frequently results from a degenerative process in older animals (usually progressive and permanent) and inflammation from myocarditis in younger ones (usually transient). Other causes of block include bacterial aortic endocarditis that extends to the interventricular septum, neoplasia, overdose of anti-arrhythmic drugs (digitalis, calcium channel blockers, β-blockers), thoracic trauma, parasites (trichinosis) and neuromuscular diseases (myasthenia gravis).

Third-degree atrioventricular block is occasionally diagnosed in older cats. It seems more common in those that have hyperthyroidism. Structural changes consistent with an underlying cardiomyopathy are frequent, and congestive heart failure is present in approximately 30 % of these cats. Because the ventricular escape rhythm frequently remains above 120 bpm, clinical signs that are recognized in dogs with atrioventricular block are not as commonly reported in cats which frequently survive beyond one year without the need of specific therapy to address the arrhythmia. However, if the escape rhythm rate in cats falls below approximately 100 bpm, congestive heart failure develops. Although cats, less frequently than dogs, have clinical signs with third-degree atrioventricular block, they are more likely to have syncope associated with paroxysmal complete atrioventricular block (see above).

The electrocardiographic characteristics of complete atrioventricular block include blocked P waves with a sinus axis that are dissociated from the QRS complexes. The number of P waves typically exceeds the number of QRS complexes. The morphology of the QRS complexes and the rate of the ventricular escape rhythm vary depending on the site of block. In dogs, the escape rhythm usually results in wide QRS complexes and a rate below 40 to 60 bpm. In cats, the escape rhythm is usually characterized by narrow QRS complexes (≤40 ms) and a rate between 80 and 140 bpm. In dogs, ventriculo-phasic sinus arrhythmia may be identified (Boxes 12.10 and 12.11). On occasion, atrial fibrillation can be associated with complete atrioventricular block. This is characterized by an absence of P waves with a regular and slow ventricular escape rhythm. Examination of the baseline can reveal a rapid undulation corresponding to fibrillation waves. However, in many cases, fibrillation waves are not visible on the electrocardiogram.

Because third-degree atrioventricular block is the most common reason for pacemaker implantation in the dog and cat, some additional clinically relevant comments concerning the evaluation of the electrocardiogram are warranted. Clinical signs related to third-degree atrioventricular block are related primarily to the bradycardia of the escape rhythm. The rate and rhythm of the ventricular escape rhythm is variable. The faster, more regular and consistent escape rhythms are more likely to persist than cease, thus giving time to prepare for pacemaker implantation on a non-emergency basis. Escape rhythms that are slow (less than 30 bpm), irregular and varying in morphology (indicating most likely different sites of origin within the ventricle) are rhythms that may stop abruptly, thus demanding emergency pacemaker implantation. Evaluation of the rhythm must me coupled with an assessment of myocardial size and function, which are intertwined with the prognosis of third-degree heart block.

Although the implantation of a single chamber pacemaker into the right ventricle is most common, there are circumstances in which individual dogs (younger, large breed, and dogs with structurally normal heart) would

Atrioventricular blocks | 271

BOX 12.10.
THIRD-DEGREE ATRIOVENTRICULAR BLOCK IN THE DOG

HEART RATE: dependent on the location of the block.
R-R INTERVAL: usually regular, except if premature beats present, or if escape rhythm from various foci.
P WAVE: present, sinus axis.
ATRIOVENTRICULAR CONDUCTION: absent (complete atrioventricular dissociation).
PQ INTERVAL: variable because of atrioventricular dissociation.
QRS COMPLEX: normal (<70 ms) or wide (>70 ms) based on the site of block and the origin of the escape rhythm.
VENTRICULO-ATRIAL CONDUCTION: usually absent.
BLOCKED BEATS: all.

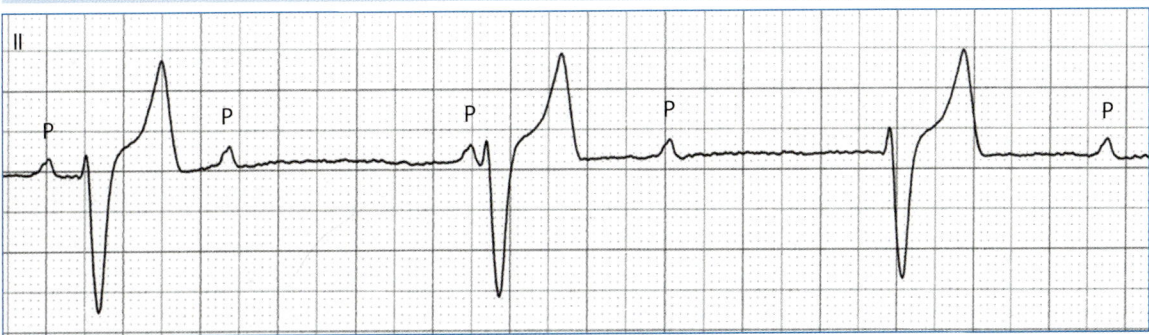

Dog, German Shepherd, female, 6 years.
Lead II - speed 50 mm/s - calibration 10 mm/1 mV.

Notes: third-degree atrioventricular block. There are normal P waves with sinus axis and a rate of 120 bpm. All P waves are dissociated from the QRS complex. The escape rhythm is ventricular with wide QRS complexes (80 ms) and a rate of 57 bpm. Ventriculo-phasic sinus arrhythmia is present, although concomitant respiratory sinus arrhythmia cannot be completely ruled-out.

BOX 12.11.
THIRD-DEGREE ATRIOVENTRICULAR BLOCK IN THE CAT

HEART RATE: dependent on the site of the block.
INTERVAL R-R: usually regular, except in the presence of premature or escape ectopic ventricular beats or rhythms with different origin.
P WAVE: present, sinus axis.
ATRIOVENTRICULAR CONDUCTION: absent (complete atrioventricular dissociation).
PQ INTERVAL: variable because of atrioventricular dissociation.
QRS COMPLEX: normal (<40 ms) or wide (>40 ms) based on the site of block site and the origin of the escape rhythm.
VENTRICULO-ATRIAL CONDUCTION: usually absent.
BLOCKED BEATS: all.

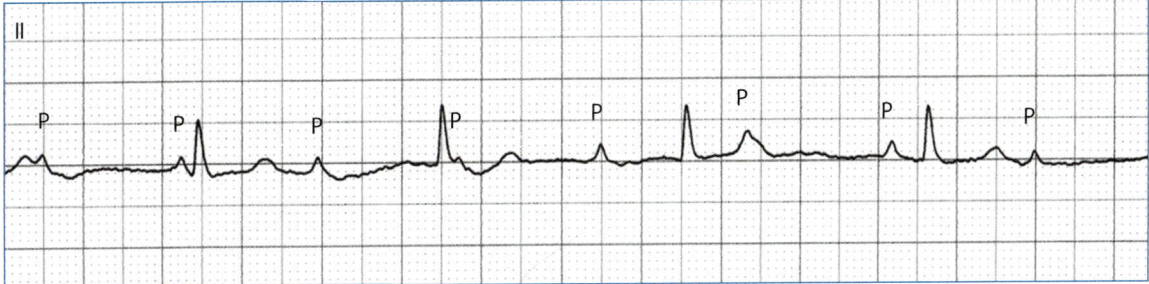

Cat, Domestic Shorthair, male, 4 years.
Lead II - speed 50 mm/s - calibration 10 mm/1 mV.

Notes: third-degree atrioventricular block. There are normal P waves with sinus axis and a rate of 180 bpm. All P waves are blocked and dissociated from the QRS complexes. The escape rhythm is ventricular with wide QRS complexes (50 ms) and firing rate of 100 bpm.

benefit from more advanced pacing methods such as dual chamber or atrial/ventricular sensed and ventricular paced devices. When these methods of pacing are under consideration it is important to closely evaluate the P waves of the electrocardiogram during third-degree atrioventricular block. The rate and rhythm of the P waves are important in the diagnosis of the underlying atrial rhythm in these cases. Some dogs may have sinus bradycardia and others may have sinus tachycardia in response to the bradyarrhythmia of a slow ventricular escape rhythm. However, some dogs may have tachyarrhythmias with an underlying atrial tachycardia coexisting with third-degree atrioventricular block. With dual chamber or atrial/ventricular sensed pacemakers tracking of atrial depolarizations/activity drives the ventricular rate. Consequently, if an atrial tachycardia is present, the ventricle could be paced at an excessively high rate. Programming methods are available to prevent this complication; however, the correct electrocardiographic diagnosis before implantation is vital to weigh the benefit of advanced pacing in light of such tachyarrhythmias. Therefore, careful examination of the atrial rate and P wave morphology is important to differentiate a sinus tachycardia from an atrial tachycardia.

Dogs with third-degree heart block may have coexisting ectopic ventricular complexes or ventricular tachycardia. These ventricular arrhythmias may be the result of the underlying disease process (e.g. myocarditis), electrical remodeling or consequences associated with a bradycardia such as early-afterdepolarizations. Polymorphic ventricular tachycardia in dogs with third degree heart block predisposes such dogs to ventricular fibrillation.

Intraventricular conduction disorders or bundle branch blocks

The penetrating portion of the distal atrioventricular bundle or bundle of His is the starting point of the intraventricular conduction system. The bundle of His extends from the nodo-Hisian portion of the atrioventricular junction to the posterior division of the left bundle branch. In dogs, the bundle of His branches out to form the right bundle branch and the two divisions of the left bundle branch (Fig. 12.5). The terminal portions of the bundle branches reach the working myocardium through a dense Purkinje network, which ensures the rapid transmission of electrical impulses to the ventricles. Based on its anatomical organization, the intraventricular conduction system of the dog can be defined as trifascicular.

Intraventricular conduction blocks are classified as anatomical or functional. Functional blocks are also called rate-dependent blocks (tachycardia-dependent or phase 3, bradycardia-dependent or phase 4). Anatomical blocks can occur at various levels along the specialized pathways of the intraventricular conduction system.

Depending on the number of branches involved, blocks can be divided into:
- monofascicular blocks,
- bifascicular blocks, and
- trifascicular blocks.

The vulnerability of the different segments of the intraventricular conduction system to conduction blocks is variable. Clinically, the right bundle branch is the most vulnerable, followed by the anterior division of the left

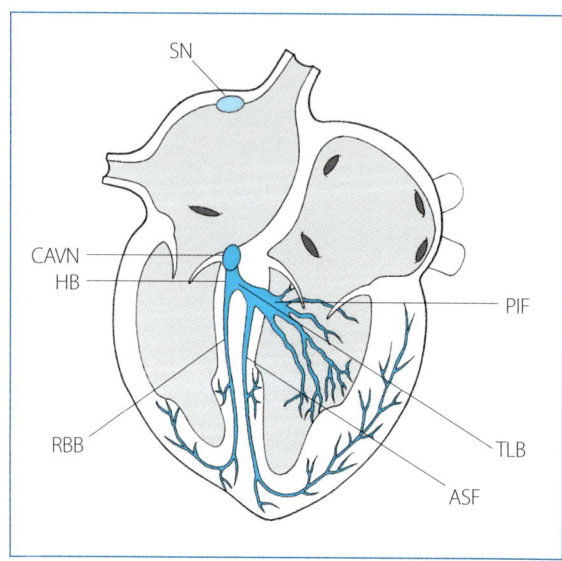

Figure 12.5. Anatomy of the atrioventricular and intraventricular conduction system. *SN*: sinus node; *CAVN*: compact atrioventricular node; *HB*: His bundle; *RBB*: right bundle branch; *TLB*: truncular portion of the left bundle branch; *PIF*: postero-inferior fascicle; *ASF*: antero-superior fascicle.

bundle branch, the posterior division of the left bundle branch, and finally the truncular portion of the left bundle branch.

The delay in intraventricular conduction caused by the block depends on its location and the extent of working ventricular myocardium that is not activated via the normal conduction pathways. The more distal the block, the smaller the mass of myocardium that is activated with delay. On the surface electrocardiogram, intraventricular blocks result in an alteration of the morphology and duration of the QRS complex. In general, widening of the QRS complex is less with blocks that only involve one fascicle than blocks that affect a bundle branch or that are associated with a diffuse lesion affecting the terminal ramifications of the conduction pathways. A bundle branch block results in the maximum prolongation of the QRS complex, as the electrical impulse, which comes from the contralateral ventricle has to travel across the interventricular septum to activate the ventricle on the side of the block. Because anatomical blocks usually occur in the presence of myocardial disease, the widening of the QRS complex is not solely dependent on the volume of myocardium that is not activated via the normal conduction pathways, but also the typical slow conduction velocity of electrical impulses in remodeled cardiac tissue.

Monofascicular blocks

Monofascicular blocks correspond to the interruption of impulse propagation in a single fascicle, but conduction is unaffected in the other portions of the conduction system. Monofascicular blocks include the:
- right bundle branch block,
- left anterior (fascicular) hemiblock or antero-superior fascicular block, and the
- left posterior (fascicular) hemiblock or postero-inferior fascicular block.

Right bundle branch block

Right bundle branch block is classified into complete or incomplete based on the site of block, and therefore the changes in QRS complex morphology and duration. In the presence of a right bundle branch block, the first vector of septal activation is normal, as the depolarization of the interventricular septum is initiated from the left bundle branch. The activation of the left ventricle that follows is also unaffected. However, the right side of the septum and the free wall of the right ventricle are activated with delay, and the activation vector is directed posterior-to-anterior and inferior-to-superior and slightly to the right. In this case, activation of the right ventricle is only possible via the ventricular working myocytes (Fig. 12.6).

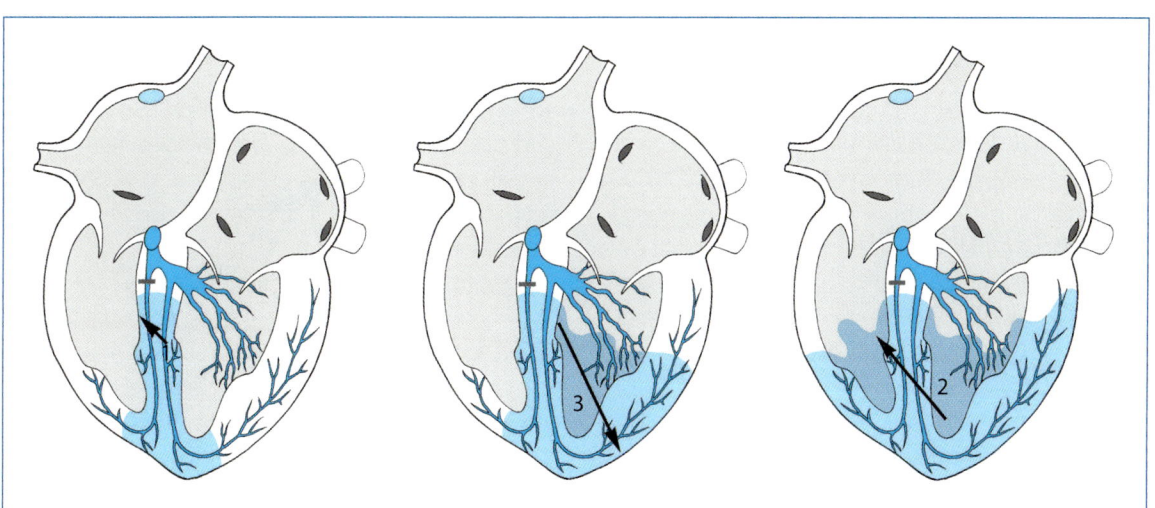

Figure 12.6. Sequence of ventricular activation during right bundle branch block. Vectors 1 and 3 have a normal direction and sequence. Vector 2, on the other hand, starts late, lasts longer and with a posterior-to-anterior, inferior-to-superior and slight rightward direction.

A right bundle branch block can occur in association with congenital heart defects (atrial septal defect, ventricular septal defect, endocardial cushion defect), degenerative and inflammatory conduction disorders, chronic degenerative valvular disease, coronary artery disease, right ventricular dilation, primary myocardial disorders, heartworm disease, chronic obstructive lung disease, hypothermia, tumors, chest trauma, or following valvuloplasty to correct pulmonic stenosis. In cats, right bundle branch block has been associated with peritoneopericardial diaphragmatic hernia. In cats with hyperkalemia electrocardiographic features of incomplete and complete right bundle branch block develop with increasing levels of serum potassium. The appearance of S waves that progressively increase in size and duration when compared to baseline electrocardiograms can assist in monitoring cats, particularly those with reperfusion injury associated with thromboembolism.

The degree and location of conduction block in the right bundle can vary with the disease process. As the conduction block of the right bundle progresses from incomplete to complete, several changes in the electrocardiogram can be noted. These alterations in the electrocardiogram include the development of S waves of increasing duration in the inferior leads (II, III, aVF), R-R' morphology in leads V_1 and aVR, duration of the QRS complex beyond the normal values and right axis shift. It should be noted that incomplete right bundle branch block can be manifested as an S wave that has a duration greater than the R wave without exceeding the normal values established for the entire QRS complex. Thus, observations of the relative contribution to the surface ECGs representation of ventricular depolarization gives evidence of progressive conduction block. Different grades of right bundle branch block have been defined based on the degree of QRS morphology alterations which may be of assistance in the evaluation of a right bundle branch block in the dog and cat:

- Grade I: the QRS complex is of normal duration and the S wave in the inferior leads (II, III, aVF) represents 40 %-50 % of the width of the QRS complex.
- Grade II: the QRS complex is of normal duration and the S wave in the inferior leads (II, III, aVF) represents more than 50 % of the width of the QRS complex. On occasion the ventricular complex has a R-R' morphology in leads V_1 and aVR.
- Grade III: the duration of the QRS complex is slightly prolonged between 70 and 80 ms in dogs and the S wave in the inferior leads (II, III, aVF) represents more than 50 % of the width of the QRS complex. In most cases the ventricular complex has a R-R' morphology in lead V_1 or aVR. The term *incomplete right bundle branch block* is also used to describe this form of intraventricular conduction disturbance resulting in a QRS complex duration that just exceeds reference values for the species considered.
- Grade IV: the duration of the QRS complex is greater than 80 ms in dogs and the S wave in the inferior leads (II, III, aVF) represents more than 50 % of the width of the QRS complex. Typically the ventricular complex has a R-R' morphology in lead V_1 or aVR (*complete right bundle branch block*).

Complete right bundle branch block is, therefore, characterized by a QRS complex with a duration exceeding 80 ms in dogs and 60 ms in cats due to a wide S wave. The QRS complex with the largest negative deflection is found in lead I, the inferior leads (II, III, and aVF) and the left precordial leads V_2 to V_6. The R wave is taller in aVR than aVL. The mean electrical axis in the frontal plane is consistent with a right axis shift which can reach −110 °. An r' wave giving the QRS complex the classical M morphology (Rr' or rR') is frequent in the right precordial lead V_1. This wave represents the second vector of delayed ventricular activation (Box 12.12). In approximately 10 % of dogs with complete right bundle branch block, there is an extreme axis deviation to approximately −80 °, there is no S wave in lead I, and the R wave is taller in aVL than aVR.

Incomplete right bundle branch block only differs from complete right bundle branch block by the duration of the QRS complex, which is less than 80 ms (Box 12.13). It should be noted that in the case of extreme right ventricular hypertrophy (e.g. severe pulmonic stenosis), electrocardiographic features of an incomplete right bundle branch block can exist in the limb leads due to the increased muscle mass rather than an actual lesion of the right bundle.

Intraventricular conduction disorders or bundle branch blocks

BOX 12.12.
COMPLETE RIGHT BUNDLE BRANCH BLOCK IN THE DOG

HEART RATE: dependent on the firing rate of the sinus node.
R-R INTERVAL: variable depending on the regularity of the sinus rhythm.
P WAVE: present, sinus axis.
ATRIOVENTRICULAR CONDUCTION: present.
PQ INTERVAL: usually normal.

QRS COMPLEX: longer than 80 ms. The mean electrical axis in the frontal plane is deviated to the right up to $-110°$; in 10 % of dogs it is around $-80°$. r' or R' waves usually present in V_1.
VENTRICULO-ATRIAL CONDUCTION: absent.
BLOCKED BEATS: no.

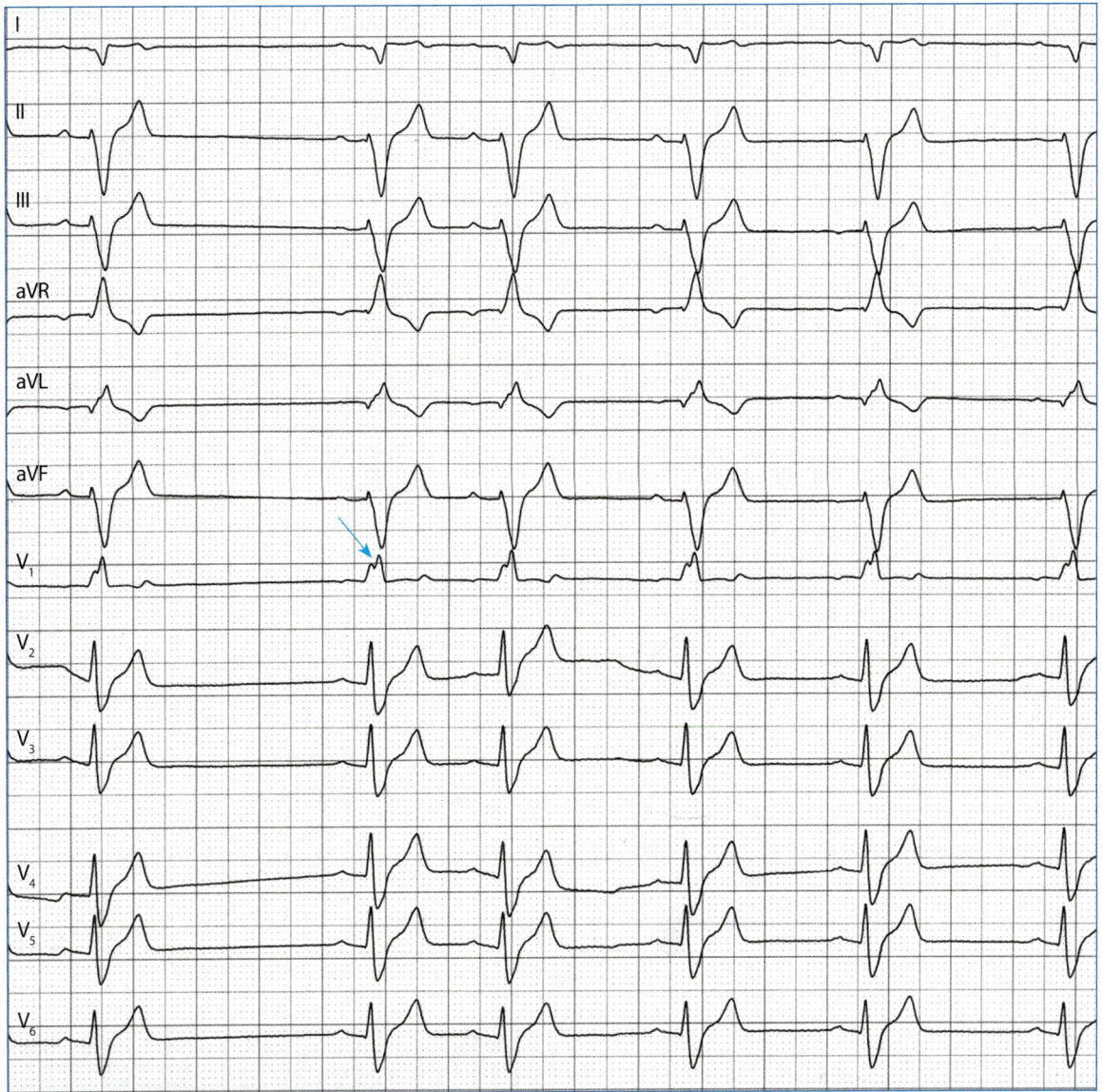

Dog, Cocker Spaniel, male, 13 years.
Twelve leads (I, II, III, aVR, aVL, aVF, V_1, V_2, V_3, V_4, V_5, V_6) - speed 50 mm/s - calibration 5 mm/1 mV.

Notes: respiratory sinus arrhythmia with a rate of 100 bpm with complete right bundle branch block. QRS complexes have an increased duration (80 ms) with a wider negative deflection in leads I, II, III, aVF, V_2, V_3, V_4, V_5, V_6. The mean electrical axis of the QRS complex in the frontal plane is deviated to the right ($-110°$). In the right precordial lead V_1 a secondary R' wave is present giving the classical M morphology to the QRS complex (rR') (arrow).

Chapter 12. Conduction disorders

BOX 12.13.
INCOMPLETE RIGHT BUNDLE BRANCH BLOCK IN THE DOG

HEART RATE: dependent on the firing rate of the sinus node.
R-R INTERVAL: variable depending on the regularity of the sinus rhythm.
P WAVE: present, sinus axis.
ATRIOVENTRICULAR CONDUCTION: present.
PQ INTERVAL: usually normal.

QRS COMPLEX: less than 80 ms. The mean electrical axis in the frontal plane is deviated to the right up to −110° and in 10 % of dogs it is around −80°. Usually r' wave present in V_1.
VENTRICULO-ATRIAL CONDUCTION: absent.
BLOCKED BEATS: no.

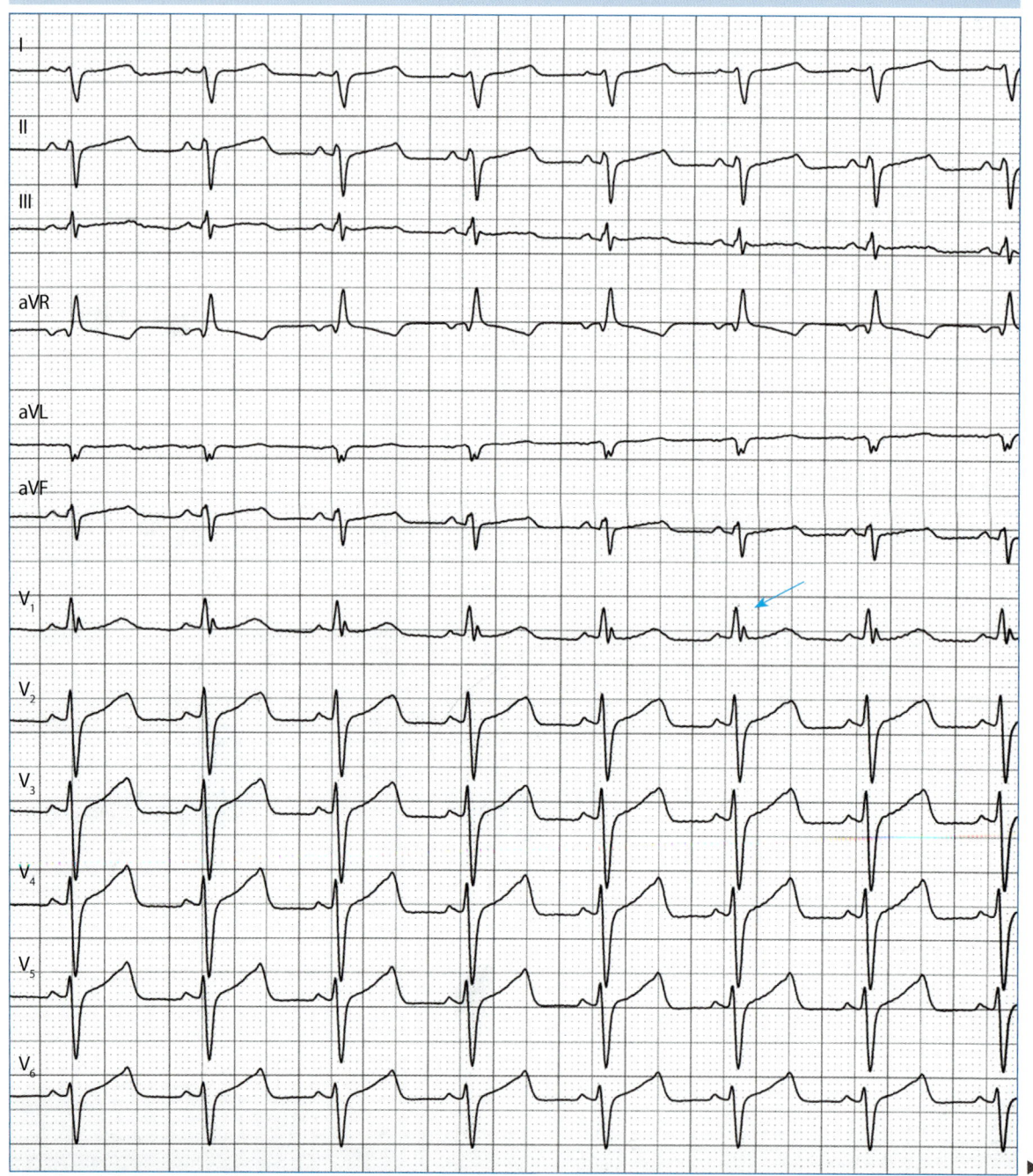

Left anterior fascicular block or left anterior hemiblock

The term hemiblock refers to a conduction disorder that involves one of the divisions of the left bundle branch. If ventricular depolarization is represented by three consecutive vectors of activation, then a left hemiblock affects the third vector. The third vector can be divided into two components, 3a and 3b (see p. 44). A *left anterior fascicular block* alters 3a, which represents the depolarization of the antero-superior portion of the left ventricle activated by the antero-superior fascicle. In addition, a block of the anterior fascicle also alters the first vector of septal activation, as this fascicle normally contributes to the depolarization of the interventricular septum. In the presence of a left anterior fascicular block, the septal vector (first vector), that results from the early activation of the posterior wall is deviated, and as a result the initial portion of the QRS complex is oriented towards +80 °/+90 °. The second vector of right ventricular depolarization is unaffected and follows a normal sequence, direction and duration. Finally, the depolarization of the antero-superior portion of the left ventricle does not occur via the anterior fascicle, but depends on the propagation of the electrical wavefront through a dense network of interconnected fibers of conduction tissue between the anterior and posterior fascicles, as well as regular working myocytes. The resulting prolongation in ventricular depolarization is so small that the duration of the QRS complex measured on an electrocardiogram recorded at standard speeds remains within normal limits, as shown experimentally in the dog by MB Rosenbaum.

Instead of a change in QRS complex duration, a left anterior fascicular block causes a marked left axis deviation in the frontal plane (Fig. 12.7).

The left anterior fascicular block is one of the most common intraventricular conduction disturbances reported in veterinary medicine, and it is especially common in cats with hypertrophic cardiomyopathy.

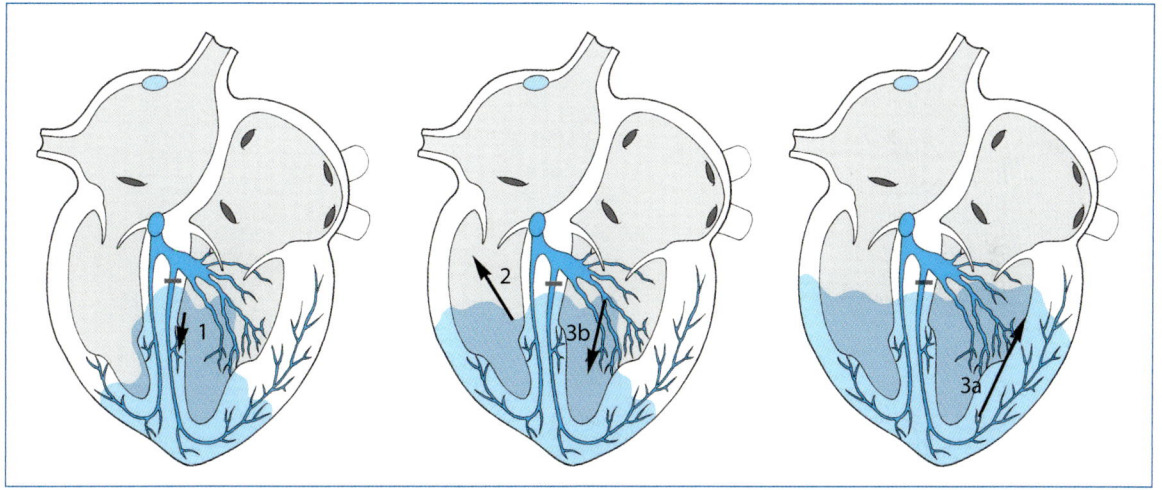

Figure 12.7. Sequence of ventricular activation during left anterior fascicular block. Vector 1 is directed downward and to the left. Vectors 2 and 3b have a normal direction and sequence. The myocardial region dependent on vector 3a is activated late with a posterior-to-anterior direction and from the apex towards the base of the left ventricle.

Dog, French Bulldog, female, 1 year.
Twelve leads (I, II, III, aVR, aVL, aVF, V_1, V_2, V_3, V_4, V_5, V_6) - speed 50 mm/s - calibration 5 mm/1 mV.

Notes: sinus rhythm with incomplete right bundle branch block. The duration of the QRS complex is normal (60 ms) with a mean electrical axis of −150 °. In the right precordial lead V_1, there is a secondary r' wave giving the QRS complex (Rr') the classical M morphology (arrow).

Chapter 12. Conduction disorders

The electrocardiographic characteristics of the left anterior fascicular block include a QRS complex with a duration of approximately 70 ms in dogs and 40 ms in cats. The mean electrical axis in the frontal plane is deviated to the left between –30 ° and –60 °. The early activation of the posterior wall of the left ventricle typically produces a qR pattern in aVL and an rS pattern in leads II, III, aVF and V_5 (Boxes 12.14 and 12.15).

Some comments with regards to the presence of S waves and left anterior fascicular block in the cat should

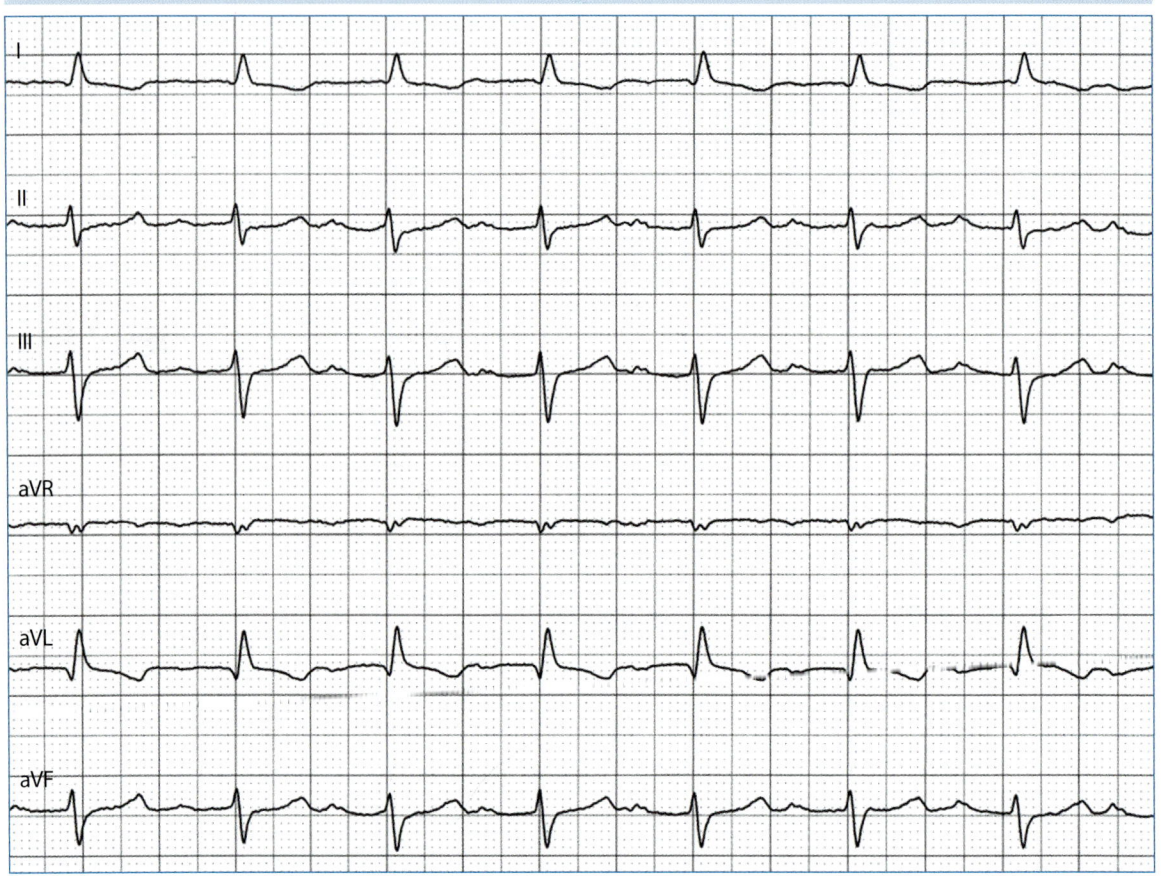

BOX 12.14.
LEFT ANTERIOR FASCICULAR BLOCK IN THE DOG

HEART RATE: dependent on the firing rate of the sinus node.
R-R INTERVAL: variable depending on the regularity of the sinus rhythm.
P WAVE: present, sinus axis.
ATRIOVENTRICULAR CONDUCTION: present.
PQ INTERVAL: usually normal.

QRS COMPLEX: approximatively 70 ms. The mean electrical axis in the frontal plane is deviated to the left between –30 ° and –60 °. qR morphology in aVL and rS pattern in leads II, III, aVF and V_5.
VENTRICULO-ATRIAL CONDUCTION: absent.
BLOCKED BEATS: no.

Dog, mongrel, male, 12 years.
Six limbs leads (I, II, III, aVR, aVL, aVF) - speed 50 mm/s - calibration 5 mm/1 mV.

Notes: sinus rhythm with a left anterior fascicular block. S waves present in the inferior leads (II, III, and aVF). In leads I and aVL the QRS complex has a qR morphology. The mean electrical axis of the QRS complex in the frontal plane is deviated to the left (–30 °). The duration of the QRS complex is normal (55 ms). There is also a first-degree atrioventricular block (PQ 160 ms).

be considered. Frequently, a requirement for the diagnosis of a left anterior fascicular block has been made that a "deep S wave" be present in leads II, III, aVF; however, the definition of "deep" has not been established. There is no proof of when the left anterior fascicle is blocked relative to the QRS morphology in cats with clinical disease. As stated above the ratio of the R wave to S wave may be a more critical point; however, examination of electrocardiograms in the cat often reveals very small complexes whereby such a criteria would be met with doubt. Just as with incomplete and complete right bundle branch block it is plausible that variation in the degree of blockade in the left anterior fascicle also can exists. In fact, some cats with overall small QRS complexes but yet an rS pattern associated with a confirmed diagnosis of cardiomyopathy may develop much deeper S waves as disease progresses. In contrast, an over-diagnosis of the left anterior fascicular block should not be made in the normal cat that simply has a small QRS complex, but with the compatible QRS pattern.

> **BOX 12.15.**
> **LEFT ANTERIOR FASCICULAR BLOCK IN THE CAT**
>
> **HEART RATE:** dependent on the firing rate of the sinus node.
> **R-R INTERVAL:** variable depending on the regularity of the sinus rhythm.
> **P WAVE:** present, sinus axis.
> **ATRIOVENTRICULAR CONDUCTION:** present.
> **PQ INTERVAL:** usually normal.
>
> **QRS COMPLEX:** approximatively 40 ms. The mean electrical axis in the frontal plane is deviated to the left between −30 ° and −60 °. qR morphology in aVL and rS pattern in leads II, III and aVF.
> **VENTRICULO-ATRIAL CONDUCTION:** absent.
> **BLOCKED BEATS:** no.

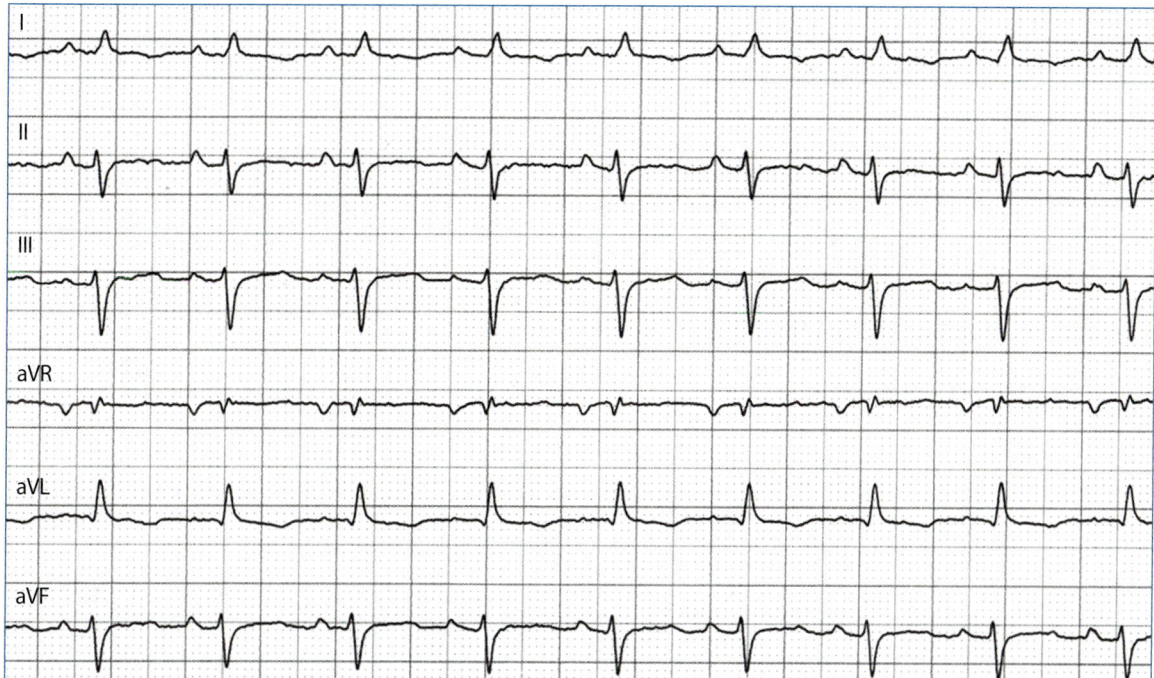

Cat, Domestic Shorthair, male, 19 years.
Six limbs leads (I, II, III, aVR, aVL, aVF) - speed 50 mm/s - calibration 10 mm/1 mV.

Notes: sinus rhythm with left anterior fascicular block. S waves are found in the inferior leads (II, III, and aVF). In leads I and aVL QRS complexes have a qR morphology. The mean electrical axis of the QRS complex in the frontal plane is deviated to the left (−40 °). The duration of the QRS complex is normal (40 ms).

Left posterior fascicular block or left posterior hemiblock

Left posterior fascicular block is less common than anterior fascicular block because the anatomical organization of the left posterior fascicle makes it less at risk of being damaged. A left posterior hemiblock alters the second component of the third vector of activation (phase 3b). As a result, the infero-posterior, apical and inflow regions of the left ventricle are not activated via the normal conduction pathways. Instead, the electrical impulse originates from the left anterior fascicle and the electrical wavefront then propagates through the regular working myocytes to depolarize the regions normally activated by the posterior fascicle. Phase 3b is slightly delayed and follows an anterior-to-posterior direction. A posterior fascicular block also alters the first septal vector of depolarization, since the activation of the septum depends predominantly on the posterior division of the left bundle. In the presence of a posterior fascicular block, early activation of the anterior wall of the left ventricle results in an axis deviation of the initial portion of the QRS complex to approximately –60 °, with evidence of R waves in lead I and aVL and Q waves in leads II, III and aVF. The second vector of right ventricular depolarization has a normal sequence, direction and duration. The block of the posterior fascicle then causes a deviation of the electrical axis towards the right in the frontal plane (between +100 ° and +120 °). The duration of the QRS complex is not significantly prolonged during a left posterior hemiblock (Fig. 12.8). It is not possible to diagnose a left posterior fascicular block from the surface electrocardiogram with certainty since minor right axis shifts can be present with right ventricular hypertrophy or as a result of the animal's chest conformation.

Bifascicular blocks

Bifascicular blocks correspond to an interruption of impulse propagation in two branches of the intraventricular conduction system.

Three types of bifascicular block can be identified on the electrocardiogram:
- left bundle branch block,
- right bundle branch block with anterior fascicular block, and
- right bundle branch block with posterior fascicular block.

Left bundle branch block

Lesions of the conduction system that result in a left bundle branch block can occur at the pre-divisional level (*classic left bundle branch block* or *truncular block*),

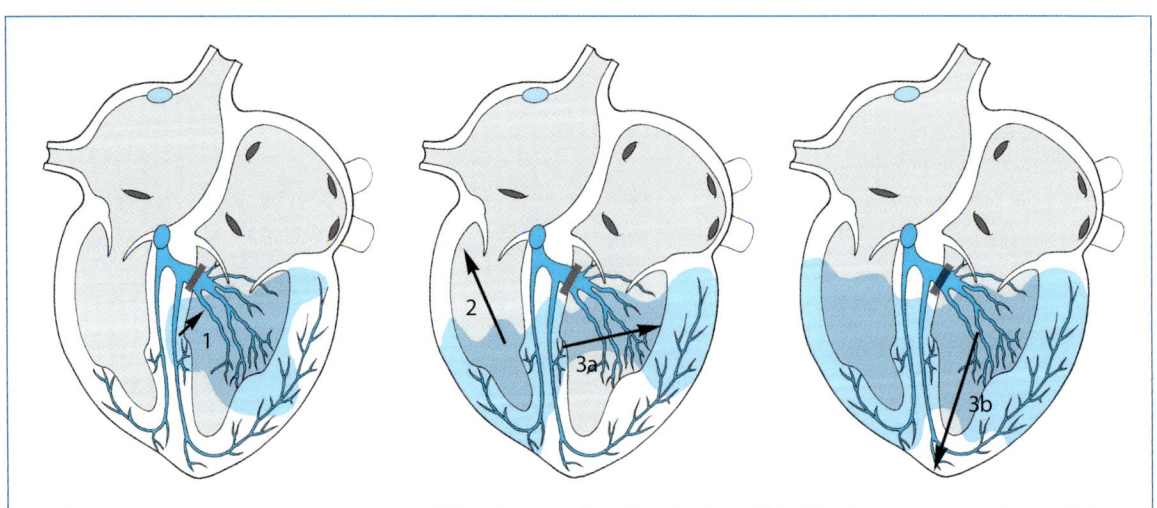

Figure 12.8. Sequence of ventricular activation during left posterior fascicular block. Vector 1 has an activation sequence directed anteriorly and to the left, vector 2 and 3a have a normal direction and sequence. The myocardial region dependent on vector 3b is activated late by the anterior fascicle and has an anterior-to-posterior direction from the base towards the apex of the left ventricle.

involve both fascicles of the left bundle branch (*post-divisional left bundle branch block*), or affect the more distal portions of its arborization. In humans with truncular and divisional left bundle branch block, a Q wave, which is the electrocardiographic representation of the first vector of ventricular depolarization, is absent in lead II. In dogs with left bundle branch block, however, it is common that a Q wave remains present in lead II. In these dogs, the Q wave probably corresponds to early electrical vectors of activation that arise from the lateral wall of the right ventricle, or it indicates that the block along the left bundle is distal enough to allow normal septal activation by the unaffected more proximal portion of the left bundle branch. The second vector of activation has a normal direction and sequence. Depolarization of the left ventricle occurs via the propagation of the electrical wavefront through the working myocardium in a right-to-left, anterior-to-posterior and superior-to-inferior direction with a marked prolongation in conduction time (Fig. 12.9).

The presence of a left bundle branch block usually indicates severe myocardial damage, for example in dogs with dilated cardiomyopathy and congestive heart failure. This conduction abnormality further deteriorates the left ventricular systolic function by worsening intra- and interventricular dyssynchrony. The concomitant presence of systolic dysfunction and left bundle branch block is associated with increased mortality in humans and dogs. Possible causes of left bundle branch block include inflammatory or degenerative diseases of the conduction tissue, cardiac hypertrophy (for example secondary to subaortic stenosis), trauma, cardiomyopathies and neoplasia.

Electrocardiographic characteristics of left bundle branch block include QRS complexes with a normal axis in the frontal plane (between +40 ° and +100 ° in dogs and between 0 ° and +160 ° in cats) and a marked increase in duration (>80 ms in dogs and >60 ms in cats) due to a wide R wave. The widest component of the QRS is positive in leads I, II, III, aVF, V_2 to V_6 and negative in leads aVR, aVL and V_1. The presence or absence of a Q wave in lead II depends on the site of block (Box 12.16).

Right bundle branch block associated with left anterior fascicular block

A left anterior fascicular block deviates the electrical axis superiorly and to the left in the frontal plane, whereas an isolated right bundle branch block deviates the axis superiorly and to the right.

When combined, the resultant electrical axis is oriented superiorly or superiorly and slightly to the left. Since a right bundle branch block does not interfere with the first septal activation vector, the classical

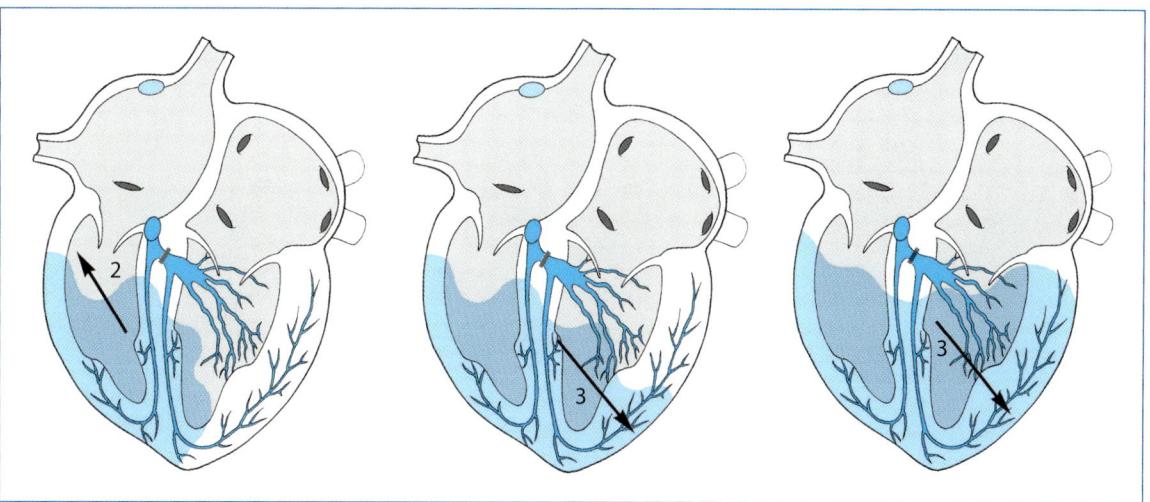

Figure 12.9. Sequence of ventricular activation during truncular left bundle branch block. The first vector is absent. Vector 2 has a normal direction and sequence of activation. The activation of the interventricular septum is delayed and oriented right-to-left. Vector 3 has a normal direction but the left ventricular mass is activated extremely late.

BOX 12.16.
LEFT BUNDLE BRANCH BLOCK IN THE DOG

HEART RATE: dependent on the firing rate of the sinus node.
R-R INTERVAL: variable depending on the regularity of the sinus rhythm.
P WAVE: present, sinus axis.
ATRIOVENTRICULAR CONDUCTION: present.
PQ INTERVAL: usually normal.

QRS COMPLEX: increased duration (>80 ms). The mean electrical axis in the frontal plane is normal. QRS complex predominantly positive in leads I, II, III, aVF, V_2 to V_6 and V_{10} and negative in leads aVR, aVL and V_1. Septal q waves in lead II usually not present but dependent on site of block.
VENTRICULO-ATRIAL CONDUCTION: absent.
BLOCKED BEATS: no.

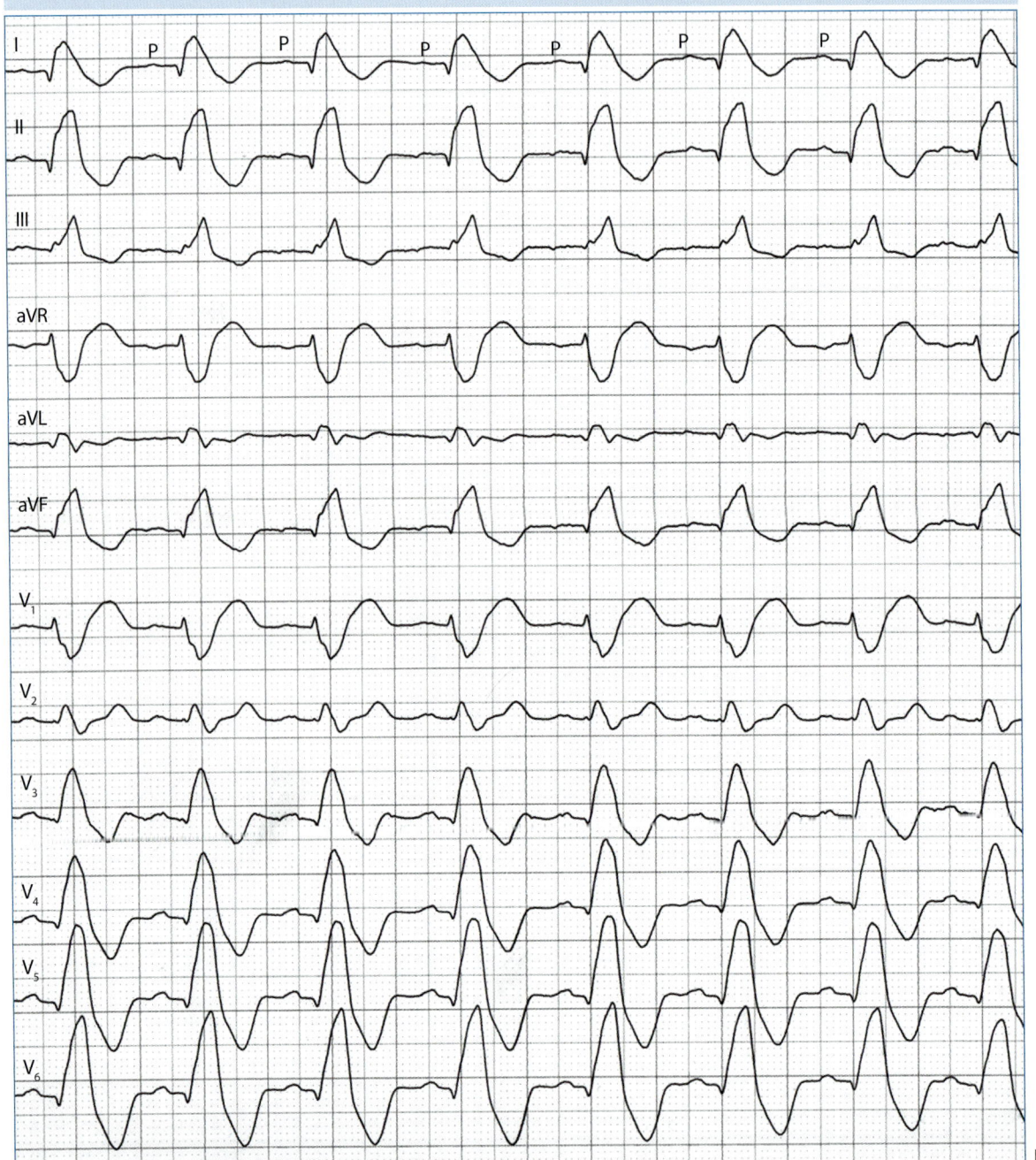

posterior-to-anterior direction of septal activation caused by a left anterior fascicular block is apparent on the electrocardiogram when the two blocks are combined. The remaining of the QRS complex has the characteristics of a right bundle branch block. Finally, the precordial leads maintain the typical features of right bundle branch block because the QRS changes resulting from an anterior fascicular block are only evident in the frontal plane.

A bifascicular block is commonly a sign of an ongoing disease process involving the conduction system, and may precede the occurrence of third-degree atrioventricular block. The etiology of this type of block is similar to that of a third-degree atrioventricular block.

The electrocardiogram of a right bundle branch block associated with a left anterior fascicular block is characterized by QRS complexes of increased duration (>80 ms in dogs and >60 ms in cats), an inferior-to-superior axis deviation between –60 ° and –90 °, and with the largest negative deflection in leads I, II, III, aVF, and V_2 to V_6.

In the right precordial lead V_1, the QRS complex usually is M shaped with two positive deflections (Rr' or rR'). The R wave is taller in aVL than in aVR and it is preceded by a q wave (Box 12.17).

Right bundle branch block associated with left posterior fascicular block

Isolated right bundle branch block deviates the electrical axis superiorly and to the right in the frontal plane, and an isolated posterior fascicular block deviates the axis inferiorly and to the right. As a result, the association of the two blocks deviates the axis to the right and superiorly or inferiorly depending on which of the two blocks has more impact on the direction of the main electrical wavefront. In the presence of a right bundle branch block combined with a left posterior fascicular block, the first vector of activation is directed upward and to the left and is responsible for the early activation of the anterolateral wall of the left ventricle; the second vector is directed upward and to the right, as a result of the late activation of the right ventricular free wall. The third vector, of greater amplitude, is directed to the right and inferiorly and corresponds to the activation of the posterior wall of the left ventricle.

A right bundle branch block associated with left posterior fascicular block can be suspected when the QRS complex has the characteristics of a complete right bundle branch block with an electrical axis deviated inferiorly and to the right, the presence of a Q wave in leads II, III and aVF, and the absence of a Q wave in leads I and aVL.

Trifascicular blocks

A *trifascicular block* is present when interruption of impulse propagation alternates between all three subdivisions of the distal atrioventricular bundle on a single or consecutive electrocardiographic tracings. The association of a bifascicular block and Mobitz type II second-degree atrioventricular block is also a form of trifascicular block, because the atrioventricular block reflects the interruption of impulse conduction in all three divisions of the distal atrioventricular bundle. Conversely, the presence first-degree atrioventricular block with a bifascicular block is not necessarily a form of trifascicular block, because the site of delayed conduction can be at the level of the compact atrioventricular node.

Trifascicular blocks result from extensive damage of the conduction system (transient in case of myocarditis) and, regardless of the etiology, tend to progress to third-degree (complete) atrioventricular block.

The electrocardiogram can display different patterns in trifascicular block: a left bundle branch block alternating with a right bundle branch block, a right bundle branch block with a left anterior fascicular block alternating with a left bundle branch block, or a bifascicular block associated with a Mobitz type II second-degree atrioventricular block (Box 12.18). These observations can be made on a single electrocardiogram, or several tracings recorded consecutively in the same animal.

Dog, Boxer, male, 8 years.
Twelve leads (I, II, III, aVR, aVL, aVF, V_1, V_2, V_3, V_4, V_5, V_6) - speed 50 mm/s - calibration 5 mm/1 mV.

Notes: sinus rhythm with a left bundle branch block. The QRS complexes have increased duration (105 ms) with normal mean electrical axis in the frontal plane (+63 °). Small Q wave present in lead II can represent the second right ventricular vector if the left bundle branch block is truncular or the first (or septal) vector if the block is postdivisional.

BOX 12.17.
RIGHT BRANCH BLOCK WITH LEFT ANTERIOR FASCICULAR BLOCK IN THE DOG

HEART RATE: dependent on the firing rate of the sinus node.
R-R INTERVAL: variable depending on the regularity of the sinus rhythm.
P WAVE: present, sinus axis.
ATRIOVENTRICULAR CONDUCTION: present.
PQ INTERVAL: usually normal.

QRS COMPLEX: exceeding 80 ms. The mean electrical axis in the frontal plane is between –60 ° and –90 °. Usually there are r' or R' wave s in V_1, and a qR complex in aVL.
VENTRICULO-ATRIAL CONDUCTION: absent.
BLOCKED BEATS: no.

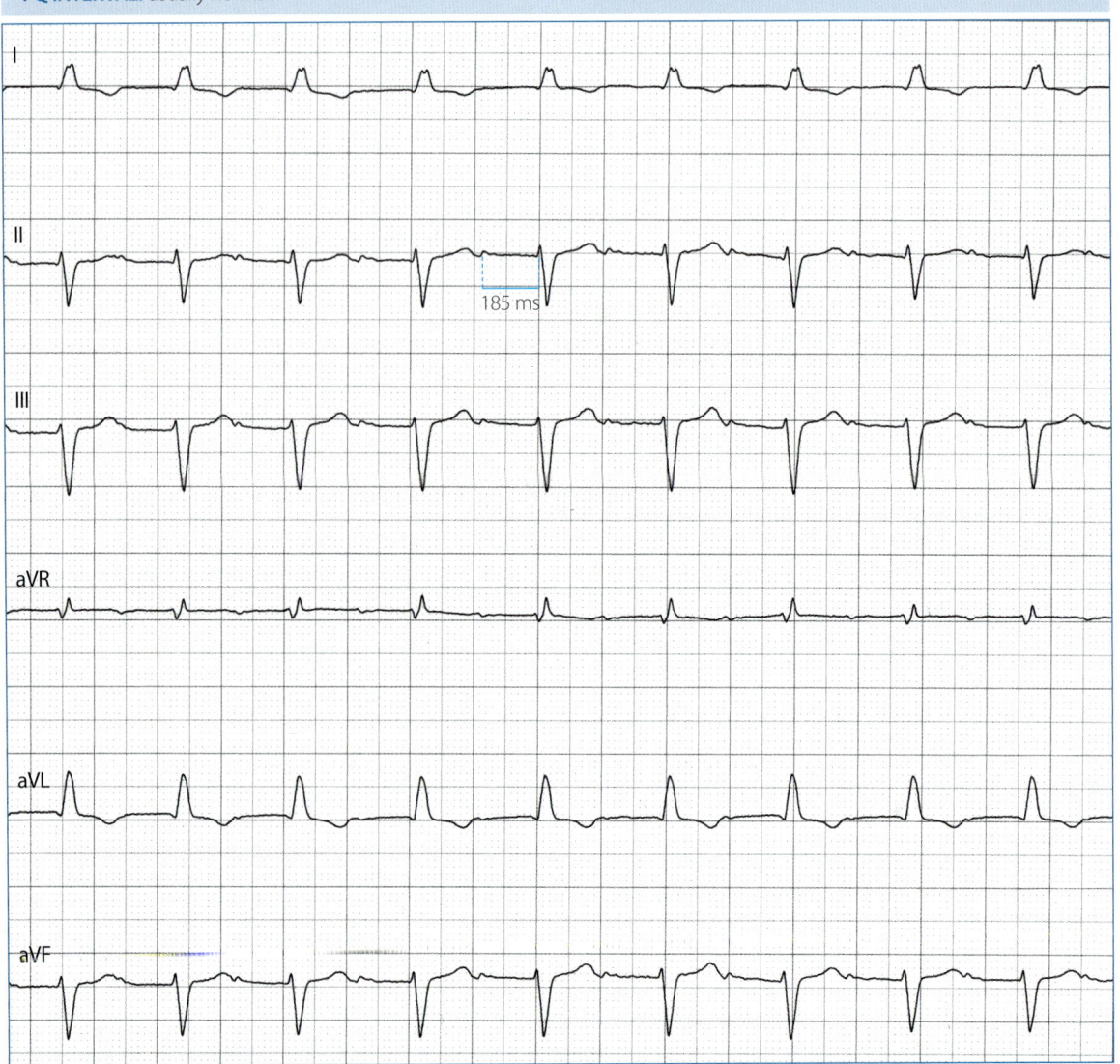

Dog, mongrel, male, 12 years.
Six limbs leads (I, II, III, aVR, aVL, aVF) - speed 50 mm / s - calibration 5 mm / 1 mV

Notes: progression of a left anterior fascicular block (Box 12.14) in a right bundle branch block associated with a left anterior fascicular block. The QRS complex has a duration of 65 ms with an increased duration of 20 ms from the initial recording. The mean electrical axis in the frontal plane is deviated (–76 °) with an additional counterclockwise shift of 30 ° compared to the previous tracing. There are obvious qR complexes in aVL, with a taller R wave in aVR. Note the concomitant presence of a first-degree atrioventricular block (PQ 185 ms).

Intraventricular conduction disorders or bundle branch blocks | 285

BOX 12.18.
TRIFASCICULAR BLOCK IN THE DOG

HEART RATE: dependent on the firing rate of the sinus node.
R-R INTERVAL: variable depending on the regularity of the sinus rhythm.
P WAVE: present, sinus axis.
ATRIOVENTRICULAR CONDUCTION: present.
PQ INTERVAL: usually normal.
QRS COMPLEX: variable morphology. The electrocardiogram can display any of the three combinations of block.
A right bundle branch block associated with a left anterior fascicular block, a right bundle branch block associated with a left posterior fascicular block, and a left bundle branch block or right bundle branch block that are found on the same electrocardiogram or at different times in the same animal. In addition it can be a bifascicular block associated with a Mobitz type II second-degree atrioventricular block.
VENTRICULO-ATRIAL CONDUCTION: absent.
BLOCKED BEATS: yes, if coexists with Mobitz type II second-degree atrioventricular block.

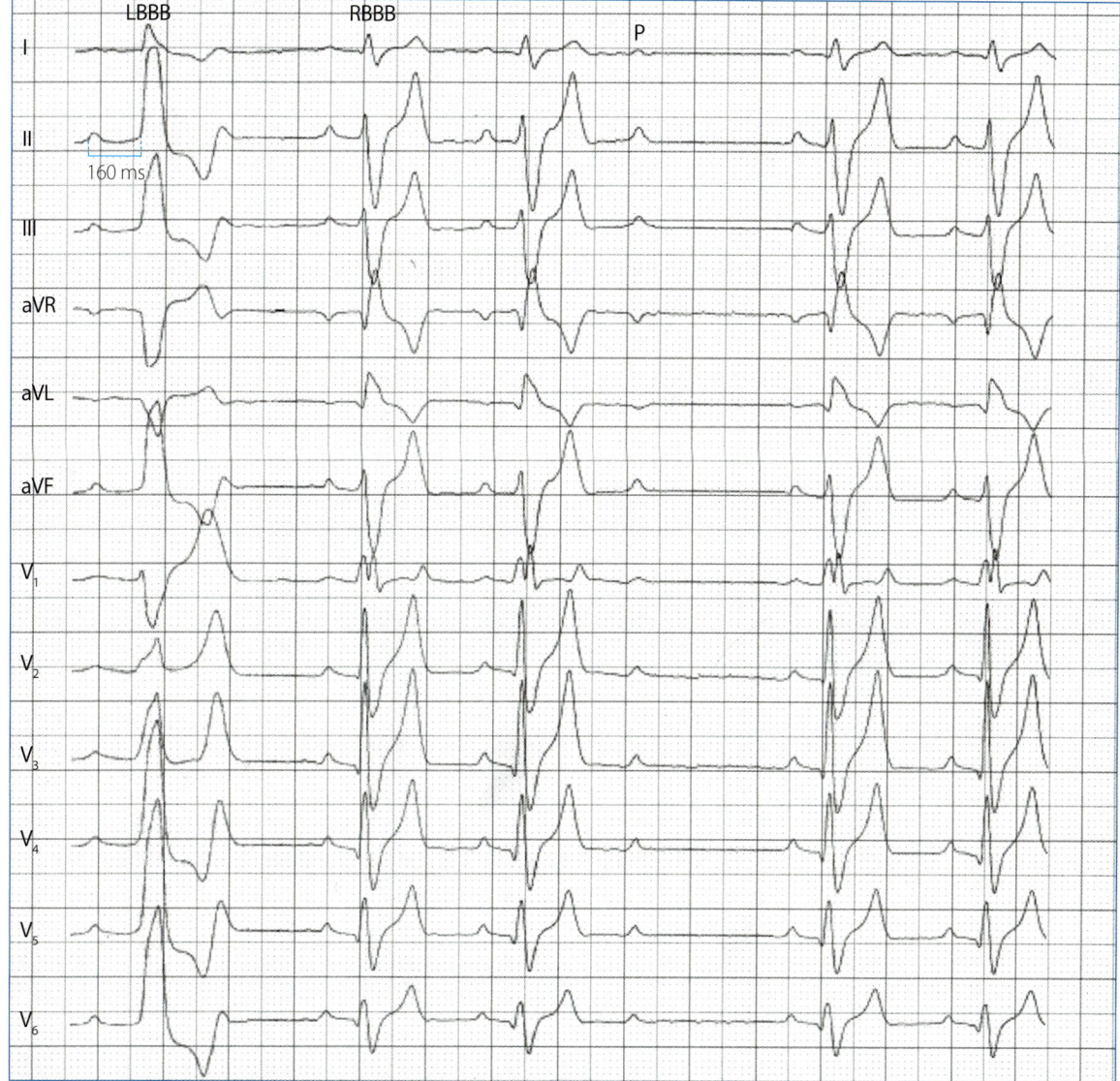

Dog, Labrador Retriever, male, 9 years.
Twelve leads (I, II, III, aVR, aVL, aVF, V_1, V_2, V_3, V_4, V_5, V_6) - speed 50 mm/s - calibration 10 mm/1 mV.

Notes: trifascicular block. A left bundle branch block (LBBB) with first-degree atrioventricular block (PQ 160 ms) alternating with a complete right bundle branch block (RBBB). Also present, a Mobitz type I (Wenckebach type) second-degree atrioventricular block (P).

Aberrant conduction

Aberrant conduction is an intraventricular conduction delay of a supraventricular impulse as a result of a functional block in one of the branches of the conduction pathways. Functional bundle branch block occurs when an impulse reaches the intraventricular conduction system before this has fully recovered from a previous depolarization. It is associated with an abrupt change in rhythm cycle length. Therefore, if a branch block is not preceded by a change in cardiac cycle length, it should not be considered to represent a form of aberrant conduction.

Two forms of aberrant conduction are recognized:
- tachycardia-dependent block or phase 3 block, and
- bradycardia-dependent block or phase 4 block.

A *tachycardia-dependent block* can be explained by the differences in the refractory period duration between different portions of the intraventricular conduction system. In healthy tissue, the refractory period of the right bundle branch is slightly longer than the left. A prolongation of the refractory period of the left bundle branch can occur in disease states that affect the left ventricle. Because the refractory period of an impulse that ends a long R-R interval is prolonged, the subsequent beat, if premature, can reach a portion of the conduction system during its refractory period while it propagates normally through other segments. As a result, the QRS complex of the early beat displays an aberrant (i.e. different from the other QRS complexes) morphology on the electrocardiogram (Figs. 12.10-12.12).

A particular type of tachycardia-dependent aberrancy is called Ashman's phenomenon, which is common during atrial fibrillation (see p. 171). Aberrancy can be distinguished from a ventricular premature beat by assessing the coupling interval. If the coupling interval is constant over several cycles it is more likely to be a ventricular premature

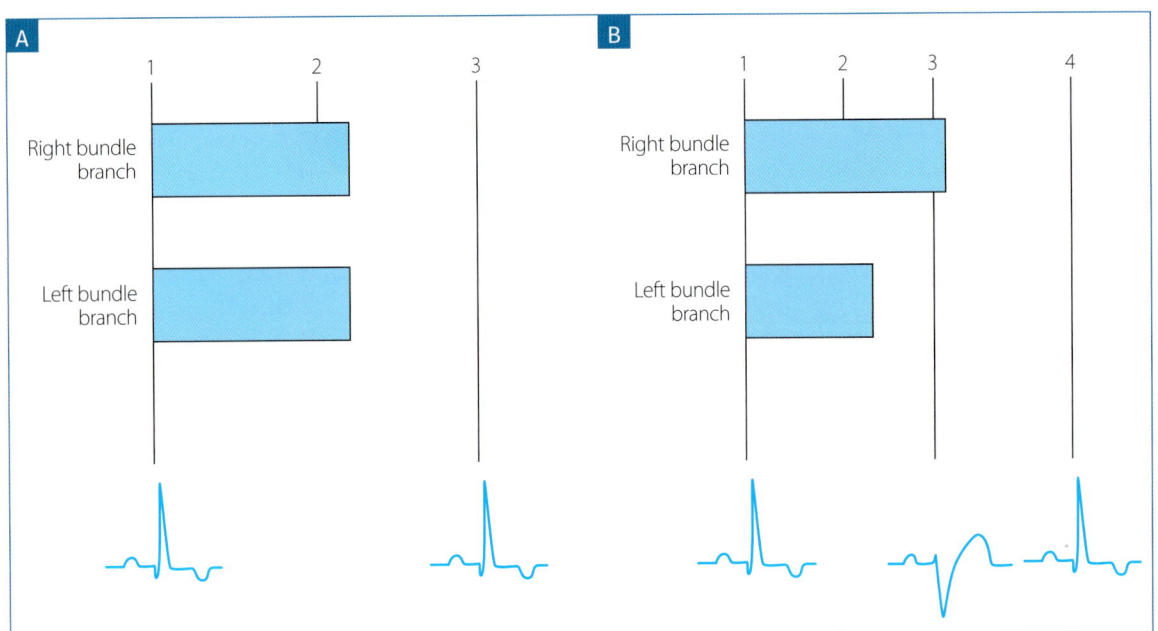

Figure 12.10. Aberrant intraventricular conduction.
A) The two branches have the same refractory period. In this case, impulses 1 and 3 fall after the refractory period and are normally conducted. Impulse 2 occurs instead when the two branches are refractory and is not conducted. B) Under normal conditions, the right bundle branch has a longer refractory period than the left bundle branch. In this situation, impulses 1 and 4 fall after the refractory period and are normally conducted. The premature impulse 2 occurs, instead, when the two branches are refractory and is not conducted. Finally, the premature impulse 3 reaches the right bundle branch during its refractory period and therefore the QRS complex displays a right bundle branch block morphology.

beat than supraventricular with aberrancy. The aberrancy of Ashman's phenomenon can go over several cycles.

A *bradycardia-dependent block* results from the slow and progressive depolarization of the membrane potential of conduction tissue cells (latent or subsidiary pacemakers) during long diastolic intervals. As the membrane potential moves towards less negative values, less sodium channels become available and the rate of rise of phase 0 of the action potential decreases, which interferes with impulse propagation. Therefore, at the end of a long cycle length (long R-R), the membrane potential of cells within one bundle branch may have already reached values at which the number of sodium channels in a closed state is not sufficient to propagate an electrical impulse. As a result, ventricular depolarization is dependent on the contralateral bundle branch.

The electrocardiographic features of aberrant conduction include a wide QRS complex with the characteristics of a left or right bundle branch block for the beat that ends a long R-R-short R-R sequence, which corresponds to tachycardia-dependent aberrancy (Fig. 12.12), or a very long R-R interval (long cycle length), which corresponds to bradycardia-dependent aberrancy. As indicated previously, a right bundle branch block pattern is more common for the aberrant beat.

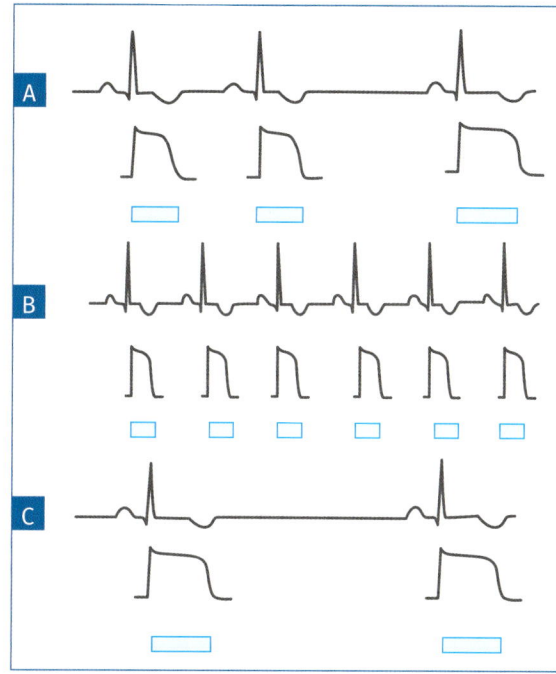

Figure 12.11. Action potential duration and refractory period in relation to heart rate variation.
A) The duration of the refractory period depends on the previous R-R interval. A short R-R interval is followed by an action potential of shorter duration and therefore the refractory period is also shorter. Conversely, a long R-R interval results in a prolonged action potential duration and refractory period.
B) During tachycardia the refractory period is shortened.
C) During bradycardia the refractory period is prolonged.

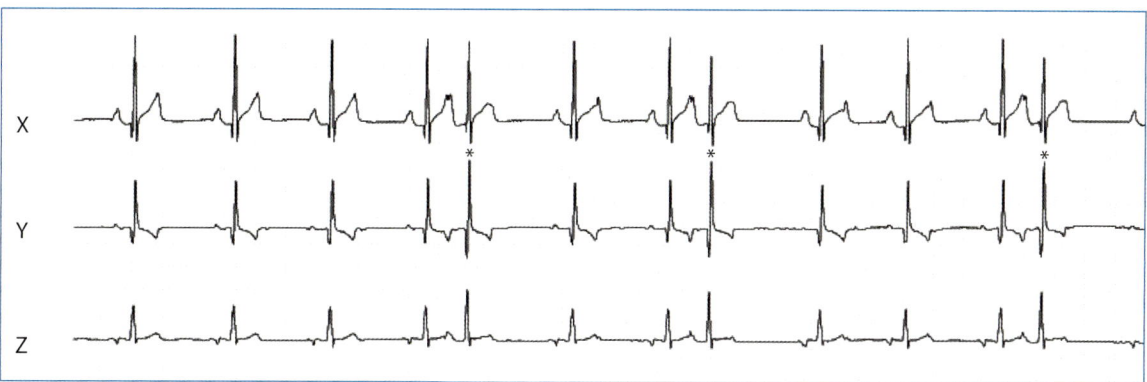

Figure 12.12. Tachycardia-dependent aberrant conduction (Dog, Brittany Spaniel, male, 11 years). Leads modified orthogonal X, Y and Z from 24-hour Holter recording. 8 s strip. The underlying rhythm is sinus with a relatively consistent sinus P-P interval that averages 615 ms (range 566-632 ms). This example demonstrates tachycardia-dependent aberrant conduction because the premature atrial ectopic beats are conducted with abnormal QRS morphology (*), but they are not preceded by a longer P-P interval (long-short effect on action potential duration) which is a type of tachycardia-dependent aberrant conduction known as Ashman's phenomenon. Note the change in morphology across the 3 orthogonal leads associated with intervals from 261 ms to 273 ms.

Linking or sustained aberrant conduction

The term *linking* refers to sustained aberrant conduction, a form of functional intraventricular block. It requires a macro-reentrant circuit constituted of the two branches with different properties: one branch is the preferential conduction pathway (dominant branch) and the other (dependent branch) has a long refractory period which impairs its ability to conduct impulses once they exceed a specific rate. Frequently, these pathways are formed by the left and right bundle branches. In the event of an abrupt variation of rate, an electrical impulse can travel down the dominant branch but is blocked within the dependent branch, which has a prolonged refractory period. However, the impulse is able to enter the dependent branch retrogradely and is again interrupted within the branch, which has not yet fully recovered from the previous depolarization, and prolongs its refractory state. As a result, the next antegrade impulse is unable to travel down the dependent branch, but conducts through the dominant branch and re-enters the dependent branch retrogradely, where once again it blocks in an area of refractory tissue. These consecutive impulses that alternatively block in an antegrade and retrograde direction in the dependent branch maintain the functional block, until a change in rate allows full recovery of the two branches of the reentrant circuit (Fig. 12.13). Although the functional block in the dependent branch of the circuit is not initially apparent on the electrocardiogram (*concealed conduction*), its effect is visible on the subsequent beat, which has aberrant morphology. In summary, each aberrant beat can be "linked" to the effect of the previous beat on the conduction properties of the dependent branch of the circuit.

Linking can be either tachycardia or bradycardia-dependent; tachycardia-dependent linking is encountered with atrial fibrillation (Fig. 12.13) and supraventricular tachycardias.

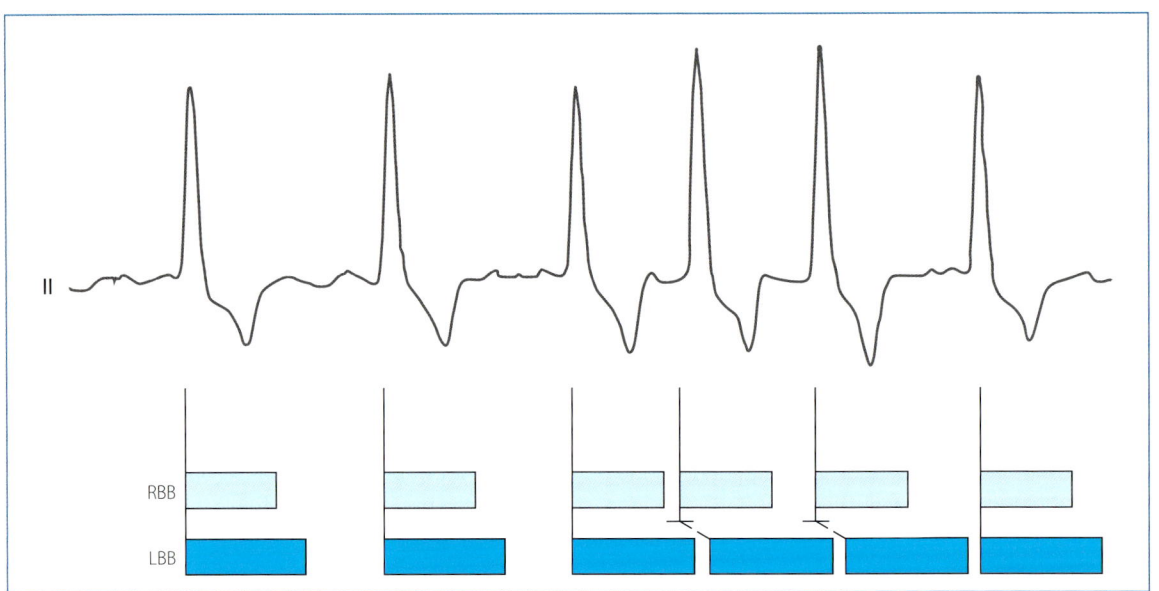

Figure 12.13. Sustained aberrant conduction or *linking* (Dog, mongrel, male 13 years. Lead II - speed 50 mm/s - calibration 10 mm/1 mV). The animal was diagnosed with atrial fibrillation and dilated cardiomyopathy which was responsible for a prolongation of the refractory period of the left bundle branch. The first three beats occur after both bundle branches have repolarized and are normally conducted. The fourth beat, because of its prematurity, occurs in the refractory period of the left bundle branch (LBB) and is then conducted along the right bundle branch (RBB) with a left bundle branch block morphology. The electrical impulse conducted along the right bundle branch (dominant arm) is conducted retrogradely along the left bundle branch (dependent arm) extending the refractory period of the latter. At this point, the fifth beat encounters the left branch when it is refractory, and is subsequently blocked (phase 3 linking). The last beat, which occurs later, reaches the ventricles at the end of the refractory period of the left bundle branch and is therefore normally conducted.

The electrocardiographic characteristics of *linking* include the presence of several consecutive beats with a wide QRS complex appearance and a left bundle branch block or right bundle branch block morphology whenever the reentrant circuit is formed by the bundle branches, and evidence of an abrupt shortening of the R-R interval before the first aberrant beat in case of tachycardia-dependent *linking* or longer than the baseline cycle length in case of bradycardia-dependent *linking*. Linking is frequently present during atrial fibrillation. It is important to be able to distinguish atrial fibrillation with aberrant intraventricular conduction from ventricular tachycardia and pre-excited atrial fibrillation. Ventricular tachycardia is frequently regular (constant R-R intervals) whereas atrial fibrillation is irregular (unless atrial fibrillation is associated with third-degree atrioventricular block). Pre-excited atrial fibrillation is usually very rapid and the QRS morphology changes, because the QRS complexes represent variable degrees of fusion between impulses travelling through the accessory pathway and the atrioventricular node (see p. 161).

Gap phenomenon and supernormal conduction

The electrocardiographic diagnosis of the gap phenomenon and supernormal conduction is challenging. Various electrophysiologic mechanisms can mimic supernormal conduction, including the gap phenomenon, rate-related changes in tissue refractoriness, dual atrioventricular node physiology, concealed conduction, or peeling back of the refractory period, which leads some electrophysiologists to prefer the term "pseudo-supernormal conduction". In contrast, others believe that supernormal conduction is an under-recognized mechanism of altered conduction.

The most common manifestation of the gap phenomenon involves impulse propagation through the atrioventricular junction. The *gap phenomenon* refers to the ability of a premature impulse to propagate through the atrioventricular node, although other premature beats with longer coupling intervals (in other words "not as premature") fail to reach the ventricles. Gap phenomenon occurs when the atrioventricular junction behaves as it is divided into two levels, and the refractory period of the distal level is longer than the refractory period of the proximal level. In this situation, most premature impulses are able to travel through the proximal level but are blocked in the distal portion of the atrioventricular node. However, an impulse with a shorter coupling interval reaches the proximal level of the atrioventricular junction during its relative refractory period. As a result, its propagation is possible but slowed down, which gives enough time for the distal level of the atrioventricular node to recover from its refractory period and conduct the impulse to the ventricles. Although the two areas of block are frequently localized within the atrioventricular junction, other portions of the conduction system can be the site of the gap phenomenon, including a proximal segment of the His Purkinje system and a distal segment of the His Purkinje system, and the atrium and the atrioventricular node (Fig. 12.14).

Supernormal conduction corresponds to a short period during the repolarization of a myocyte when a stimulus is able to trigger membrane depolarization, although the same intensity impulse would fail to trigger an action potential if it occurred slightly before or after the supernormal phase (see p. 14). Supernormal conduction is not "better" conduction (for example faster conduction) than normal, but it is a time when impulse conduction is not expected.

Supernormal intraventricular conduction can occur during sinus rhythm, supraventricular tachycardia or atrial fibrillation. A prerequisite to supernormal conduction is a functional bundle branch block (QRS complexes conducting with aberrancy because of an elevated heart rate) during baseline rhythm. Beats that occur during the supernormal period display a normal QRS morphology or a lesser degree of aberrancy. Supernormal conduction is associated with the following situations:
- premature atrial ectopic beats during sinus rhythm with bundle branch block (Fig. 12.15),
- narrow and wide QRS complex alternans during supraventricular tachycardia, and
- narrow QRS complexes during atrial fibrillation with bundle branch block.

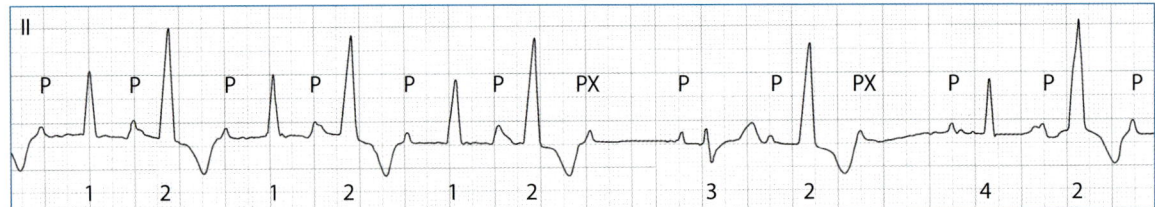

Figure 12.14. Gap phenomenon (Cat, unknown age, Lead II - speed 50 mm/s - calibration 10 mm/1 mV).
Four different QRS complexes are identified in this electrocardiogram (labeled as 1, 2, 3 and 4) recorded from a cat with hypertrophic cardiomyopathy. The underlying rhythm is sinus rhythm with a constant P-P interval of 355 ms which corresponds to a heart rate of approximately 169 bpm. The R-R interval varies because of a variable PR interval (there is no Q wave). The QRS complex labeled as "1" has a duration of 50 ms with a preceding PR interval of approximately 180 ms. The QRS complex labeled as "2" has a duration of 65 ms with a preceding PR interval of approximately 100 ms (this is estimated because of the appearance of the P wave on top of the T wave). Additionally the QRS and T wave are larger for the complexes labeled as "2". QRS complexes "1" and "2" represent varying degrees of left bundle branch block. When atrioventricular block occurs (PX) the left bundle branch has more time to recover as the atrioventricular node distal to the point of the complete block does. This results in improved atrioventricular conduction evidenced by a shorter PR interval (80 ms) and faster conduction through the left bundle branch with a narrower QRS complex (40 ms) (QRS complex "3"). The second blocked P wave (PX) is followed by a conducted P wave with a longer PR interval of 140 ms. The conduction delay in the atrioventricular node coupled with the previous block has permitted more time for the distal conduction to recover resulting in a narrow upright QRS complex compatible with incomplete left bundle branch block (QRS complex "4"). This electrocardiogram is an example of the gap phenomenon because block or increased conduction time in the atrioventricular node results in narrower QRS complexes (QRS complexes "3" and "4"), reflecting improved conduction through the left bundle. This is in contrast to the left bundle branch block that occurs when conduction through the AV node is more rapid and the electrical impulse reaches the left bundle during its refractory period (QRS complexes "1" and "2"). Therefore, examination of this ECG demonstrates that a more proximal block permits recovery and less conduction delay of the more distal conduction system while improved proximal conduction results in increasing degrees of conduction delay or block in the distal conduction system, and thus, shows gap phenomenon.

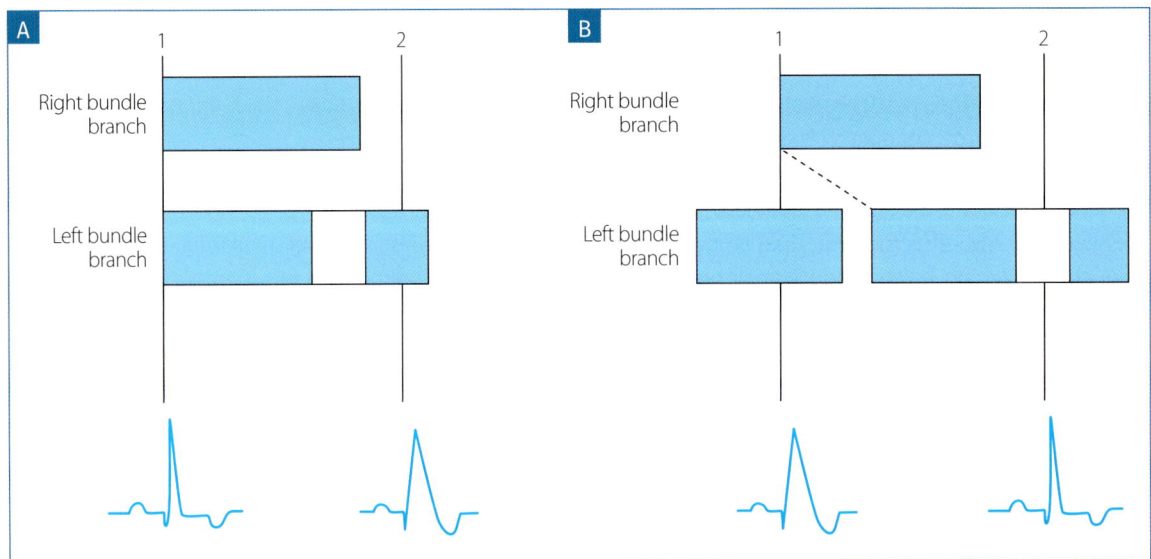

Figure 12.15. Supernormal conduction along the right bundle branch for a premature atrial ectopic beat during sinus rhythm conducted with left bundle branch block. A) The first beat is normally conducted. The next premature atrial ectopic beat (2) enters the right bundle branch in its excitable phase, while the left bundle branch is still refractory, and therefore the QRS complex displays a left bundle branch block morphology. B) The basic rhythm is sinus with a left bundle branch block. Activation of the left bundle branch is delayed and occurs retrogradely from an impulse originating from the right bundle branch. This retrograde activation further delays the refractory period of the left bundle branch allowing the next beat (2) to reach the left bundle branch during the supernormal period and to conduct normally or with only a minor degree of aberrancy compared to the baseline rhythm.

Supernormal conduction likely explains narrow and wide QRS complex alternans (although other mechanisms are also possible) during supraventricular tachycardia with regular R-R intervals. It occurs when the refractory period of the left bundle branch is delayed compared to that of the right bundle branch. First, an antegrade impulse blocks in the left bundle but travels down the right bundle and re-enters the left bundle retrogradely where it is again stopped; this event corresponds to the linking phenomenon previously described. The timing of the next impulse is such that it reaches the area of block in the left bundle branch during the supernormal phase of the tissue and is able to conduct antegradely; because it also conducts down the right bundle branch, the resulting QRS complex is narrow. The subsequent impulse reaches the left bundle branch before its full recovery from the previous depolarization resulting in the return of the functional block.

In this example, the prolongation of the refractory period of the left bundle branch caused by the linking phenomenon allowed the electrical impulse to reach the area of slow conduction in the left bundle during its supernormal period (Fig. 12.16). If the impulse had reached the area of block sooner or later, it would have been unable to propagate.

The occasional presence of narrow QRS complexes during atrial fibrillation conducted with bundle branch block is another example of supernormal conduction. Usually, when a short R-R interval follows a long R-R interval, aberrant intraventricular conduction occurs as the impulse reaches the ventricles when some of the pathways are still in their refractory state (*Ashman's phenomenon*) (see p. 171). However, if the QRS complex ending a shorter R-R interval is more narrow than QRS complexes occurring when the heart rate is slower or faster, it can reflect supernormal conduction.

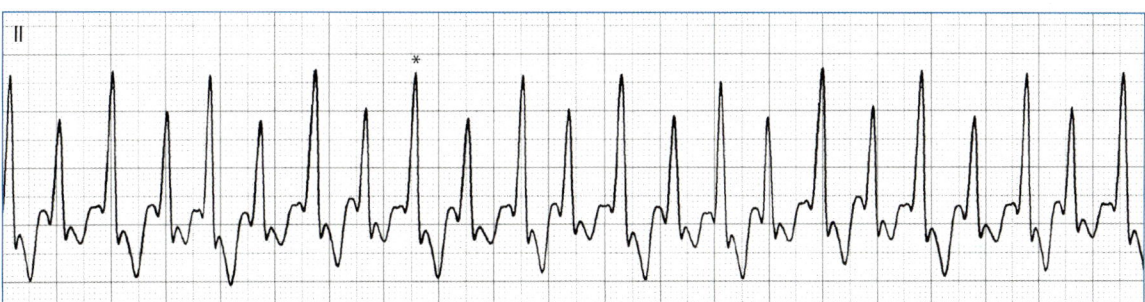

Figure 12.16. Supernormal conduction during orthodromic atrioventricular reciprocating tachycardia (Dog, Great Dane, male, 6 months. Lead II - speed 50 mm/s - calibration 20 mm/1 mV).
The underlying rhythm is an orthodromic atrioventricular reciprocating tachycardia mediated by a right postero-septal accessory pathway. Note the presence of QRS complexes with a duration of 75 ms alternating with QRS complexes with a duration of 80 ms and different morphology (*). The complexes with normal morphology are conducted during the supernormal period, while the wide QRS complexes reach the ventricles during the refractory period of the left bundle branch. There is also a beat-to-beat cycle length alternans from 180 ms to 200 ms suggestive of the presence of a dual physiology of the atrioventricular node.

Suggested readings

1. Abbott JA, King RR. Third-degree atrioventricular block following non-penetrating chest trauma in a dog. *J Small Anim Pract* 1993; 3:377-380.
2. Baron Toaldo M, Critelli M, Santilli RA. ECG of the month. Pacemaker implantation in a dog with trifascicular block. *J Am Vet Med Assoc* 2011; 239:438-440.
3. Benjamin J, Scherlag BJ, ElSherif N, et al. Experimental model for study of Mobitz type II and paroxysmal atrioventricular block. *Am J Cardiol* 1974; 34:309-317.
4. Billen F, Israël N. Syncope secondary to transient atrioventricular block in a German Shepherd dog with dilated cardiomyopathy and atrial fibrillation. *J Vet Cardiol* 2006; 8:63-68.
5. Blumenthal SR1, Vonderhaar MA, Tilley LP, Pulliam CL, Gordon BE. P-wave duration in a clinically normal hound population. *Lab Anim Sci* 1996; 46:211-214.
6. Bolton GR, Ettinger SJ. Right bundle branch block in the dog. *J Am Vet Med Assoc* 1972; 160:1104-1119.

7. Branch CE, Robertson BT, Williams JC. Frequency of second-degree atrioventricular heart block in dogs. *Am J Vet Res* 1975; 36:925-929.
8. Buchanan JW, Botts RP. Clinical effects of repeated cardiac punctures in dogs. *J Am Vet Med Assoc* 1972; 161:814-818.
9. Castellanos AI, Interian A Jr, Cox MM, Myerburg RJ. Alternating Wenckebach periods and allied arrhythmias. *Pacing Clin Electrophysiol.* 1993; 16:2285-300.
10. Castellanos AI, Cox MM, Fernandez PR, Interian A Jr, Mayor M, Ravina T, Myerburg RJ. Mechanisms and dynamics of episodes of progression of 2:1 atrioventricular block in patients with documented two-level conduction disturbances. *Am J Cardiol* 1992; 15:70:193-9.
11. Chastain CB, Riedesel DH, Graham DL. Ventricular septal hemangiosarcoma associated with right bundle branch block in a dog. *J Am Vet Med Assoc* 1974; 165:177-179.
12. Church WM, Sisson DD, Oyama MA, et al. Third degree atrioventricular block and sudden death secondary to acute myocarditis in a dog. *J Vet Cardiol* 2007; 9:53-57.
13. De Micheli A, Medrano GA, Sodi-Pallares D. Electrovectorcardiographic study of branch blocks in dogs in the light of the ventricular activation process. *Acta Cardiol* 1963; 18:483-514.
14. Detweiler DK. The dog electrocardiogram: a critical review. In MacFarlane PW, Veitch Lawrie TD, eds. Comprehensive Electrocardiology. Theory and practice in health and disease. New York, NY: Pargamon Press 1993; 1267-1329.
15. Elizari MV, Lázzari JO, Rosenbaum MB. Phase-3 and phase-4 intermittent left bundle branch block occurring spontaneously in a dog. *Eur J Cardiol* 1973; 1:95-103.
16. Elizari MV, Schmidberg J, Atienza A, et al. Clinical and Experimental Evidence of Supernormal Excitability and Conduction. *Current Cardiology Reviews* 2014; 10: 202-221.
17. Gallagher JJ, Ticzon AR, Wallace AG, et al. Activation studies following experimental hemiblock in the dog. *Circ Res* 1974; 35:752-763.
18. Guimond C, LeBlanc RA, Pelletier B, et al. Supernormal conduction and atrial echo beats in the dog. *Eur Heart J* 1981; 2:499-507.
19. Hackett TB, Van Pelt DR, Willard MD, et al. Third degree atrioventricular block and acquired myasthenia gravis in four dogs. *J Am Vet Med Assoc* 1995; 206:1173-1176.
20. James TN, Isobe JH, Urthaler F. Correlative electrophysiological and anatomical studies concerning the site of origin of escape rhythm during complete atrioventricular block in the dog. *Circ Res* 1979; 45:108-119.
21. James TN, Robertson BT, Waldo AL, et al. De subitaneis mortibus. XV. hereditary stenosis of the his bundle in pug dogs. *Circulation* 1975; 52:1152-1160.
22. Kaneshige T, Machida N, Itoh H, et al. The anatomical basis of complete atrioventricular block in cats with hypertrophic cardiomyopathy. *J Comp Pathol* 2006; 135:25-31.
23. Kaneshige T, Machida N, Yamamoto S, et al. A histological study of the cardiac conduction system in canine cases of mitral valve endocardiosis with complete atrioventricular block. *J Comp Pathol* 2007; 136:120-126.
24. Kellum HB, Stepien RL. Third-degree atrioventricular block in 21 cats (1997-2004). *J Vet Intern Med* 2006; 20:97-103.
25. Lazzara R, Yeh BK, Samet P. Functional anatomy of the canine left bundle branch. *Am J Cardiol* 1974; 33:623-632.
26. Leininger SR. Right bundle-branch block in a dog. *Mod Vet Pract* 1984; 1:33-36.
27. Moise S. Right bundle branch block in a dog with sinus tachycardia. *J Am Vet Med Assoc* 1984; 184:1458-1459.
28. Oxford EM, Giacomazzi FB, Moise NS, et al. Clinical and electrocardiographic presentations of transient trifascicular block in three cats. *J Vet Cardiol 2018*; doi.org/10.1016/j.jvc.2018.02.002
29. Rishniw M, Tobias AH, Marks SL, et al. ECG of the month. High-grade second-degree AV block and right bundle-branch block in a cat. *J Am Vet Med Assoc* 1994; 205:425-427.
30. Robotham GR. Right bundle branch block in the dog. *Canine Pract* 1979; 6:67-70.
31. Rosenbaum MB, The Hemiblocks: Diagnostic criteria and Clinical Significance. *Am Heart J* 1970; 70:141-146.
32. Rosenbaum MB, Elizari MV, Lazzari JO. Gli emiblocchi. Edizioni Piccin Padova (I). 1976; 2-134.
33. Rosenbaum MB, Elizari MV, Lazzari JO, et al. Intraventricular trifascicular blocks. Review of the literature and classification. *Am Heart J* 1969; 78:450-459.
34. Santilli RA, Porteiro Vázquez DM, Vezzosi T, et al. Long-term intrinsic rhythm evaluation in dogs with atrioventricular block. *J Vet Intern Med* 2016; 30:58-62.
35. Santilli RA, Battaia S, Perego M, et al. Bartonella-associated inflammatory cardiomyopathy in a dog. *J Vet Cardiol* 2017; 19:74-81
36. Schrope DP, Kelch WJ. Signalment, clinical signs, and prognostic indicators associated with high-grade second- or third-degree atrioventricular block in dogs: 124 cases (January 1, 1997-December 31, 1997). *J Am Vet Med Assoc* 2006; 228:1710-1717.
37. Sleeper MM, Bissett S, Craig L. Canine trichinosis presenting with syncope and AV conduction disturbance. *J Vet Intern Med* 2006; 20:1228-1231.
38. Spear JF, Moore EN. Supernormal excitability and conduction in the His-Purkinje system of the dog. *Circ Res 1974*; 35:782-792.
39. Spear JF, Moore EN. Supernormal conduction in the canine bundle of His and proximal bundle branches. *Am J Physiol* 1980; 238:H300-306.
40. Tyzka LS, Houston D, Stauffer S, et al. Exercise in electrocardiography [right bundle branch block in a cat]. *Can Vet J* 1992; 33:137-138.
41. Troy GC, Turnwald GH. Atrial fibrillation and abnormal ventricular conduction presented as right bundle branch block in a dog with an atrial septum primum defect. *J Am Vet Med Assoc* 1979; 14:417-420.
42. VanOpstal JM, Verduyn SC, Leunissen HDM, et al. Electrophysiological parameters indicative of sudden cardiac death in the dog with chronic complete AV-block. *Cardiovasc Res* 2001; 50:354-361.
43. Watt TB. Features of fascicular block imposed upon existing right bundle branch block in the dog and baboon. *Am J Cardiol* 1977; 39:1000-1007.
44. Watt TB Jr, Freud GE, Durrer D, et al. Left anterior arborization block combined with right bundle branch block in canine and primate hearts. An electrocardiographic study. *Circ Res* 1968; 22:57-63.

CHAPTER 13

Electrocardiographic changes secondary to systemic disorders and drugs

Cardiac impulse formation and propagation can be affected by metabolic and electrolyte abnormalities, various diseases, and drugs (e.g. antiarrhythmic agents, sedatives). The timely identification of these changes is critical to prevent initiation of arrhythmias and deterioration of cardiac function.

Hypoxia

Hypoxia triggers hyperventilation and activation of the adrenergic system secondary to stimulation of the carotid body chemoreceptors. Therefore, the typical response to hypoxia is sinus tachycardia and tachypnea. However, the effect is different if the ventilation rate is maintained constant, or during apnea (upper airway obstruction, diving reflex). In this situation, hypoxia results in an increase in peripheral vascular resistance and vagally-mediated bradycardia.

Hypoxia can result in alterations of the ST segment and T wave morphology (Fig. 13.1). Severe hypoxia can trigger premature ventricular ectopic beats progressing to ventricular tachycardia, or sinus bradycardia, which can deteriorate into cardiac arrest.

Electrolytic disorders

The three electrolytes that are critical for normal electrical impulse formation and propagation are potassium, calcium and magnesium. The impact of electrolyte imbalances on the characteristics of the action potential are usually difficult to predict because ion channel properties are influenced by extra- and intracellular electrolyte concentrations.

Hyperkalemia

Hyperkalemia is a frequent complication of hypoadrenocorticism (Addison's disease), urinary tract obstruction or rupture, oliguric and anuric renal failure, and the reperfusion phase following aortic thromboembolism. Intra- and extracellular potassium concentration is the most important contributor to the membrane resting potential. Hyperkalemia causes the resting membrane potential to shift to less negative values, and as a result it leads to a decrease in the slope of phase 0 of the action potential. In addition, hyperkalemia is associated with a shortening of the action potential duration, because the activity of the channels responsible for the repolarizing current I_{Kr} increases in the presence of elevated extracellular potassium concentration. This effect is opposite to what would be expected if potassium exchange across the cell membrane was only determined by concentration gradients. As plasma potassium concentration rises, it initially increases the excitability of the cardiomyocytes as it brings the resting membrane potential closer to the threshold potential for depolarization. As hyperkalemia worsens, the resting membrane potential can reach values above the threshold potential keeping the myocytes in a depolarized state and preventing the formation of subsequent action potentials (loss of excitability) (Fig. 13.2). These changes are reversible once potassium levels return to normal values.

The effects of hyperkalemia on the cardiomyocytes and the electrocardiogram also depend on calcium concentration. Specifically, hypocalcemia amplifies the effect of hyperkalemia on the cardiac action potential. Alternatively, it diminishes the depolarizing effects of hypokalemia.

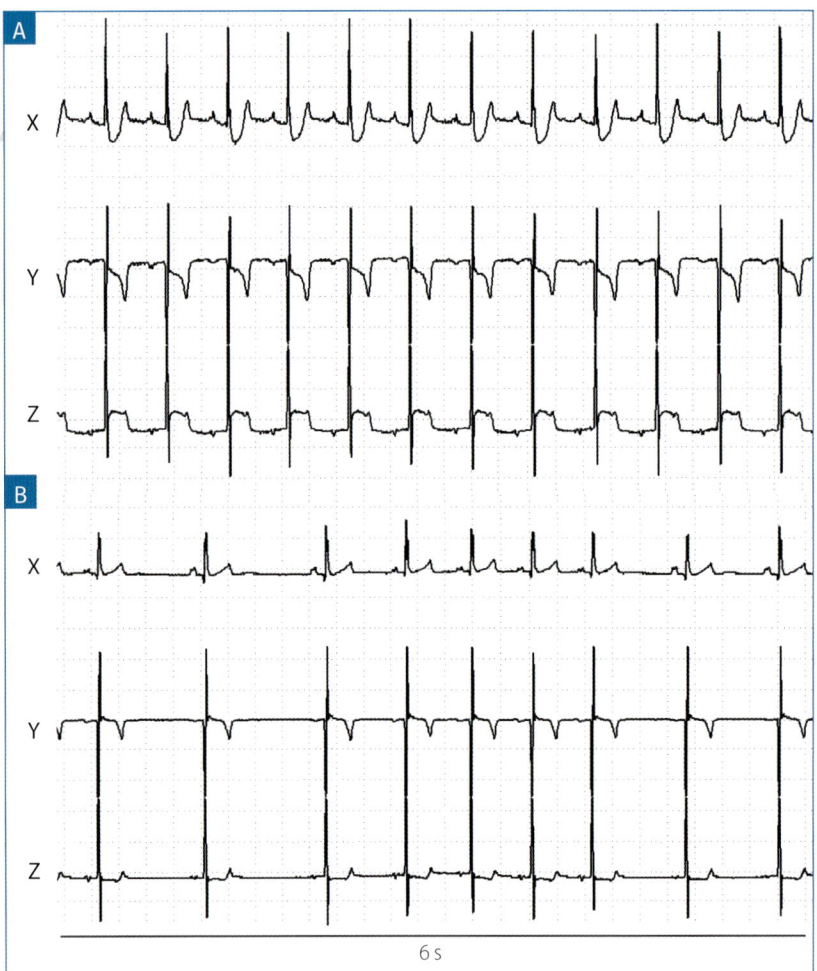

Figure 13.1. Leads X, Y and Z from a Holter recording in a syncopal dog with ST segment alteration due to hypoxia caused by severe pulmonary hypertension (systolic pulmonary artery pressure 160 mmHg). A) Syncope was triggered by excitement causing sinus tachycardia and ST segment depression (X, Y), or elevation (Z) depending on the lead. B) When the dog was not excited, a sinus arrhythmia was present with a normal ST segment.

The atrial myocardium seems to be the most sensitive tissue to the effects of hyperkalemia, followed by the ventricular myocardium and finally, the myocytes forming the conduction system. However, QRS complexes of cats with reperfusion injury following thromboembolism often display S waves and a right axis shift suggestive of incomplete or complete right bundle branch block as an initial alteration of the electrocardiogram associated with hyperkalemia. This finding of course could be the consequence of multiple factors due to reperfusion injury.

Alterations of the electrocardiogram usually occur when serum concentration of potassium reaches 6 to 6.5 mmol/L. The T wave shape becomes tall and peaked ("tented" T wave) with symmetrical ascending and descending branches. The QT interval is shortened. In addition, it causes a delay in intra-atrial impulse propagation with a prolongation of the P wave duration and a reduction of its amplitude.

Moderate hyperkalemia (approximately 6.5 to 8.5 mmol/L) results in sinus bradycardia, a more pronounced reduction in P wave amplitude (Fig. 13.3), a broadening of the QRS complex, a prolongation of the PQ interval occasionally leading to atrioventricular block, and ST segment depression in the inferior leads (II, III, aVF).

Severe hyperkalemia (8.5 and 10 mmol/L) results in the progressive interruption of atrial myocardium depolarization. However, conduction persists within the cells of the preferential pathways between left and right atrium and between sinus and atrioventricular node.

Electrolytic disorders | 295

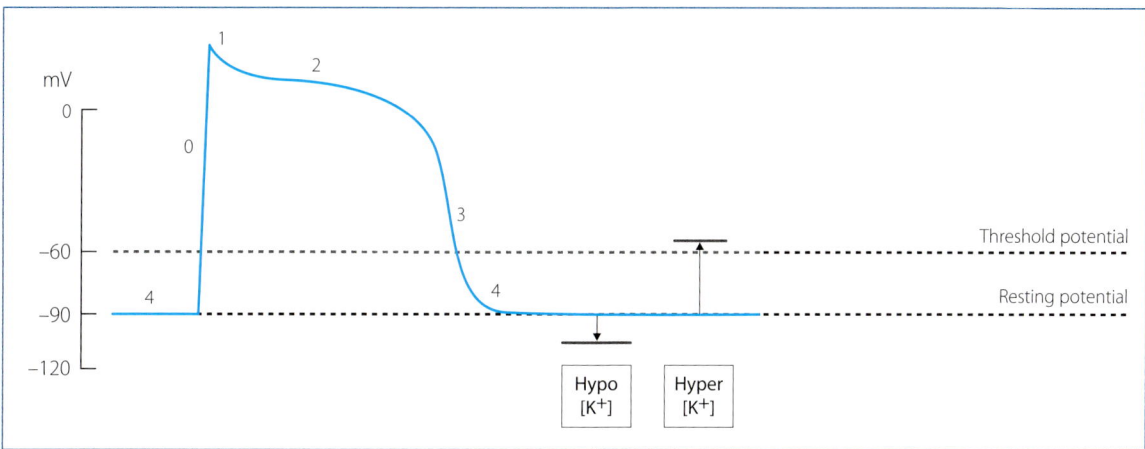

Figure 13.2. Electrocardiographic changes during variations of potassium plasma concentrations. Effects of hypo- and hyperkalemia on the resting transmembrane potential. In the presence of hyperkalemia the transmembrane potential decreases towards the threshold membrane potential. Conversely, hypokalemia results in a shift of the transmembrane potential towards more negative values (hyperpolarization).

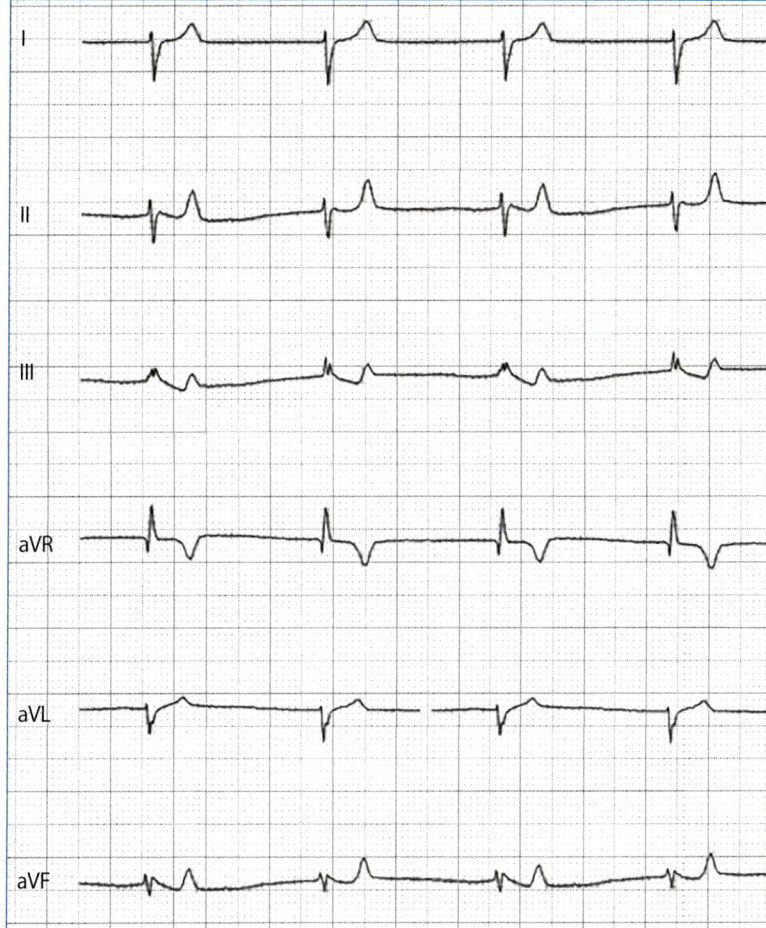

Figure 13.3. Six-lead electrocardiogram recorded from a cat - speed 50 mm/s - calibration 10 mm/1 mV - with a potassium concentration of 7.0 mmol/L. P waves are absent, T waves are peaked and evidence exists of an incomplete right bundle branch block (S waves in leads I, II and aVF are present with a right axis shift).

The rhythm observed on the electrocardiogram is described as a *sino-ventricular rhythm* and is characterized by an absence of P waves (Fig. 13.4).

Extreme hyperkalemia (>10 mmol/L) can result in atrial and ventricular asystole, possibly ventricular flutter and fibrillation. Holter recordings of cats wit reperfusion injury secondary to cardiomyopathy and thromboembolism indicate that death frequently occurs because of ventricular asystole and not ventricular fibrillation (Fig. 13.5). The electrical activity of the sinus node, the region of the *crista terminalis* and the Bachmann's bundle do, however, remain unchanged.

Hypokalemia

Hypokalemia induces a shift of the resting membrane towards more negative values (hyperpolarization) and a decrease in cell excitability and conduction velocity. In addition, it is associated with an increase in action potential duration, possibly because extracellular potassium concentration impacts the activity of the transmembrane potassium channels. By delaying repolarization, hypokalemia promotes ectopies from early after-depolarization. Finally, it increases the automaticity of the Purkinje fibers (Fig. 13.2).

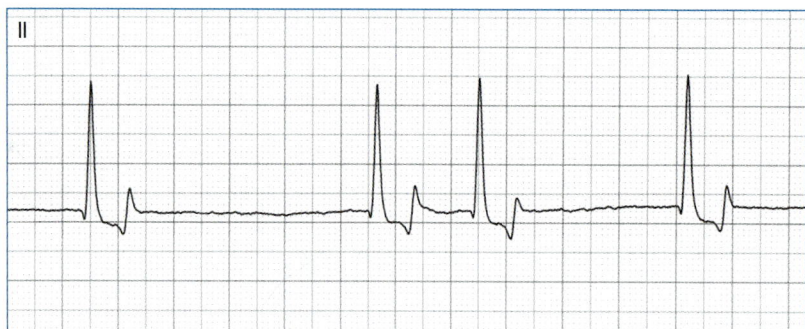

Figure 13.4. Sino-ventricular rhythm during Addisonian crisis (Dog, Bull Terrier, male, 5 years. Lead II - speed 50 mm/s - calibration 10 mm/1 mV). The basic rhythm is a sino-ventricular rhythm characterized by the absence of atrial depolarization (P waves) due to high potassium serum levels, which maintain the atrial myocytes in a constant state of depolarization. Note the characteristic presence of irregular R-R intervals.

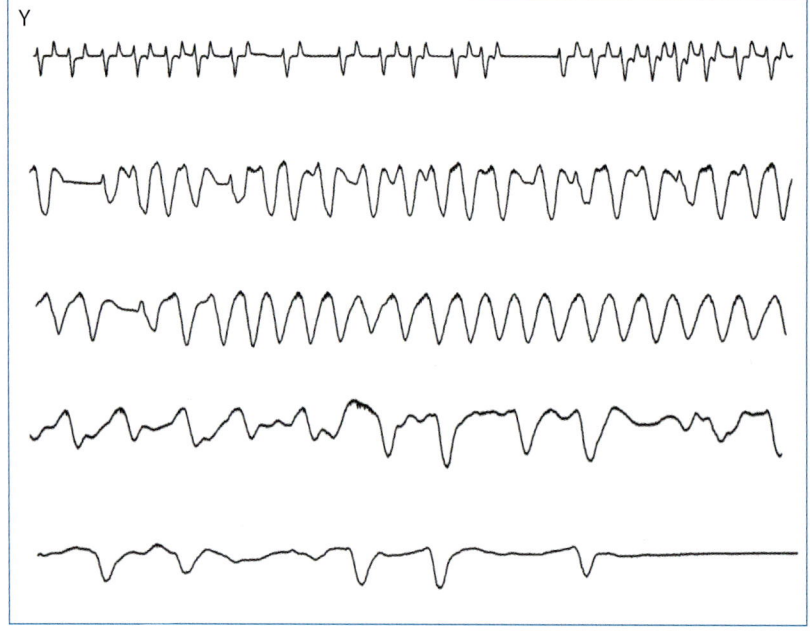

Figure 13.5. Segments of a continuous electrocardiogram recorded from a cat suffering from reperfusion injury because of severe thromboembolism associated with cardiomyopathy (Lead Y from a 24-hour electrocardiographic recording full disclosure image). Potassium was 9.6 mmol/L. This recording shows the electrocardiographic features of severe hyperkalemia. The top tracing shows an irregular rhythm with no P waves, deep S waves and spiked T waves. This progresses to a wide QRS complex that continues to have an irregular rhythm. It is difficult to know if this portion of the electrocardiogram is a conduction abnormality of supraventricular origin or a ventricular rhythm. A faster more regular rhythm similar to ventricular flutter is seen before the heart rate slows dramatically and asystole follows.

Electrocardiographic changes secondary to hypokalemia are related to its effects on electrical impulse conduction and action potential repolarization. Impaired conduction with severe hypokalemia can affect the duration of the P wave, prolong the PQ interval or result in atrioventricular block, and increase QRS complex duration. Delayed repolarization is reflected by QT interval prolongation, broad and biphasic T waves with diminished amplitude, the presence of U waves and ST segment deviation. In animals with structural heart disease, hypokalemia can significantly increase the risk of ventricular tachycardia and ventricular fibrillation.

Hypercalcemia and hypocalcemia

The effect of hypercalcemia (total calcium serum concentration usually exceeding 12 mg/dL in dogs and 11 mg/dL in cats) and hypocalcemia (concentrations below 6.5 mg/dL in both dogs and cats) is on the action potential duration.

Hypercalcemia causes a decrease in the action potential duration of the ventricular myocytes, which is reflected by a shortening of the QT interval on the electrocardiogram.

Hypocalcemia causes a prolongation of phase 2 (plateau) of the action potential and QT interval prolongation on the electrocardiogram.

Hypomagnesemia

Hypomagnesemia may result from inadequate dietary intake or excessive loss of magnesium due to diuretic therapy. Electrophysiological changes secondary to hypomagnesemia are due to the interactions of this ion with potassium and calcium. Hypomagnesemia increases the concentration of cytosolic calcium and prevents the accumulation of intracellular potassium.

The electrocardiographic changes from hypomagnesemia are not well characterized. Hypomagnesemia can cause a prolongation of the action potential duration and conduction times; therefore PQ, QT intervals and QRS complex duration increase. In some cases, a U wave may become apparent. Rarely, hypomagnesemia promotes the occurrence of premature ventricular ectopic beats and it can increase the risk for polymorphic ventricular tachycardias.

Pericardial diseases

The accumulation of fluid in the pericardial space may be manifested on the electrocardiogram in two ways: electrical alternans and a reduction in QRS complex amplitude (Fig. 13.6).

Electrical alternans refers to beat-to-beat P wave, QRS complex and/or T wave voltage alternation, as well as PQ and ST segment deviation. It is QRS complex alternans that is most commonly identified on the electrocardiogram. The mechanism with pericardial effusion is the continuous swinging of the heart in the pericardial sac towards and away from the recording electrodes. Electrical alternans has been reported to occur in approximately a third of dogs with pericardial effusion. It is likely that it is more common when a large volume of effusion is present. It should be remembered that the other cause of alternating QRS amplitude is some rapid rate supraventricular tachycardias.

Low-voltage (low amplitude) QRS complexes is another common feature of pericardial effusion. It can be associated with electrical alternans. The reduction in QRS complex amplitude is thought to be associated with the volume of pericardial effusion: for example, the typical small amount of blood that accumulates in the pericardial space during an acute hemorrhage is usually not sufficient to affect the amplitude of QRS complexes; conversely, the large volume of sero-hemorrhagic fluid that characterizes idiopathic pericardial effusion is more likely to affect the size of the QRS complexes. Pleural effusion, a pneumothorax or a thick layer of subcutaneous fat also interfere with the transmission of the electrical activity to the surface electrodes of the electrocardiogram and can be associated with small amplitude QRS complexes.

Abdominal diseases

Abdominal diseases, including gastric dilation-volvulus, splenic masses, and pancreatitis are frequently associated with ventricular arrhythmias (Fig. 13.7). Gastric dilatation-volvulus is a medical and surgical emergency. Preoperative ventricular arrhythmias have been reported to be a negative prognostic indicator. However, arrhythmias are more common post-operatively. The main trigger for

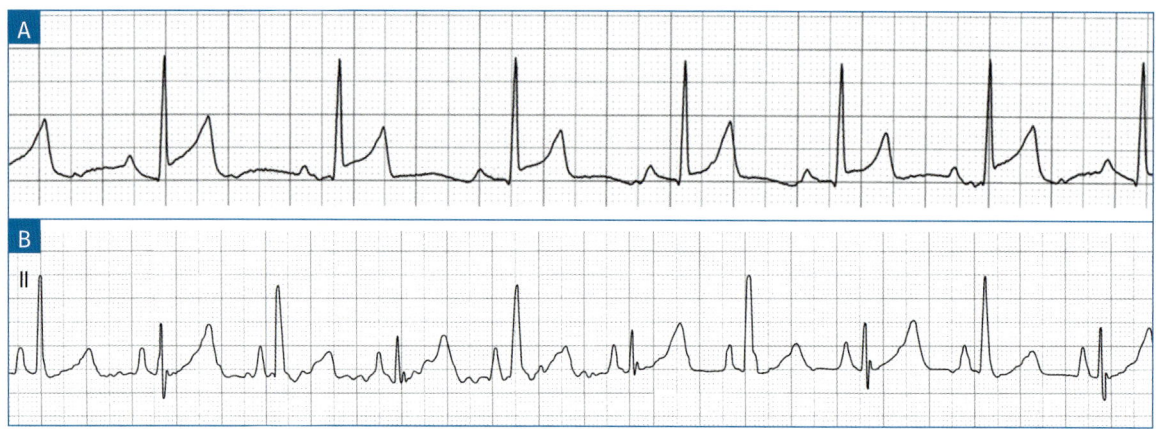

Figure 13.6. Electrocardiographic changes during pericardial effusion.
A) Dog, German Shepherd, male, 10 years. Lead II - speed 50 mm/s - calibration 10 mm/1 mV.
The basic rhythm is a sinus rhythm with a rate of 120 bpm. Note the presence of a beat-to-beat variation of ST segment elevation (from 0.2 mV to 0.3 mV) and the PQ segment depression.
B) Dog, Labrador Retriever, male, 9 years, with pericarditis and cardiac tamponade. Lead II - speed 25 mm/s - calibration 5 mm/1 mV. Electrical alternations of the QRS complex and T wave is evident. Note as the QRS amplitude decreased the T wave amplitude increased. In some instances, the T wave may actually change in polarity. Alternans of the P wave is not apparent. This electrocardiogram represents an alternating morphology and size with every other beat and is the classic characterization of electrical alternans. It is possible however to have alternations at different ratios such as 3:1 or 4:1.

arrhythmias after surgery is the sequence of a period of tissue ischemia followed by reperfusion, which leads to the release of circulating myocardial depressant factors, including cytokines and possibly platelet exosomes. The most common arrhythmia is an accelerated idioventricular rhythm with an average firing rate within 10 % the underlying sinus rate, and frequent fusion and capture beats (see p. 210). Arrhythmias occur soon after surgery, usually do not cause hemodynamic instability and resolve spontaneously within 72 hours. Other rhythm abnormalities include isolated premature ventricular beats or periods of allorhythmia (ventricular bigeminy, trigeminy, quadrigeminy), ventricular tachycardia with the largest negative deflection in the inferior leads (II, III, aVF) and left precordial leads (V_2-V_6), suggesting a left ventricular origin because of the right bundle branch block morphology, and finally sinus or atrial tachycardia. Atrial fibrillation can develop in these dogs given the combination of triggers (atrial premature complexes) and modulating factors (stress/high sympathetic tone coupled with medications that increase parasympathetic tone such as narcotics). Additionally, most dogs with gastric volvulus are large breeds making them more predisposed to atrial fibrillation because of a larger atrial mass. When atrial fibrillation develops perioperatively or intraoperatively it usually resolves soon after return of normal autonomic balance; however, if it is noted acutely treatment with intravenous lidocaine is often effective in this specific situation.

The same type of arrhythmias is occasionally detected in systematically ill animals with large splenic and liver masses, pancreatitis, and after trauma (e.g., hit-by-car with large muscular contusions).

Chronic respiratory diseases

Chronic respiratory diseases such as chronic obstructive pulmonary disease, interstitial pulmonary fibrosis, or chronic upper airway obstruction can induce electrocardiographic changes secondary to hypervagotonia and right heart chamber remodeling when pulmonary hypertension is present. These changes include sinus bradycardia, pronounced respiratory sinus arrhythmia, and on occasion alterations of the P wave and QRS morphology that reflect right atrial and right ventricular enlargement (Fig. 13.8). Although tall P waves may be identified, right atrial enlargement may not be present in dogs with respiratory disorders.

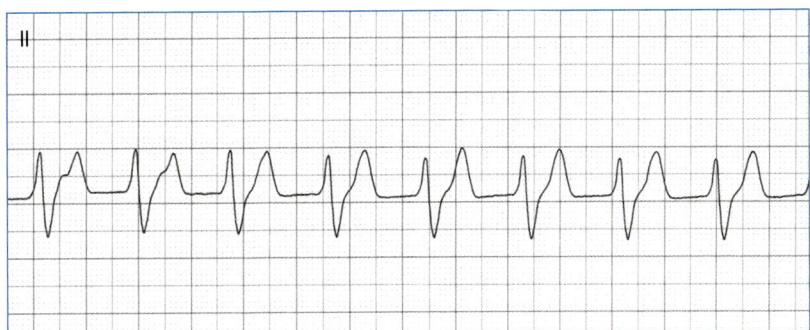

Figure 13.7. Accelerated idioventricular rhythm after gastric dilation-torsion volvulus (Dog, Labrador Retriever, female, 11 years. Lead II - speed 50 mm/s - calibration 10 mm/1 mV).
The basic rhythm is an accelerated idioventricular rhythm with a rate of 160 bpm. Note the presence of wide QRS complexes (80 ms) conducted with a right bundle branch block morphology and regular R-R intervals.

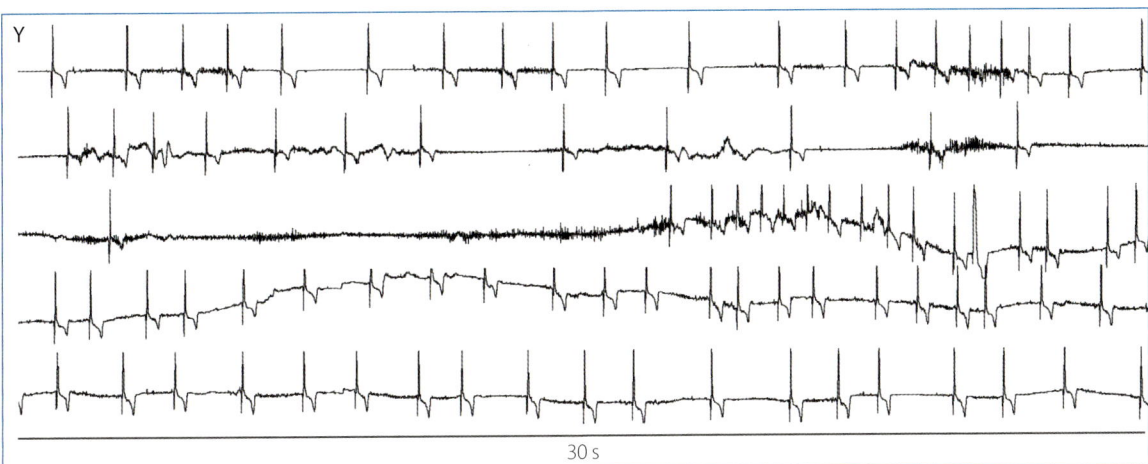

Figure 13.8. Continuous electrocardiographic recording made during 24-hour Holter monitoring (lead Y) of a 4-year old Cavalier King Charles Spaniel with a history of syncope during sleep. The dog would make a sharp noise while sleeping and become limp. Although motion artifact is apparent in this recording, its presence is not distracting but informative. During this time the dog would have sharp movements and become flaccid. The owners reported the dog snored loudly during sleep. Multiple episodes of marked bradycardia with pauses were documented during sleep as shown here. An oral examination revealed an elongated soft palate, which was corrected surgically. After surgery, the owners reported no further episodes. The post-pause increase in the heart rate was a physiologic response to the severe drop in cardiac output, hypotension and hypoxia.

Endocrine diseases

Hyperthyroidism leads to sinus tachycardia in addition to structural and functional cardiac changes and congestive heart failure. Most affected cats have electrocardiographic abnormalities that include sinus tachycardia, increased QRS voltage (>0.9 mV in lead II), supraventricular tachycardia, ventricular or intra-ventricular conduction disturbances (right bundle branch block and left anterior fascicular block) (Fig. 13.9). The increased QRS voltage is not only because of the myocardial hypertrophy (due to the trophic effect of thyroxin) but the decrease in body fat and muscle. Supraventricular and ventricular arrhythmias associated with thyrotoxicosis are triggered by an increased sensitivity to catecholamines. Most of these arrhythmias resolve spontaneously after hyperthyroidism is treated.

Hypothyroidism is associated with a dysfunction and reduction in the number beta-adrenergic receptors. Hypothyroidism also alters the function of the cardiac sarcomere. Thus, a lowered thyroid hormone concentration leads to a reduction in myocardial contractility and the discharge rate of the sinus node. Electrocardiographic changes include sinus bradycardia, atrioventricular conduction disturbances, low-voltage QRS complexes, inversion of T wave polarity. Hypothyroidism could be

Drugs

Drugs, including antiarrhythmic agents, sedatives and anesthetics, can alter pacemaker cell automaticity, cause conduction and repolarization abnormalities, or be pro-arrhythmic.

Antiarrhythmic drugs

All anti-arrhythmics and digoxin have the potential to affect the appearance of the electrocardiogram. The changes described below are not automatically seen with treatment because most often they are dose dependent.

Class I drugs
Quinidine
Quinidine is a class IA antiarrhythmic agent (sodium channel blocker), which decreases the rate of phase 0 depolarization. It also prolongs the refractory period of the atrial, ventricular and Purkinje cells, and depresses spontaneous automaticity of pacemaker cells by reducing phase 4 depolarization and moving all the threshold membrane potential to less negative values. Finally, it has a vagolytic effect, which counter-balances its impact on spontaneous automaticity and prevents a reduction in the rate of sinus node depolarization, as well as increasing atrioventricular conduction conduction velocity. Quinidine overdose results in an increase in the duration of the PQ interval, the QRS complex and the QT interval. As any drug that delays repolarization, it increases the risk of triggered activity-induced arrhythmias.

Procainamide
Procainamide is a class IA antiarrhythmic drug (sodium channel blocker) with electrophysiological properties that are similar to quinidine. The electrocardiographic findings associated with procainamide overdose include an increase in QRS complex and QT interval duration.

Lidocaine
Lidocaine is a class IB antiarrhythmic drug (sodium channel blocker), which decreases the rate of phase 0 depolarization (decreased automaticity). It also shortens the duration of the action potential of cardiomyocytes without reducing their refractory period via a mechanism known as post-repolarization refractoriness. Post-repolarization refractoriness results from the blockade of sodium channels which remain unavailable for a period of time after completion of the action potential despite the membrane potential returning to resting values. This effect is also amplified at elevated heart rates (use-dependence). Lidocaine has more effect on ventricular myocytes, but it can also successfully terminate some supraventricular arrhythmias, including vagally-induced atrial fibrillation. Electrocardiographic changes associated with lidocaine can include a decrease in QT interval duration and, with toxic doses, an increase in the duration of the PQ and QT intervals, sinus bradycardia, and various degrees of atrioventricular block.

Mexiletine
Mexiletine is a class IB antiarrhythmic drug (sodium channel blocker) and an analogue of lidocaine. In dogs, no effects on the sinus automaticity and conduction intervals have been noted.

Class II drugs
Beta-blockers
Beta-blockers are class II antiarrhythmic drugs that decrease the rate of the sinus node discharge and decrease conduction through the atrioventricular junction. They also decrease the automaticity of ectopic foci. The electrocardiographic findings associated with the use of β-blockers include an increase in PQ interval duration. Overdose of beta-blockers causes an increase of P wave, PQ interval, QRS complex and QT interval duration associated with sinus bradycardia and various degrees of atrioventricular block. Beta-blockers can also depress the spontaneously depolarization of subsidiary ventricular pacemakers.

Class III drugs
Class III antiarrhythmic drugs include amiodarone and sotalol. They prolong the duration of atrial and ventricular action potential and atrioventricular conduction. Both amiodarone and sotalol are responsible for an increase in PQ and QT intervals. At high doses some class III antiarrhythmics may cause the appearance of a U wave in addition to prolonging the QT interval (Fig. 13.12). On occasion, the prolongation of the plateau phase of the action potential can lead to early after-depolarizations and polymorphic ventricular tachyarrhythmias (torsade des pointes). It is known as a proarrhythmic effect.

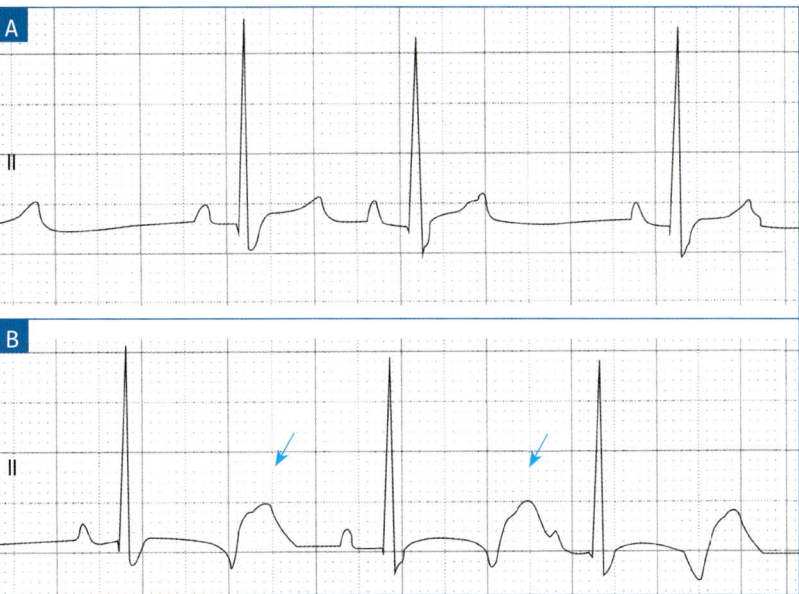

Figure 13.12. Lead II electrocardiogram - speed 50 mm/s - calibration 10 mm/1 mV) recorded from a dog before and after treatment with a class III antiarrhythmic drug with potent potassium channel blocking properties.
A) Electrocardiogram recorded before treatment shows a QT interval of ~ 200 ms and a PQ interval of ~ 90 ms.
B) Electrocardiogram recorded after treatment shows a QT interval of ~300 ms, a QU interval of ~ 400 ms and a PQ interval of ~90 ms. In addition to the PQ interval remaining relatively constant the heart rate is not different before and after treatment. However, because of the prolongation of repolarization the QT interval is prolonged and a U wave has developed (arrows).

Class IV drugs

Calcium channel blockers (verapamil, diltiazem) are responsible for a decrease of the sinus rate and a reduction in atrioventricular conduction velocity. Calcium channel blockers prolong the PQ interval. Overdose can result in second or third-degree atrioventricular block and an increase in the duration of both QRS complexes and QT interval.

Digoxin

At therapeutic doses digoxin reduces the slope of phase 4 in pacemaker cells, decreases the upstroke velocity (phase 0) of the action potential, as well as its amplitude and duration. Electrocardiographic changes associated with digoxin administration include a reduction of the sinus rate, prolongation of the PQ interval and a shortening of the QT interval. A toxic dose of digoxin can cause atrioventricular blocks of different degree, sinus bradycardia, junctional premature ectopic beats, junctional rhythm, nonparoxysmal junctional tachycardia, focal atrial tachycardia, premature ventricular ectopic beats, and bidirectional ventricular tachycardia. Digoxin-induced ventricular tachyarrhythmias are initiated by delayed after-depolarization (triggered activity) as a result of intracellular calcium accumulation. Coving of the ST segment is also a feature of digoxin overdose.

Anticholinergics

Anticholinergic drugs, such as atropine and glycopyrrolate are used to increase sinus rate. Due to their parasympatholytic effect, they cause an increase in the firing rate of the sinus node and a decrease in atrioventricular conduction time. The increase in heart rate is associated with an increase in myocardial oxygen consumption, which can predispose to the development of supraventricular and ventricular arrhythmias in animals with pre-existing cardiac disease.

The treatment effect of atropine is dependent on the route of administration and dose. When atropine is administered intravenously the heart rate is greater than when administered intramuscularly or subcutaneously. In general, higher doses produce faster heart rates with a maximum increase in rate with doses of 0.04-0.06 mg/kg. In dogs, as judged by heart rate variability, the parasympathetic system most often is suppressed at the 0.04 mg/kg dose. Under experimental conditions in dogs, whereby vagal tone was increased with the administration of opioids, low doses of atropine (0.01 mg/kg) resulted in a brief slowing of the sinus rate. The degree of slowing was minimal and may not be clinically important. This initial slowing at low doses is hypothesized to be the result of initial blockade of presynaptic inhibitory muscarinic (M_2) receptors (high-affinity) that lead to an increase in the release of acetylcholine which slows the sinus rate. Then, after a brief time, blockade of postsynaptic muscarinic receptors (low-affinity) are blocked and the parasympatholytic effects dominate with a faster sinus rate. Clinically, the effect more often observed with the administration of atropine occurs at the usual therapeutic doses whereby there is not a slowing of the sinus rate but of the ventricular rate because of temporary atrioventricular block which is rarely of concern. This can occur regardless of the route of administration, although it may be more profound with intravenous treatment. The mechanism for atrioventricular blockade after administration of atropine is hypothesized to be due to the varied distribution of muscarinic receptor subtypes within the atrioventricular and sino-atrial nodes (Fig. 13.13).

Drugs used for sedation

The cardiovascular and electrophysiological effects and interactions of drugs used for sedation, pre-anesthesia and anesthesia are varied and complex. It is beyond the scope of this writing to address the multitude of pathways that may cause changes to the electrocardiogram because of electrophysiological alterations that occur during induction and maintenance of anesthesia. However, sedation of animals is frequently required to perform examinations in cardiology. Thus, the electrophysiological effects of drugs commonly used for the sedation of dogs and cats and the resulting electrocardiographic changes are addressed herein.

With respect to the numerous drugs used for sedation the physiological responses are most often highly dependent on the following: dosage, route of administration, underlying rhythm, cardiac status and the interplay of cardiovascular reflexes coupled to the central nervous system effects. The medications used in the sedation of dogs and cats are grouped based on their mechanism of action; however, as is true for all classifications of drugs, individual variation exists. Another important clinical point is that the sedation of fractious, anxious or uncooperative dogs and cats is often achieved with a combination of drugs from different categories. Combining drugs together can in some circumstances provide better sedation and any side effects can be counterbalanced. Finally, the balance of the sympathetic and parasympathetic system in the individual animal can be critical to the response to a particular drug. The following drug descriptions provide information concerning the drug classifications and Table 13.1 summarizes the effects on heart rate and atrioventricular conduction for specific drugs.

Figure 13.13. Continuous six-lead electrocardiogram - speed 50 mm/s - calibration 5 mm/1 mV- after the administration of intramuscular atropine at 0.04 mg/kg in a dog with sinus bradycardia. The dog had upper airway obstruction. To determine the chronotropic competency of this dog before undergoing soft palate resection, atropine was given to suppress the parasympathetic system. Three time points during the 52 min recording are shown in each frame. The vertical line in the heart rate (frequency) (HF) tachogram shown above the electrocardiograms indicates these three time points. Note time (minutes) is shown on the X-axis of the tachogram and electrocardiogram. This continuous recording shows several consistent features that characterize the electrocardiogram of a dog treated with atropine.
A) Pronounced sinus arrhythmia exists 36 s after the intramuscular administration of atropine. Note on the heart rate tachogram and the variability in the R-R intervals. This is indicated by the fluctuation and spread (single arrow) of the heart rate. Between 25 and 30 min the variability in the R-R intervals decreases causing the spread of R-R intervals to be narrower so that the deflections in variability are so small that it appears as a more singular line (double arrow).
B) Sinus arrhythmia persists 15 min after the administration of atropine, but the P-P intervals are not as long. In addition, second-degree heart block is present with a single P wave that is not conducted. This second-degree heart block occurs with a faster sinus rate (see text for explanation). The PQ interval preceding the block P wave has a slight increase in duration (intervals from left to right before block: 100 ms, 90 ms, 90 ms, 110 ms). Note the increasing heart rate evidenced on the tachogram. The majority of dogs given atropine will have second-degree heart block associated with an increase sinus rate. This rhythm is followed shortly thereafter by an even faster sinus rate without atrioventricular block.
C) Sinus rhythm with a heart rate of 135 bpm is present 35 min after the administration of intramuscular atropine. The parasympathetic effect of this anticholinergic drug has resulted in an increased number of impulses arising from the sinus node and an increased atrioventricular conduction through the atrioventricular node (PQ interval 80 ms). The relatively constant P-P and R-R intervals (low heart rate variability) are evident in the measurement of the electrocardiographic deflections and are shown in the heart rate tachogram as a more singular line.

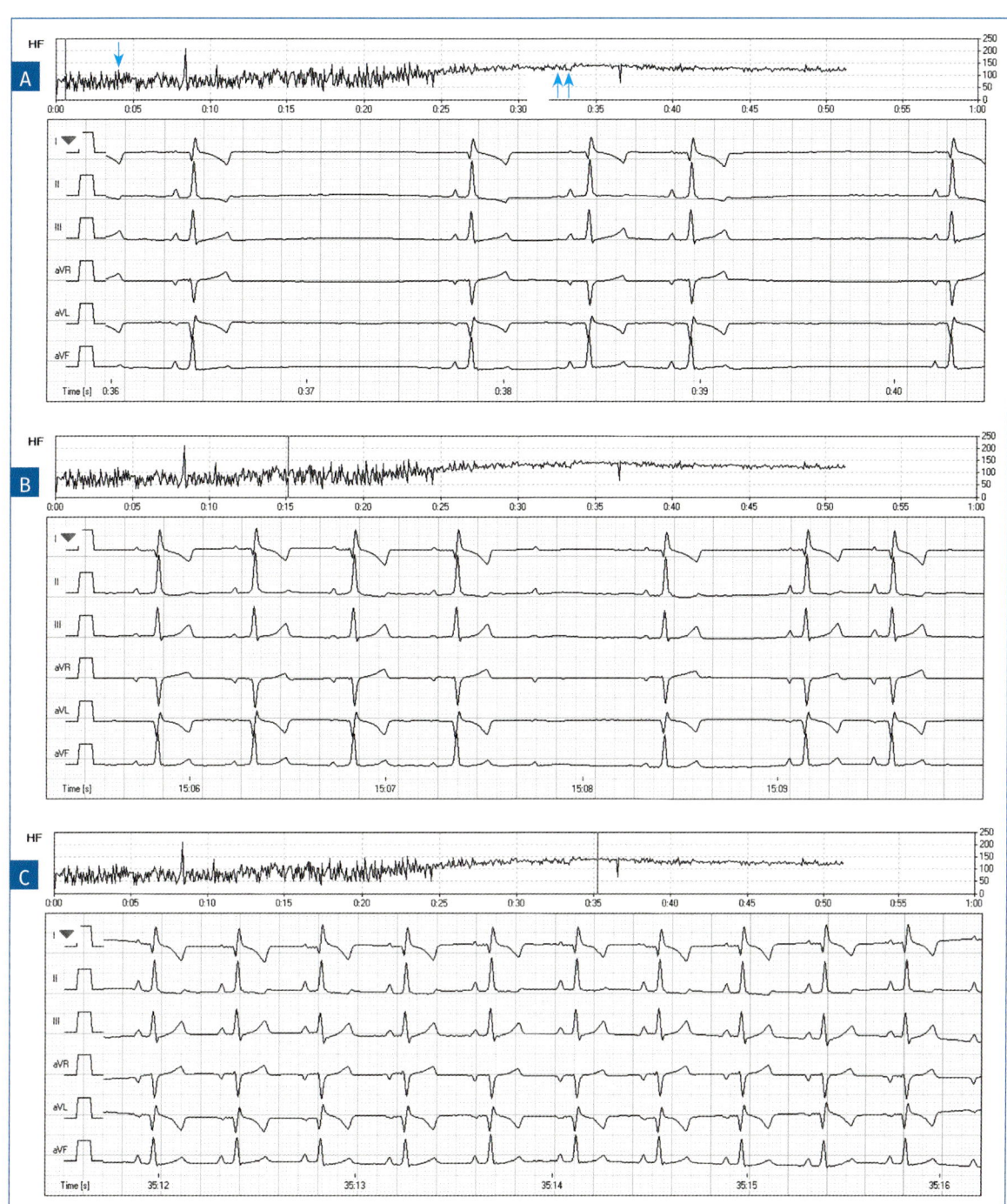

Drug	Classification	Effect on heart rate	Mechanism for heart rate effect
Alfaxalone	Neuroactive steroid Enhances action of GABA at GABA$_A$ receptor	Initially may increase rate when given IV Less effect on rate when given IM	Initial drop in blood pressure Dose-dependent
Acepromazine	Phenothiazine Alpha-1 adrenergic blocker	Variable	Dose-dependent effect on heart rate Increased rate with high dose and vasodilation Decreased rate with sedative effect The heart rate may not change with the two mechanisms having a balancing effect on rate
Buprenorphine	Partial mu-agonist opioid	Decrease in rate or no change	Parasympathomimetic
Butorphanol	Mu-antagonist/ kappa-agonist opioid	Decrease in rate or no change	Parasympathomimetic
Dexmedetomidine	Alpha-2 adrenergic agonist Some alpha-1 adrenergic effects	Decrease in rate	Reflex response to vasoconstriction Sympatholytic
Diazepam	Benzodiazepine	Possible decrease if sedated, but possible increase if patient becomes dysphoric, usually very small change	Depends on response
Gabapentin	Antiepileptic	Uncommon increase in rate	
Hydromorphone	Mu-agonist opioid	Decrease in rate	Parasympathomimetic
Ketamine	Dissociative (N-mehyl-D-aspartate receptor inhibitor and others)	Increase in rate	CNS stimulation with increased sympathetic output
Methadone	Mu-agonist opioid	Decrease in rate	Parasympathomimetic
Midazolam	Benzodiazepine	Increase in rate when given IV if causes dysphoria or a little vasodilation; no change more usual	Reflex response to vasodilation

Can be used in combination with	Comments
Opioids	Sedation can be heavy, large volume required for IM injection
Usually opioids but many other drugs can be combined with it (benzodiazepines, alpha-2 adrenergic agonist, ketamine)	Be aware of effect on blood pressure as hypotension may develop May be beneficial to sedate dogs with degenerative valve disease if normal blood pressure
Acepromazine Alfaxalone Alpha-2 adrenergic agonist Benzodiazepines	Mostly analgesic effects; usually combined with sedative drug
Acepromazine Alfaxalone Alpha-2 adrenergic agonist Benzodiazepines	Commonly used alone with success and commonly combined with other drugs
Opioids (commonly with butorphanol and methadone) Benzodiazepines Alfaxalone Ketamine (not recommended due to potential for severe hypertension)	Bradycardia as common side effect but usually not severe Treatment for bradycardia-dependent on blood pressure Hypertension- do not give anticholinergics Hypotension- may give anticholinergics Atipamezole may be used to reverse sedative effects but be VERY CAUTIOUS as can cause severe hypotension, seizures (only give IM)
Opioids Dexmedetomidine Ketamine	Many prefer midazolam now over diazepam May cause dysphoria and increase anxiety in cats and dogs but occasionally works well May be use in very ill old cats and dogs with better effect Do not give IM-propylene glycol very irritating, not absorbed as well May be use in very ill old cats and dogs with better effect Do not give IM-propylene glycol very irritating, not absorbed as well
Do not combine with morphine	May be given at home to decrease anxiety and fear before travel and admission to clinic
Acepromazine Alfaxalone Alpha-2 adrenergic agonist Ketamine (not commonly)	Can cause emesis, dysphoria, hyperactivity and hyperthermia
Benzodiazepines (midazolam) or propofol for heavy sedation to general anesthesia	Ketamine may be dangerous to some cats with cardiomyopathy Caution if combined with alpha-2 adrenergic agonist because of hypertension
Acepromazine Alfaxalone Alpha-2 adrenergic agonist Ketamine	Vomiting uncommon compared to other opioids Good pain relief in cats with thromboembolism Because it can cause panting and dysphoria, if used in respiratory distress can make monitoring of breathing pattern difficult Likely best for pain relief rather than sedation also because panting can disrupt echocardiographic examinations or procedures
See diazepam	More commonly used than diazepam because can be given IM May cause hyperexcitability

Drug	Classification	Effect on heart rate	Mechanism for heart rate effect
Morphine	Mu-agonist opioid	Decrease in rate; increase in rate if histamine release results in vasodilation	Parasympathomimetic; histamine release resulting in vasodilation
Propofol	Enhances action of GABA	Increase in rate when given as bolus too fast	Reflex response to hypotension Avoid hypotension with slow administration
Tramadol	Mu agonist opioid and inhibitor of reuptake of serotonin and norepinephrine	Minimal	Minimal
Trazodone	Antianxiety, serotonin receptor antagonist, reuptake inhibitor of serotonin	High doses decrease in rate	Hypotension

Phenothiazines

Phenothiazines block alpha-1 adrenergic receptors. Acepromazine is the most common phenothiazine derivative used in veterinary medicine. This group of drugs can potentially cause peripheral vasodilation and a mild increase in heart rate as a compensatory mechanism. However, the sedative effect can reduce heart rate, and thus, counter the increase in heart rate. The individual animal's pre-sedation state and the drug dose contribute to the heart rate response. Acepromazine has the potential to reduce the risk of arrhythmias associated with adrenergic stimulation during anesthesia.

Alpha-2 agonists

Alpha-2 adrenergic receptors agonists are potent sedatives. Dexmedetomidine is one of the most commonly used in this category. The main cardiovascular effect of alpha-2 agonists is bradycardia, with atrioventricular block and sino-atrial block. The effects immediately after injection correspond to reflex bradycardia in response to systemic vasoconstriction. Later on, bradycardia is the result of a reduction in centrally-mediated sympathetic outflow.

Dexmedetomidine and other alpha-2 adrenergic receptor agonists may be combined with midazolam, propofol, and opioids; however, careful monitoring of heart rate and ideally blood pressure is recommended (Fig. 13.14). Bradycardia can be a serious side effect. Controversy and varied opinions on the treatment of this side effect exist. Clinical management of bradycardia after sedation with dexmedetomidine is highly dependent on the systemic blood pressure at that time. Initially, the bradycardia may be reflex induced because of an increase in blood pressure; however the sedative effects and bradycardia may result in a decreased cardiac output and hypotension. Therefore, one of the most important things that can be done in the cardiac patient is to measure the blood pressure in order to determine the correct therapy. For example, if hypotension coexists with bradycardia anticholinergics are indicated, but if hypertension is present they may not be. The effects of dexmedetomidine can be reversed in dogs with the alpha-2 adrenergic receptor blocker, atipamezole hydrochloride; however, anesthesiologists warn of the strong hypotensive effects of this drug.

Can be used in combination with	Comments
Acepromazine Alfaxalone Alpha-2 adrenergic agonist Ketamine (not commonly)	Can cause emesis Can induce histamine release when given intravenously If given IV, dilute and get slowly
Ketamine (side effects counteract) Opioids Benzodiazepines	Can only be given IV but can control depth of sedation Good choice for short duration procedures (e.g. pericardiocentesis) Pay attention to any respiratory depression with or without other drugs and have oxygen and airway equipment available; intubation recommended if CNS depression needed is deeper than conscious sedation
Trazodone	Be aware of Serotonin Syndrome which can result in anxiety, hyperthermia, tremors etc. when combined with other medications that can increase serotonin levels such as trazodone
Tramadol	High dose can cause sedation and hypotension Careful when using with NSAIDS (gastrointestinal bleeding) Phenothiazine can increase plasma concentrations of trazodone

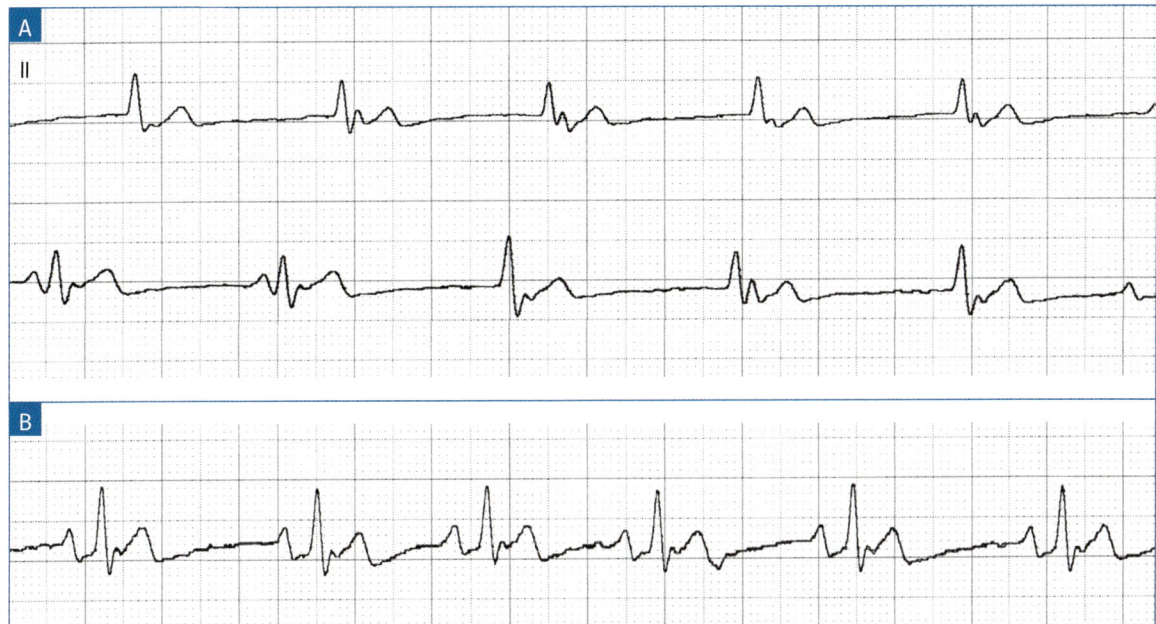

Figure 13.14. A monitoring lead II electrocardiogram - speed 50 mm/s - calibration 10 mm/1 mV - recorded from a cat that was sedated with dexmedetomidine and butorphanol.
A) A marked bradycardia is present (85 bpm). An escape rhythm from the atrioventricular junction is evident, but also positive P waves likely of sinus origin move before, within and after the QRS complex.
B) The cat was given propofol; however, the administration of this additional sedative was controversial. The heart rate did increase to 105 bpm. The cat recovered uneventfully. However, if the cat was hypotensive this could have caused problems. Determination of the blood pressure during the bradycardia is an important diagnostic evaluation when dogs and cats are sedated with alpha-2 adrenergic agonist, or with any drugs.

Opioids

Opioids can provide analgesia or sedation. The potency of these actions vary with the specific drug, route of administration and dosage. Opioids have a vagotonic effect that is dose-dependent and leads to a decrease in heart rate and, potentially, to prolongation of the PQ interval due to slowed atrioventricular conduction. Potent μ-agonist opioids (e.g. methadone, morphine, fentanyl) have the most profound bradycardic effect. This negative chronotropic effect depends on a central parasympathetic accentuation. Respiratory suppression is more common when opioids are used for sedation than when they are used for pain control. Although this class of drugs causes the cardiovascular effect of bradycardia with the associated increase in the QT interval, the other cardiac consequences are minimal. Opioids are commonly used in combination with other drugs. Importantly, the amount of sedation when drugs are combined also depends on the specific opioid used.

Parasympathetic system activation by opioids can serve as a trigger for vagally-associated atrial fibrillation in large breed dogs. An increase in vagal tone results in a shortening of the action potential duration (via the Ik_{Ach} current) in the atrial myocardium. However, because the distribution of cholinergic receptors is heterogeneous on the surface of the atria, the result is an amplification of dispersion of refractoriness within the myocaridum that promotes reentrant arrhythmias, such as atrial fibrillation. This type of atrial fibrillation has the potential to resolve once the opioids have been cleared from the body; however, it responds the majority of the time to treatment with intravenously administered lidocaine (2 mg/kg) as one or 2 doses when treated within a short time frame.

Dissociative anesthetics

Ketamine administration activates the sympathetic nervous system resulting in sinus tachycardia. In critically ill animals, adrenergic stimulation may not occur and fails to compensate the negative inotropic effects of the drug, resulting in a decrease in cardiac output and blood pressure. Ketamine increases myocardial oxygen consumption, which could increase the risk of arrhythmias in animals with preexisting cardiac disease. Theoretically, in cats with hypertrophic cardiomyopathy the higher heart rate would decrease diastolic coronary perfusion time which is detrimental to the increased muscle mass. Such a circumstance could result in decompensation.

Suggested readings

1. Allely MC, Ungar A. Interactions of beta-adrenoceptor antagonists and thyroid hormones in the control of heart rate in the dog. *Br J Pharmacol* 1985; 86:393-398.
2. Arnsdorf MF, Schreiner E, Gambetta M, et al. Electrophysiological changes in the canine atrium and ventricle during progressive hyperkalemia: electrocardiographical correlates and the in vivo validation of in vitro predictions. *Cardiovasc Res* 1977; 11:409-418.
3. Aroch I, Ohad DG, Baneth G. Paresis and unusual electrocardiographic signs in a severely hypomagnesemic, hypocalcemic lactating bitch. *J Small Anim Pract* 1998; 39:299-302.
4. Brunson CE, Abbud E, Osman K, et al. Osborn (J) wave appearance on the electrocardiogram in relation to potassium transfer and myocardial metabolism during hypothermia. *J Investig Med* 2005; 53:434-437.
5. Chah QT, Braly G, Bouzouita K, et al. Effects of hypokalemia on the various parts of the conduction system of the dog heart in situ. *Naunyn Schmiedebergs Arch Pharmacol* 1982; 319:178-183.
6. Chiba S, Kubota K, Hashimoto K, et al. Effect of hyperpotassemia on AV conduction in dog heart in situ. *Tohoku J Exp Med* 1972; 107:197-198.
7. Copland VS, Baskins SC, Patz JD. Cardiovascular and pulmonary effects of atropine reversal of oxymorphone-induced bradycardia in dogs. *Vet Surg* 1992; 21:414-417.
8. El Kassimi FA, Al-Mashhadani S, Abdullah AK, et al. Adult respiratory distress syndrome and disseminated intravascular coagulation complicating heart stroke. *Chest* 1986; 90:571-574.
9. El Shahawy M, Stefadouros MA, Carr AA, et al. Direct effect of thyroid hormone on intracardiac conduction in acute and chronic hyperthyroid animals. *Cardiovasc Res* 1975; 9:524-531.
10. Fox PR, Peterson ME, Broussard JD. Electrocardiographic and radiographic changes in cats with hyperthyroidism: comparison of populations evaluated during 1992-1993 vs. 1979-1982. *J Am Anim Hosp Assoc* 1999; 35:27-31.
11. Foster PR, Elharrar V, Zipes DP. Accelerated ventricular escapes induced in the intact dog by barium, strontium and calcium. *J Pharmacol Exp Ther* 1977; 200:373-383.
12. Freeman KP, Monlux AW, Heald D, et al. Bradycardia associated with meningioma in a dog. *J Am Vet Med Assoc* 1985; 187:838-839.
13. Gidlewski J, Petrie JP. Pericardiocentesis and principles of echocardiographic imaging in the patient with cardiac neoplasia. *Clin Tech Small Anim Pract* 2003;18:131-134.
14. Goel BG, Hanson CS, Han J. A-V conduction in hyper- and hypothyroid dogs. *Am Heart J* 1972; 83:504-511.
15. Goldberg LI. Effects of hypothermia on contractility of the intact dog heart. *Am J Physiol* 1958; 194:92-98.
16. Hanton G, Yvon A, Provost JP, et al. Quantitative relationship between plasma potassium levels and QT interval in beagle dogs. *Lab Anim* 2007; 41:204-217.
17. Hariman RJ, Chen CM. Effects of hyperkalemia on sinus nodal function in dogs: sino-ventricular conduction. *Cardiovasc Res* 1983; 17:509-517.
18. Hashimoto K, Suzuki Y, Chiba S. Influence of calcium and magnesium ions on the sino-atrial node pacemaker activity of the canine heart. *Tohoku J Exp Med* 1974; 113:187-196.
19. Hirayama Y, Saitoh H, Atarashi H, et al. Electrical and mechanical alternans in canine myocardium in vivo. Dependence on intracellular calcium cycling. *Circulation* 1993; 88:2894-2902.
20. Homma S, Gillam LD, Weyman AE. Echocardiographic observations in survivors of acute electrical injury. *Chest* 1990; 97:103-105.
21. Keyes ML, Rush JE, Rand W, et al. Ventricular arrhythmias in dogs with splenic masses. *J Vet Emer Crit Care* 1993; 3:33-38.
22. Kienle RD, Bruyette D, Pion PD. Effects of thyroid hormone and thyroid dysfunction on the cardiovascular system. *Vet Clin North Am Small Anim Pract* 1994; 24:495-507.
23. King JM, Roth L, Haschek WM. Myocardial necrosis secondary to neural lesions in domestic animal. *J Am Vet Med Assoc* 1982; 15:144-148.
24. Maaravi Y, Weiss AT. The effect of prolonged hypothermia on cardiac function in a young patient with accidental hypothermia. *Chest* 1990; 98:1019-1020.
25. MacDonald KA, Cagney O, Magne ML. Echocardiographic and clinicopathologic characterization of pericardial effusion in dogs: 107 cases (1985-2006). *J Am Vet Med Assoc* 2009; 235:1456-1461.
26. Makenzie G, Barnhart M, Kennedy S, et al. A retrospective study of factors influencing survival surgery for gastric dilatation volvulus syndrome in 306 dogs. *J Am Anim Hosp Assoc* 2010; 46:97-102.
27. Malik R, Zunino P, Hunt GB. Complete heart block associated with lupus in a dog. *Aust Vet J* 2003; 81:398-401.
28. Mebazaa A. Are platelets a "forgotten" source of sepsis-induced myocardial depressing factor(s)?. *Critical Care* 2008; 12:110-111.
29. Mendes GM, Selmi AL. Use of a combination of propofol and fentanyl, alfentanyl or sufentanyl for total intravenous anesthesia in cats. *J Am Vet Med Assoc* 2003; 223:1608-1613.
30. Miller TL, Schwartz DS, Nakayama T, et al. Effects of acute gastric distention and recovery on tendency for ventricular arrhythmia in dogs. *J Vet Intern Med* 2000; 14:436-444.
31. Moïse NS, Pariaut R, Gelzer AR, et al. Cardioversion with lidocaine of vagally associated atrial fibrillation in two dogs. *J Vet Cardiol* 2005; 7:143-148.
32. Muir WW. Gastric dilatation-volvulus in the dog, with emphasis on cardiac arrhythmias. *J Am Vet Med Assoc* 1982; 180:739-742.
33. Muir WW. Thiobarbiturate-induced dysrhythmias: the role of heart rate and autonomic imbalance. *Am J Vet Res* 1977; 38:1377-1381.

34. Murrell JC, Hellebrekers LJ. Medetomidine and dexmedetomidine: a review of cardiovascular effects and antinociceptive properties in the dog. *Vet Anaesth Analg* 2005; 32:117-127.
35. Murrell JC, Wesselink Van Notten R, Hellebrekers LJ. Clinical investigation of remifentanyl and propofol for the total intravenous anaesthesia of dog. *Vet Rec* 2005; 156:804-808.
36. Nakayama T, Nakayama H, Miyamoto M, et al. Hemodynamic and electrocardiographic effects of magnesium sulfate in healthy dogs. *J Vet Intern Med* 1999; 13:485-490.
37. Norman BC, Côté E, Barrett KA. Wide-complex tachycardia associated with severe hyperkalemia in three cats. *J Feline Med Surg* 2006; 8:372-378.
38. Orton EC, Muir WW. Isovolumic indices and humoral cardioactive substance assay during clinical and experimentally induced gastric dilatation-volvulus in dogs. *Am J Vet Res* 1983; 44:1516-1520.
39. Pasławska U, Noszczyk-Nowak A, Kungl K, et al. Thyroid hormones concentrations and ECG picture in the dog. *Pol J Vet Sci* 2006; 9:253-257.
40. Pariaut R, Moïse NS, Koetje BD, et al. Lidocaine converts acute vagally associated atrial fibrillation to sinus rhythm in German Shepherd dogs with inherited arrhythmias. *J Vet Intern Med* 2008; 22:1274-1282.
41. Pariaut R, Moïse NS, Koetje BD, et al. Evaluation of atrial fibrillation induced during anesthesia with fentanyl and pentobarbital in German Shepherd dogs with inherited arrhythmias. *Am J Vet Res* 2008; 69:1434-1445.
42. Wellstein A, Pitschner HF. Complex dose-response curves of atropine in man explained by different functions of M1- and M2- cholinoreceptors. *Naunyn Schmiedebergs Arch Pharmacol* 1988; 338:19-27.
43. Racker DK. Sinoventricular transmission in 10 mM K^+ by canine atrioventricular nodal inputs: superior atrionodal bundle and proximal atrioventricular bundle. *Circulation* 1991; 83:1738-1753.
44. Rishniw M, Tobias AH, Stinker BK, et al. Characterization of chronotropic and dysrhythmogenic effects of atropine in dogs with bradycardia. *Am J Vet Res* 1996; 57:337-341.
45. Rishniw M, Kittleson MD, Jaffe RS, et al. Characterization of parasympatholytic chronotropic responses following intravenous administration of atropine to clinically normal dogs. *Am J Vet Res* 1999; 60:1000-1003.
46. Rush JE, Hamlin RL. Effects of graded pleural effusion on QRS in the dog. *Am J Vet Res* 1985; 46:1887-1891.
47. Seliskar A, Nemec A, Roskar A, et al. Total intravenous anaesthesia with propofol or propofol/ketamine in spontaneously breathing dogs premedicated with medetomidine. *Vet Rec* 2007; 160:85-91.
48. Uilenreef JJ, Murrell JC, McKusick BC, et al. Dexmedetomidine continuous rate infusion during isoflurane anaesthesia in canine surgical patients. *Vet Anaesth Analg* 2008; 35:1-12.
49. Wallis DE, Littman WJ, Scanlon PJ, et al. The effects of elevated intracranial pressure on the canine electrocardiogram. *J Electrocardiol* 1987; 20:154-161.

CHAPTER 14

Electrocardiography and pacing

Basic components of the pacemaker

Permanent pacing is performed via the implantation of a lead positioned in contact with the endocardium or the epicardium. The lead is connected to a pulse generator frequently implanted in a subcutaneous pocket of the neck, behind the shoulder or within the muscle layers of the abdominal wall for epicardial pacemakers implanted surgically (Fig. 14.1).

The pulse generator is made of two components: an electronic circuit and a power source of lithium-based electrochemical batteries. These components are sealed inside a hermetic titanium casing. The electronic circuit controls three main functions: the pacing intervals, the electrical pulse amplitude and the function of sensing the intrinsic cardiac rhythms. Modern devices are equipped with numerous other features that include complex electronic components for programming and telemetry, filtering and protection of the devices against electrical interference, storage of events and the ability to adjust the pacing rate to the activity level during exercise (*rate response*). The pulse generator also contains an electromagnet that allows the pacemaker to function temporarily in an asynchronous mode when a magnet is placed in close proximity.

The generator is the source of electrical stimuli that are transmitted to the heart via the pacing lead, which is composed of four basic elements: the electrode, the conductor, the insulator and the connector. There are two types of electrodes: bipolar or unipolar (monopolar) (Fig. 14.1). The unipolar electrode is characterized by a cathode positioned at the lead tip and an anode formed by the surface of the generator. The electrical current for unipolar pacing is, therefore, completed over a large

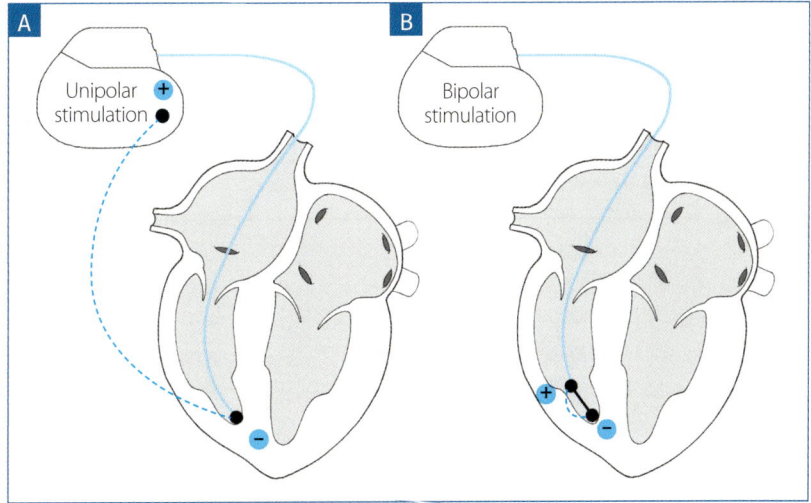

Figure 14.1. Unipolar and bipolar pacing. A) With unipolar pacing the pulse generator serves as the anode and the cathode is located at the tip of the pacing lead. The electrical current travels between the generator and the lead tip within the body. B) With bipolar pacing the anode and cathode are located at the tip of the pacing lead. The electric circuit is confined to the right ventricle.

circuit. In contrast, the electrical current associated with bipolar pacing travels over a short distance because both the cathode and anode electrodes are close to the tip of the lead. Because of the greater distance between the poles of the circuit, the unipolar systems are more subject to interference from extracardiac electrical potentials than the bipolar systems, where the electrical circuit is confined within a cardiac chamber.

Leads are described as epicardial or endocardial (also called *transvenous*) based on their placement on the surface of the heart or inside a cardiac chamber via a transvenous approach. Endocardial leads can be further classified as active or passive depending on the modality of fixation to the cardiac chamber. Active fixation leads have a helix that screws directly into the myocardium (Fig. 14.2A). Passive fixation leads have a tip that is designed to act as an anchor and secure it to the trabeculae of the cardiac chambers (Fig. 14.2B). The lead conductor is made of an alloy of platinum and iridium and joins the electrode to the proximal connector. A layer of insulation, made of silicone, polyurethane or both, prevents the dispersion of the current as it travels along the lead. To complete the circuit, the proximal portion of the lead is formed by a connector, which is attached to the generator.

Pacing modes

Pacing modes are described by an international four letter code system:
- the first letter indicates the paced chamber (A: atrium; V: ventricle; D: both);
- the second letter indicates the chamber in which the intrinsic myocardial potential is detected (A: atrium; V: ventricle; D: both; O: none);
- the third letter indicates the function modality (I: inhibited; T: trigger; D: double functioning modality ; O: no function performed);
- the fourth letter indicates the programmability characteristics (P: simple programmability; M: multiple programmability; C: telemetry communication; R: rate modulation; O: no programmability).

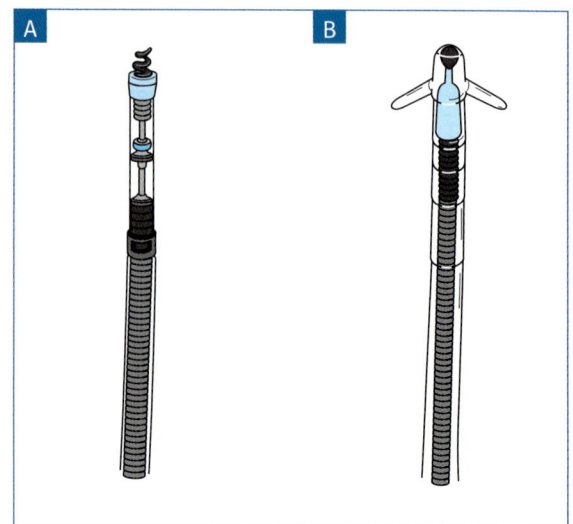

Figure 14.2. Two types of endocardial lead fixation. A) Active fixation lead. B) Passive fixation lead.

On the electrocardiogram, the stimulus artifact generated during unipolar pacing appears as a rapid and large deflection (*spike*) (Fig. 14.3A) when compared to bipolar pacing (Fig. 14.3B). Depending on the filters used during the recording of the electrocardiogram the pacing spikes during bipolar pacing may be difficult to identify. After each *spike* an atrial or ventricular capture should be present; in other words, a P wave or a QRS complex with variable duration and morphology depending on the site of the lead placement.

Single-chamber pacing

This pacing mode corresponds to the implantation of a single lead within one chamber, atrium or ventricle. The lead is used to pace (stimulate the myocardium) and sense the underlying rhythm (detect the intrinsic rhythm). Most pacemakers are programmed so that when a spontaneous beat is detected, pacing from the pacemaker is inhibited (letter code I). The most commonly used single-chamber pacing modes include:
- AAI pacing,
- VVI pacing,
- VVIR pacing, and
- VDD pacing.

Figure 14.3. A) Ventricular pacing in unipolar mode (Dog, Great Dane, male, 7 years old. Lead II - speed 50 mm/s - calibration 10 mm/1 mV). Unipolar pacing results in large amplitude spikes (arrows) in from of each ventricular paced beat (QRS complexes) on the surface electrocardiogram.
B) Ventricular pacing in bipolar mode (Dog, Kurzhaar, male, 8 years old. Lead II - speed 50 mm/s - calibration 5 mm/1 mV. Bipolar pacing results in small amplitude spikes (arrows) followed by ventricular capture (QRS complexes). On occasion, the spikes from bipolar pacing are not visible on the electrocardiogram if filters used to remove artifacts are turned on.

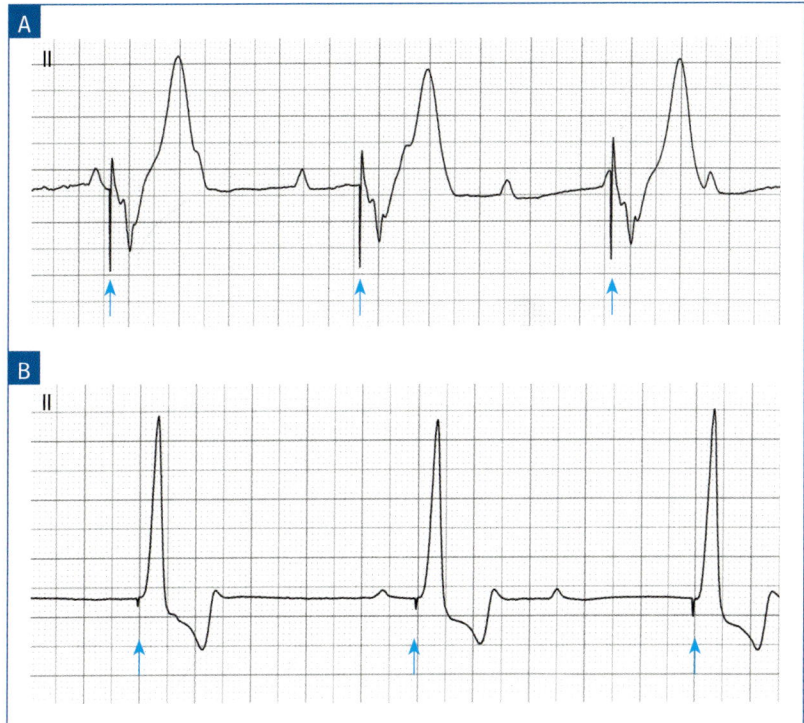

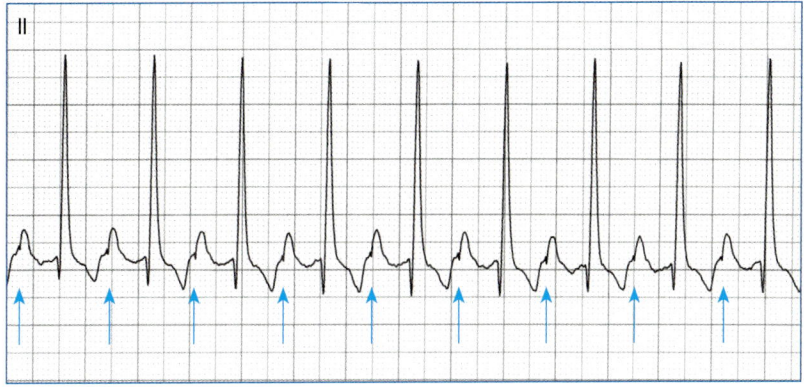

Figure 14.4. Atrial pacing in AAI mode (Dog, Dachshund, male, 8 years old. Lead II - speed 50 mm/s - calibration 10 mm/1 mV).
Bipolar pacing with a single-chamber pacemaker in AAI mode. Note the low amplitude spikes (arrows) characteristic of bipolar stimulation followed by atrial capture (P wave). The programmed atrial rate is 180 to perform an atrial pacing threshold and each stimulated P wave is followed by a sensed QRS complex with a PQ interval of 140 ms.

AAI pacing allows for the detection (*sensing*) and stimulation (*pacing*) of the atrial chamber only, through an electrode usually positioned in the right atrial appendage. Atrial pacing occurs in the absence of an intrinsic atrial rhythm, or when the sensed atrial rate is below the programmed lower rate limit (Fig. 14.4). This type of programmability is indicated for animals with sinus node dysfunction (sick sinus syndrome) that do not have concurrent atrioventricular conduction abnormalities.

VVI pacing allows for detection and stimulation of the ventricular myocardium only. For VVI pacing the electrode is most commonly placed in the apex of the right ventricle. The ventricular pacing only occurs with the absence of an intrinsic ventricular rhythm, or when the sensed ventricular rate is below the programmed lower rate limit (Fig. 14.5). This pacing modality is the most commonly used in dogs with atrioventricular conduction abnormalities.

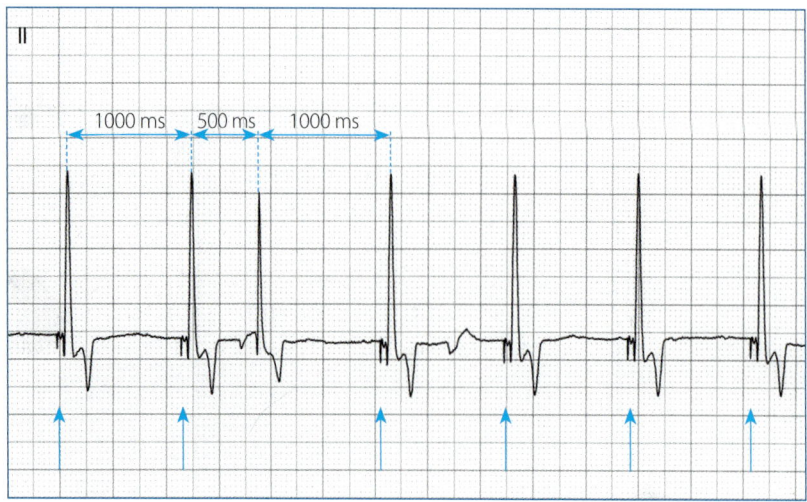

Figure 14.5. Ventricular pacing in VVI mode (Dog, Border Collie, male, 4 years old. Lead II - speed 25 mm/s - calibration 10 mm/1 mV).
Bipolar pacing with a single-chamber pacemaker rhythm in VVI mode. Note the low amplitude spikes (arrows) characteristic of bipolar stimulation followed by ventricular capture (QRS complex). The programmed ventricular rate is 60 bpm (cycle length of 1000 ms). The third beat is an atrial ectopic beat that occurs 500 ms after the last paced beat. This beat is appropriately sensed by the pacemaker and inhibits pacing for a period of 1000 ms until pacing resumes at the programmed rate.

Hysteresis is another programmable function with single-chamber pacing. It is designed to favor intrinsic beats over paced beats. It is achieved by slightly delaying the lower pacing rate after every sensed intrinsic beat in order to give an opportunity (a "second chance") for another intrinsic beat. Whenever hysteresis is turned on, the interval between a sensed beat and a paced beat is longer than the interval between two paced beats on the electrocardiogram (Fig. 14.6). Hysteresis is useful in animals with sinus node dysfunction or second-degree atrioventricular block, as it decreases the number of "non-physiological" paced beats whenever an underlying sinus rhythm with a rate above the programmed hysteresis rate but below the lower pacing rate is present.

VDD pacing involves the placement of a single lead designed with two electrodes. The distal electrode is positioned at the apex of the right ventricle. The second electrode is located more proximally on the lead, such that it "floats" within the right atrial chamber. The electrode in the ventricle can pace and sense. The floating electrode within in the right atrium only senses atrial events. The sensed atrial depolarizations (P waves) trigger ventricular pacing after a programmed atrioventricular interval. It is theoretically an advantage over VVI pacing because it preserves the physiological sequence of contraction of the cardiac chambers (*atrioventricular synchrony*). With the VDD mode it is possible to select a upper racking rate (upper limit of spontaneous atrial

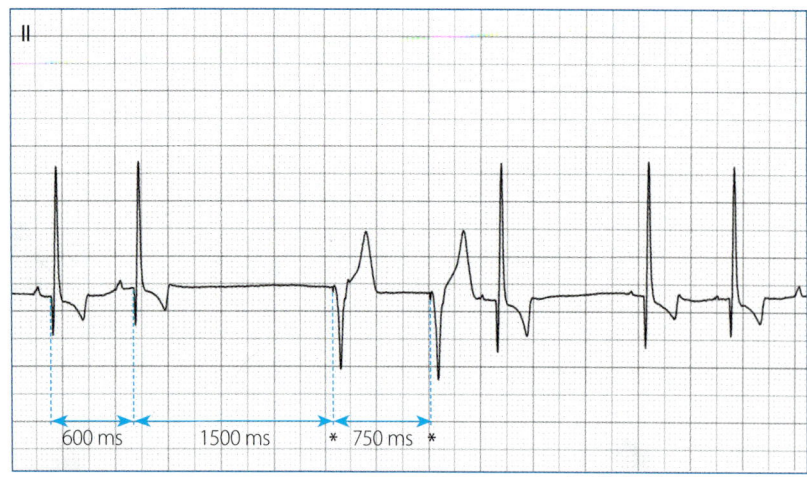

Figure 14.6. Ventricular pacing in VVI mode with hysteresis function activated (Dog, mixed breed, male, 10 years. Lead II - speed 25 mm/s - calibration 10 mm/1 mV).
Bipolar pacing in VVI mode with a programmed ventricular rate of 80 bpm (cycle length of 750 ms) and hysteresis set at 40 bpm (cycle length of 1500 ms). The second sinus beat is appropriately sensed and followed by a pause of 1500 ms, which is interrupted by a paced beat (*) because no intrinsic beat is detected during that period of time. Pacing (*) resumes at a rate of 80 bpm until another intrinsic beat is sensed.

depolarizations that are "followed" and permitted to trigger a ventricular paced beat). Depending on the relationship of the programmed rate and atrioventricular interval pacing can result in a 2:1 conduction ratio or higher (Fig. 14.7). VDD pacing is used in dogs with abnormalities of the atrioventricular conduction system but with normal sinus node activity.

With single-chamber pacing the rate can be altered in response to exercise to optimize cardiac output. With VDD pacing mode it is not necessary to program a ventricular pacing rate that adapts to exercise as long as the sinus node is chronotropically competent. The programmability of the heart rate in response to exercise is identified with the letter R added to the three letter codes AAI, VVI (AAIR, VVIR). Several types of activity sensors are used to detect the onset and offset of exercise. Sensors include motion and ventilation sensors, but also sensors of QT interval, temperature, blood pH and venous oxygen level.

Dual-chamber pacing

In the *DDD pacing* mode, one lead is placed in the right atrial appendage to detect the intrinsic electrical activity and stimulate the atrial myocardium, and a second lead is placed in the apex of the right ventricle to detect the intrinsic electrical activity and stimulate the ventricle. Thus, DDD pacing permits both sensing and pacing of the atrium and ventricle. The third letter D indicates that if an intrinsic rhythm is detected in either the atrium or the ventricle, pacing is inhibited in that location, but if an intrinsic rhythm is detected in the atrium, it will trigger an atrioventricular delay followed by ventricular pacing.

Advanced programming knowledge is required for this type of pacing in order to have proper tracking of spontaneous atrial depolarizations and to prevent tracking during excessively high atrial rates that may occur with supraventricular tachycardias (Fig. 14.8). DDD pacing is used in dogs with sinus node dysfunction and atrioventricular conduction abnormalities, particularly in young dogs with hearts large enough to accommodate two leads.

Biventricular pacing

This modality allows simultaneous stimulation of both ventricles: the right by implanting an apical endocardial electrode, and the left ventricle via an epicardial electrode placed in a lateral coronary vein (a tributary of the great cardiac vein). The use of this modality is restricted to large dogs with left bundle branch block and interventricular dyssynchrony or dogs with drug-resistant rapid ventricular response rates during atrial fibrillation that necessitated radiofrequency ablation of the atrioventricular node.

The main goal of biventricular pacing is to improve cardiac output by decreasing the delay between right and left ventricular chamber contraction that exists in the presence of a left bundle branch block. The left ventricular stimulation is programmed to start soon after right ventricular pacing, which appears on the surface electrocardiogram as a QRS complex of shorter duration compared to the baseline QRS complex (Fig. 14.9).

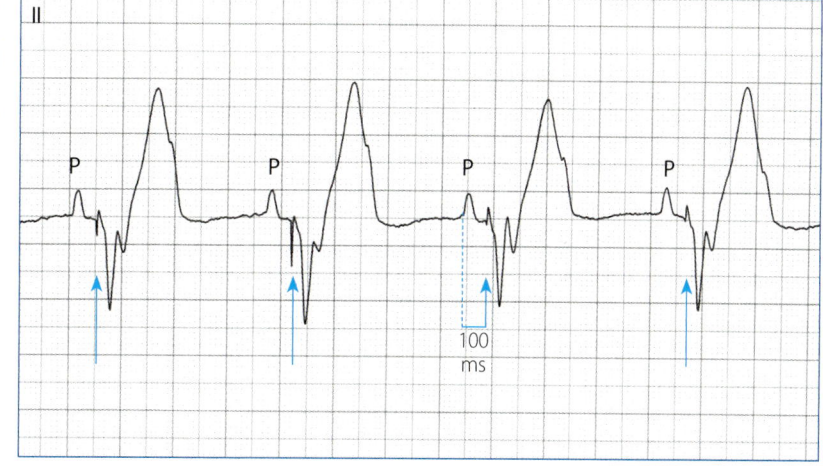

Figure 14.7. Ventricular pacing in VDD mode (Dog, Dogue de Bordeaux, male, 6 years old. Lead II - speed 50 mm/s - calibration 10 mm/1 mV). An intrinsic atrial rhythm (P waves) is sensed and followed by the *spikes* (arrows) and QRS complexes of paced beats. The programmed atrioventricular interval (AVI), which corresponds to the PQ interval, is 100 ms.

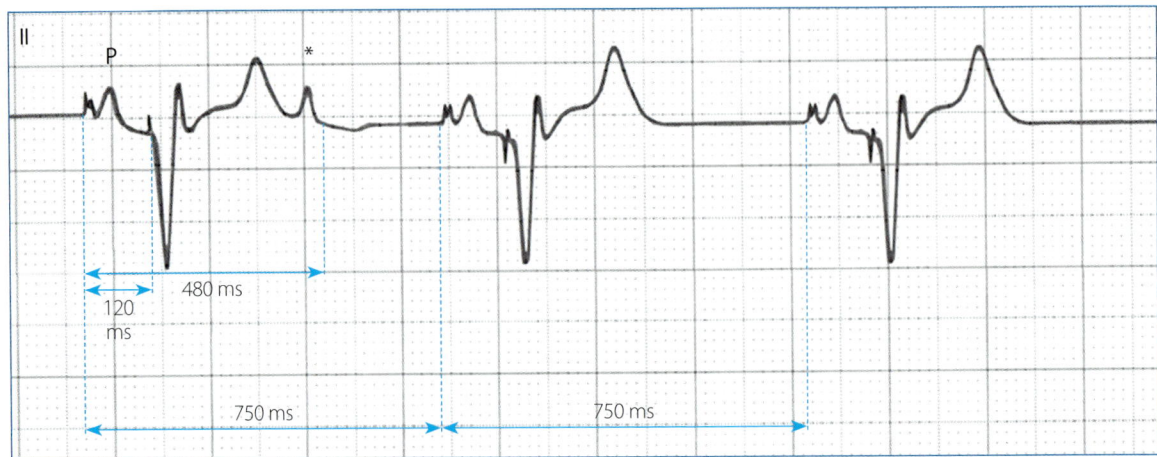

Figure 14.8. Atrial and ventricular pacing in DDD mode (Dog, Rottweiler, female, 5 years. Lead II - speed 50 mm/s - calibration 10 mm/1 mV). The paced AV interval is set at 120 ms; the atrial pacing rate is set at 750 ms, the total atrial refractory period is programmed at 480 ms. The first beat corresponds to atrial followed by ventricular pacing with a AV interval of 120 ms. The next P wave (*) is a spontaneous impulse likely originating from the dog's sinus node. It is sensed during the programmed total atrial refractory period, and therefore does not reset the pacing cycle, as this is the rule for any sensed event during the refractory period. In the absence of another spontaneous beat following the end of total atrial refractory period, atrial pacing resumes at a rate of 80 bpm (750 ms) followed by ventricular paced complexes.

Pacemaker malfunction

Pacemaker malfunction occurs because of errors during the implantation process, defective equipment or improper programming. Reported complications associated with the implantation technique and the equipment include lead dislodgement, increased pacing threshold secondary to exit block, lead perforation of the right atrium or ventricle, lead fracture or insulation break, and pulse generator battery depletion. Complications associated with pacemaker programming include undersensing and oversensing of the underlying cardiac rhythm and non-cardiac electrical interference.

The electrocardiographic signs of pacemaker malfunction can be divided into four categories:
- absence of pacing spikes and capture,
- presence of pacing spikes and failure to capture,
- presence of pacing spikes with detection (oversensing or undersensing) problems, and
- presence of pacing spikes and capture at a rate that markedly exceeds the programmed pacing rate (*runaway phenomenon*).

Absence of pacing spikes and capture

The absence of spikes and the corresponding atrial or ventricular capture (Fig. 14.10) may be due to:
- pulse generator component malfunction,
- battery depletion,
- loose connection between the pulse generator and the pacing lead,
- lead fracture, and
- detection (oversensing) of extracardiac myopotentials (in particular with unipolar pacing), or electromagnetic interference.

It is important to remember that the filters used to limit artifacts during the recording of an electrocardiogram can also eliminate the low amplitude pacing stimuli associated with bipolar pacing. It is therefore recommended to evaluate the electrocardiogram without excessive filtering whenever pacing spikes are not visible in order to confirm their absence.

Presence of spikes and failure to capture

Failure to capture (*loss of capture*) refers to the absence of an atrial or ventricular depolarization (P wave or QRS

Figure 14.9. Resynchronization with biventricular pacing (Dog, Napolitan Mastiff, male, 4 years old. Lead II - speed 50 mm/s - calibration 5 mm/1 mV).
A) Single right ventricular chamber pacing. The QRS complex has a duration of 117 ms.
B) Single left ventricular chamber pacing. The QRS complex has a duration of 125 ms.
C) Biventricular pacing. The QRS complex has a duration of 100 ms.

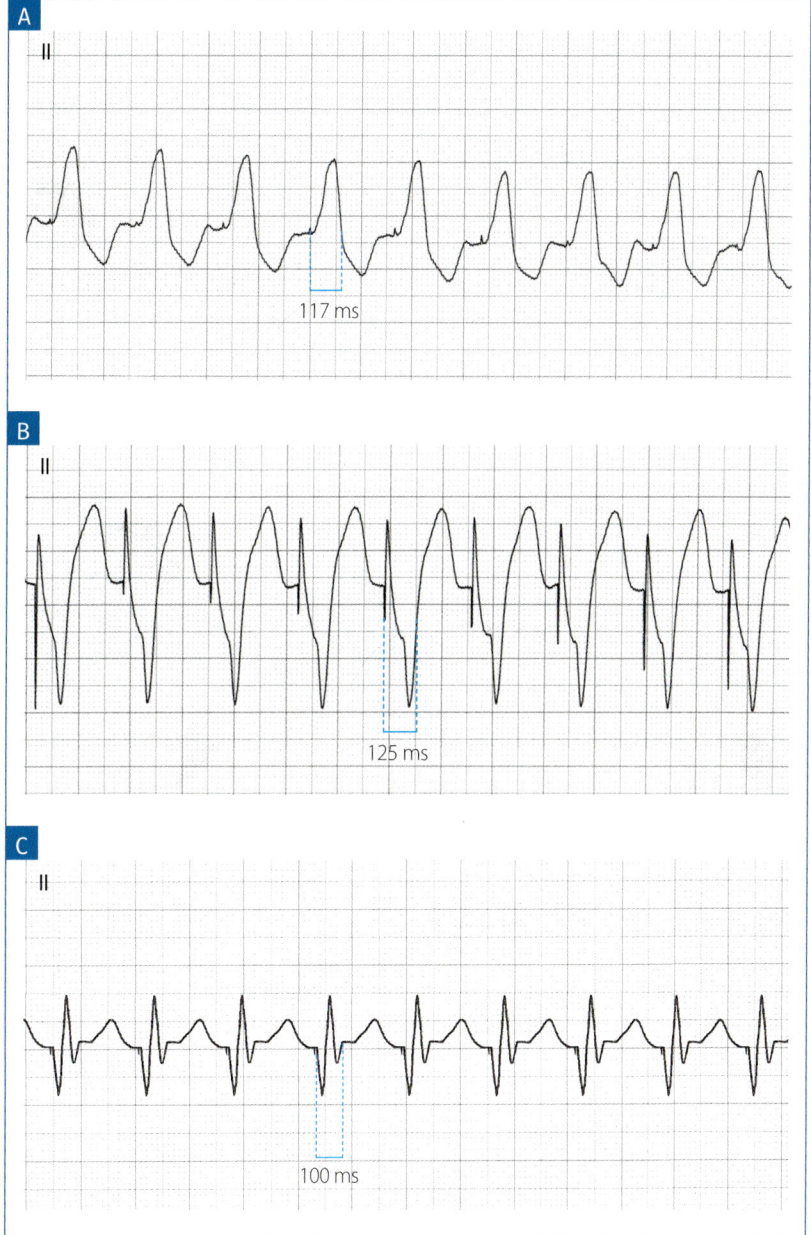

complex after a pacing spike on the electrocardiogram) in response to an electrical impulse above pacing threshold from the pulse generator. Failure to capture can result from:

- pacing lead fracture or insulation defect. Lead fracture results in a rise in lead impedance, and an insulation defect causes a drop in lead impedance;

- a rise in pacing threshold associated with tissue reaction at the electrode-endocardium interface. An acute inflammatory response around the lead tip can develop after implantation and trigger an increase in pacing threshold within the first 6-8 weeks after implantation. Nowadays, this complication is rare because a small amount of steroids (*steroid eluting lead*)

Chapter 14. Electrocardiography and pacing

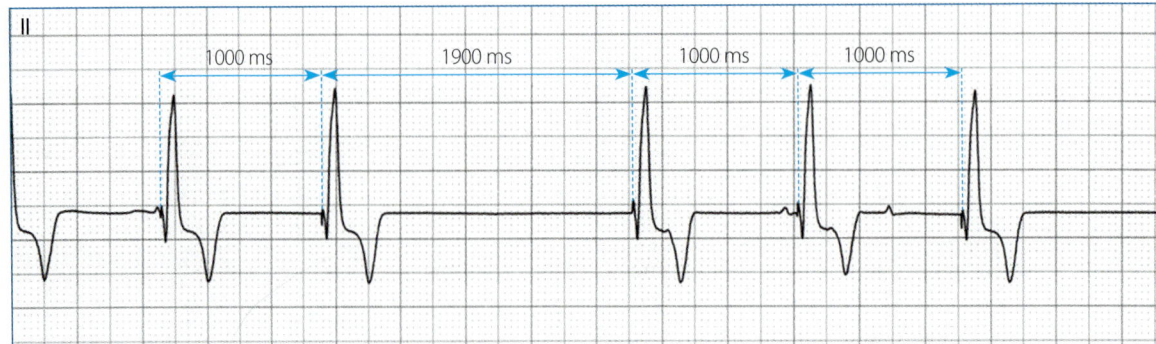

Figure 14.10. Pacemaker malfunction characterized by the absence of spikes and ventricular capture in a dog with single chamber ventricular pacing (Dog, German Shepherd, female, 6 years. Lead II - speed 25 mm/s - calibration 5 mm/1 mV). Ventricular bipolar pacing in VVI mode with a pacing rate of 60 bpm (cycle length of 1000 ms). The first two QRS complexes are preceded by a pacing spike at a rate of 60 bpm, followed by a 1900 ms pause and the absence of pacing spikes. After the pause, pacing resumes at the programmed rate. The most common causes of intermittent absence of pacing spikes and ventricular capture include oversensing of extra-cardiac myopotentials, electromagnetic interference, end-of-life of the pulse generator battery or component malfunction, a loose connection at the junction between the generator and the lead, and partial lead fracture.

is embedded in the tip of most pacing leads to limit the inflammatory response post-implantation. Elevation of the pacing threshold beyond the initial maturation phase can be caused by electrolyte (hyperkalemia) and acid-base (acidosis) disturbances, the use of class 1C anti-arrhythmic drugs and progressive myocardial fibrosis secondary to cardiomyopathies;
- electrode dislodgement during the first month after implantation, or microdislodgement, when the displacement of the lead is not visible on radiographs;
- cardiac perforation by the tip of the pacing lead.

Pacing in the absence of capture is diagnosed on the electrocardiogram by the presence of pacing spikes not followed by a P wave or a QRS complex (Fig. 14.11).

Presence of spikes with under- or oversensing

Inappropriate detection of intrinsic beats is called *undersensing*, and erroneous recognition of cardiac or extracardiac myopotentials is called *oversensing*.

Undersensing

Undersensing corresponds to a failure to recognize ("sense") the intrinsic cardiac electrical events (P waves or QRS complexes) by the pacemaker, which delivers pacing stimuli irrespective of the underlying rhythm. Undersensing is usually caused by inadequate programming of the sensitivity (too low sensitivity), low amplitude myocardial impulses secondary to structural cardiac disease below the sensitivity threshold of the pacemaker, pacing lead dislodgment; lead fracture or insulation break, and finally, asynchronous pacing mode (VOO).

On the electrocardiogram, paced beats compete with the underlying rhythm, and behave like a parasystolic focus (Fig. 14.12).

Oversensing

Oversensing corresponds to the detection of cardiac or extracardiac events that typically should not be recognized ("*sensed*") and subsequently inhibit pacing. Electrical signals identified incorrectly as cardiac potentials include electromagnetic interference, skeletal myopotentials, or electrical activity caused by a lead fracture or insulation break. Oversensing of the P waves, QRS complexes and T waves can occur if the sensitivity (sensitivity too high) or refractory period of the pacemaker is inadequately programmed.

On the electrocardiogram, oversensing is characterized by the absence of pacing activity at times when pacing stimuli should be delivered based on the

Pacemaker malfunction | 321

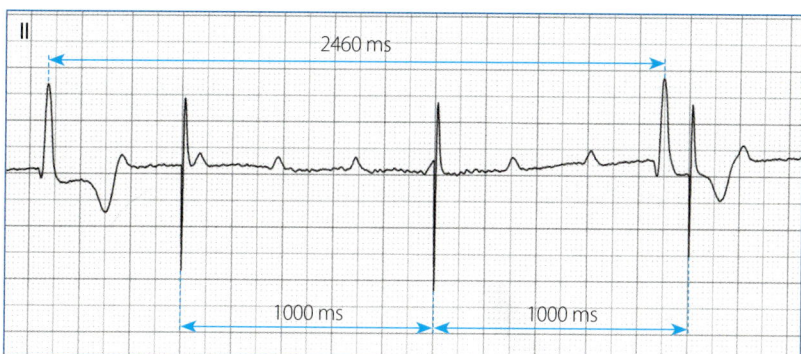

Figure 14.11. Pacemaker malfunction characterized by the presence of spikes and no capture (Dog, English Bulldog, male, 8 years old. Lead II - speed 50 mm/s - calibration 10 mm/1 mV).
Unipolar ventricular pacing in VVI mode with a programmed ventricular rate of 60 bpm (cycle length of 1000 ms). The underlying rhythm is a third-degree atrioventricular block with an escape rhythm (ventricular rate 26 bpm; cycle length of 2460 ms). The spikes are visible (arrows) with regular cycle length (1000 ms) and no capture. The third pacing spikes, which occurs between the QRS complex and the T wave of a ventricular escape beat shows that the failure to capture is associated with a failure to appropriately sense the intrinsic rhythm. Common causes of pacing failure in the presence of pacing spikes include lead dislodgement, perforation of the right ventricle by the pacing lead, pacing threshold exceeding programmed pulse amplitude, and lead fracture or insulation defect.

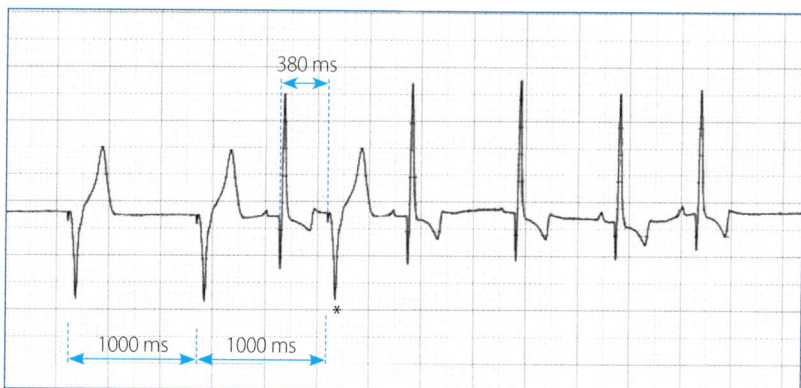

Figure 14.12. Pacemaker malfunction with undersensing (Dog, mixed breed, male, 10 years. Lead II - speed 25 mm/s - calibration 10 mm/1 mV).
Bipolar pacing in VVI mode with a pacing rate programmed at 60 bpm (cycle length of 1000 ms). The first two beats are ventricular paced beats with a cycle length of 1000 ms. Then a sinus beat occurs followed by another paced ventricular beat (*) just 380 ms later, indicating that the spontaneous sinus beat was undersensed. A properly programmed pacemaker would have "recognized" the sinus QRS complex and delayed ventricular pacing by 1000 ms. The subsequent four sinus beats are adequately sensed as indicated by the absence of paced complexes.

programmed pacing rate (Fig. 14.13). It reflects the inhibition of pacing activity by oversensed electrical signals. In some pacemaker models, sensing of rapid repetitive events over a short period of time can activate noise reversion, a pacemaker algorithm that switches the pacing mode to asynchronous (for example VOO if the pacemaker was programmed in the VVI mode). Noise reversion is a safety feature designed to maintain pacing activity whenever electrical interference affects the sensing function of the pacemaker. Newer pacemaker models are better protected against environmental electromagnetic interference (for example, magnetic resonance imaging-safe pulse generators are now available) and do not include the noise reversion algorithm.

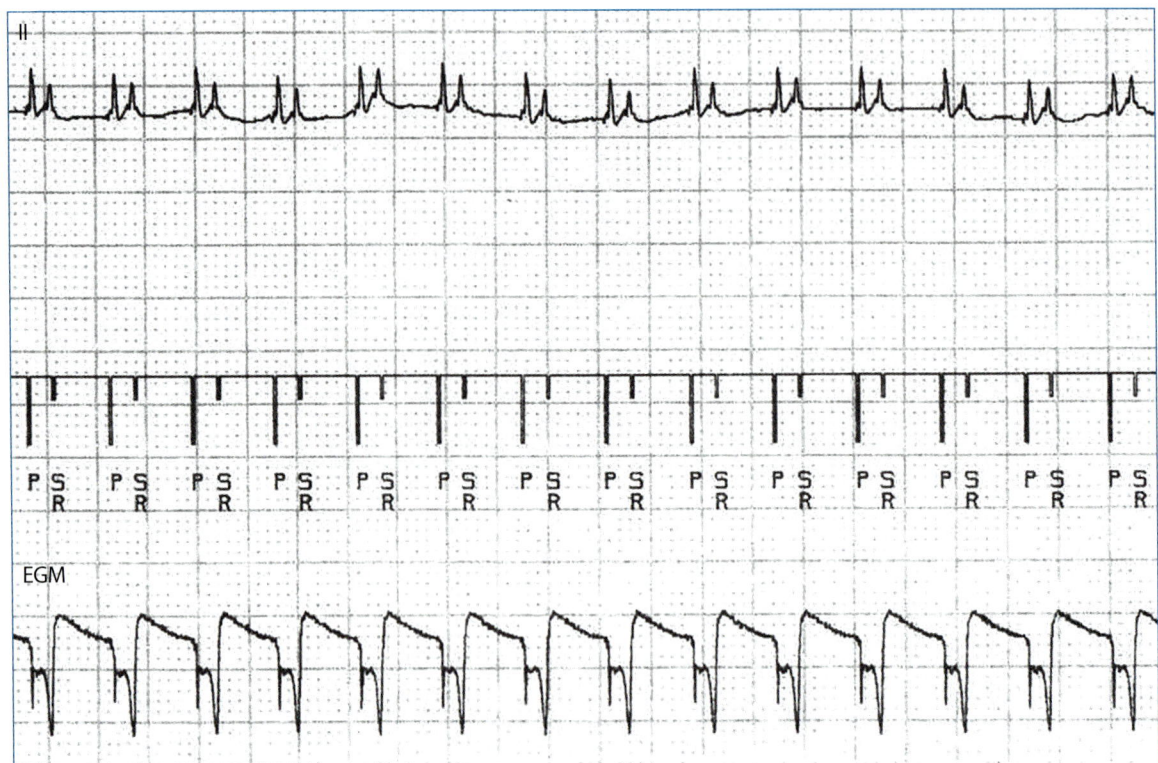

Figure 14.13. Pacemaker malfunction with T-wave oversensing (Lead II - speed 25 mm/s - calibration 10 mm/ 1mV). Programming pacemaker strip of a dog with sinus node dysfunction. A ventricular pacing lead was positioned in the right ventricle. Small pacing artifacts are seen in the ECG (top strip) just before the R wave. The marker channel (middle strip) indicates when pacing occurs (P). The T wave amplitude is high in this dog, and it is sensed by the pacemaker. Because this sensed event occurs during the programmed refractory period, and it is indicated as a sensed refractory event (SR). The electrogram or EGM (bottom strip) shows the pacing artifact and the deflections corresponding to the QRS and T wave on the surface electrocardiogram. A sensitivity test should be performed to determine the inherent R wave amplitude and then adjust the value of the sensitivity parameter to avoid T-wave oversensing. During tachycardia the T wave amplitude usually increases in dogs and if multiple refractory sensed events occur over a short period of time a common programming problem known as noise reversion can occur. The preferred method to correct noise reversion is to adjust the sensitivity parameter before making any change in the duration of the programmed refractory period.

Presence of pacing spikes and capture at a rate that markedly exceeds the programmed pacing rate (runaway phenomenon)

The runaway phenomenon is a rare pacemaker malfunction associated with end-of-life of the battery. It is characterized by intermittent bursts of extremely rapid low amplitude pacing spikes. In some cases, the pacing stimuli fail to stimulate the cardiac chambers resulting in a loss of capture; in other cases, the pacing stimuli trigger a rapid tachycardia that can be fatal.

On the electrocardiogram the runaway phenomenon is characterized by the presence of intermittent bursts of pacing *spikes* of decreasing amplitude with a rate of approximately 2,000 stimuli per minute, with or without evidence of atrial or ventricular capture.

Suggested readings

1. Bellenger CR, Ilkiw JE, Nicholson AI, et al. Transvenous pacemaker leads in the dog: an experimental study. *Res Vet Sci* 1990; 49(2):211-215.
2. Bonagura JD, Helphrey ML, Muir WW. Complications associated with permanent pacemaker implantation in the dog. *J Am Vet Med Assoc* 1983; 182(2):149-155.
3. Bulmer BJ, Oyama MA, Lamont LA, Sisson DD. Implantation of a single lead atrioventricular synchronous (VDD) pacemaker in a dog with naturally occurring 3rd-degree atrioventricular block. *J Vet Intern Med* 2002; 16(2):197-200.
4. Bulmer BJ, Sisson DD, Oyama MA, et al. Physiologic VDD versus nonphysiologic VVI pacing in canine third-degree atrioventricular block. *J Vet Intern Med* 2006; 20(6):1287-1290.
5. Cervenec RM, Stauthammer CD, Fine H, Kellihan HB, Scansen BA. Survival time with pacemaker implantation for dogs diagnosed with persistent atrial standstill. *J Vet Cardiol* 2017; 19:240-246.
6. Cobb MA, Nolan J, Brownlie SE, et al. Use of a programmable, activity-sensing, rate regulating pacemaker in a dog. *J Small Anim Pract* 1990; 31(8):398-400.
7. Darke PGG, Been M, Marks A. Use of a programmable, "physiological" cardiac pacemaker in a dog with total atrioventricular block (with some comments on complications associated with cardiac pacemakers). *J Small Anim Pract* 1985; 26(6):295-303.
8. Darke PGG, McAreavey D, Been M. Transvenous cardiac pacing in 19 dogs and one cat. *J Small Anim Pract* 1989; (9):491-499.
9. Domenech O, Santilli R, Pradelli D, et al. The implantation of a permanent transvenous endocardial pacemaker in 42 dogs: A retrospective study. *Med Sci Monit* 2005; 11(6):BR168-BR175.
10. Ferasin L, Faena M, Henderson SM, et al. Use of a multi-stage exercise test to assess the responsiveness of rate-adaptive pacemakers in dogs. *J Small Anim Pract* 2005; 46(3):115-120.
11. Fox PR, Moise NS, Woodfield JA, et al. Techniques and complications of pacemaker implantation in four cats. *J Am Vet Med Assoc* 1991; 199(12):1742-1753.
12. Hervé D, Troger JC. Retrospective study of the implantation of eighteen cardiac pacemakers in the dog. *Pract Med Chir Anim Comp* 2003; 38(2):161-166.
13. Hildebrandt N, Stertmann WA, Wehner M, et al. Dual chamber Pacemaker implantation in dogs with Atrioventricular block. *J Vet Intern Med* 2009; 23: 31-38.
14. Johnson MS, Martin MWS, Henley W. Results of pacemaker implantation in 104 dogs. *J Small Anim Pract* 2007; 48(1):4-11.
15. Lombard CW, Tilley LP, Yoshioka M. Pacemaker implantation in the dog: survey and literature review. *J Am Anim Hosp Assoc* 1981; 17(5):751- 758.
16. Oyama MA, Sisson DD, Lehmkuhl LB. Practices and outcome of artificial cardiac pacing in 154 dogs. *J Vet Intern Med* 2001; 15(3):229-39.
17. Prosek R, Sisson DD, Oyama MA. Runaway pacemaker in a dog. *J Vet Intern Med* 2004; 18(2):242-244.
18. Roberts DH, Tennant B, Brockman D, et al. Successful use of a QT-sensing rate-adaptive pacemaker in a dog. *Vet Rec* 1992; 130(21):471-472.
19. Sisson DD, Thomas WP, Woodfield J, et al. Permanent transvenous pacemaker implantation in forty dogs. *J Vet Intern Med* 1991; 5(6):322- 331.
20. Moïse NS, Estrada A: Noise Reversion in Paced Dogs. *J Vet Cardiol* 2002; 4 (2):13-21.
21. Wess G, Thomas WP, Berger DM, et al. Applications, complications, and outcomes of transvenous pacemaker implantation in 105 dogs (1997- 2002). *J Vet Intern Med* 2006; 20(4):877-884.

Guided interpretation of electrocardiographic tracings

TRACING 1 - Sinus rhythm with complete right bundle branch block 326

TRACING 2 - Atrial fibrillation with truncular left bundle branch block 327

TRACING 3 - Sinus tachycardia with ventricular quadrigeminy 328

TRACING 4 - Sinus rhythm with complete right bundle branch block and a prolonged ventricular pause secondary to paroxysmal atrioventricular block 329

TRACING 5 - Sinus rhythm with delayed intraventricular conduction, occasional atrial ectopies and a run of inferior right atrial ectopic rhythm originating from the coronary sinus 330

TRACING 6 - Pacemaker malfunction with loss of capture and undersensing 331

TRACING 7 - Focal atrial tachycardia arising from the *Crista terminalis* 332

TRACING 8 - Sinus rhythm with signs of intra-atrial conduction delay and a run of non-sustained monomorphic ventricular tachycardia 333

TRACING 9 - Sinus rhythm with electrocardiographic signs of right ventricular enlargement 334

TRACING 10 - Sinus rhythm with ventricular pre-excitation 335

TRACING 11 - Sinus rhythm with first-degree atrioventricular block, 2:1 second-degree atrioventricular block and ventriculo-phasic sinus arrhythmia 336

TRACING 12 - Focal junctional tachycardia with isorhythmic atrioventricular dissociation and type I synchronization 337

TRACING 13 - Third-degree atrioventricular block and escape rhythm originating from two different ectopic foci 338

TRACING 14 - Orthodromic atrioventricular reciprocating tachycardia 339

TRACING 15 - Sinus rhythm with Mobitz type II second-degree atrioventricular block 340

TRACING 1
DOG, MONGREL, FEMALE, 3 YEARS OLD

Twelve leads (I, II, III, aVR, aVL, aVF, V_1, V_2, V_3, V_4, V_5, V_6) - speed 50 mm/s - calibration 5 mm/1 mV

The dominant rhythm is a sinus rhythm with a rate of 125 bpm. The P waves are normal in morphology, amplitude and duration (amplitude of 0.3 mV, duration of 40 ms). Their mean electrical axis in the frontal plane is +80°.
The PQ interval has a normal and fixed duration of 100 ms.
The QRS complex is wide (approximately 80 ms) with a mean electrical axis in the frontal plane deviated to the right and equal to −165°. The QRS complexes include a deep S wave in the inferior leads (II, III, and aVF) and in the left precordial leads (from V_2 to V_6). The R wave is more positive in aVR than aVL. The QRS complex in lead V_1 has the characteristic M (or rR') morphology.
The QT interval measures 300 ms, which is prolonged for an underlying heart rate of 125 bpm. The ST segment is elevated in the inferior leads (II, III and aVF) and in all the left precordial leads (from V_2 to V_6).
The P-P and R-R intervals are regular (470 ms).
The presence of S waves in the inferior leads (II, III, and aVF) that represent more than 50 % of the duration of the QRS complex, the duration of the QRS complex greater than 80 ms and an rR' morphology in lead V_1 supports the diagnosis of complete right bundle branch block. The elevation of the ST segment and QT prolongation reflect alterations in ventricular repolarization following the abnormal sequence of depolarization, and have no clinical significance.

Electrocardiographic diagnosis: Sinus rhythm with complete right bundle branch block.

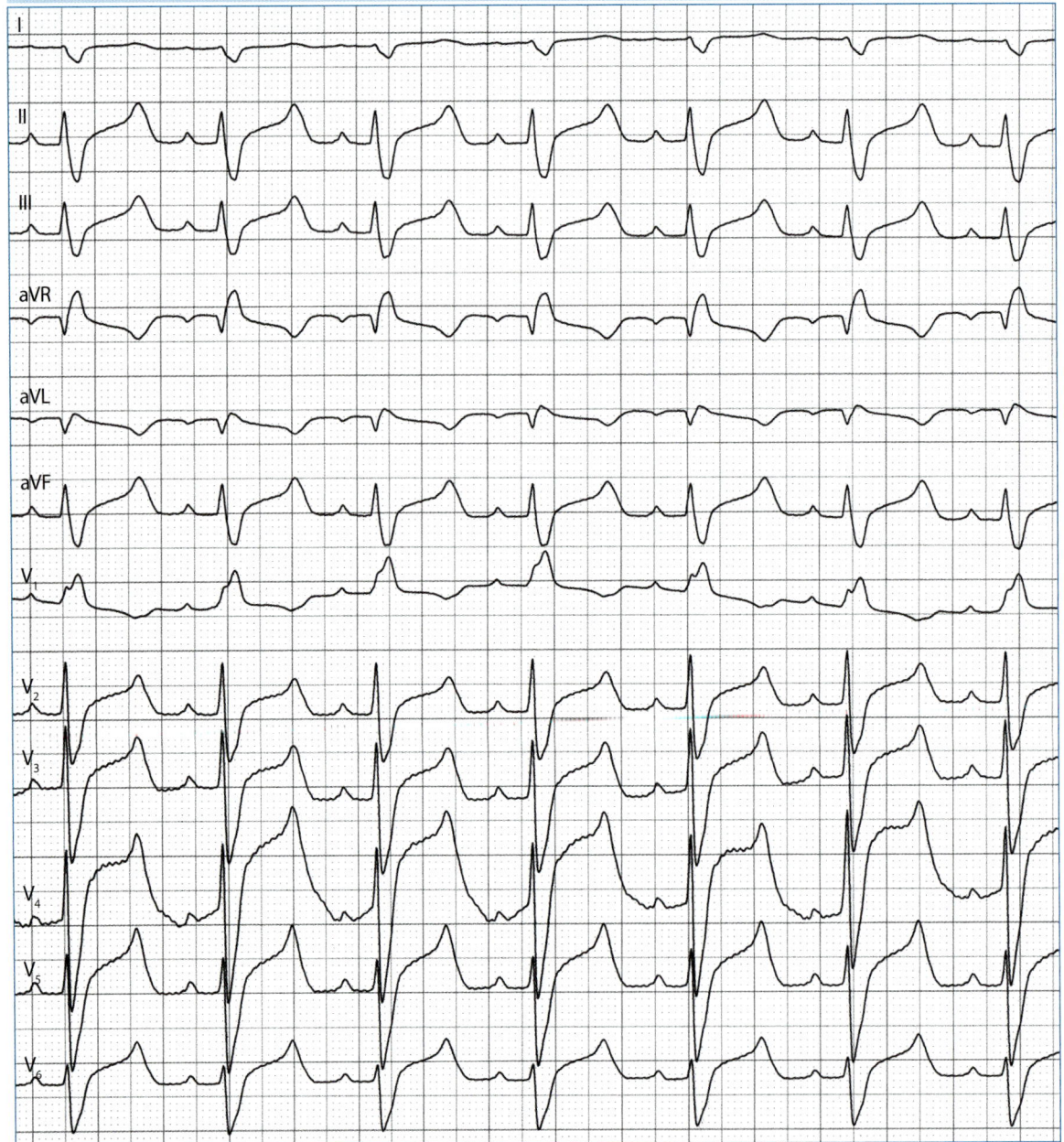

TRACING 2
DOG, AKITA INU, FEMALE, 1 YEAR OLD

Twelve leads (I, II, III, aVR, aVL, aVF, V_1, V_2, V_3, V_4, V_5, V_6) - speed 50 mm/s - calibration 5 mm/1 mV

The dominant rhythm is a wide QRS complex (QRS duration of approximately 90 ms) and irregular (variable R-R intervals between 210 and 310 ms) tachycardia with an average rate of 220 bpm.
There are no visible P waves. Subtle undulations of the baseline suggesting the presence of fibrillation waves or artifacts.
The QRS complexes have an increased duration (90 ms) and a mean electrical axis of +86° in the frontal plane.
The QT interval is normal (approximately 210 ms).
The ST segment is slightly depressed in the inferior leads (II, III, and aVF).
In the presence of a sustained and irregular wide QRS complex tachycardia and the absence of visible P waves, the electrocardiogram must be evaluated further to differentiate between monomorphic ventricular tachycardia, atrial fibrillation conducted with a left bundle branch block, and finally, pre-excited atrial fibrillation. The concordance of QRS morphology between limb and precordial leads (in other words QRS morphology is consistent with a left bundle branch block in the limb leads and in the chest leads) and the presence of precordial discordance does not support the diagnosis of monomorphic ventricular tachycardia. The absence of a delta wave, a QRS duration of 90 ms, a very fast heart rate and a pronounced beat-to-beat variation of QRS complex morphology does not support the presence of pre-excitation. Thus, the diagnosis is atrial fibrillation conducted with a left bundle branch block. The absence of Q waves in lead I suggests that the site of block is pre-divisional (truncular portion of the bundle). Note the delayed intrinsicoid deflection (R wave onset to peak duration) in the left precordial leads (from V_2 to V_6) suggesting severe myocardial disease. The beat-to-beat variation in QRS morphology likely reflects rate-dependent aberrant conduction.

Electrocardiographic diagnosis: Atrial fibrillation conducted with truncular left bundle branch block.

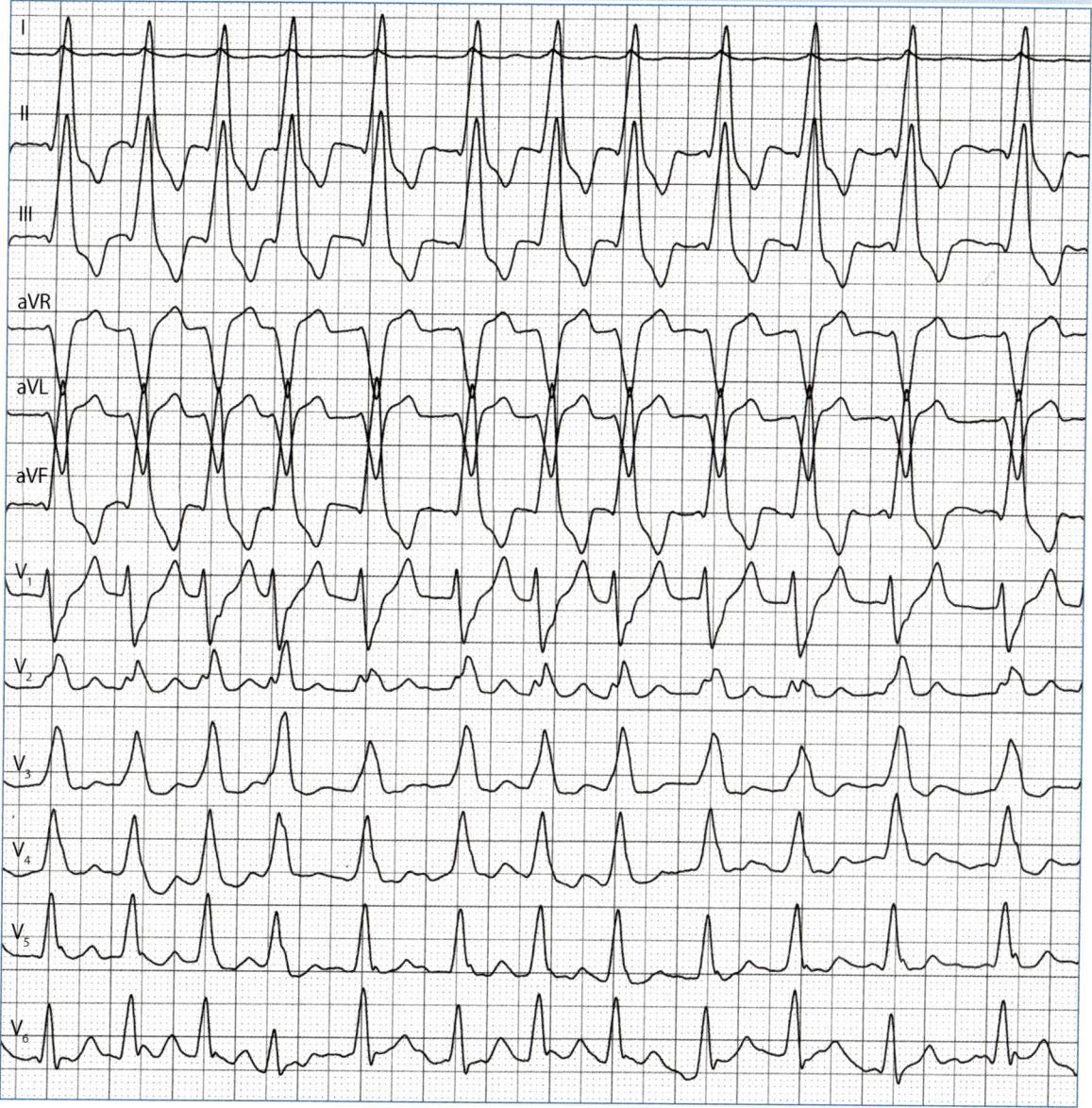

TRACING 3

DOG, NEAPOLITAN MASTIFF, MALE, 5 MONTHS OLD

Twelve leads (I, II, III, aVR, aVL, aVF, V$_1$, V$_2$, V$_3$, V$_4$, V$_5$, V$_6$) - speed 50 mm/s - calibration 5 mm/1 mV

On this electrocardiogram, the underlying rhythm is sinus in origin. The average heart rate is approximately 180 bpm, which is consistent with sinus tachycardia.

The P waves are normal in morphology, amplitude and duration (amplitude of 0.3 mV, duration of 40 ms). Their mean electrical axis is +90° in the frontal plane.

The PQ interval has a normal and fixed duration of 80 ms.

The QRS complexes during sinus rhythm have normal morphology, amplitude and duration (60 ms) with a mean electrical axis of +92° in the frontal plane. The QT interval is normal (179 ms).

The ST segment is isoelectric in all leads during sinus rhythm.

The fourth and the eighth QRS complexes differ markedly from the sinus beats: they are wider (80 ms) with a large negative deflection in the inferior leads (II, III, and aVF) and in the left precordial leads (V$_3$-V$_6$), and the largest positive amplitude in lead aVR, consistent with a right bundle branch block morphology. In this particular case, since the dog is dolicomorphic and lead V$_1$ (positioned in the fifth right intercostal space) is recording ventricular depolarization originating from the left ventricle (note that the QRS in V$_1$ is also positive also during sinus rhythm), the precordial discordance/concordance rule cannot be used to determine the origin of the wide QRS complexes. In addition, the interval between these beats and the preceding sinus beat is shorter than the average R-R interval. These two characteristics support the diagnosis of ventricular premature beats (also referred to as VPCs, PVCs). They are followed by a pause that can be described as fully compensatory because the sum of the interval preceding the premature beat (180 ms) and the interval following the premature beat (460 ms) is equal to twice the interval between two sinus (320 ms). The repetitive pattern of three sinus beats followed by one ventricular premature beats is called ventricular quadrigeminy.

Electrocardiographic diagnosis: Sinus tachycardia with ventricular quadrigeminy.

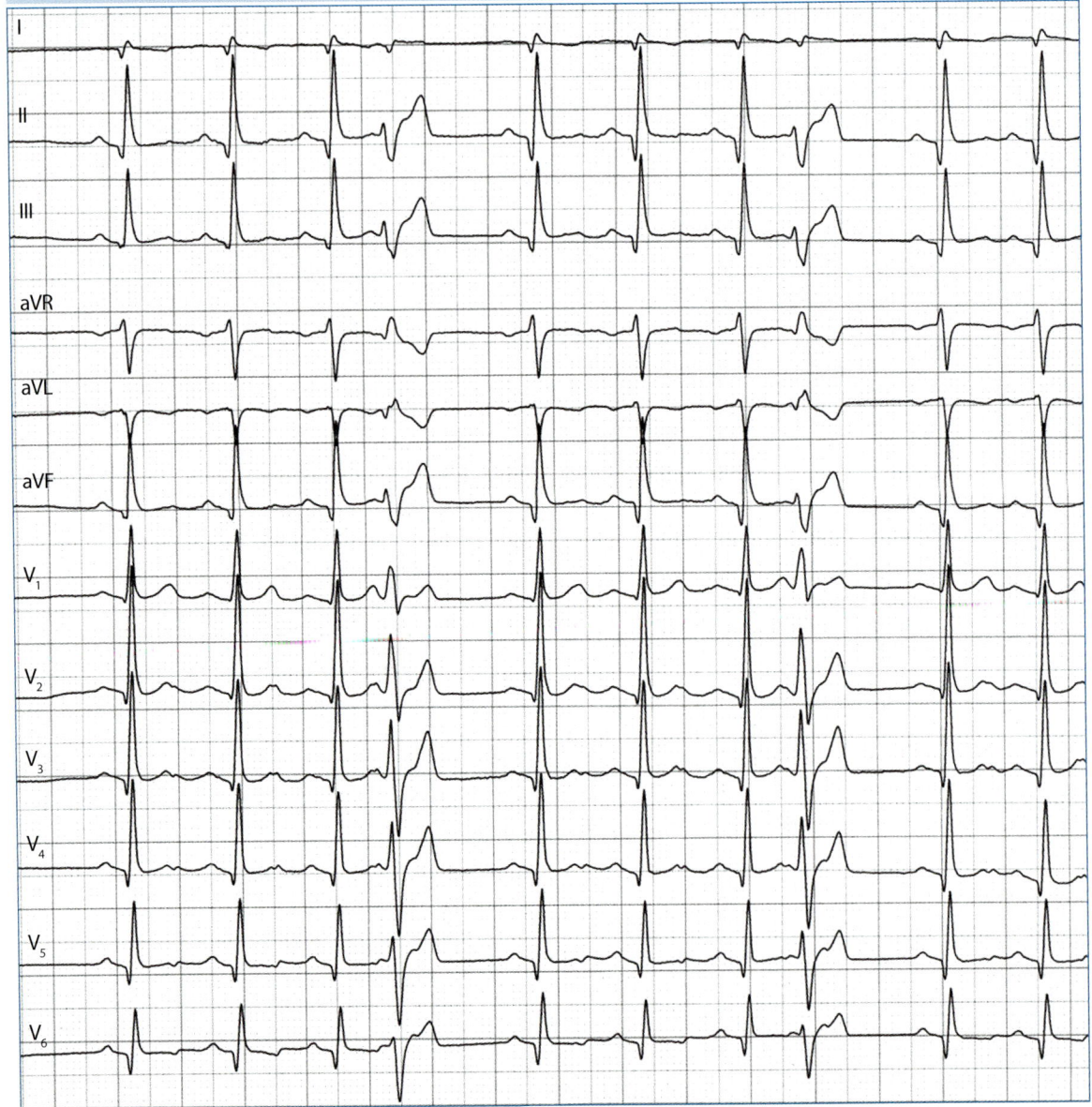

TRACING 4

CAT, DOMESTIC SHORTHAIR, FEMALE, 15 YEARS OLD

Six limb leads (I, II, III, aVR, aVL, aVF) - speed 50 mm/s - calibration 10 mm/1 mV

The initial rhythm is a sinus rhythm with a rate of 165 bpm. The P waves are normal in morphology, amplitude and duration (amplitude of 0.2 mV, duration of 30 ms). Their mean electrical axis is +68 ° in the frontal plane.
The PQ interval has a normal and fixed duration of 60 ms.
The QRS complexes are wide (>50 ms) with deep S waves in the inferior leads (II, III, and aVF) and a pronounced R wave in aVR. Their mean electrical axis is deviated to the right (−160 °). This is consistent with a complete right bundle branch block.
The QT interval is normal (200 ms).
The ST segment is normal in all leads.

The P-P and R-R intervals are regular (370 ms).
After the first four beats there are sinus P waves not followed by QRS complexes, indicating a paroxysmal atrioventricular block, which results in a prolonged ventricular pause. The presence of a bundle branch block followed by paroxysmal atrioventricular block suggests an inflammatory or degenerative process affecting the atrioventricular and intraventricular conduction tissue.

Electrocardiographic diagnosis: Sinus rhythm with complete right bundle branch block and prolonged ventricular pause caused by paroxysmal atrioventricular block.

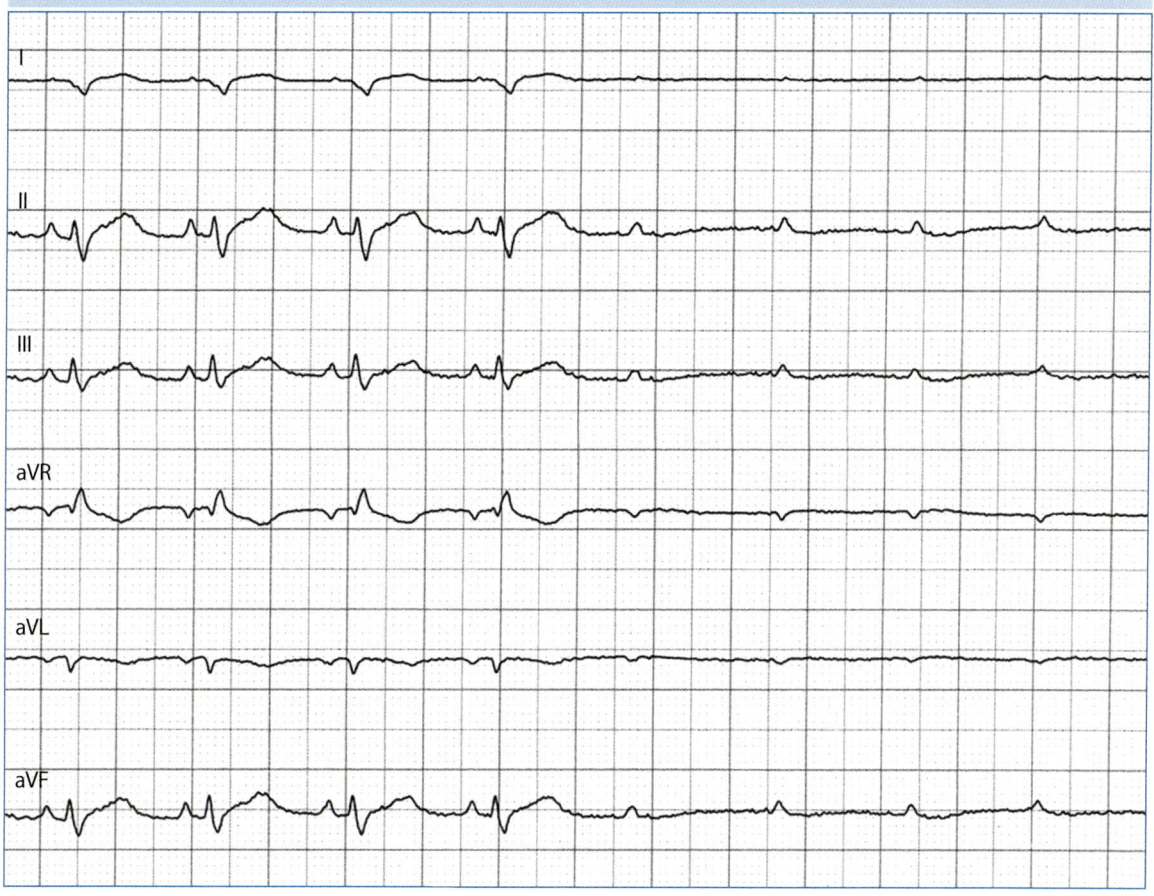

TRACING 5

DOG, GERMAN SHEPHERD, FEMALE, 5 YEARS OLD

Twelve leads (I, II, III, aVR, aVL, aVF, V_1, V_2, V_3, V_4, V_5, V_6) - speed 25 mm/s - calibration 5 mm/1 mV

The initial rhythm is a sinus rhythm with a rate of 110 bpm. Sinus P waves are normal in morphology, amplitude and duration (amplitude of 0.4 mV, duration of 40 ms) with a mean electrical axis of +80 °. The PQ interval is constant and normal with a duration of 120 ms.
The QRS complex has a normal morphology and increased duration (80 ms); the mean electrical axis is +83 °.
The QT interval is normal (240 ms) and is, therefore, of normal duration. The ST segment is isoelectric in all leads.
The P-P and R-R intervals are irregular.
The fourth, sixth, seventh, eighth, ninth and tenth beat display P' waves that differ from the sinus P waves, and their morphology is slightly variable. All P' waves are negative in leads II, III, aVF, positive in leads I and aVR, with maximum positive amplitude in aVL. Their mean electrical axis is approximately −65 °. P'Q intervals are variable (160 to 200 ms). All these features are consistent with ectopic P' wave originating from the inferior region of the right atrium. The P' wave of the sixth and seventh beats share some characteristics of the sinus P waves and the other P' waves, which suggests that they are fusion beats. The occurrence of a sequence of more than three ectopic beats with a mean ventricular rate of 125 bpm and prolonged (60 ms) bifid P' waves is consistent with an inferior right atrial ectopic rhythm originating from the region of the coronary sinus. Increasing in duration of the QRS complex with normal axis is likely to be an index of intraventricular conduction delay or left ventricular enlargement.

Electrocardiographic diagnosis: Sinus rhythm with intraventricular conduction delay, occasional atrial ectopies and a run of inferior right atrial ectopic rhythm originating from the coronary sinus.

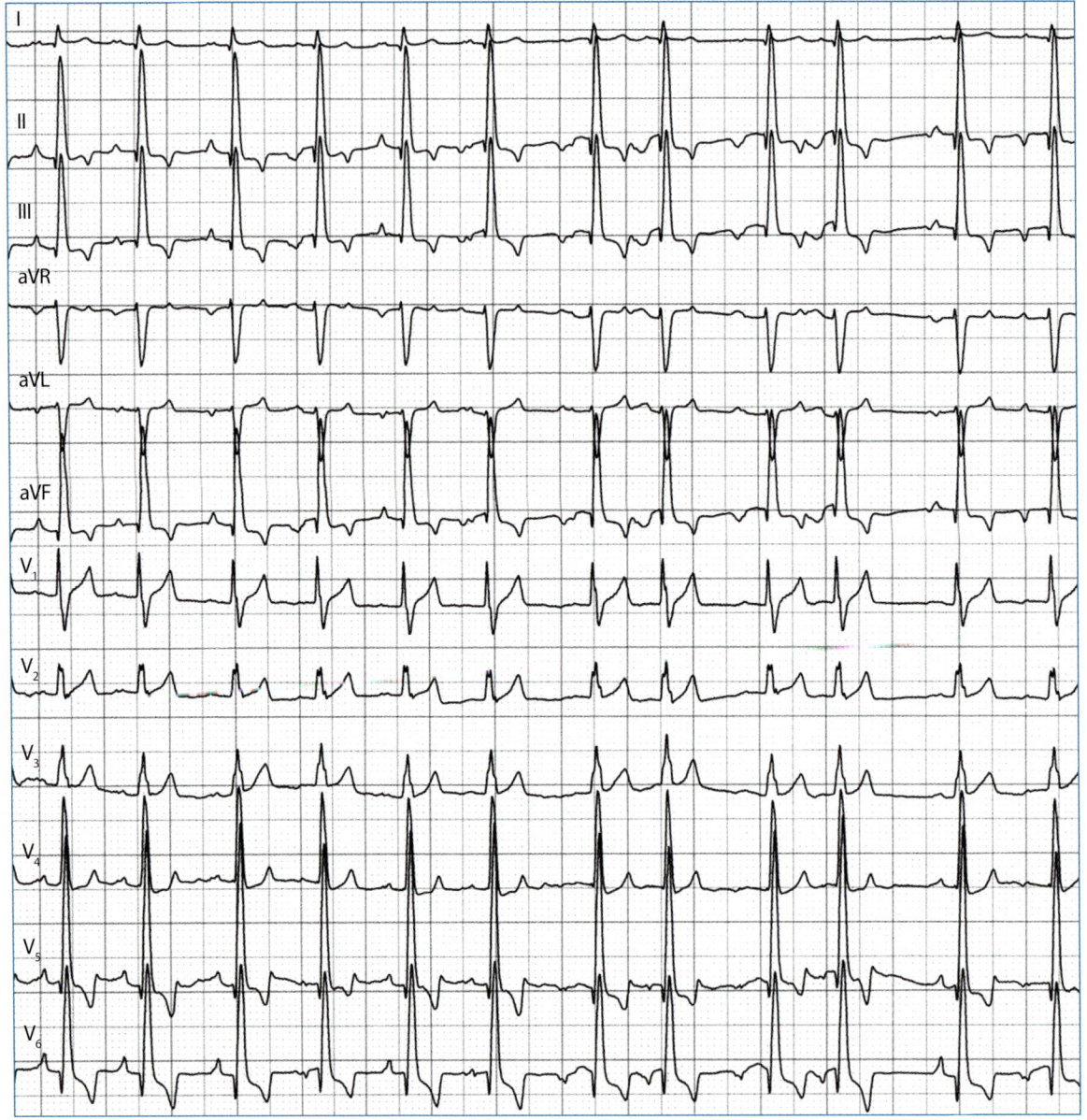

TRACING 6
DOG, GERMAN SHEPHERD, MALE, 6 YEARS OLD

Six limb leads (I, II, III, aVR, aVL, aVF) - speed 50 mm/s - calibration 5 mm/1 mV

Ventricular pacemaker implanted in VVI mode and a pacing rate of 60 bpm.

The dominant rhythm is a wide QRS complex (90 ms) rhythm with a rate of 60 bpm.

The QRS complexes have a right bundle branch block morphology (wide negative deflection in the inferior leads and wide positive deflection in aVR) and a mean electrical axis of –90 °. There are no visible P waves. The ventricular rhythm is an escape rhythm, or idioventricular rhythm.

Narrow vertical signals occurring at a rate of 43 to 60 bpm are visible and consistent with pacing spikes of a unipolar pacemaker. The spikes are not followed by QRS complexes indicating a failure to capture the ventricles. In addition the irregularity of the pacing spikes suggests an intermittent failure to sense the intrinsic ventricular rhythm. Indeed the first ventricular beat (QRS complex) is appropriately detected and followed by a pacing spike after an interval of 1000 ms (60 bpm), which corresponds to the programmed pacing rate. However, the interval between the second QRS complex and the subsequent spike is shorter than 1000 ms, indicating that the QRS complex was not sensed by the pacemaker. Any spontaneous beat (QRS complex) should reset the pacemaker timing cycle. The combination of failure to capture and failure to sense suggest electrode dislodgement.

Electrocardiographic diagnosis: Pacemaker malfunction with loss of capture and undersensing.

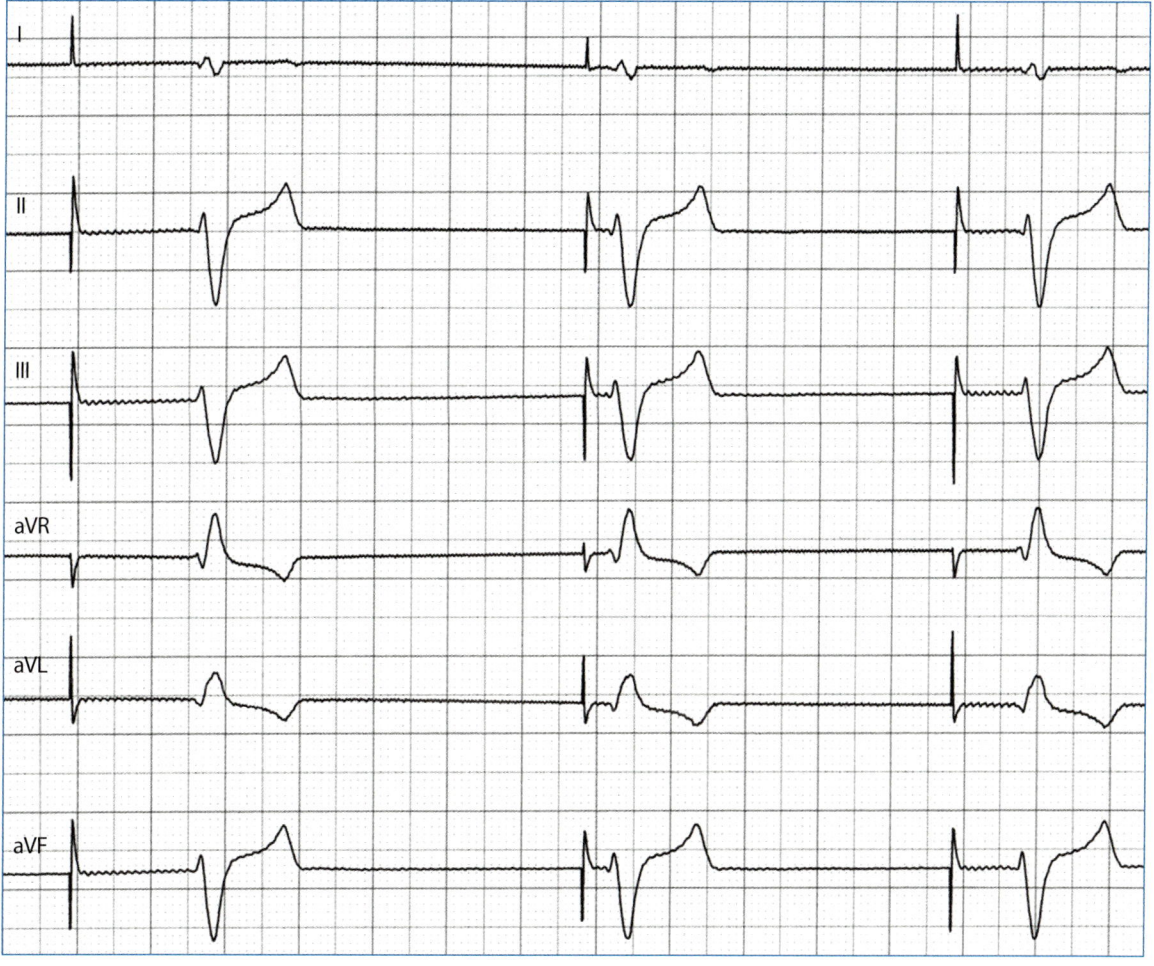

TRACING 7

DOG, GERMAN SHEPHERD, FEMALE, 12 YEARS OLD

Twelve leads (I, II, III, aVR, aVL, aVF, V$_1$, V$_2$, V$_3$, V$_4$, V$_5$, V$_6$) - speed 50 mm/s - calibration 5 mm/1 mV

The dominant rhythm is a narrow QRS complex tachycardia at a rate of 230 bpm. The R-R intervals of the tachycardia are mostly regular but there are occasional irregularities (cycle-length irregularities).
Some P' waves with positive polarity in leads II, III and aVF, negative in aVR and aVL, and slightly positive in lead I (superior-to-inferior axis of +78 °) are visible within the descending limb of the preceding T wave (camel sign). These P' waves are most visible in the last two complexes from the right where the RP'/ P'R ratio is 1.4.

The QRS complexes have normal amplitude and duration (50 ms) and a mean electrical axis of +100 °. The QT interval is normal (230 ms). The ST segment is isoelectric in all leads.
A supraventricular tachycardia with a ventricular rate >180 bpm and cycle length irregularities, P' wave with a superior-to-inferior axis, and a RP'/P'R>0.7 ratio are consistent with a focal atrial tachycardia originating from the superior right atrial region (*crista terminalis*).
Electrocardiographic diagnosis: Focal atrial tachycardia.

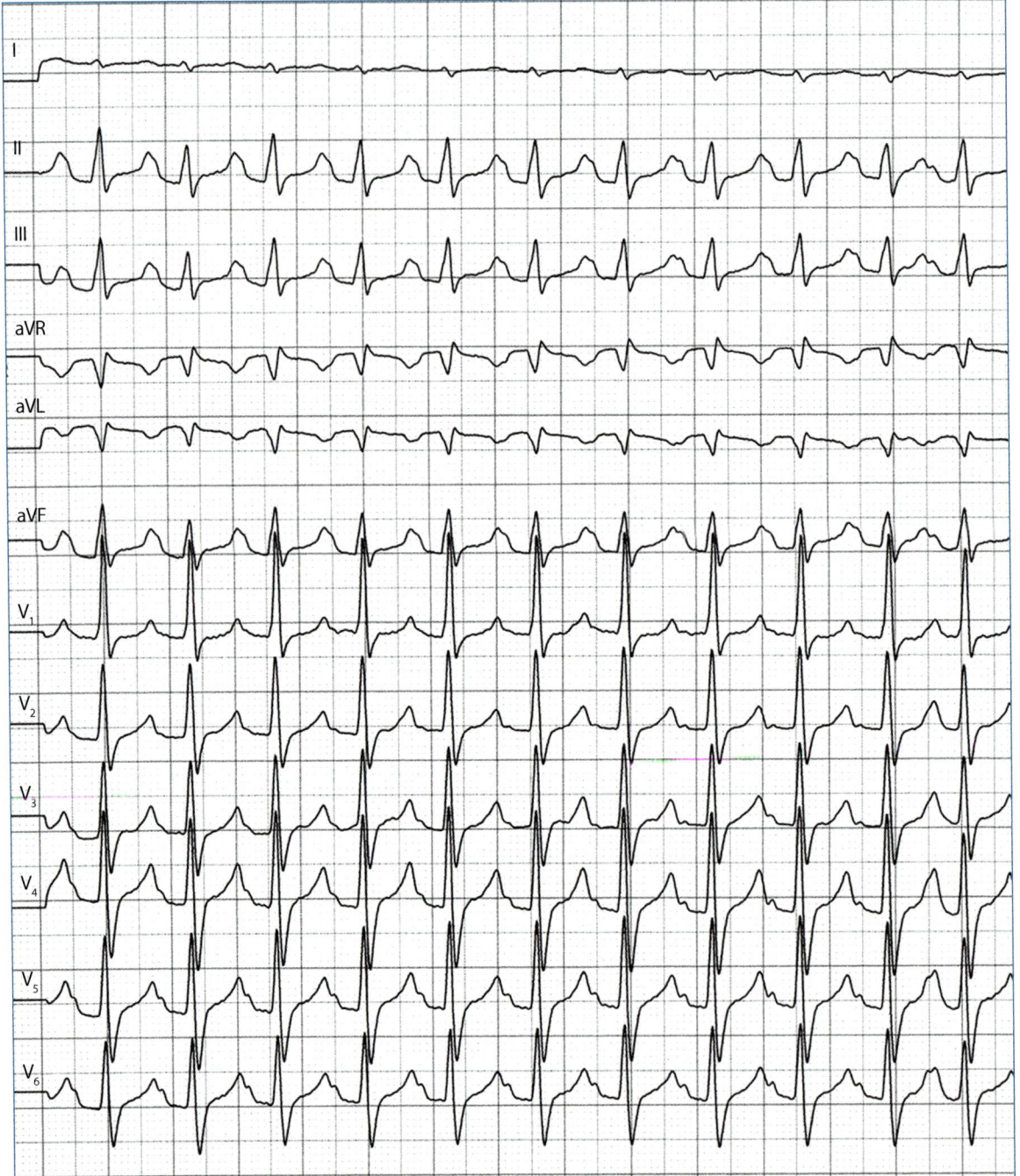

TRACING 8
DOG, MIXED BREED, FEMALE, 12 YEARS OLD

Twelve leads (I, II, III, aVR, aVL, aVF, V_1, V_2, V_3, V_4, V_5, V_6) - speed 50 mm/s - calibration 5 mm/1 mV

The initial rhythm is a sinus rhythm with a rate of 150 bpm. The P waves have normal morphology, mildly increased amplitude and duration (amplitude of 0.4 mV, duration of 50 ms) and bifid morphology (more evident in last two sinus P waves). Their mean electrical axis in the frontal plane is +80°. The presence of wide and bifid P waves is suggestive of left atrial enlargement or intra-atrial conduction delay. The PQ interval has a normal and fixed duration of 85 ms. The QRS complex of the sinus beats has normal duration (50 to 60 ms) and amplitude with a mean electrical axis of +63 °. The QT interval is normal (approximately 190 ms). The ST segment is isoelectric in all leads.

Following the second sinus beat, the rhythm is interrupted by five similar wide QRS complexes (80 ms) conducted with a right bundle branch block morphology (large negative deflection in the inferior leads II, III, and aVF, and an electrical axis of −80 ° to +85°). There is discordance between the limb leads and precordial leads (in other words, the morphology of the QRS complexes in the precordial leads is not consistent with a right bundle branch block), and there is positive precordial concordance in the precordial leads (in other words, the QRS complex polarity is positive in the six precordial leads). The rate of the wide QRS complex rhythm is 200 bpm and it is regular. During the tachycardia, some P waves are visible but they are not associated with the QRS complexes (atrioventricular dissociation). The eighth beat has an intermediate morphology between the sinus beats and the ventricular beats, and corresponds to a fusion beat. A regular wide QRS complex tachycardia with precordial concordance, signs of atrioventricular dissociation and fusion beats has all the characteristics of a monomorphic ventricular tachycardia. It is non-sustained because it lasts less than 30 s.

Electrocardiographic diagnosis: Sinus rhythm with signs of intra-atrial conduction delay and a run of non-sustained monomorphic ventricular tachycardia.

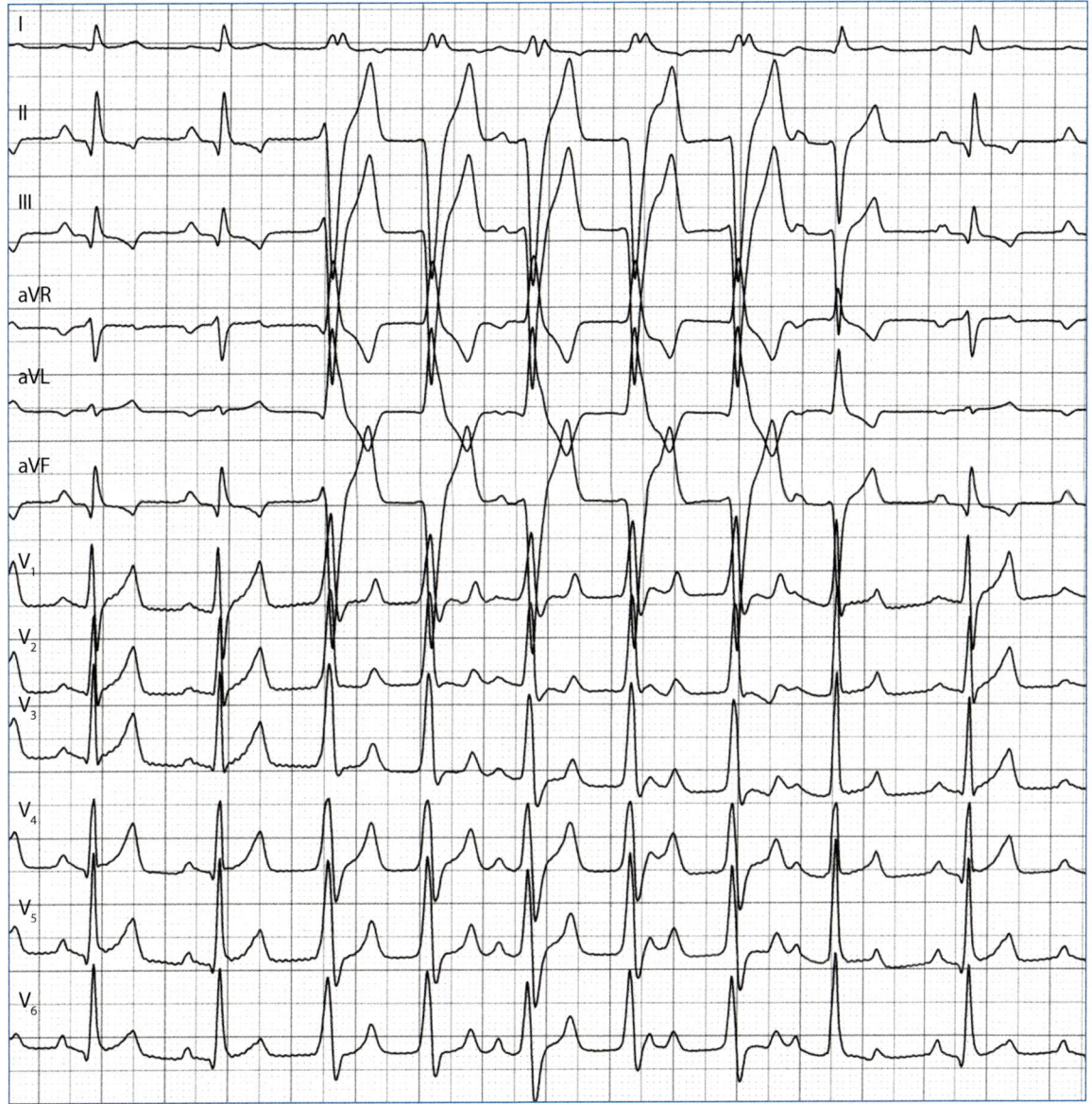

TRACING 9

DOG, DOGUE DE BORDEAUX, FEMALE, 1 YEAR OLD

Twelve leads (I, II, III, aVR, aVL, aVF, V_1, V_2, V_3, V_4, V_5, V_6) - speed 50 mm/s - calibration 5 mm/1 mV

The dominant rhythm is a sinus rhythm with a rate of 120 bpm. The P waves are normal in morphology, amplitude and duration (amplitude of 0.3 to 0.4 mV, duration of 40 ms). Their mean electrical axis is +80°. The PQ interval has a normal and fixed duration of 90 ms.
QRS complexes have a normal duration (60 ms) and their mean electrical axis is shifted to the right (−150°). The QT interval is normal (200 to 210 ms). The ST segment is isoelectric in all leads.

The P-P and R-R intervals are regular (500 ms).
The QRS complex amplitude in lead I (S>0.05 mV), lead II (S>0.35 mV), V_2 (S>0.8 mV) and V_4 (S>0.7 mV), the R/S ratio in V_4 <0.87 and the right axis deviation of the mean electrical axis support the diagnosis of right ventricular enlargement.

Electrocardiographic diagnosis: Sinus rhythm with electrocardiographic signs of right ventricular enlargement.

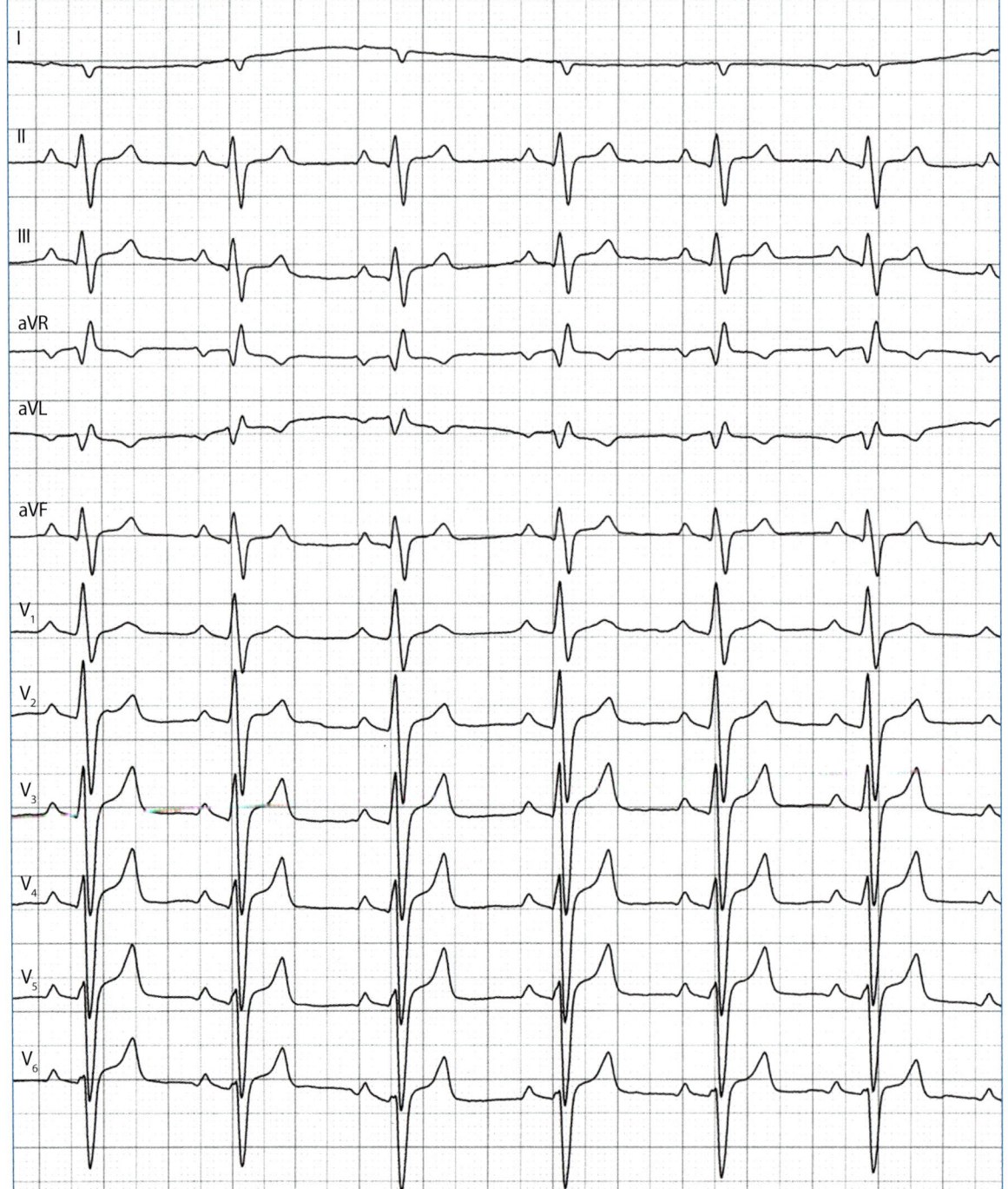

TRACING 10
DOG, LABRADOR RETRIEVER, MALE, 2 YEARS OLD

Twelve leads (I, II, III, aVR, aVL, aVF, V_1, V_2, V_3, V_4, V_5, V_6) - speed 50 mm/s - calibration 5 mm/1 mV

The dominant rhythm is a sinus rhythm with a rate of 140 bpm. The P waves are normal in morphology, amplitude and duration (amplitude of 0.35 mV, duration of 40 ms). Their electrical axis is +70°.
The PQ interval is short and measures approximately 50 ms.
QRS complexes have increased duration (>70 ms), their mean electrical axis is slightly deviated to the left (+ 10°) and there is an alteration of their initial portion that is more obvious as a slurring of the ascending branch in the left precordial leads (delta wave).
QT interval is normal (190 ms).
The ST segment is isoelectric in all leads.
The P-P and R-R intervals are regular (460 ms).
The combination of a short PQ interval followed by a QRS complex with a slight increase in duration and a delta wave and a T wave that is opposite polarity to that of the δ wave supports the diagnosis of ventricular pre-excitation.
During ventricular pre-excitation, the atrial wavefront of depolarization reaches the ventricles first via the accessory pathway resulting in a shortening of the PQ interval. The QRS complex is results from the depolarization of a portion of the ventricles by the accessory pathway and the other part by the normal conduction pathways once the atrial wavefront has crossed the atrioventricular node. Note that the presence of the delta wave is more obvious in the left precordial leads than the limb leads.
Electrocardiographic diagnosis: Sinus rhythm with ventricular pre-excitation.

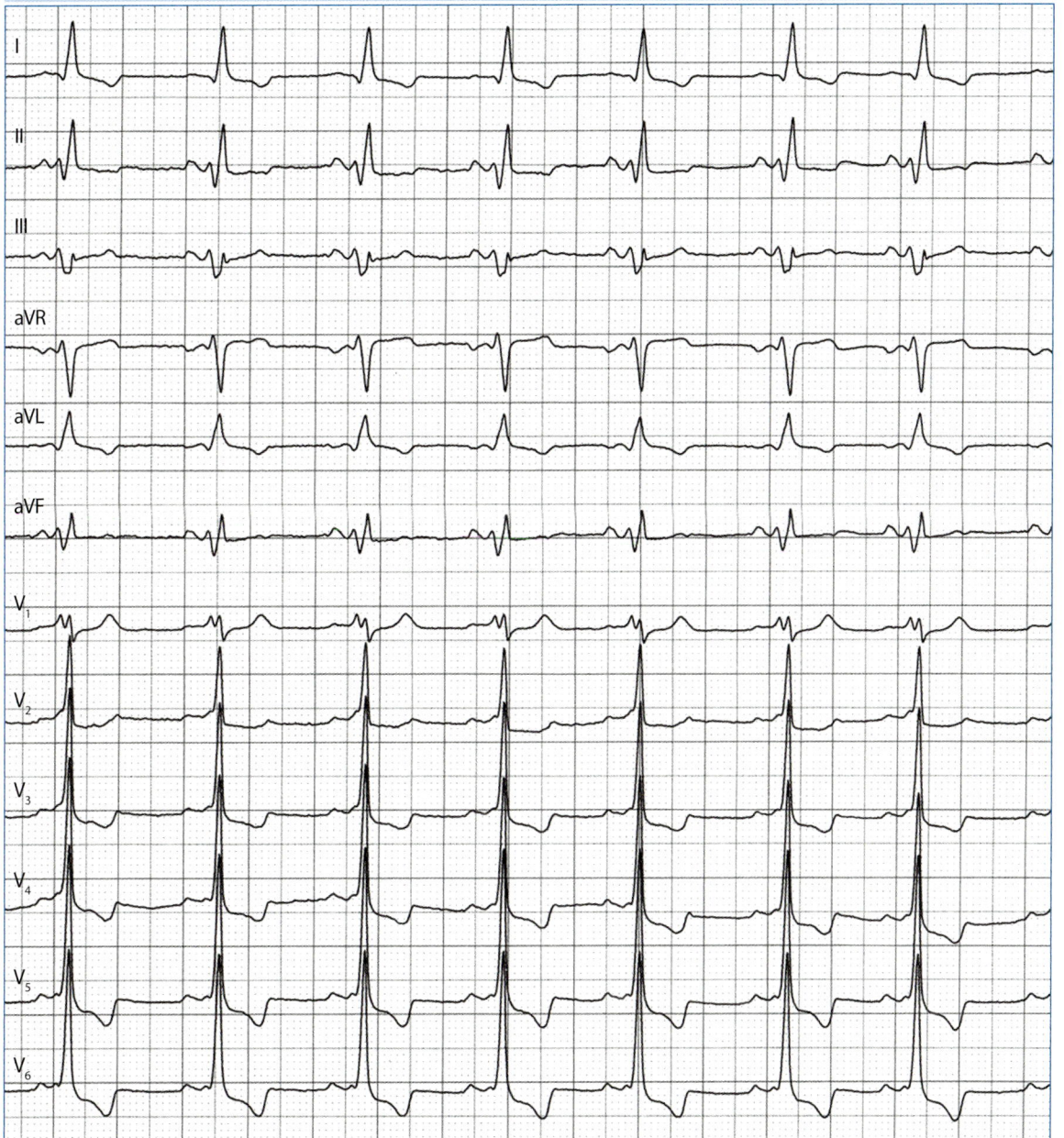

TRACING 11
DOG, MIXED BREED, MALE 11 YEARS OLD

Twelve leads (I, II, III, aVR, aVL, aVF, V$_1$, V$_2$, V$_3$, V$_4$, V$_5$, V$_6$) - speed 50 mm/s - calibration 5 mm/1 mV

The dominant rhythm is a sinus rhythm with an average atrial rate of 80 bpm and a ventricular rate of 40 bpm. The P waves are normal in morphology, amplitude and duration (amplitude of 0.3 mV, duration of 40 ms). Their mean electrical axis is +61°.
The PQ interval of the two beats visible on the tracing is prolonged with a fixed duration of 200 ms.
QRS complexes have normal morphology, amplitude and duration (40 to 50 ms) and a mean electrical axis of +80°. The QT interval slightly exceeds the reference values (252 ms), which is expected when the heart rate is 40 bpm.
The ST segment is isoelectric in all leads.

The first and the third P waves are followed by a QRS complex, while the second and fourth are blocked. The atrioventricular conduction ratio is constant and equal to 2:1, in other words every other P wave is blocked. This is characteristic of 2:1 second-degree atrioventricular block. In addition, the P-P interval is variable: it is shorter when the P-P interval includes a QRS complex, and it is longer when there is no QRS complex between the two P waves. This is consistent with ventriculo-phasic sinus arrhythmia. The PQ interval of the conducted beats is prolonged, which indicates first-degree atrioventricular block.
Electrocardiographic diagnosis: Sinus rhythm with first-degree atrioventricular block, 2:1 second-degree atrioventricular block and ventriculo-phasic sinus arrhythmia.

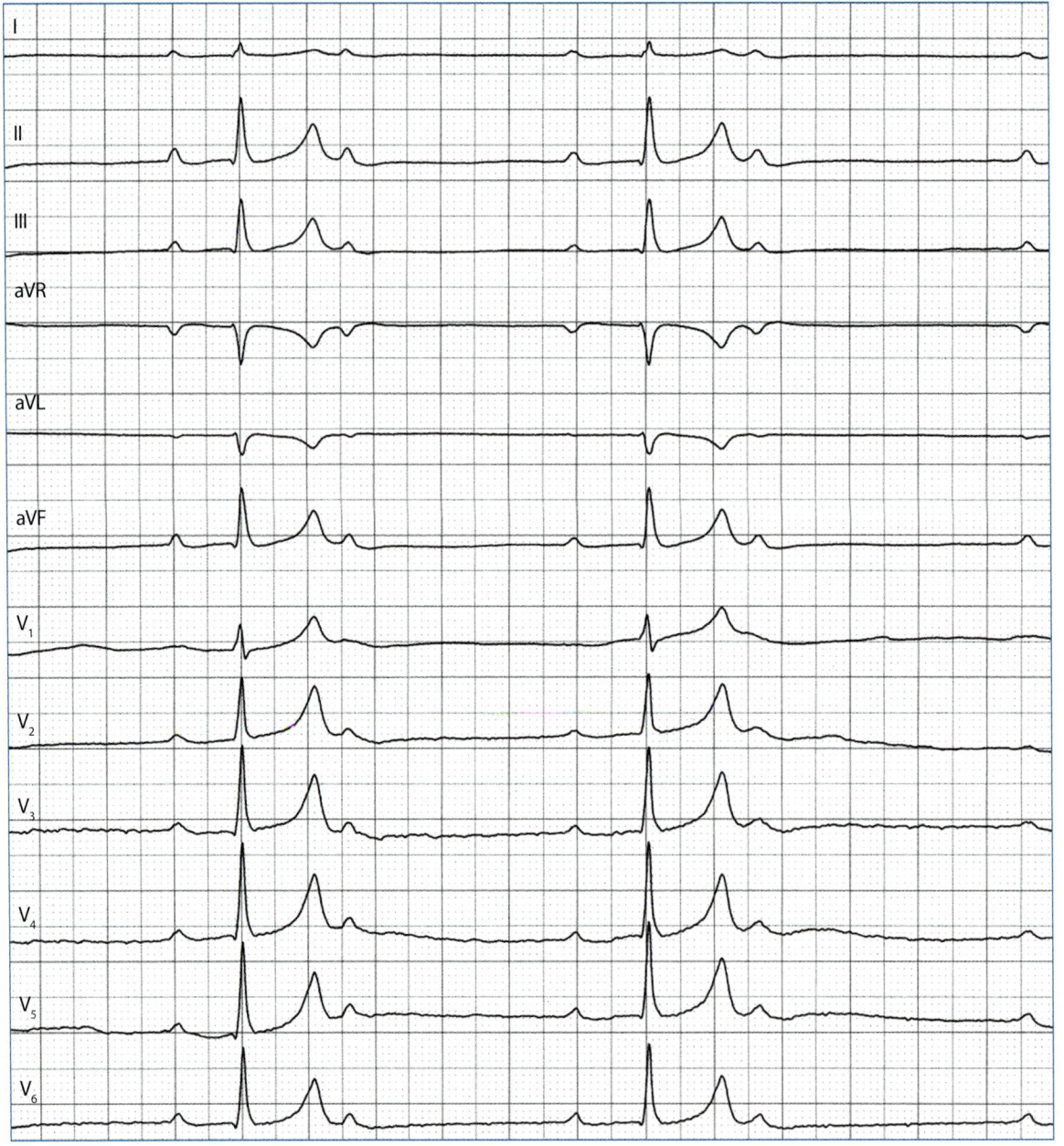

TRACING 12
DOG, LABRADOR RETRIEVER, MALE, 1 YEAR OLD

Twelve leads (I, II, III, aVR, aVL, aVF, V_1, V_2, V_3, V_4, V_5, V_6) - speed 50 mm/s - calibration 5 mm/1 mV

The rhythm is characterized by narrow QRS complexes (40 ms), regular R-R intervals and a rate of 130 bpm. Their mean electrical axis is +90°. The QT interval is normal (190 ms). The ST segment is isoelectric in all leads.

Occasional P waves are visible and appear to have normal morphology, amplitude and duration (amplitude of 0.30 mV, duration of 40 ms). Their mean electrical axis is +80°.

The P waves are dissociated from the QRS complexes. The morphology and duration of the QRS is consistent with an origin in the nodo-Hisian (or junctional) region. On the left portion of the tracing the P waves are not visible because they overlap with the QRS complexes. Subsequently they appear in front of the QRS complex as the discharge rate of the sinus node decreases slightly. This pattern is called atrioventricular isorhythmic dissociation. It occurs when two contemporary rhythms have similar discharge rates: for example a sinus rhythm that depolarizes the atria in an anterograde direction and an ectopic junctional or ventricular rhythm that depolarizes the ventricles. The progressive shift of the P wave from the right to left of the QRS complex corresponds to isorhythmic atrioventricular dissociation with type I synchronization.

Overall, the presence of narrow QRS complexes with regular R-R intervals and a rate between 100 and 160 bpm, combined with isorhythmic atrioventricular dissociation is characteristic of focal junctional tachycardia.

Electrocardiographic diagnosis: Focal junctional tachycardia with isorhythmic atrioventricular dissociation and type I synchronization.

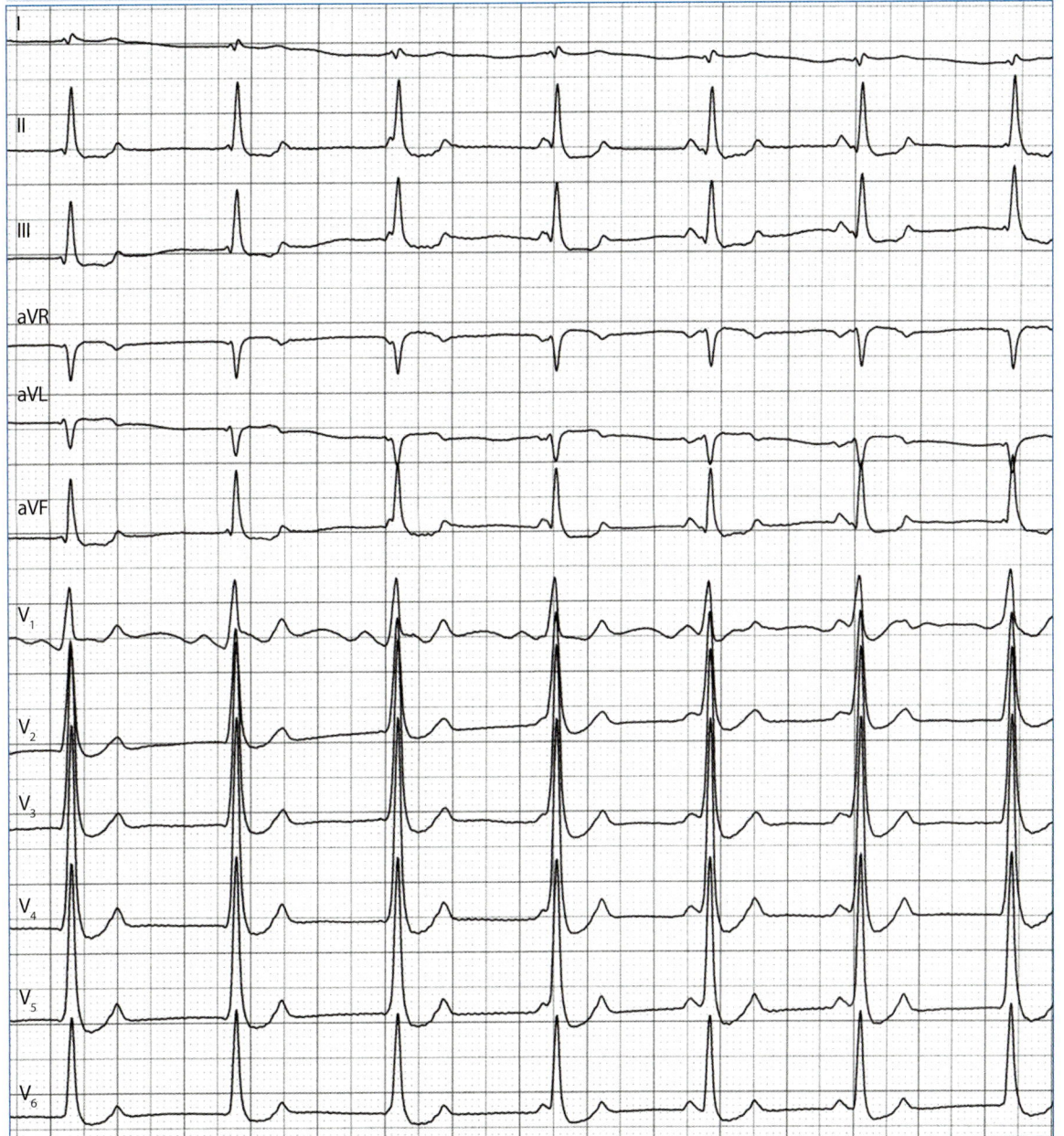

TRACING 13

DOG, BEAGLE, MALE, 7 YEARS OLD

Twelve leads (I, II, III, aVR, aVL, aVF, V_1, V_2, V_3, V_4, V_5, V_6) - speed 50 mm/s - calibration 5 mm/1 mV

The dominant ventricular rhythm is formed by wide QRS complexes (100 ms) depolarizing the ventricles at a rate of 40 bpm.

The P waves are normal in morphology, amplitude and duration (amplitude of 0.4 mV, duration of 40 ms). Their mean electrical axis is +52°. PQ intervals are variable and range from 130 ms to 200 ms.

The QRS complexes have increased duration and a right bundle branch block morphology. The two QRS complexes that are visible on the tracing have different morphology particularly in the precordial leads, which suggests a different origin within the ventricles. The QT interval lasts 260 ms and is therefore prolonged. The ST segment is isoelectric all leads.

The P-P and R-R intervals are regular and measure 300 ms and 1700 ms, respectively. The P waves are likely dissociated from the QRS complexes because the PQ interval is variable and they are many more P waves than QRS complexes. In addition, the slow ventricular rhythm formed by wide QRS complexes is consistent with a ventricular escape rhythm.

Electrocardiographic diagnosis: Third-degree atrioventricular block and escape rhythm originating from two different ectopic foci.

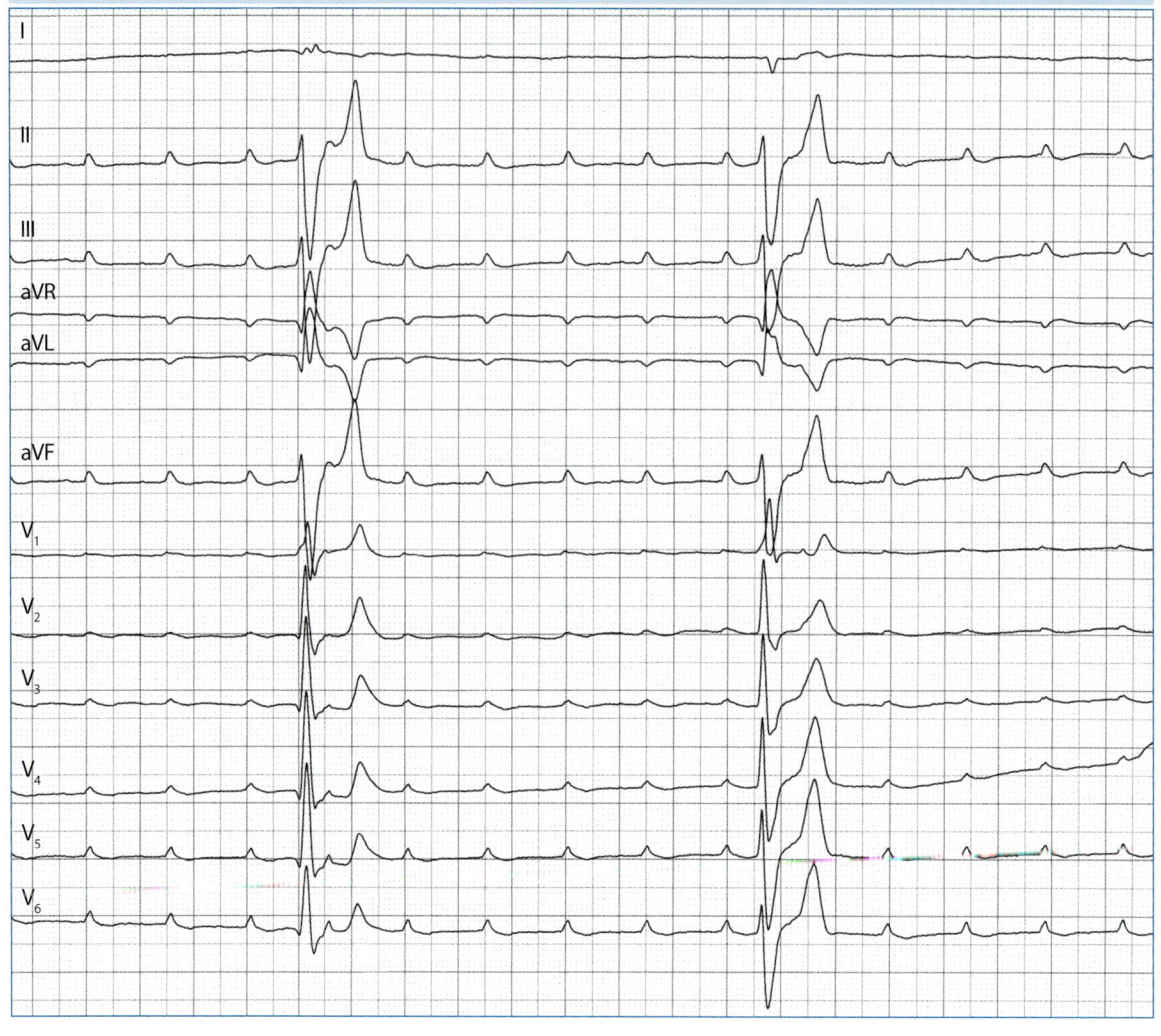

TRACING 14
DOG, LABRADOR RETRIEVER, MALE, 2 YEARS OLD

Twelve leads (I, II, III, aVR, aVL, aVF, V_1, V_2, V_3, V_4, V_5, V_6) - speed 50 mm/s - calibration 5 mm/1 mV

The first two beats are sinus with a rate of 125 bpm. The P waves are normal in morphology, amplitude and duration (amplitude of 0.3 mV, duration of 40 ms) with mean electrical axis of +60°. The PQ interval is normal with a fixed duration of 100 ms.

The QRS complexes of the two sinus beats have normal morphology, amplitude and duration (approximately 45 ms) with a mean electrical axis of +94 °. The QT interval is normal (170 ms). The ST segment is isoelectric in all leads.

The second sinus beat is followed by a premature and wide QRS complex (90 ms) with a right bundle branch block morphology (larger negative deflection in the inferior leads II, III and aVF and in left precordial leads). No visible P wave in front of the QRS complex. It is consistent with a ventricular premature beat.

Subsequently, there is the onset of a narrow QRS complex tachycardia with regular R-R intervals (200 ms).

The first beat of the tachycardia that ends the postextrasystolic pause is not preceded by a P wave and it, therefore, likely corresponds to a junctional escape beat. During the tachycardia there are P'waves with negative polarity in leads II, III and aVF and equally positive polarity in aVR and aVL (inferior- to-superior axis of –90 °) with the initial part of the ST segment. The RP'/ P'R ratio is 0.5 (measured at the sixth beat of the narrow QRS complex tachycardia).

During the tachycardia, the QRS complexes have normal morphology, amplitude and duration and a mean electrical axis of +94 °. Beat-to-beat variation in R wave amplitude greater than 1 mm is visible in lead aVF (electrical alternans).

There is an elevation of the ST segment in lead aVR.

The combination of a ventricular rate above 180 bpm, P'waves with an inferior-to-superior axis, electric alternans in at least one of the twelve leads and a RP'/P'R ratio <0.7 supports the diagnosis of orthodromic atrioventricular reciprocating tachycardia.

Electrocardiographic diagnosis: Orthodromic atrioventricular reciprocating tachycardia.

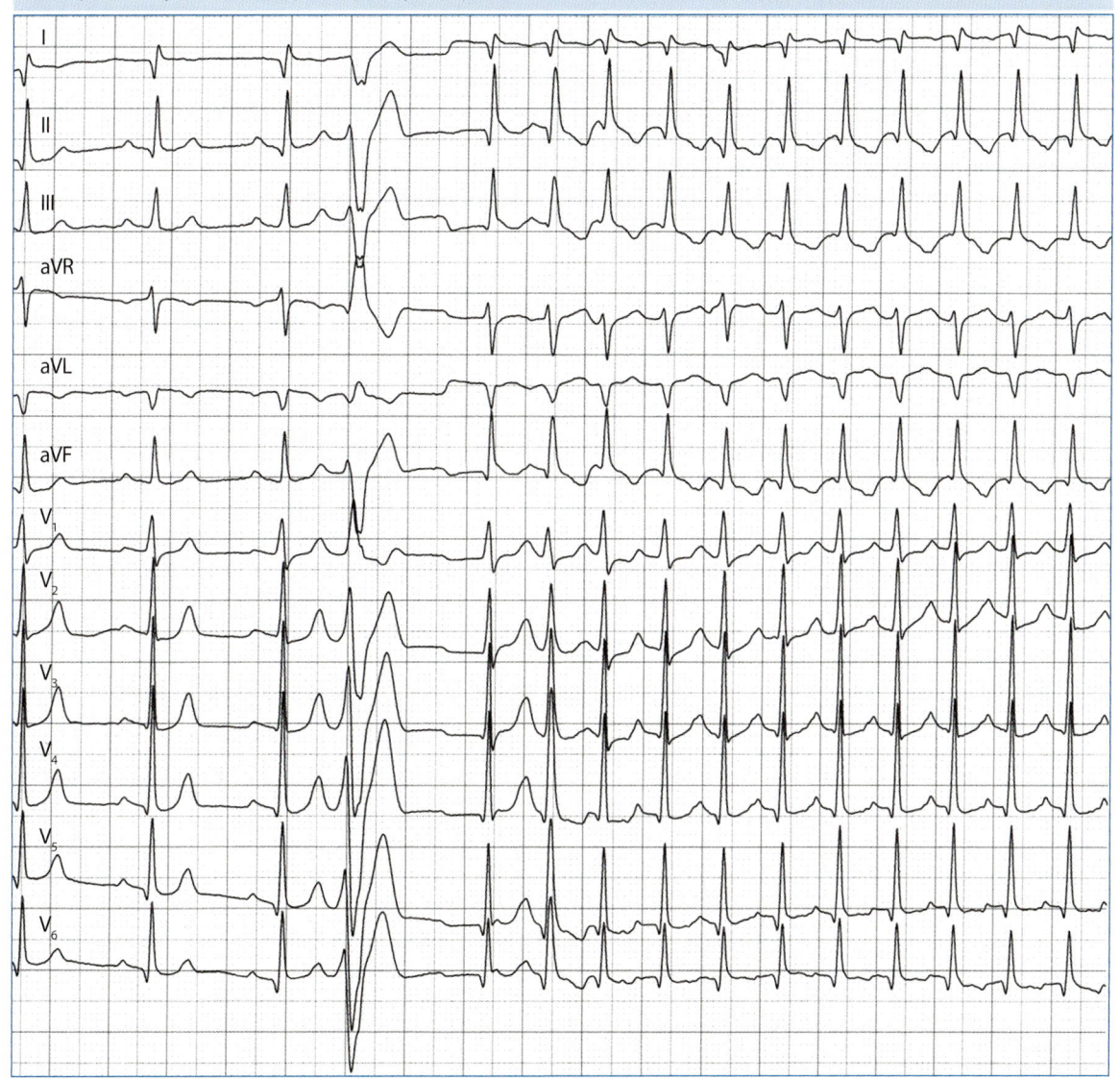

TRACING 15

DOG, YORKSHIRE TERRIER, MALE, 12 YEARS OLD

Twelve leads (I, II, III, aVR, aVL, aVF, V_1, V_2, V_3, V_4, V_5, V_6) - speed 50 mm/s - calibration 5 mm/1 mV

The dominant rhythm is a sinus rhythm with a rate of 140 bpm. The P waves have normal morphology, amplitude and duration (amplitude of 0.3 mV, duration of 30 ms). The mean electrical axis of the P wave is +60°.
The PQ interval has a normal and fixed duration of approximately 90 ms.
The QRS complexes have normal morphology, amplitude and duration (30 to 40 ms) and a mean electrical axis in the frontal plane of +90°.
The QT interval is normal (180 ms).

The ST segment is isoelectric in all leads.
The P-P and R-R intervals are regular (310 ms).
After the fourth beat a P wave with sinus axis is not followed by a QRS complex, supporting the diagnosis of second-degree atrioventricular. The PQ interval before the blocked P wave has the same length (approximately 90 ms) as the other conducted P waves. The block can, therefore, be further described as Mobitz type II second-degree atrioventricular block.

Electrocardiographic diagnosis: Sinus rhythm with Mobitz type II second-degree atrioventricular block.

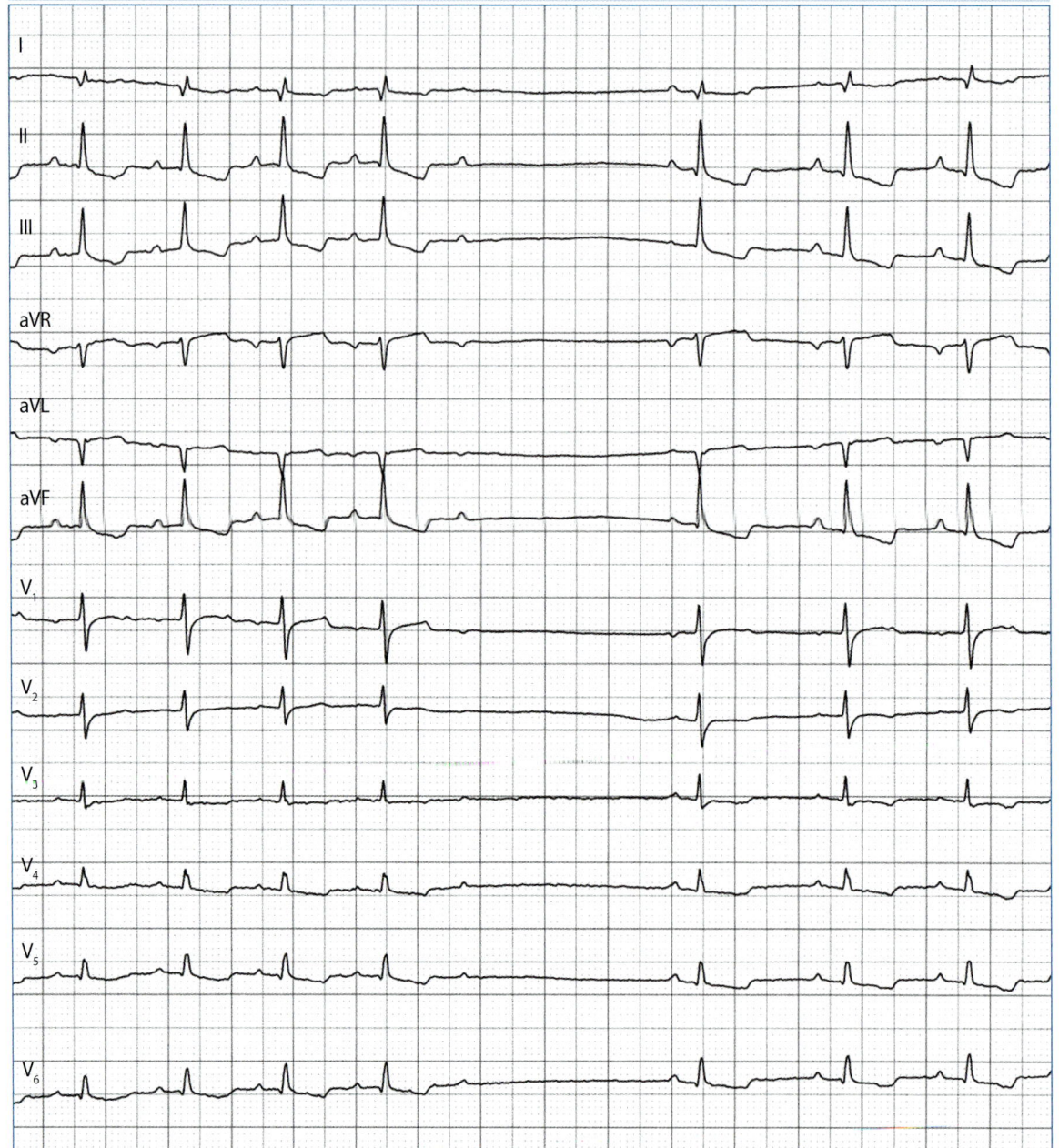

Alphabetical index

A

Abdominal diseases 297
Aberrant conduction 132, 171, 172, 175, 179, 232, 286, 288, 288, 327
Abnormal automaticity 93, 94, 141, 163, 206, 210, 230
Acepromazine 306, 307, 308, 309
Action potential 9, 10, 11, 12, 13, 14, 16, 18, 19, 46, 47, 54, 55, 56, 57, 62, 94, 95, 96, 97, 99, 101, 112, 118, 119, 174, 185, 212, 219, 225, 287, 289, 293, 296, 297, 301, 302, 303, 310
Addison's disease 254
Alfaxalone 306, 307, 309
Alpha-2 agonists 244, 308
Amiodarone 58, 259, 302
Antiarrhythmic 125, 163, 207, 228, 230, 293, 302, 303
Anticholinergic 121, 146, 303, 304, 307, 308
Antidromic atrioventricular reciprocating tachycardia 103, 161
Ashman's phenomenon 171, 178, 179, 286, 287, 291
Asystole 115, 119, 236, 241, 254, 255, 296
Atrial dissociation 65, 142, 143
Atrial ectopic beat 103, 120, 131, 132, 133, 134, 139, 140, 141, 143, 287, 289, 290, 316
Atrial ectopic rhythm 103, 325, 330
Atrial enlargement 43, 51, 83, 84, 85, 86, 131, 156, 163, 168, 174, 175, 186, 196, 298, 333
Atrial fibrillation 8, 17, 58, 65, 77, 93, 100, 101, 103, 104, 118, 119, 120, 123, 127, 131, 145, 154, 161, 166, 168, 172, 174, 175, 176, 177, 178, 179, 181, 184, 205, 230, 232, 233, 235, 252, 261, 270, 286, 288, 289, 298, 300, 302, 310, 317, 325, 327
Atrial flutter 8, 17, 65, 93, 97, 100, 101, 103, 104, 120, 123, 127, 142, 145, 166, 167, 168, 169, 170, 171, 172, 173, 174, 181, 182, 183, 184, 185, 230, 265, 266
Atrial parasystole 103, 141, 142, 143
Atrial rate 47, 91, 166, 168, 171, 172, 181, 185, 214, 265, 272, 315, 317, 336
Atrial repolarization 39, 40, 43, 51, 55, 84, 85
Atrial standstill 8, 102, 103, 119, 120, 178, 219, 239, 252, 253, 254, 255
Atrial tachycardia 8, 17, 58, 93, 95, 97, 103, 104, 120, 127, 131, 145, 146, 163, 164, 165, 166, 167, 172, 174, 179, 181, 182, 183, 184, 185, 224, 230, 249, 264, 266, 272, 298, 303, 325, 332
Atrionodal bundles 1, 4, 5, 44
Atrioventricular bundle 1, 4, 5, 6, 7, 16, 43, 44, 149, 151, 203, 272, 283
Atrioventricular conduction 1, 4, 9, 13, 16, 17, 18, 44, 51, 85, 102, 110, 111, 112, 114, 118, 120, 137, 151, 153, 154, 155, 159, 165, 166, 169, 170, 171, 172, 173, 181, 183, 184, 185, 197, 198, 263, 264, 266, 267, 268, 269, 290, 299, 301, 302, 303, 304, 310, 315, 317, 336
Atrioventricular junction 1, 4, 5, 6, 11, 16, 44, 62, 63, 64, 76, 80, 94, 95, 102, 103, 127, 135, 140, 141, 149, 151, 199, 210, 248, 254, 262, 264, 266, 270, 272, 289, 301, 302, 309
Atrioventricular node 1, 2, 3, 4, 5, 6, 7, 8, 9, 10, 14, 15, 16, 17, 18, 19, 20, 41, 44, 51, 64, 78, 80, 93, 94, 99, 102, 103, 104, 110, 114, 119, 127, 128, 131, 132, 135, 140, 141, 144, 145, 146, 148, 149, 150, 151, 154, 155, 156, 158, 159, 161, 163, 171, 175, 176, 177, 178, 179, 185, 186, 191, 196, 197, 240, 253, 258, 259, 260, 263, 264, 265, 266, 272, 283, 289, 290, 291, 294, 304, 317, 335
Atrioventricular reciprocating tachycardia 8, 17, 58, 93, 100, 101, 102, 103, 104, 135, 145, 154, 156, 158, 159, 160, 161, 181, 182, 183, 184, 185, 194, 291, 325, 339
Atrioventricular synchrony 17, 112, 115, 316
Atropine 189, 250, 253, 303, 304

B

Bachmann's bundle 1, 2, 4, 41, 42, 44, 253, 259, 262, 296
Bailey's hexaxial system 25, 28, 29, 59
Benzodiazepines 306, 307, 309
Beta-blockers 302
Bezold-Jarisch reflex 72, 236, 240, 241, 243, 251
Biatrial enlargement 51, 86

Bidirectional ventricular tachycardia 103, 104, 204, 220, 221, 303
Bifascicular block 272, 280, 283, 285
Bigeminy 120, 140, 178, 198, 220, 221, 224, 227, 298
Bipolar lead 21, 24, 25, 28, 33
Biventricular pacing 317, 319
Bowditch effect 105, 106
Bradyarrhythmia 93, 102, 119, 228, 239, 272
Bradycardia-dependent block 99, 286, 287
Breathing artifacts 64, 65
Bretylium 96
Bundle branch block 55, 56, 62, 72, 104, 141, 156, 159, 171, 172, 178, 179, 180, 190, 191, 192, 200, 207, 208, 209, 210, 211, 212, 213, 214, 216, 218, 220, 221, 225, 227, 228, 229, 231, 232, 233, 234, 235, 246, 259, 263, 265, 266, 268, 269, 272, 273, 274, 275, 276, 277, 279, 280, 281, 282, 283, 284, 285, 286, 287, 288, 289, 290, 291, 294, 295, 298, 299, 300, 317, 325, 326, 327, 328, 329, 331, 333, 338, 339
Buprenorphine 306
Butorphanol 306, 307, 309

C

Calipers 47, 62, 63
Cardiomyopathy 8, 58, 87, 93, 108, 112, 119, 131, 155, 161, 165, 168, 174, 186, 187, 192, 202, 206, 209, 212, 216, 222, 226, 227, 228, 229, 230, 231, 236, 240, 243, 270, 277, 279, 281, 288, 290, 296, 307, 310
Cavotricuspid isthmus-dependent atrial flutter 167, 168, 169, 172
Coronary sinus 2, 3, 4, 5, 6, 8, 9, 13, 16, 103, 104, 127, 128, 131, 133, 145, 146, 154, 163, 168, 325, 330
Coumel's triangle 206
Couplet/s 118, 120, 123, 140, 178, 196, 198, 212, 218, 220, 221, 224, 225, 226, 227, 228, 236
Coupling interval 105, 107, 109, 118, 120, 124, 139, 141, 143, 178, 194, 195, 197, 200, 201, 213, 214, 221, 227, 236, 286, 289

Crista terminalis 2, 3, 4, 8, 9, 132, 145, 163, 168, 172, 253, 296, 325, 332
Cushing's reflex 240, 241, 300

D

Damping effect 54
Delayed after-depolarization 95, 96, 97, 210, 212, 217, 220, 225, 231, 303
Dexmedetomidine 306, 307, 308, 309
Diazepam 306, 307
Digoxin 56, 163, 189, 220, 244, 302, 303
Diltiazem 303
Diphasic wave 41
Dual-chamber pacing 317

E

Early after-depolarization 95, 96, 97, 98, 216, 217, 219, 225, 296, 302
Einthoven triangle 25
Electrical alternans 58, 158, 159, 160, 161, 162, 181, 297, 298, 339
Electrical axis 29, 47, 52, 58, 59, 60, 61, 62, 63, 66, 87, 88, 89, 90, 91, 104, 131, 132, 133, 137, 139, 151, 159, 191, 192, 199, 206, 210, 211, 234, 249, 274, 275, 276, 277, 278, 279, 281, 282, 283, 284, 326, 327, 328, 329, 330, 331, 332, 333, 334, 335, 336, 337, 338, 339, 340
Electrical interference 38, 64, 65, 313, 318, 321
Electrocardiograph 21, 35, 36, 37, 38, 39, 65
Electrocardiographic ruler 62, 63
Electrocution 301
Electrode placement 63, 64, 66, 67
Electromechanical dissociation 103, 239, 256, 257
Enhanced normal automaticity 93, 94, 95, 145, 151
Equivalent dipole theory 21, 24

F

fibrillation 8, 12, 17, 58, 65, 77, 93, 100, 101, 103, 104, 113, 118, 119, 120, 123, 125, 127, 131, 145, 154, 161, 166, 168, 169, 172, 174, 175, 176, 177, 178, 179, 180, 181, 184, 194, 204, 205, 215, 220, 221, 222, 223, 227, 230, 232, 233, 235, 236, 252, 254, 256, 261, 270, 272, 286, 288, 289, 291, 296, 297, 298, 300, 301, 302, 310, 317, 325, 327
Fibrous trigone 1, 4, 5, 6
First-degree atrioventricular block 75, 262, 263, 278, 283, 284, 285, 325, 336
Focal atrial tachycardia 8, 93, 103, 104, 127, 135, 145, 163, 164, 165, 166, 167, 174, 181, 182, 183, 184, 185, 230, 303, 325, 332
Focal junctional tachycardia 81, 97, 103, 149, 150, 151, 152, 153, 181, 182, 184, 185, 325, 337

G

Gabapentin 306
Gap junctions 2, 3, 14, 230, 252
Gap phenomenon 289, 290
Glycopyrrolate 303

H

Heart rate variability 77, 78, 79, 80, 122, 123, 249, 303, 304
His bundle 1, 2, 4, 6, 7, 10, 16, 18, 93, 104, 127, 135, 149, 189, 203, 253, 263, 265, 266, 272
Hisian ventricular beats 191
Holter 33, 36, 50, 57, 74, 76, 77, 78, 79, 94, 120, 121, 122, 123, 124, 125, 146, 172, 174, 204, 208, 214, 216, 221, 224, 227, 234, 236, 239, 241, 243, 249, 251, 252, 260, 269, 287, 294, 296, 299
Hydromorphone 306
Hyperadrenocorticism 241
Hyperaldosteronism 300
Hypercalcemia 19, 55, 97, 297
Hyperthermia 301, 307, 309
Hyperthyroidism 35, 87, 163, 270, 299, 300
Hypocalcemia 19, 58, 218, 293, 297
Hypokalemia 19, 56, 58, 95, 97, 163, 217, 218, 293, 295, 296, 297
Hypomagnesemia 56, 58, 97, 218, 297
Hypothermia 10, 55, 95, 96, 239, 243, 254, 256, 274, 301
Hypothyroidism 95, 189, 230, 299
Hypoxia 96, 110, 239, 254, 256, 293, 294, 299
Hysteresis 125, 316

I

Idioventricular rhythm 43, 93, 95, 103, 113, 189, 191, 198, 203, 204, 205, 207, 210, 211, 212, 213, 214, 223, 230, 231, 234, 249, 257, 298, 299, 300, 331
Inferior fascicle 1, 2, 4, 6, 7, 45, 62, 262, 272
Inferior nodal extension 1, 4, 5, 16
Inter-atrial block 142, 259
Internodal tracts 1, 4, 5, 44
Intra-atrial block 142, 259
Intracranial diseases 300
Intraventricular block 103, 120, 230, 231, 259, 273, 288
Intraventricular conduction system 1, 7, 51, 145, 151, 155, 207, 272, 280, 286
Ischemia 11, 35, 51, 56, 58, 95, 100, 156, 189, 210, 222, 230, 231, 298, 301
Ischemic cardiomyopathy 206, 222, 230

J

Junctional ectopic beat 103, 131, 132, 135
Junctional ectopic rhythm 103, 156

K

Kent fibers 8
Ketamine 306, 307, 309, 310, 312

L

Ladder diagram 62, 63, 64
Lidocaine 224, 298, 302, 310
Linear conductor theory 24
Linking 73, 178, 180, 288, 289, 291
Lone atrial fibrillation 127, 174, 175
Longitudinal dissociation 6, 16, 146, 149

M

Macroreentrant atrial tachycardia 103, 145
Methadone 306, 307, 310
Mexiletine 228, 302
Midazolam 306, 307, 308
Mobitz type I 264, 265, 266, 267, 268, 283, 285, 291, 325, 340
Mobitz type II 264, 265, 268, 283, 285, 291, 325, 340
Morphine 307, 308, 310
Multifocal atrial tachycardia 103, 145, 166, 167
Muscle artifacts 64, 65, 66
Myocarditis 56, 86, 131, 163, 165, 168, 174, 189, 206, 222, 228, 230, 270, 272, 283, 301

N

Negative wave 24, 28, 43, 53, 54, 58
Non-paroxysmal junctional tachycardia 93, 95, 103, 104, 145, 149, 151, 153

O

Opioids 119, 174, 244, 259, 264, 303, 307, 308, 309, 310
Orthodromic atrioventricular reciprocating tachycardia 17, 58, 100, 103, 154, 156, 158, 159, 160, 181, 182, 183, 184, 185, 194, 291, 325, 339
Orthogonal bipolar lead system 33
Osborn wave 55, 301
Overdrive suppression 13, 15, 71, 94, 95, 150, 198, 200, 241, 250
Oversensing 318, 320, 322

P

Pacemaker cells 1, 9, 10, 14, 15, 41, 71, 94, 95, 135, 145, 189, 194, 195, 203, 245, 247, 250, 252, 253, 270, 301, 302, 303
Pacemaker malfunction 121, 318, 320, 321, 322, 325, 331
Pacing modes 314
Parasystole 103, 141, 142, 143, 194, 200, 201
Paroxysmal atrial tachycardia 165
Paroxysmal atrioventricular block 269, 325, 329
Paroxysmal sustained atrial tachycardia 165

Pericardial diseases 297
Permanent junctional reciprocating tachycardia 16, 103, 154, 159, 161, 162, 163, 181, 182, 183, 184, 185
Pleomorphism 207, 208, 210, 212, 213, 214, 216, 234
P mitrale 85
Poincaré plot 77, 79, 123, 124, 249, 251
polymorphic ventricular tachycardia 93, 96, 98, 103, 104, 204, 216, 217, 218, 219, 220, 221, 222, 223, 224, 225, 226, 227, 228, 237, 272, 297
Positive wave 24, 26, 46, 54, 58, 156
Precordial concordance 209, 232, 233, 234, 235, 333
Precordial lead/s 24, 25, 26, 28, 30, 31, 32, 37, 45, 47, 49, 52, 53, 54, 55, 56, 64, 87, 121, 131, 190, 192, 194, 207, 208, 209, 218, 225, 227, 228, 229, 231, 232, 233, 234, 235, 274, 275, 277, 283, 298, 326, 327, 328, 333, 335, 338, 339
Procainamide 96, 302
Propofol 307, 308, 309
Propranolol 222, 250
Proximal atrioventricular bundle 1, 4, 5, 6, 16, 44, 149
Pulmonary vein atrial tachycardia 165
Pulseless electrical activity 103, 239, 256, 257
Purkinje network 2, 7, 8, 15, 18, 43, 47, 99, 189, 210, 272

Q

Quadrigeminy 120, 140, 198, 298, 325, 328
Quinidine 58, 96, 302

R

Reentry 12, 93, 96, 99, 100, 101, 102, 131, 146, 163, 165, 167, 169, 172, 174, 194, 206, 210, 212, 216, 227, 252
Ryanodine 11, 96, 107, 109, 252

S

Second-degree atrioventricular block 75, 77, 81, 97, 151, 153, 163, 164, 165, 166, 167, 184, 244, 245, 262, 263, 264, 265, 266, 267, 268, 269, 283, 285, 325, 336, 340
Self limiting atrial tachycardia 165

Sick sinus syndrome 246, 247, 251, 259, 315
Sino-atrial block 103, 218, 219, 244, 245, 247, 249, 254, 259, 260, 261, 300, 308
Sino-ventricular rhythm 102, 103, 239, 253, 254, 255, 296
Sinus arrest 94, 102, 103, 114, 126, 135, 174, 218, 219, 239, 244, 245, 246, 247, 249, 250, 251, 252, 254, 259, 300
Sinus arrhythmia 18, 47, 48, 50, 52, 55, 57, 71, 72, 73, 74, 75, 76, 77, 78, 81, 84, 94, 105, 106, 120, 140, 190, 196, 197, 199, 239, 244, 245, 247, 249, 250, 251, 252, 259, 263, 264, 265, 266, 268, 269, 270, 271, 275, 294, 298, 304, 325, 336
Sinus rate 71, 75, 94, 95, 96, 103, 106, 110, 111, 146, 150, 203, 204, 205, 210, 212, 225, 241, 250, 252, 259, 264, 268, 298, 303, 304
Sinus rhythm 43, 48, 49, 50, 51, 52, 71, 72, 73, 74, 75, 76, 77, 78, 80, 81, 85, 86, 88, 89, 90, 94, 95, 100, 104, 105, 107, 108, 110, 117, 118, 120, 122, 123, 131, 135, 136, 139, 140, 142, 149, 150, 155, 156, 157, 166, 172, 174, 181, 183, 185, 195, 196, 197, 200, 203, 204, 205, 210, 212, 213, 214, 215, 216, 218, 219, 220, 226, 227, 232, 234, 239, 245, 246, 249, 250, 259, 260, 262, 263, 266, 267, 268, 269, 275, 276, 277, 278, 279, 282, 283, 284, 285, 289, 290, 298, 300, 301, 304, 316, 325, 326, 328, 329, 330, 333, 334, 335, 336, 337, 340
Sinus standstill 102, 103, 138, 178, 239, 246, 247, 248, 249, 254, 260, 261
Sinus tachycardia 72, 86, 91, 93, 94, 95, 97, 103, 110, 111, 126, 145, 146, 147, 148, 181, 182, 184, 190, 198, 240, 241, 243, 262, 268, 272, 293, 294, 299, 300, 301, 310, 325, 328
Slurring 55, 87, 90, 176, 335
Sotalol 96, 228, 235, 302
Spikes 115, 314, 315, 316, 317, 318, 320, 321, 322, 331
Splintering 156
Spontaneous automaticity 1, 11, 14, 15, 302
Sulcus terminalis 2
Supernormal conduction 200, 289, 290, 291
Supraventricular tachycardia 51, 56, 85, 95, 97, 103, 104, 109, 112, 119, 126, 145, 146, 159, 161, 163, 166, 181, 182, 184, 185, 203, 209, 231, 232, 233, 234, 235, 250, 252, 264, 288, 289, 291, 297, 299, 300, 317, 332
Sustained aberrant conduction 288
Syncope 35, 72, 112, 119, 121, 125, 126, 212, 218, 227, 228, 240, 241, 243, 247, 251, 252, 269, 270, 294, 299

T

Tachycardia-dependent block 98, 286
Takahashi's lead system 26, 30, 31
Thebesian's ostium 6
Third-degree atrioventricular block 43, 64, 71, 81, 116, 119, 127, 175, 178, 199, 219, 230, 257, 259, 262, 270, 271, 272, 283, 289, 301, 303, 321, 325, 338
Torsade de pointes 57, 58, 96, 103, 104, 204, 216, 217, 218, 219, 220, 225
Tramadol 308, 309
Trazodone 308, 309
Trifascicular block 272, 283, 285
Trigeminy 120, 140, 198, 227, 298
Triggered activity 94, 95, 96, 131, 149, 151, 163, 165, 166, 174, 189, 191, 194, 200, 206, 210, 212, 216, 217, 227, 302, 303

Triplet 120, 140, 178, 198, 212, 218, 224, 225, 226, 227, 228, 236

U
Undersensing 318, 320, 321, 325, 331

V
Valve annuli 1
Vasovagal reflex 240
Venous ostia 1
Ventricular arrest 103, 239, 254, 255, 257
Ventricular arrhythmia 96, 97, 98, 100, 117, 124, 194, 189, 194, 203, 214, 218, 219, 222, 224, 225, 226, 227, 228, 229, 230, 231, 235, 236, 237, 247, 272, 297, 299, 300, 302, 303
Ventricular depolarization 18, 39, 40, 41, 43, 44, 45, 46, 51, 53, 58, 59, 61, 64, 86, 87, 132, 151, 154, 155, 156, 159, 177, 189, 210, 254, 256, 264, 274, 277, 280, 281, 287, 318, 328
Ventricular ectopic beats 17, 56, 100, 103, 156, 158, 175, 178, 189, 190, 191, 192, 193, 194, 195, 196, 198, 199, 203, 204, 206, 212, 217, 218, 219, 220, 221, 227, 228, 230, 236, 293, 297, 303
Ventricular enlargement 54, 55, 56, 62, 86, 87, 88, 89, 90, 91, 175, 195, 298, 325, 330, 334
Ventricular fibrillation 8, 12, 103, 104, 113, 118, 125, 194, 204, 215, 220, 221, 222, 227, 230, 236, 254, 256, 272, 296, 297, 301
Ventricular flutter 103, 204, 210, 215, 217, 296
Ventricular hypertrophy 56, 107, 121, 230, 274, 280
Ventricular parasystole 194, 200, 201
Ventricular repolarization 12, 39, 40, 46, 47, 56, 57, 59, 155, 194, 217, 225, 326

Ventricular tachycardia 8, 17, 58, 65, 71, 72, 81, 93, 95, 96, 97, 98, 100, 101, 103, 104, 107, 113, 119, 120, 124, 125, 127, 161, 178, 179, 180, 194, 198, 203, 204, 205, 206, 207, 208, 209, 210, 211, 212, 214, 215, 216, 217, 218, 219, 220, 221, 222, 223, 224, 225, 226, 227, 228, 229, 230, 231, 232, 234, 235, 236, 240, 241, 243, 251, 272, 289, 293, 297, 298, 300, 303, 325, 327, 333
Ventriculo-atrial conduction 16, 17, 113, 138, 149, 150, 158, 159, 161, 163, 182, 184, 191, 197, 210, 213, 214, 216, 217, 247, 248, 261
Verapamil 303

W
Wandering pacemaker 3, 18, 48, 50, 51, 52, 62, 75, 76, 77, 78, 80, 84, 106, 121
Wenckebach 103, 110, 151, 153, 163, 164, 166, 167, 184, 264, 265, 266, 267, 285
Wiggers 221, 222, 223
Wilson's lead system 30